Emergency Medicine

Updated Mega Edition for Students and Practitioners

Fifth Edition

Emergency Medicine

Updated Mega Edition for Students and Practitioners

Fifth Edition

SN Chugh MD, MNAMS, FICP, FIACM, FICN, FISC, FIMSA

Former
Senior Professor of Medicine
Pt BD Sharma Postgraduate Institute of Medical Sciences
and
Pro Vice-Chancellor
Pt BD Sharma University of Health Sciences
Rohtak, Haryana

Ashima Chugh MD

Ex-Senior Resident
GB Pant Hospital
New Delhi

CBSPD

CBS Publishers & Distributors Pvt Ltd

New Delhi • Bengaluru • Chennai • Kochi • Kolkata • Lucknow • Mumbai
Hyderabad • Jharkhand • Nagpur • Patna • Pune • Uttarakhand

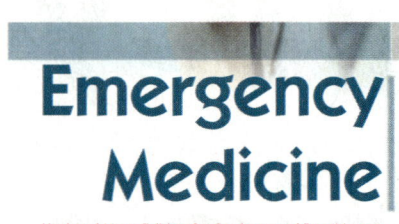

Emergency Medicine

Updated Mega Edition for Students and Practitioners

Fifth Edition

ISBN: 978-93-88327-95-4

Fifth Edition: 2019
Reprint: 2021, 2023, **2024**
Fourth Edition: 2014
Reprint: 2014, 2016, 2017

Published by Satish Kumar Jain and produced by Varun Jain for

CBS Publishers & Distributors Pvt Ltd

4819/XI Prahlad Street, 24 Ansari Road, Daryaganj, New Delhi 110 002, India

Ph: 011-23289259, 23266861, 23266867   Website: www.cbspd.com
                                              e-mail: delhi@cbspd.com

Corporate Office: 204 FIE, Industrial Area, Patparganj, Delhi 110 092, India
Ph: 011-49344934   Fax: 011-49344935
                          e-mail: publishing@cbspd.com; publicity@cbspd.com

Branches

- **Bengaluru:** Seema House 2975, 17th Cross, K.R. Road, Banasankari 2nd Stage, Bengaluru 560 070, Karnataka, India
  Ph: +91-80-26771678/79   Fax: +91-80-26771680   e-mail: bangalore@cbspd.com
- **Chennai:** 7, Subbaraya Street, Shenoy Nagar, Chennai 600 030, Tamil Nadu, India
  Ph: +91-44-26680620, 26681266   Fax: +91-44-42032115   e-mail: chennai@cbspd.com
- **Kochi:** 42/1325, 1326, Power House Road, Opposite KSEB, Power House, Ernakulum 682018, Kochi, Kerala, India
  Ph: +91-484-4059061–67   Fax: +91-484-4059065   e-mail: kochi@cbspd.com
- **Kolkata:** 147, Hind Ceramics Compound, 1st Floor, Nilgunj Road, Belghoria, Kolkata 700056, West Bengal, India
  Ph: +91-33-25330055/56   e-mail: kolkata@cbspd.com
- **Lucknow:** Basement, Khushuma Complex, 7 Meerabai Marg (behind Jawahar Bhawan), Lucknow 226001, UP, India
  Ph: +91-522-4000032   e-mail: tiwari.lucknow@cbspd.com
- **Mumbai:** PWD Shed, Gala No. 25/26, Ramchandra Bhatt Marg, Next JJ Hospital Gate No. 2, Opp. Union Bank of India, Noorbaug, Mumbai 400009, Maharashtra, India
  Ph: +91-22-66661880/89   e-mail: mumbai@cbspd.com

Representatives

- **Hyderabad** 0-9885175004
- **Patna** 0-9334159340
- **Jharkhand** 0-9811541605
- **Pune** 0-9664372571
- **Nagpur** 0-8692091830
- **Uttarakhand** 0-9716462459

Printed at: Goyal Offset Works Pvt. Ltd., Haryana (INDIA)

Preface to the Fifth Edition

After the success of the fourth edition, we are overwhelmed to write this updated and revised fifth edition of the book. We had positive feedback about the popularity of the book from the undergraduate and postgraduate students who have gone through the fourth edition.

Keeping in mind the suggestions of our colleagues and students, we have altered the text and added a few new emergencies. Now, this book is complete in all aspects for emergency treatment of most of serious patients. Wherever necessary, we have changed a few figures also.

After going through the fifth edition, we are convinced that it will cater to the needs of students and will apprise them about the recent advances made in the field of emergency management.

This book is most useful to private practitioners who deal with the emergency cases. After going through this book, they can update their knowledge by sitting in their clinics.

We are thankful to the CBS Publishers & Distributors, who have taken so much pain to bring out this colourful fifth edition.

SN Chugh
Ashima Chugh

Preface to the First Edition

Most of the clinical conditions present acutely as an emergency and patient lands in the casualty and accidental department of a hospital or an institution. Every physician has to handle the emergency situations in clinical practice, while resident staff deals with them in a hospital. The clinical efficiency and capabilities of a doctor/physician depend on the current knowledge and acquaintance with the recent advances in medicine. For every physician it is a must to be well-versed with the emergencies and equipment/procedure required for that. Every physician is duty-bound to refer the patient to an institution if the necessary facility/equipment/expertise is not available.

To write a book on emergency as a single-handed physician is a formidable and challenging task. Nobody will accept the challenge of writing a book unless or until he/she possesses the knowledge to deal with the acute medical conditions. To write a book by multiple authors has become not only customary but also essential because it is not possible for one author to deal with such a fast-changing subject of medicine.

Having a very long experience of teaching undergraduate and postgraduate students, I decided to write this book on the request of my resident staff and students. I have the blessings of my teachers as well as my colleagues, Dr Harpreet Singh, Dr HK Aggarwal, Professor of Medicine, to write the necessary book. They assured me necessary help and even helped me whenever I needed.

My sole purpose of writing this book was to teach the undergraduate and postgraduate students the necessary management of emergencies through this book which is handy, concise and updated. I think it will be useful to the students and practising physicians and will make them acquainted with necessary decisions to be taken in emergency situations.

SN Chugh

A Request

Dear Students/Physicians,

The fifth edition of my book *Emergency Medicine* is a revised and updated mega edition, containing the comprehensive text of all common emergencies in the coloured boxes and tables that soothe one's eyes. The text has been prepared after consultation with my colleagues and resident staff. I have added a few new emergencies on the request of students and practitioners. The success of this edition depends entirely on the students and readers. I have made every effort to provide detailed information to the readers on each and every emergency; yet if there is any lapse on my part, I may be excused. Comments and suggestions from the readers will be appreciated if sent to the publisher directly (*email*: publishing@cbspd.com).

SN Chugh

Contents

SECTION 1
Emergencies in Pulmonary Medicine

SECTION 2
Emergencies in Gastroenterology and Hepatology

SECTION 3
Emergency Related to Infections

SECTION 4
Emergencies in Cardiology

SECTION 5
Emergency in Neurology

Contents

Section 6
Emergencies in Haematology

Section 7
Emergencies in Endocrinology and Metabolism

Section 8
Emergencies in Nephrology

Section 9
Poisonings as Emergencies

SECTION 10
Emergencies in Internal Medicine

SECTION 11
Emergencies Related to Acid–Base and Electrolyte Disturbance

SECTION 12
Skin Emergencies

Emergencies in Pulmonary Medicine

- Severe or Massive Haemoptysis
- Community-Acquired and Hospital-Acquired Pneumonia
- Acute Severe Bronchial Asthma
- Acute Respiratory Distress Syndrome (ARDS)
- Pulmonary Venous Thromboembolism
- Pneumothorax
- Asphyxia
- Chronic Obstructive Pulmonary Disease (COPD) with Acute Exacerbation
- Type II Acute Respiratory Failure
- Acute Empyema Thoracis
- Pulmonary Hypertension and Cor Pulmonale

Severe or Massive Haemoptysis

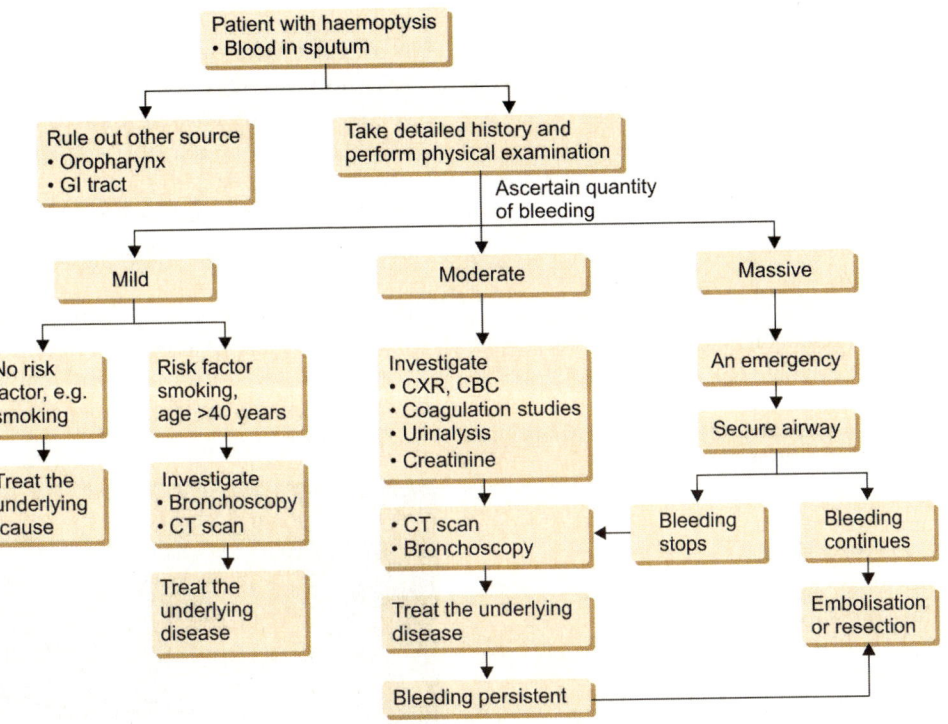

Fig. 1.1: Decision-making analysis of patient with haemoptysis

MASSIVE HAEMOPTYSIS

Definition

Massive haemoptysis is defined as expectoration of more than 200 ml of blood in 24 hours. Massive haemoptysis can represent acute life-threatening emergency, should be subjected to appropriate diagnostic tests to find out the specific cause. Expectoration of even small amount of blood is a frightening symptom. Large amounts of blood can fill the airways and alveolar spaces, not only seriously disturbing the alveolar gas exchange but also causing choking or suffocation.

Pseudohaemoptysis means the blood expectorated is not coming from the lungs; is actually coming from upper respiratory tract (sinus, nares, pharynx or mouth) initiating the coughing with blood.

Causes

Although there are a large number of causes of haemoptysis (Box 1), but common causes encountered in clinical practice are (i) bronchitis, (ii) bronchiectasis, (iii) pneumonia, (iv) tuberculosis, (v) lung abscess and (vi) bronchogenic carcinoma, etc.

Clinical Work-up/Evaluation

It includes:
1. History
2. Physical examination
3. Laboratory investigations

History

- First ascertain weather patient has haemoptysis, pseudohaemoptysis or haematemesis.
- Now concentrate on the the duration, character (blood-tinged purulent sputum / pink frothy sputum or pure blood) and precipitating factors of haemoptysis provide helpful diagnostic clues:
  - The purulent sputum streaked with blood and fever suggests an infection as the cause (Fig. 1.2).
  - Haemoptysis lasting more than 24 hours despite appropriate treatment of infection suggests an endobronchial lesion such as tuberculosis or cancer as the causes of bleeding.

Box 1   Causes of haemoptysis
1. Diseases of bronchi
• Bronchial adenoma
• Bronchial carcinoma, metastatic cancer
• Acute or chronic bronchitis
• Bronchiectasis, advanced cystic fibrosis
• Foreign body
2. Diseases of lung parenchyma
• Tuberculosis
• Suppurative pneumonia
• Lung abscess
• Trauma
• Parasitic, e.g. lung flukes
• Fungal, e.g. aspergilloma, actinomycosis
• Wegener's granulomatosis, microscopic polyangitis
• Pulmonary endometriosis (catamenial haemoptysis)—a rare cause
3. Lung vascular disease
• Pulmonary embolism
• Goodpasture's syndrome
• Polyarteritis nodosa
• AV malformation
• Inhalation injury, e.g. toxic chemical, ilicit substances
4. Cardiovascular diseases
• Acute left ventricular failure
• Mitral stenosis
• Aortic aneurysm
5. Haematological diseases
• Anticoagulants therapy/thrombolytic agents
• Thrombocytopenia
• Leukaemia
• Haemophilia
6. Iatrogenic
• Bronchoscopy
• Pulmonary artery rupture during catheterisation

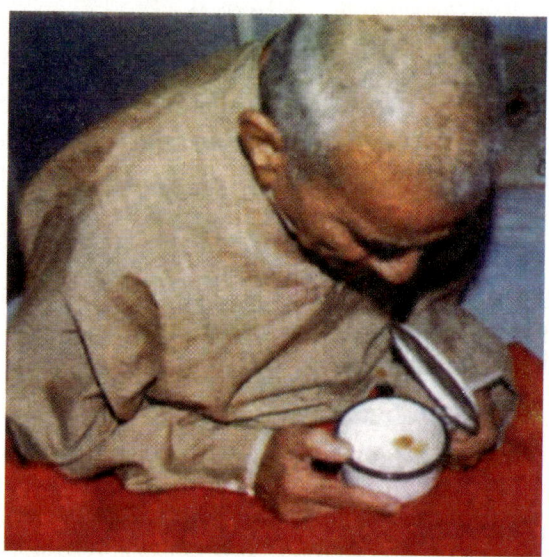

Fig. 1.2: Haemoptysis in a patient with pneumonic consolidation. Note the blood stained sputum

- Expectoration of frank blood in smokers over the age of 40 years suggests a bronchogenic carcinoma.
- Recurrent haemoptysis of small amounts of blood over a period of years suggest underlying bronchial adenoma.
- Fever, recurrent pneumonias with haemoptysis indicate bronchiectasis as the underlying cause. If sputum fetid, then lung abscess may be the underlying cause.
- If haemoptysis is due to cardiovascular cause, then associated symptoms such as dyspnoea, orthopnoea, paroxysmal nocturnal dyspnoea (PND) help in the diagnosis.
- Monthly haemoptysis in a woman suggests catamenial haemoptysis (lung endometriosis).
- If haemoptysis is associated with pain chest and wheezing in a patient with deep vein thrombosis, then possibility of acute pulmonary embolism is most likely.
- Chronic cough (>2 years) with mucopurulent or purulent sputum streaked with blood indicates chronic obstructive puomonary disease (COPD), and if there is recent change in colour or quantity of sputum or haemoptysis indicate acute exacerbation.
- History of drugs such as anticoagulants should also be taken.
- History of any procedure.

Physical Examination

A thorough physical examination should be done to find out the underlying cause (listed in Box 1). Look for, i.e.
- Finger clubbing (common in bronchiectasis, lung cancer and lung abscess).
- Signs of malignancy, i.e. cachexia, hepatomegaly, lymphadenopathy.
- Signs of consolidation and pleurisy indicate pneumonia or a pulmonary infarct.
- Signs of airway obstruction (rhonchi/wheezes) indicate COPD. Localised/diffuse crackles indicate parenchymal lung disease.

- Systemic signs such as rash, purpura, haematuria, splinter haemorrhage for systemic vascular diseases. Look for signs of mitral valve disease and signs of left heart failure (crackles and rales at the lung bases).

Diagnostic Evaluation

- *Blood count:* Total leucocytes count and differential leucocyte count to be done for any evidence of infection. Haemoglobin estimation and platelet count to be done for severity of blood loss and anaemia, and bleeding disorder.
- *Urine examination, blood urea and serum creatinine* for systemic diseases such as polyarteritis nodosa, Goodpasture's syndrome or vasculitis.
- *Coagulation studies* to identify the correctable haematological abnormalities.
- *Chest X-ray* is mandatory, provides valuable informations for pulmonary congestion (oedema), pneumonia (consolidation), tuberculosis (a cavity), lung abscess (a cavity with fluid and air), pulmonary infarcts (multiple peripheral triangular shadows), lung cancer (a big solid lesion with atelectasis), etc. The chest X-ray has its limitations. It has been reported that 30% of chest X-ray of the patients with haemoptysis may be normal.
- *CT scan:* It is particularly useful in investigating peripheral lesions seen on chest X-ray which may not be accessible to bronchoscopy and facilitates accurate percutaneous needle biopsy, if indicated.
- *Sputum examination* by Gram and acid-fast stains (along with corresponding culture) is indicated. In suspected mass lesion, sputum may be examined for malignant cells.
- *Fibreoptic bronchoscopy* is particularly useful for localising the site of bleeding and for visualisation of endobronchial lesions. When bleeding is massive, rigid bronchoscopy is often preferable than fibreoptic because of better airways control and efficient suction capabilities.
  Bronchoscopy may not be necessary when other tests have pinpointed the bleeding

site and is also not recommended in mild haemoptysis which is likely to be due to acute respiratory infection (tracheo-bronchitis, pneumonia). In patients suspected of bronchiectasis, high resolution computed tomography (HRCT) is now the procedure of choice instead of bronchography.

Angiography: CT pulmonary angiography may be necessary in patients suspected of pulmonary embolism with pre-existing lung disease where ventilation perfusion scan is difficult to interpret.

Ventilation perfusion (V/Q) lung scan: It is useful in establishing the diagnosis of suspected thromboembolic disease.

Management

The rapidity of bleeding and its effect on gas exchange determines the urgency of management. Establish the diagnosis first, and find out the cause if bleeding is mild and gas exchange is preserved; but if there is massive haemoptysis, then to maintain adequate gas exchange, following steps may be taken:

1. Bed-rest, mild sedation and cough suppression may help the bleeding to subside.
2. If origin of the blood is known and is limited to one lung, the bleeding lung should be placed in the dependent position so that blood is not aspirated into unaffected lung.
3. Oxygen supplementation is guided by blood gas analysis, is needed to correct hypoxaemia. With massive (large volume) haemoptysis, the need to control the airway and maintain adequate gas exchange, endotracheal intubation and mechanical ventilation may be necessary.
4. Blood volume should be replaced by blood transfusions, if necessary. Coagulopathies should be treated with transfusion of the appropriate coagulation factors and platelets.
5. Resuscitation of shock by fluids, blood transfusion and drugs, if necessary. Most patients of haemoptysis resolve with treatment of infection, inflammation or with removal of offending stimulus.
6. In massive, i.e. large volume haemoptysis, if there is danger of flooding of the lung with blood contralateral to the side of haemorrhage despite the proper positioning, isolation of right and left bronchi from each other can be achieved with specially designed double lumen endotracheal tube.
7. Endoscopic balloon tamponade is done to occlude the bronchus having the bleeding site by inserting a balloon catheter through a bronchoscope after direct visualisation of bleeding site, and by inflating the balloon. This technique not only prevents the aspiration of blood into unaffected areas but also may promote tamponade (compression) the bleeding site and stoppage of bleeding.
8. Other available techniques to control the bleeding in massive haemoptysis include *laser photocoagulation, embolotherapy* and *surgical resection* of the involved area of lung. Haemoptysis due to bleeding from an endobronchial tumour can be stopped temporarily by coagulating the bleeding site by laser therapy (neodymium:Yttrium-aluminium-garnet—Nd:YAG). Embolotherapy, is an angiographic procedure in which a vessel proximal to the bleeding site is cannulated and gel foam is injected to occlude the vessel like an embolus. Surgical resection of the involved part is indicated only in life-threatening haemoptysis not responding to other measures or can be done electively when the disease is localised and haemoptysis is recurrent.

Community-Acquired and Hospital-Acquired Pneumonia

COMMUNITY-ACQUIRED PNEUMONIA (CAP)

Definition

Pneumonia is an acute inflammation of the lung parenchyma by infective or non-infective process presenting with features of consolidation on clinical and radiological examination. It may be *community acquired, hospital acquired* and *ventilator-associated*. It is a leading cause

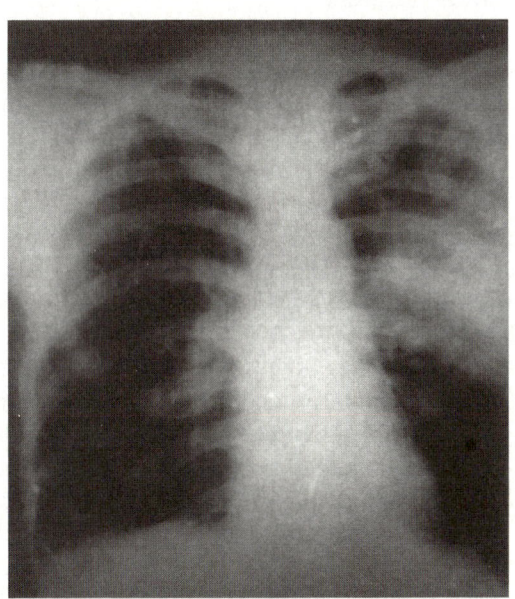

Fig. 2.1: Chest X-ray showing consolidation left mid-zone. Note the homogenous opacity

of death and morbidity in the developing as well as in developed countries. It is one of the most common causes for hospital admission in adults and children.

Community-acquired pneumonia refers to pneumonia occurring in young healthy adults in a community. Infection is usually spread by droplets inhalation and, most patients affected are previously well. Cigarette *smoking, alcoholism,* and *corticosteroid* or *immunosuppressive therapy* all impair mucociliary clearance and immune defense and predispose to it.

Causative Pathogens

The potential pathogens in CAP include bacteria, fungi, virus and protozoa. Newly identified pathogens include metapneumoviruses, the coronoviruses and methicillin-resistant staphylaccoccus aures (MRSA).

Identification of the aetiological microorganism is of prime importance, since, this is key to start the antimicrobial therapy. However, despite intensive investigations the causative organism is not isolated in a large number of cases and, therefore, the initial antimicrobial therapy is empirical and is based on (i) the setting in which infection was acquired (Box 2), (ii) the clinical presentation, (iii) pattern of radiological findings, (iv) result of Gram staining of the sputum, and (v) current trend of susceptibility of the suspected pathogens to antimicrobial agents. However, multidrug resistant pathogens are being incriminated as the cause over the past decade. When the causative organism is found, then specific antibiotic therapy can be chosen. The common pathogens causing community-acquired pneumonia are given in Box 1 and different settings, i.e. out-patient as well as in-hospital (hospital-acquired pneumonia) are given in Box 2.

Box 1	Causative pathogens responsible for community-acquired pneumonia
Common	*Uncommon*
• Streptococcus pneumoniae	• Legionella species
• Mycoplasma pneumoniae	• Staphylococcus aureus
• H. influenzae	• Coxiella burnetti/Chlamydia
• Respiratory viruses, e.g. influenzae, parainfluenzae	• Oral anaerobes
	• Fungal

Box 2	Pathogens causing community-aquired pneumonia (CAP) in different settings		
Out patient	*Non-ICU*	*ICU*	
• Streptococcus pneumoniae	S. pneumoniae	S. pneumoniae	
• Mycoplasma	M. pneumoniae	S. aureus	
• H. influenzae	Chlamydia	Legionella spp.	
• C. pneumoniae	H. influenzae	Gram negative baccilli	
• Respiratory viruses	Logionella spp.	H. influenzae	
		Respiratory viruses	

The *predisposing factors* to community-acquired pneumonia are:
1. Alcoholism
2. Chronic obstructive pulmonary disease and/or smoking
3. Recent attack of influenza
4. Old age
5. Structural lung disease, e.g. bronchiectasis, lung abscess

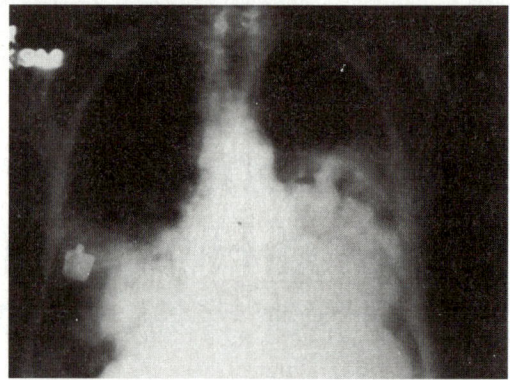

Fig. 2.2: Bilateral consolidation due to community. acquired pneumonia. Note the homogenous opacities in the mid and lower zones of both the lungs

6. Contact with sick bird (*Chlamydia* species) and rabbit (*Francisella tulasencis*), sheep, goat and cat (*Coxiella burnetti*)
7. Poor orodental hygiene (oral anaerobes)
8. Travelling (endemic mycosis)
9. Dementia, stroke, epilepsy and unconsciousness

Clinical Features

Community-acquired pneumonia (CAP) may present as *lobar pneumonia* which is a radiological and pathological term referring to a homogenous consolidation (clinical term) of one or more lobes (Figs 2.1 and 2.2) often associated with pleural inflammation. *Bronchopneumonia* refers to a more patchy alveolar consolidation associated with bronchial and bronchiolar inflammation often affecting both the lower lobes.

1. **Typical presentation:** The 'typical' pneumonia syndrome presents with sudden onset of fever with chills and/or sweats, non-productive or productive cough with mucoid or purulent sputum, hemoptysis, and in some cases, pleuritic chest pain. The most common pathogen is *S. pneumoniae*. Severely ill patients may have septic shock and an evidence of organ failure or any other complication.

2. **Atypical presentation:** It is characterised by a gradual onset, dry cough,

extrapulmonary symptoms (headache, myalgia, fatigue, sore-throat, nausea, vomiting and diarrhoea) and minimal findings on chest examination despite abnormal chest X-ray (no correlation between physical and radiological findings). The causative organisms include *Mycoplasma pneumoniae, L. pneumophila, P. carinii*, anaerobes, etc. Certain viruses (influenza), and tuberculosis also produce atypical manifestations of pneumonia. In immunocompromised host, *Pneumocystis carinii* is the most common pathogen. These patients have concurrent infections with other opportunistic pathogens such as pulmonary and frequently extrapulmonary, oral thrush due to *Candida* or extensive perineal ulcers due to herpes simplex virus.

Physical findings are:
- Fever or hypothermia, tachycardia and arterial gas desaturation.
- An increased respiratory rate and use of accessory muscles of respiration.
- Palpation reveals increased or decreased vocal fremitus (pleural effusion).
- Percussion reveals dull percussion note on the area involved.
- Auscultation reveals crackles, bronchial breath sounds. A pleural rub may be heard over the area involved.

Diagnosis

Sudden onset of fever, productive cough, haemoptysis and pleuritic chest pain are classical tetrad of pneumonia.

Confirmation is done with consolidation of lung seen on chest X-ray.

Differential Diagnosis

The differential conditions to be kept in mind are:
1. Acute bronchitis
2. Chronic bronchitis with acute excerbation
3. Heart failure
4. Pulmonary embolism
5. Hypersensitivity pneumonia
6. Radiation pneumonitis

Investigations

1. *Chest X-ray:* It is helpful
   i. To confirm the presence and location of pulmonary infiltrates. Most pulmonary pathogens produce focal lesions. Multiple areas of involvement suggest hematogenous spread. Diffuse lesions in immunocompromised host suggest infection by *P. carinii* and viral infections
   ii. To assess the extent of lung involvement
   iii. To detect pleural and lymph node (hilar lymphadenopathy) involvement and pulmonary cavitation
   iv. To assess the response to antimicrobial therapy
   v. To rule out other conditions that simulate pneumonia on X-ray

   Usually chest X-ray shows *reticular pattern* in *Mycoplasma* infection, *homogenous localised opacity* and *air bronchogram* are seen in *S. pneumoniae* infection.

2. *Sputum examination:* It remains the mainstay of the diagnosis but its specificity is decreased because it gets contaminated during expectoration with bacteria that colonise the upper respiratory tract. It has low sensitivity also. However, an acceptable sample should have less than 10 epithelial cells and more than 25 leukocytes per low power field. Sputum should be examined by **Gram staining** which may show *gram-positive diplococci* in pneumococcal pneumonia and *gram-negative bacilli* in hospital-acquired pneumonia. **Ziehl-Neelsen** stain for *Mycobacterium tuberculosis* (AFB) must be done, as well as **Giemsa staining** for *P. carinii*. Sputum culture should also be done.

   Expectorated sputum is easily collected from patients with a vigorous cough but may be scanty in patients with atypical pneumonia, in elderly and in patients with disturbed sensorium. In such a situation, sputum can be induced with ultrasonic nebulization of 3% saline. For patients admitted to ICU and intubation a deep seated suction aspirate or bronchoalveolar lavage sample may be obtained for culture.

3. *Blood culture:* It is useful if pneumonia is associated with bacteremia, neutropenia, asplenia, liver disease and immunocompromised state, only 5–14% blood culture are positive in hospitalised patients and *S. pneumoniae* is the common pathogen isolated.

4. *Blood test: Total and differential leucocyte* count and *ESR* may suggest an evidence of infection.

5. *Biochemical tests* include blood glucose, urea, serum creatinine, electrolyte bilirubin.

6. *Antigen tests:* Two commercially available tests for *pneumococcal* and *Legionella* antigens are positive in urine with 90–99% sensitivity and specificity. Other antigen tests include rapid test for influenzae virus and direct fluorescent antibody test for influenza and respiratory syncytial virus.
Serological tests: These tests are sometimes helpful. They depend on the host immune response and usually become positive later in the course of the disease. They are:
   - Indirect immunofluorescence test (IgA, IgM 4–6 fold rise in antibody titre suggests *M. pneumoniae* infection).
   - *PCR (polymerase chain reaction) amplify DNA or RNA of pathogens hence, is useful to detect Legionella. mycoplasma and S. pneumoniae.*
   - Indirect fluorescent antibody test for Legionella.
   - Microimmunofluorescence for *C. psittaci.*

7. *ECG:* It shows myocarditis in *C. burnetti* infection.

8. *Invasive diagnostic procedures:* These may be occasionally required to obtain the pulmonary material sometimes to establish the diagnosis. These are:
   - Transtracheal aspiration
   - Percutaneous transthoracic lung puncture and aspiration
   - *Fibreoptic bronchoscopy.* Either bronchoalveolar lavage of aspirated material after brushing or transbronchial lung biopsy specimens may be obtained
   - Open lung biopsy

9. *Other tests:* If empyema is a clinical consideration, pleural aspiration is indicated. Pleural fluid culture is generally considered diagnostic of the aetiology of pneumonia

10. *Arterial blood gas* or oxygen saturation

11. *Biomarkers of severe inflammation*, i.e. C-reactive-protein (CRP) and procalcitonin levels increase due to acute phase reactants to bacterial pathogens

Management

Assessment of Severity and Decision to Hospitalise

Most of the patients with pneumonia can be treated on out-patient basis. The criteria for hospital admission include:

1. Leucopenia (WBC <5000 cells/ml) not attributed to a known cause.

2. *S. aureus*, gram-negative organism or anaerobes as the suspected cause of pneumonia.

3. Presence of complications, e.g. empyema thoracis, meningitis, endocarditis.

4. Inability to take oral medication or altered mental status.

5. Failure of outpatient management, e.g. treatment compliance is poor.

Nowadays, there are two set criteria; pneumonia severity index (PSI) is a prognostic model used to identify the patients at lower risk and CURB-65 is used to assess the severity of illness.

1. The PSI uses points for 20 variables and classifies patients into 5 classes, advocates admission for class 4 and 5 patients.

2. **CURB**-65 include 5 variables, i.e. **C** for confusion, **U** for urea >7 mmol/L, **R** for respiratory rate >30 min, **B** blood pressure <90/60 mmHg and 65 denotes the age. This criteria is practicable and easy to

remember, hence, extensively been used to assess the severity and mortality. The score O carries least mortality while score 5 carries highest mortality. The patients with score 1 and above should be hospitalised and with score >3 admitted to ICU.

Neither PSI nor CURB-65 is ideal for determining the need for ICU care. The severity criteria proposed by infectious diseases Society of America and American Thoracic Society guidelines are better-suited for this purpose. However, septic shock and/or respiratory failure in emergency department is an obvious indication for ICV care.

The plan of management of community-acquired pneumonia includes:

1. To decide whether patient needs outhospital or in-hospital treatment (read the criteria).
2. To determine the most likely organism depending on the age and choice of empirical therapy.
3. To determine the prevalence of antibiotic resistance pattern in the community.
4. Associated illness or comorbidity.

Outpatient Management

Pneumonia in an otherwise healthy adult is most likely to be due to *Mycoplasma pneumoniae*, *S. pneumoniae* or *Chlamydia pneumoniae*, hence, empirical therapy with azithromycin (Box 3) remains the treatment of choice. Erythromycin (500 mg every 6 hourly) or doxycycline (100 mg every 12 hourly) is another option. Fluoroquinolones can also be used but has borderline activity against pneumococci *in vitro*.

In older patients with underlying chronic respiratory disease, *Legionella pneumophilia*, *H. influenzae* organisms should be considered in addition to above mentioned organisms. In older patients or adult outpatients with pre-existing respiratory disease with typical presentation of pneumonia, either a *fluoroquinolone plus* the β-lactamase inhibitor *amoxicillin* and *clavulanic acid* can be used. For *Mycoplasma* and *Legionella pneumoniae*, a cephalosporin is the

drug of choice. The duration of therapy for such pneumonia is 2 to 3 weeks; the long duration is frequently recommended to prevent relapse.

Pneumonia due to *anaerobes* is treated with clindamycin (300 mg 6 hourly or 450 mg 8 hourly for 7 to 10 days) with amoxycillin (500 mg 8 hourly) plus metronidazole (500 mg 6 hourly) or with amoxycillin/clavulanic acid combination.

The outpatient treatment is summarised in Box 3.

Box 3 Outpatient empirical treatment for community-acquired pneumonia (US/Canadian approach)	
Without cardiopulmonary and/or comorbid condition and no antibiotic in past 3 months	*With cardiopulmonary and/or comorbid condition and antibiotic in past 3 months*
• Newer macrolide (clarithromycin 500 mg bid oral or azithromycin 500 mg OD then 250 mg OD oral)	• Antipneumococcal fluoroquinolones, e.g. levofloxacin 750 mg oral daily or moxifloxacin 400 mg or gemifloxacin 320 mg oral daily • Beta-lactam (high dose amoxicillin 1 g tid) or amoxicillin and clavulanate 2 g bid
• Doxycycline 100 mg bid orally	• Third generation cephalosporin (ceftriaxone, cefpodoxime 200 mg oral bid) or cefuroxime 500 mg bid plus a macrolide.

In-hospital Management (non-ICU and ICU)

1. *Antibiotic therapy:* The hospitalised patients must undergo prompt microbial evaluation and receive empirical antimicrobial therapy based on Gram's staining of the sputum and knowledge of the current antimicrobial sensitivity. Parenteral antibiotic therapy is mandatory. The empirical therapy for hospitalised patient depends on ICU and non-ICU basis (Box 4). Therapy with a macrolide or a fluoroquinolone within previous

3 months is associated with increased chances of infection with resistant strains of *S. pneumoniale*, hence a fluoroquinolone based regimen should be used for patients recently given a macrolide (Box 3). On improvement, therapy can be switched from intravenous to oral agents to complete 7–10 days course of antibiotics.

The antibiotic therapy to be modified after culture and sensitivity report of sputum. If sputum production is scanty and patient's condition is critical, invasive methods may be used to procure the pulmonary specimen for isolation of pathogens.

Management of bacteremic pneumococcal pneumonia includes a combination therapy (a azithromycin + amoxycillin clavulanate). This combination has synergistic effect and better tolerance.

Antibiotic under special circumstances is chosen on the basis of organism.

I. If *Pseudomonas* is considered to be the cause for CAP patient in ICU, an anti-pneumococcal anti-pseudomonas β-lactam (piperacillin/tazobactam 4.5 g I.V. 6 hourly, cefepime 1–2 g I.V. 12 hourly, imipenem 500 mg I.V. 6 hourly, meropenem 1g I.V. 8 hourly plus a fluoroquinolone (ciprofloxacin or levofloxacin IV).
  - The above β-lactams *plus* an aminoglycoside (amikacin/tobramycin and azithromycin).
  - The above β-lactams plus an aminoglycoside plus anti-pneumococcal fluoroquinolone.

II. If methicillin resistant *aureus* (MRSA) is the cause then add linezolid 600 mg I.V. 12 hourly or vancomycin 1 g I.V. 12 hourly.

2. *Adequate hydration and oxygen therapy:* Oxygen should be administered to all the hypoxaemic patients and high concentration (>35%) should be used in all patients who do not exhibit hypercapnia associated with COPD. Assisted ventilation may be considered if patient remains hypoxaemic despite O_2 therapy.

3. *Treatment of hypotension:* Inspite of treatment with I.V. fluids patient remains in hypotension, adrenal insufficiency may be suspected and patient should be put on inotropic support and glucocorticoids if needed.

4. *Treatment of pleural pain:* To relieve pain parenteral pethidine (50–100 mg) or morphine (5–10 mg) may be used with utmost caution in patient's with poor respiratory function.

5. *Physiotherapy* with relief of pleural pain, patient should be encouraged to cough efficiently to help in mucus clearance and to improve gas exchange.

6. *Immunomodulatory therapy* with drotrecogin alfa (activated) may be considered in patients with severe septic shock and high APACHE II score >25.

Box 4	Empirical antibiotic therapy for hospitalised patients (US/Canadian approach)	
In patients non ICU	*In patients ICU*
• Fluoroquinolone, e.g. moxifloxacin 400 mg orally or I.V. or levofloxacin 750 mg oral or I.V. or gemifloxacin 320 mg oral or I.V. • A β-lactam (cefotaxime 1–2 g I.V. 8 hourly), ceftriaxone 1–2 g I.V. OD) ampicillin 1–2 g I.V. 4–6 hourly *plus* a macrolide, e.g. clarithromycin or azithromycin oral, in special circumstance I.V. azithromycin, 1 gm stat then 500 mg once daily.	• A β-lactam (cefotaxine 1–2 g I.V. 8 hourly, ceftriaxone 2 g I.V. OD) ampicillin sulbactam 2 g I.V. 8 hourly *plus* • Azithromycin or a fluoroquinolone (gemifloxacin 320 mg orally or IV)

NOSOCOMIAL PNEUMONIA (HOSPITAL ACQUIRED AND VENTILATOR ASSOCIATED)

Definition

Hospital-acquired pneumonia (HAP) develops more than 48 hrs after admission to the hospital and *Ventilator Associated Pneumonia (VAP)* develops in mechanically ventilated patients more than 48 hrs after endotracheal intubation.

CAP vs Nosocomial Pneumonia (HAP/VAP)

Nosocomial pneumonia differs from community: acquired pneumnia (CAP) by three underlying factors:

1. Different infections and causes
2. Different antibiotic susceptibility patterns with higher rates of drug resistance.
3. Poor underlying health status of patients predisposing them to risk for more severe infection.

Pathogenesis

Colonisation of the pharynx (by instrumentation, endotracheal intubation, use of broad spectrum antibiotics) and possibly the stomach (gastric microbial overgrowth due to elevation of pH by use of antacids, H_2-receptors blocks and proton-pump inhibitors) with bacteria is the key factor in pathogenesis of nosocomial pneumonia.

Within 48 hrs of admission, 75% of seriously all hospitalised patients have their upper respiratory tract colonised with organisms from hospital environment. Impaired cellular and mechanical defense in the lungs of hospitalised patients also increase the risk of infection after aspiration.

Predisposing factors

1. Advanced ages
2. Mulnutrition
3. Altered state of consciousness
4. Defective swallowing
5. Underlying pulmonary and systemic diseases.

MICROBIOLOGY

The microbiology of HAP and VAP is more or less same. The most common organisms responsible for them are given in Box 5.

Box 5 Microbiology of nosocomial pneumonia

Hospital-acquired Pneumonia (HAP)	Ventilaor-associated Pneumonia (VAP)
• *S. aureus* (both methicilline sensitive *S. aureus* and methicillin-resistant *S. aureus* MRSA) • *P. aeruginosa* • *Enterobacter* species, *K. pneumoniae* and *E coli.*	• *Acinetobacter* species • *Stenotrophomonas maltophilia* • Anaerobes

Note: Mycobacteria, fungi, chlamydiae, viruses are uncommon causes of nosocomial pneumonia

Clinical Features

The symptoms and signs of nesocomial pneumonias are nonspecific such as *fever, chest pain, hemophysis* and *purulent sputum.* *Chest X-rays* show progressive pulmonary opacity in most cases. The **clinical signs** are same as in CAP.

Differential Diagnosis

The conditions include:

- Heart failure
- Atelectasis
- Aspiration pneumonia
- ARDS
- Pulmonary embolism
- Pulmonary haemorrhage.

Investigations

- **Blood exam** for leucocytosis and FSRIC reactive protein
- **Blood culture** from two different sites to isolate the organism.
- **Arterial blood gas analysis** to define the severity of illness and need for assisted ventilation.
- **Thoracentesis** of pleural fluid if present.

Imaging Studies

Chest X-rays/CT scan to determine the lung involvement and its complications.

Special Investigations

In HAP patients who subsequently need mechanical ventilation, secretions obtained from spontaneous expectoration, sputum induction, nasotracheal suction fluid and endotracheal aspiration should be **cultured**.

- For patients with suspected VAP, endotracheal aspiration using sterile suction catheter should be obtained from lower respiratory tract for **culture**.

Management

- **Supportive case** includes O_2 administration, fluid therapy, fever management, skin

---

Table 2.1   Risk factors for multidrug resistant (MDR) pathogens, methicillin-resistant S. aureus (MRSA) and Pseudomonas and other gram-negative bacilli in patients with HAP and VAP pneumonias (Nosocomial pneumonias)

1. Risk factors for MDR pathogens

- Antibiotic therapy in preceding 90 days
- Septic shock, ARDS preceding VAP
- Five or more days in hospital prior to HAP/VAP
- Acute renal replacement therapy prior to HAP/VAP onset
- Treatment in a unit where >10% of gram-negative organisms are resistant to monotherapy or in a unit where local antibiotic sensitivity rates are not known

2. Risk factors for MRSA

- Antibiotic therapy in preceding 90 days
- Renal replacement therapy in the preceding 30 days
- Use of gastric acid suppressants, i.e. PPIs
- Positive culture or prior MRSA colonisation
- Hospitalisation in a unit where prevalence of MRSA is not known or in a unit where >20% of S. aureus organisms are MRSA.

3. Risk factors for Pseudomonas and other gram-negative organisms

- Antibiotic therapy in the preceding 90 days
- Structural lung disease, e.g. COPD, cystic fibrosis, bronchiectasis, etc.
- Recent hospitalisation and instrumentations
- Positive culture for P. aeruginosa in the past year.

---

care, etc. (Read care of patients in RICV—Respiratory Intensive Care Unit)

- **Antibiotic treatment:** The initial treatment of HAP and VAP is usually empirical based on risk factors for MRSA and multiple drug-resistant pathogens (Table 2.1).

Treatment of Ventilator-induced Pneumonia

1. **Empirical therapy:** In patients without risk factors for MDR pathogens, treatment with an antibiotic is same as for community-acquired pneumonia (CAP). The antibiotics used are:
   - *Ceftriaxone* (2 g I.V. daily) or *cefotaxime* 2 g I.V. 8 hrly.

   or

   Ampicillin or *sulbactam* 3 g I.V. 6 hrly

   or

   Ertapenem (1 g I.V. daily)
   Majority of these patients are treated with a single antibiotic.
   In patients with risk factors for MDR pathogens, the standard treatment recommended includes three antibiotics; two directed at *P. arrogenosa* and one at MRSA. The antibiotics used are:

   a. *A β-lactam*
      - *Ceftazidine* (2 g I.V. 8 hrly) or *cefopime* (2 g I.V. 8–12 hrly or *piperacillin Tazobactum* (4.5 g I.V. 6 hrly) *or imipenem* (500 mg I.V. 6 hrly)
      plus

   b. A second agent active against gram-negative pathogens, i.e.
      - *Gentamicin* or *tobramycin* (7 mg/kg I.V. daily) or *amikacin* (20 mg/kg/I.V. daily) or *Ceprofloxacin* (400 mg/I.V. 8 hrly) or *levofloxacin* (750 mg I.V. daily)
      plus

   c. An agent active against gram-positive bacterial pathogens, i.e.
      - *Linezolid* (600 mg I.V.–12 hrly) or *Vancomycin* (15 mg/Kg 12 hrly)

2. **Specific therapy:** Once the aetiologic diagnosis is made, broad-spectrum empirical therapy is modified to treat the know pathogen. For patients with MDR risk factors, antibiotic regimens can be reduced to a single agent or to two-drug combination instead of three-drug combination in most of the cases. If the clinical pulmonary infection score (CPIS) which includes fever, lencocytosis, oxygenation, chest radiograph and tracheal aspirate improve over the first 3 days, antibiotics should be stopped after 8 days. so as to avoid emergence of antibiotic-resistant strain.

The major controversy regarding specific therapy for VAP concerns the need to improve on the antibiotic regimen for *Pseudomonas infection*. The results of combination therapy are limited and treatment failures are common. The high rates of clinical failure and death due to VAP caused by *P. aeruginosa* despite combination therapy indicate that better regimens are needed such as *aerosolised antibiotics*.

3. **Supportive treatment** is same as CAP.

Treatment of Hospital-acquired Pneumonia (HAP)

The treatment of HAP in nonintubated patients both inside and outside the ICU is similar to VAP. The lower freqency of MDR pathogens and better host's immunity allows monotherapy in a large population of cases of HAP than of VAP.

The only pathogen that are more common to non VAP population are anaerobes because of greater risk of microaspirations by nonintubated patients and lower oxygen tensions in the lower respiratory tract, hence target therapy against anaerobes is indicated.

Diagnosis of HAP in nonintubated patients is more difficult because lower respiratory tract samples are more difficult to obtain. In addition, many of the underlying respiratory diseases that predispose to HAP are associated with inability to cough adequently. The blood culture in HAP are infrequently positive.

Despite these difficulties, the prognosis in HAP is better than that of VAP. The antibiotic failure is also lower in HAP than in VAP.

Acute Severe Bronchial Asthma

Note: In asthmatic patients recordings of PEF <200 L/min indicate *severe disease* and values of <100 L/min indicate *life-threatening asthma*.

ACUTE SEVERE BRONCHIAL ASTHMA

Definition

Acute severe bronchial asthma (previously called status asthmaticus) is used to describe life-threatening episodes of asthma during which the patient is distressed by severe breath-lessness, cough, wheeze and other symptoms of asthma due to severe airway obstruction resulting in use of accessory muscles of respiration; and response to maintenance therapy fails and aggressive therapy becomes necessary.

Acute episodes of severe bronchial asthma are one of the most common respiratory emergencies seen in clinical practice, hence, it is essential to recognise them early with early institution of therapy.

Precipitating Factors

A stable patient of asthma develops an acute severe attack (acute excerbation) either due to omission or inadequacy of the maintenance drug treatment. Other factors that push the patient into acute attack or excerbation are given in Box 1.

Box 1 Risk factors and triggers for asthma
I. Endogenous factors
• Genetic predisposition
• Atopy
• Obesity
• Airway hypersensitivity
• Menstrual cycles can precipitate asthma called catamenial asthma
II. Environmental factors
• Indoor and outdoor allergens
• Passive smoking
• Occupational sensitizers at workplace
• Infection, i.e. Mycoplasma, Chlamydophila or viral (rhinovirus)
TRIGGERS
• Allergens (inhaled allergens, house dust mites, exposure to pets)
• Gastroesophageal reflux
• Upper respiratory infections (rhinitis, sinusitis, postnasal discharge)
• Exercise-induced and hyperventilation
• Cold air or air pollutants (SO_2), changes in weather
• Drug, e.g. beta-blockers, aspirin
• Irritants (household sprays, paint fumes)
• Stress and emotional disturbance

Clinical Features

The clinical features result due to acute severe reversible airway obstruction resulting in dyspnoea at rest, use of extra-respiratory muscles for respiration and fall in pulse pressure on inspiration (*pulsus paradoxus*).

Box 2 Clinical features of acute severe asthma

Symptoms
- Severe respiratory distress, cough and wheezing Dyspnoeic at rest
- Feeling of heaviness/tightness of chest due to increase in anteroposterior diameter of chest
- Inability to complete the sentences without becoming breathless and may become cyanotic.
- Inability to get out of bed or get proper sleep.

Signs
- Tachypnoea (respiratory rate >25/min) and tachycardia (HR >100/min)
- Hunched shoulders, use of accessory muscles and indrawing of intercostal spaces
- Wheezing becomes extensive and high-pitched (may become absent in severe attack)
- Silent chest—breath sounds may be inaudible
- Pulsus paradoxus due to reduced cardiac return as a result of hyperinflated lungs. This sign may become absent if the patient's breathing is shallow as it requires a large negative intrathoracic pressure to produce it.

There is loss of adventitial breath sounds and wheezing becomes high-pitched and may even become absent. The clinical features are given in Box 2.

In extreme situations, wheezing may lessen markedly or even disappear, cough may become ineffective and patient may develop gasping type of respiration. These findings indicate excessive mucus plugging and impending suffocation. Central cyanosis develops and chest becomes silent and bradycardia may occur. All these are ominous signs.

Life-threatening features include:
- Severe dyspnoea
- Inability to speak
- Central cyanosis
- Reduced or altered consciousness
- Silent chest
- Bradycardia
- PEF <100 L/min

Investigations

Investigations are done to grade the severity and to identify the complications (e.g. atelectasis, spontaneous pneumothorax, pneumonia, etc.). These are:

1. **Chest X-ray:** It is done to see any evidence of infection, e.g. pneumonia or complications such as atelectasis or pneumothorax.

2. **Peak expiratory flow rate (PEFR):** It is useful to assess the severity. PEFR <40% of predicted value or his/her personal best suggests severe obstruction (Fig. 3.1). Majority of patients with acute severe asthma have PEFR less than 100 L/min and find difficulty in blowing into peak flowmeter.

3. **Arterial gas analysis:**
   - Presence of hypoxaemia (PaO_2 <6Q mmHg) indicates a very serious state.
   - Acidosis (pH <7.38) and hypercapnia ($PaCO_2$ >40 mmHg) indicate fear of impending respiratory failure. In fact, $PaCO_2$ is generally low during an acute attack (hypocapnia), due to hyperventilation hence, rise in $PaCO_2$ even to normal or above is an ominous sign.

4. **Other tests:**
   - TLC and DLC for an evidence of infection.

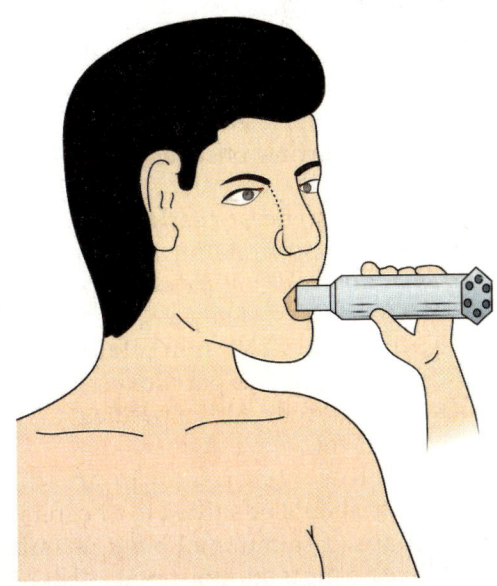

Fig. 3.1: Peak flow measurement: Peak flowmeter

- Blood biochemistry and serum electrolytes to assess the effect of an acute attack.
- ECG to look for ischaemic changes as a result of hypoxaemia, right heart strain and arrhythmias.

Differential Diagnosis

Acute attack of bronchial asthma must be differentiated from cardiac asthma (acute left ventricular failure). Other conditions that simulate an acute attack of asthma are:

- **Pulmonary embolism**
- **Acute upper respiratory obstruction** (suffocation by tumour or laryngeal oedema).
- **Hypersensitivity pneumonia** (eosinophilic pneumonias).
- **Vocal cord dysfunction** presenting with severe laryngospasm or laryngotracheal hyper-reactivity.
- **Endobronchial disease** such as foreign body aspiration, a neoplasm or bronchial stenosis. These conditions produce localised persistent wheezing with paroxysmal attacks of coughing.

Management

Aims and Objectives

- Early recognition and early institution of therapy so as to prevent death.
- Correction of hypoxaemia.
- To overcome airflow obstruction as early as possible.
- To reduce recurrences or early relapse.
- Removal of the precipitating factor.
  1. *Treatment in accidental and emergency:*
     - The patient is initially assessed. Tachycardia (HR >110/min), tachypnoea (>25/min), pulsus paradoxus, inability to speak, PEFR <40% of predicted value indicate severe asthma.
     - If PEFR is <100 L/min in an adult, patient should be shifted to a hospital.
     - Nebulised salbutamol 5 mg or terbutaline 2.5 mg is administered 2–4 hourly or as required (Fig. 3.2). These drugs can

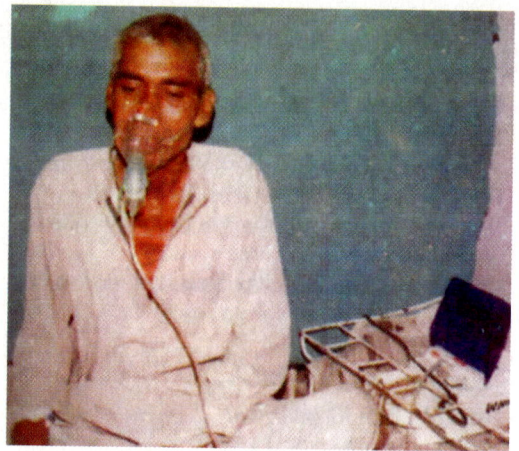

Fig. 3.2: Patient of acute severe asthma being nebulised at the bedside

    be administered by inhalation (metered dose inhaler with spacer).
- Short course of prednisolone 40 mg orally or hydrocortisone 200 mg IV
- Oxygen—high flow (40–60%).
- Maintain I.V. access and take chest X-ray.
- Sedatives should be avoided.

2. *Treatment in hospital (respiratory ICU):*
   - Proper hydration of the patient with I.V. fluids.
   - The patient is reassessed after admission to the hospital for severity and life-threatening situation.
   - Oxygen therapy 40–60% to achieve SaO_2>90% is continued.
   - The PEFR is measured and if asthma is under control, then continue nebulised salbutamol or terbutaline 4 hourly, prednisolone 40–60 mg/day for 2 days or hydrocortisone IV.

If features of severity persist (Fig. 3.3).
- Add ipratropium bromide 0.5 mg to the nebulised salbutamol/terbutaline.
- Continue nebulised salbutamol/terbutaline treatment every 15–30 min if necessary, reduce to 4 hourly once clear response to treatment occurs. In critically ill patients with impending respiratory failure, *I.V. beta-agonist (salbutamol, terbutaline)* may be used.

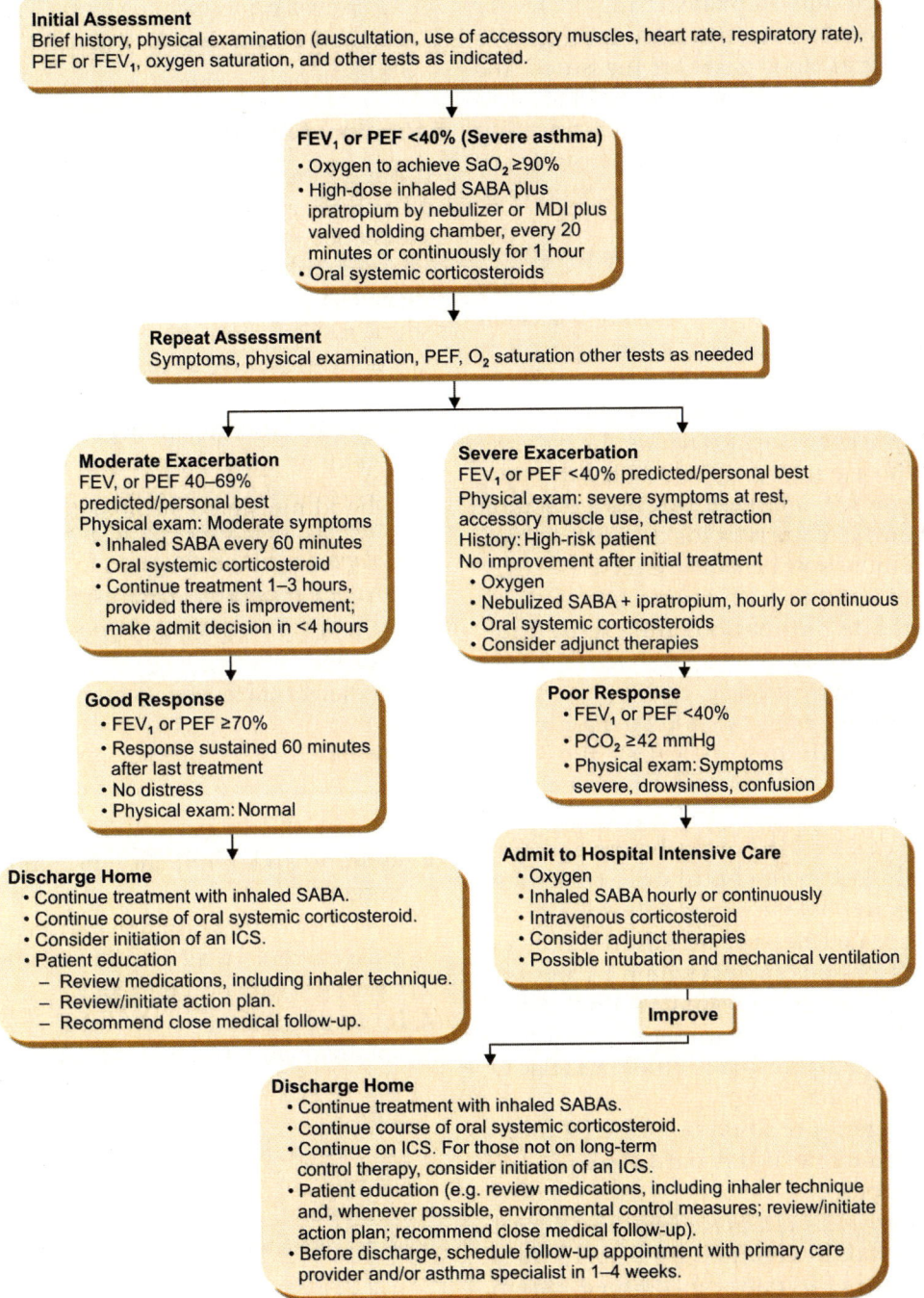

Initial Assessment
Brief history, physical examination (auscultation, use of accessory muscles, heart rate, respiratory rate), PEF or FEV$_1$, oxygen saturation, and other tests as indicated.

FEV$_1$ or PEF <40% (Severe asthma)
- Oxygen to achieve SaO$_2$ ≥90%
- High-dose inhaled SABA plus ipratropium by nebulizer or MDI plus valved holding chamber, every 20 minutes or continuously for 1 hour
- Oral systemic corticosteroids

Repeat Assessment
Symptoms, physical examination, PEF, O$_2$ saturation other tests as needed

Moderate Exacerbation
FEV, or PEF 40–69% predicted/personal best
Physical exam: Moderate symptoms
- Inhaled SABA every 60 minutes
- Oral systemic corticosteroid
- Continue treatment 1–3 hours, provided there is improvement; make admit decision in <4 hours

Severe Exacerbation
FEV$_1$ or PEF <40% predicted/personal best
Physical exam: severe symptoms at rest, accessory muscle use, chest retraction
History: High-risk patient
No improvement after initial treatment
- Oxygen
- Nebulized SABA + ipratropium, hourly or continuous
- Oral systemic corticosteroids
- Consider adjunct therapies

Good Response
- FEV$_1$ or PEF ≥70%
- Response sustained 60 minutes after last treatment
- No distress
- Physical exam: Normal

Poor Response
- FEV$_1$ or PEF <40%
- PCO$_2$ ≥42 mmHg
- Physical exam: Symptoms severe, drowsiness, confusion

Discharge Home
- Continue treatment with inhaled SABA.
- Continue course of oral systemic corticosteroid.
- Consider initiation of an ICS.
- Patient education
  - Review medications, including inhaler technique.
  - Review/initiate action plan.
  - Recommend close medical follow-up.

Admit to Hospital Intensive Care
- Oxygen
- Inhaled SABA hourly or continuously
- Intravenous corticosteroid
- Consider adjunct therapies
- Possible intubation and mechanical ventilation

Improve

Discharge Home
- Continue treatment with inhaled SABAs.
- Continue course of oral systemic corticosteroid.
- Continue on ICS. For those not on long-term control therapy, consider initiation of an ICS.
- Patient education (e.g. review medications, including inhaler technique and, whenever possible, environmental control measures; review/initiate action plan; recommend close medical follow-up).
- Before discharge, schedule follow-up appointment with primary care provider and/or asthma specialist in 1–4 weeks.

FEV$_1$: forced expiratory volume in 1 second; ICS: inhaled corticosteroid; MDI: metered-dose inhaler; PEF: peak expiratory flow; SABA: short-acting β$_2$-agonist, SaO$_2$: oxygen saturation.

Fig. 3.3: Management of asthma exacerbations; emergency department and hospital-based treatment. Adapted from National Asthma Education and Prevention Program. Expert Panel Report 3: Guidelines for the Diagnosis and management of Asthma National institute of Health, Pub No. 08-4051 Bethesda, MD, 2007.

- Magnesium sulphate (25 mg/kg I.V. or by nebuliser up to maximum 2.0 g).
- Arterial blood gases are measured; the $PaCO_2$ greater than 6 kPa and PaO_2 less than 8 kPa alongwith deteriorating consciousness (confusion, drowsiness, coma) are indications for intubation and mechanical ventilation with 100% O_2.
- *Antibiotics:* Mycoplasma and Chlamydophilia infection predisposes to acute exacerbation. Antibiotics are indicated in the presence of infection (purulent sputum, leucocytosis). Amoxycillin or one of the macrolides is adequate.
- *Intravenous aminophylline:* In patients who are refractory to inhaled therapy, slow I.V. infusion of aminophylline and systemic steroids in acute asthma demonstrate beneficial effect.
- For asthma with respiratory failure, initiate intubation and ventilation straightway.

Monitoring of treatment
- *PEFR recordings* should be made every 15–30 minutes to assess the early response and as and when required basis. In hospital, PEFR values should be charted 4–6 hourly, before and after inhaled bronchodilator treatment throughout the period of hospital stay.
- Repeated measurement of arterial blood gas tensions and pH within 1–2 hours is necessary in all patients if first arterial sample shows features of life-threatening situation ($PaO_2 < 8$ kPa and $PaCO_2 > 6$ kPa and rising).
- Oxygen saturation by pulse oximetry is valuable in all patients to assess response.

3. *Recovery phase of asthma:* Aggressive treatment should continue for 7 to 10 days; thereafter, it may be stepped down. Physio-therapy and expectorants to assist expectoration may be useful at this stage. Oral corticosteroids should be continued for 2 weeks then substituted by steroids inhalers for maintenance.

4. *Correction of precipitating factor:* Triggering or provoking agents must be avoided (Fig. 3.3).

Refractory Asthma

Although most patients with asthma are controlled with appropriate medication. Persistence of asthmatic symptoms despite maximum inhaled therapy is termed as *refractory asthma*. The causes or factors that make the asthma resistant are:

1. Poor compliance or non compliance with medication.
2. Exposure to high, ambient levels of allergens or unidentified occupational agents.
3. Gastroesophageal reflux.
4. Chronic infection with *mycoplasma* or *Chlamydophila pneumoniae*.
5. Drugs, e.g. beta blockers, aspirin, NSAIDs.
6. Systemic diseases, e.g. hyper or hypothyroidism.
7. Premenstrual tenson worsens asthma.

Treatment

1. Correct use of inhalers to improve compliance.
2. Identify and eliminate the underlying trigger.
3. Low dose of theophylline may be helpful. Most patients may require maintenance treatment with oral steroids.
4. In some patients with allergic asthma omalizumab (anti-IgE) is effective particularly when there are frequent exacerbations.
5. A few patients may get benefit with infusion of beta-agonists (salbutamol or terbutaline).
6. Anti-TNF therapy may also be effective.

Corticosteroid-resistant Asthma

It is defined as failure to respond to a high dose of oral prednisolone (40 mg OD over 2 weeks). There are several mechanisms involved in steroid-resistant asthma such as reduction in circulating monocytes and lymphocytes, an increase in spliced form of steroid receptors GR-β, an abnormal histone acetylation, a defect in IL-10 production.

Brittle Asthma

Chaotic variations in lung functions despite appropriate therapy is called brittle asthma.

1. **Type 1 brittle asthma:** There is variation in pattern of asthma and it responds to either oral steroids or infusion of β_2-agonists.

2. **Type 2 brittle asthma:** These have normal or near normal lung function but unpredictable. They may not respond to steroids or inhaled bronchodilator. These patients respond to subcutaneous adrenaline administration. This asthma may result in death.

Acute Respiratory Distress Syndrome (ARDS)

ACUTE RESPIRATORY DISTRESS SYNDROME (ARDS)

Diagnostic Criteria

Acute onset dyspnoea following medical or surgical disorder:

1. Inspired oxygenation PaO_2/FiO_2 ratio <200 mmHg.
2. Normal pulmonary capillary wedge pressure (PCWP) <18 mm with normal left atrial pressure.

Step	Goals and limits
Start volume/pressure cycled ventilation	• Tidal volume ≤6 ml/kg • Plateau pressure <30 cm H₂O • RR ≤35 per minute
Oxygenate	• FiO_2 ≤0.6 • PEEP ≤10 cm H₂O • SaO_2 88–95%
Minimize acidosis	• PH ≥7.30 • RR ≤35 per minute
Diuresis	• MAP ≥65 mmHg • Avoid hypoperfusion

A Algorithm for management of severe ARDS

3. Bilateral diffuse pulmonary infiltrates.

Evidence based step-wise initial management of ARDS is shown in Fig. 4.1A

Definition

Acute respiratory distress syndrome is defined as an acute hypoxic respiratory failure resulting

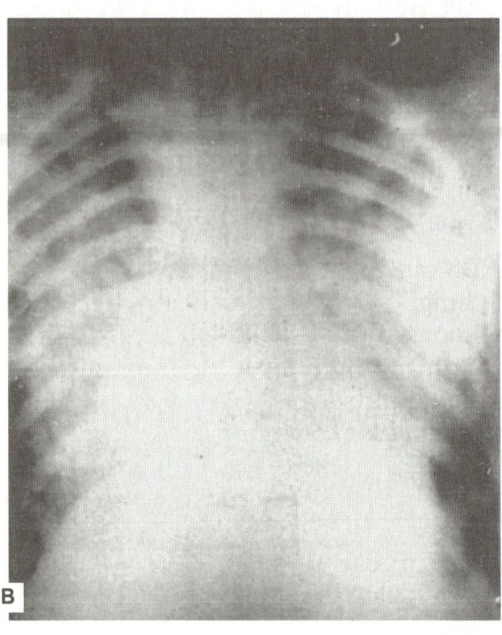

B

X-ray chest AP view: Non-cardiogenic pulmonary oedema (adult respiratory distress syndrome)

Fig 4.1A and B: Acute respiratory distress syndrome (ARDS). (A) Diagnostic criteria and algorithm for management of ARDS; (B) Radiological appearance—pulmonary oedema with normal cardiac shadow

from a systemic or pulmonary insult without any evidence of heart failure. It is characterised by extensive bilateral pulmonary infiltrates, rapid onset dyspnoea, refractory hypoxaemia, stiff lung (decreased compliance) and respiratory distress / failure.

It is an emergency and carries a high mortality rate (40–60%).

Recently European–American consensus conference defined ARDS as a condition of acute onset with following features:

i. Impaired oxygenation (it is defined as a ratio of PaO_2 to the fraction of inspired O_2 (FiO_2) that is <200 mmHg. It is further used to categorise ARDS into mild (200–300 mmHg] moderate (100–200 mmHg) and severe <100 mmHg by Berlin definition)

ii. Chest X-ray showing diffuse bilateral lung infiltrates.

iii. Pulmonary capillary wedge pressure (PCWP) is normal, i.e. less than or equal to 18 mmHg when measured and no clinical evidence of left atrial hypertension to exclude cardiogenic pulmonary oedema. This is also called '*noncardiogenic pulmonary oedema*'.

Causes

ARDS can occur as a non-specific reaction of the lungs to a wide variety of insults direct (pulmonary insult) or indirect (systemic insult) including shock, sepsis, embolism, trauma, inhalation of toxic gases and smoke, etc. (Box 1). Pneumonia is a common cause of ARDS.

Pathophysiology

ARDS can be considered as the earliest manifestation of a generalised inflammatory reaction and irrespective of its cause, evolves through the following phases:

1. **Exudative phase (*non-cardiogenic pulmonary oedema*):** This is the early phase of ARDS; occurs within 24–96 hours following a precipitating event. It is characterised by endothelial injury, denudation of type I epithelial cells, increase in

Box 1 Causes of acute respiratory distress syndrome
Systemic insults (indirect injury)
• Trauma, head injury
• Shock, sepsis
• Pancreatitis
• Repeated blood transfusions
• Disseminated intravascular coagulation (DIC)
• Burns
• Drugs, e.g. opiates, aspirin, phenothiazines, tricyclic antidepressant, nitrofurantoin, amiodarone, paraquat
• Thrombotic thrombocytopenic purpura
• Cardiopulmonary bypass
Pulmonary insults (direct injury)
• Aspiration of gastric contents
• Embolism, e.g. thrombus, fat, air and amniotic fluid.
• Miliary tuberculosis
• Diffuse pneumonia, acute eosinophilic pneumonia, cryptogenic pneumonia
• Near drowning
• Toxic gas inhalation, e.g. CO, NO_2, PH_3, chlorine, SO_2, ammonia, hyperbaric O_2
• Lung contusion
• Radiation exposure
• High altitude pulmonary oedema
• Lung re-expansion or reperfusion

vascular permeability, release of inflammatory cytokines and hyaline membrane formation. There is decreased surfactant production. It usually lasts for 3–7 days. The clinical hallmarks of this phase are bilateral pulmonary infiltrates (*noncardiogenic pulmonary oedema*), dyspnoea and marked hypoxaemia.

2. **Proliferative phase (*stage of development of pulmonary hypertension*):** By 3–7 days, patient who survives the initial phase progresses to proliferative stage. Necrotic type I cells are replaced by type II epithelial cells which proliferate and form new alveolar epithelium. Interstitial and alveolar oedema starts decreasing and these spaces are filled with RBCs, inflammatory cells and cellular debris. This phase is characterised by worsening hypoxaemia (cyanosis) as a result of pulmonary shunting of blood and development of pulmonary hypertension as a result of

hypoxic vasoconstrictive response and microthrombi formation.

3. **Fibrotic phase:** After about 7–10 days of onset of ARDS, activated fibroblasts accumulate in the interstitial spaces. Subsequently fibrosis sets in with loss of elastic tissue and obliteration of the lung vasculature. This may slowly resolve or may result in lung destruction which may be irreversible.

Clinical Features

In addition to the clinical manifestations of the provoking medical or surgical condition, the patients usually develop *unexplained dyspnoea, dry cough, labored breathing*, and may become *agitated* and *disoriented* usually after 24–72 hours of precipitating event. *Tachypnoea, tachycardia* and *cyanosis* appear later. *Fine crackles* are heard throughout both lung fields.

Investigations

Investigations are done to find out the treatable underlying cause such as infections and to assess the progress of the disease.

1. **Chest X-ray (Fig. 4.1B):** The radiological features become evident by about 12 hours after the clinical onset of type I respiratory failure (ARDS). Initially, patchy ill-defined opacities or infiltrates may become apparent throughout the lungs, sparing the costophrenic angles. Later, the chest X-ray shows bilateral, diffuse shadowing with an alveolar pattern and air bronchogram is frequently visible which distinguishes it from cardiogenic pulmonary oedema, and last of all it may progress to the picture of complete 'white out'. Heart size remains normal. After about a week, the lungs remain diffusely abnormal suggestive of interstitial and air-space fibrosis.

2. **Arterial blood gas analysis:** It shows characteristic of type I respiratory failure, i.e.:
   - Refractory hypoxaemia (PaO_2 <60 mmHg/or <8.0 kPa).

   - Hypocapnia ($PaCO_2$ <6.6 kPa).
   - Alkalosis (pH >7.39).

3. **CT scan:** CT scan of the chest reveals diffusely distributed non-uniform ground glass opacification or consolidation. As the disease progresses, reticular appearance becomes evident indicating interstitial fibrosis. Complications of ARDS such as small pneumothorax, pneumomediastinum and interstitial emphysema become evident on CT.

4. **Measurement of pulmonary capillary wedge pressure (PCWP)** by Swan-Ganz catheter is less than 18 mmHg. The cardiac index is >2.1 L/min.

5. **Bronchoalveolar lavage** may reveal increased number of polymorph leucocytes.

Differential Diagnosis

Several conditions stimulate clinical and radiological findings of ARDS, hence, have to be differentiated. These are:

1. **Cardiogenic pulmonary oedema** (acute left ventricular failure). The PCWP is elevated (>18 mmHg).

2. **Diffuse alveolar haemorrhage:** There is haemoptysis, fall in haemoglobin, frothy red fluid on bronchoscopy and haemosiderin laden macrophages—a characteristic finding, may be seen in the bronchoalveolar lavage fluid.

3. **Metastatic carcinomatosis.**

Management

Attempts should be made to establish the cause of ARDS and institute the specific therapy to treat it, if treatable (sepsis aspiration, trauma). The other steps of management are:

1. **General measures:**
   - Procure pulmonary and systemic I.V. access for haemodynamic monitoring and fluid therapy.
   - Arterial O_2 saturation and arterial blood gas analysis must be monitored for progress.

- Adequate nutrition should be ensured through enteral feeding.
- If sepsis is the cause, empirical antibiotic therapy may be begun followed by specific therapy depending on the culture and sensitivity reports.
- Prophylaxis against pulmonary embolism (anti-coagulants), GI bleed (H_2 blockers) aspiration (proper position) and infections.

2. **Fluid restriction and diuretics:** Try to maintain low CVP (<4 mmHg) or PCWP (<10 mmHg) for few days by fluid restriction and diuretics. This management strategy will minimise the left atrial filling pressure and reduce interstitial oedema. *Transfusion of blood* or *packed red cells* is indicated if the patient is anaemic (Hb <7 g%).

3. **Oxygen therapy:** The simplest method and the lowest inspired fraction of O_2 (FiO_2) should be used to achieve a PaO_2 of 60 mmHg (O_2 saturation of about 90%). Initially spontaneous ventilation using a face mask with high flow rate can be used to improve PaO_2 without increasing FiO_2. If a FiO_2 more than 0.6 then PEEP or inverse ratio ventilation (inspiratory time is more than expiratory time) must be considered.

4. **Mechanical ventilation (assisted ventilatory support):** In ARDS, adequate oxygenation is usually not achieved with these less invasive measures listed above. Mechanical ventilatory support after endotracheal intubation is initially started with volume cycled mechanical ventilators with *low tidal volumes*. To begin with, the initial ventilator setting could be FiO_2 as 1.0 (or a lower value that can achieve a PaO_2 >60 mmHg and oxygen saturation >90%), low tidal volume 6 ml/kg body weight, PEEP less than or equal to 5 cm of water and inspiratory flow 760 L/min. High PEEP may be applied to increase the lung volume and keep the alveoli open. PEEP is applied in small increments of 3–5 cm

H_2O up to a maximum of 15 cm H_2O to achieve maximum oxygen saturation of >90% with low non-toxic FiO_2 levels (<0.6). Ventilatory rate of 20–25 breaths/minute is needed to keep $PaCO_2$ and pH normal. A multicentric trial has shown low mortality rates when low tidal volumes were used.

Airway pressure release ventilation (*inverse ratio ventilation*) and *high frequency ventilation* are other newer methods of ventilation to improve oxygenation.

5. **Other ventilatory strategies:** High frequency ventilation or partial liquid ventilation and lung replacement therapy with extracorporal membrane oxygenation has yield promising results in selected patients.

6. **Prone position:** In situations where maximal PEEP with FiO_2 of 1.0 does not supply sufficient oxygen, placing the patient in the prone position has been found helpful.

7. **Neuromuscular blockade:** In severe ARDS early neuromuscular blockade increased the rate of survival and ventilator free days, hence to be used to facilitate mechanical ventilation.

8. **Pharmacological treatment:**
   i. *Corticosteroids therapy:* To reduce potentially deleterious pulmonary inflammation steroids have been used with limited benefit.
   ii. *Recent reports using nitric oxide* (NO) inhalation (5–80 parts per million) or prostacycline (PGI_2) as a selective pulmonary vasodilator showed promising results on initial evaluation. They neither improved survival nor decreased the time of duration of ventilation, hence, not recommended now in ARDS.
   iii. *Certain antioxidants* (N-acetylcysteine, glutathione, vitamin E) have been tried to overcome free radical-mediated injury without much success.

Pulmonary Venous Thromboembolism

PULMONARY EMBOLISM

Definition

Lungs are connected to the venous side of circulation, hence, act as a first filter for a variety of diverse materials gaining access to venous circulation, thus, is a common site for embolism. In strict sense, *pulmonary embolism* represents formation of a clot or thrombus in the venous circulation, its dislodgement and propagation through venous circulation and ultimately its lodgement in pulmonary circulation. Clinically, it is defined as acute haemodynamic disturbance due to occlusion of pulmonary vasculature due to an embolus or emboli.

A great majority of patients die within first few hours of the embolic episode due to inadequate therapy because the diagnosis is either missed or delayed.

Causes

Thrombus and many other substances can embolise pulmonary circulation. The causes of pulmonary embolism are given in Table 5.1. The common sites of venous thrombosis are represented in Fig. 5.1A.

The most common cause of pulmonary embolisation is deep vein thrombosis (DVT) which constitutes 90–95% of patients, out of which 70–80% originate from the veins of

Table 5.1	Causes of pulmonary embolism
1. Thrombotic	

- Deep vein thrombosis
- Congestive heart failure
- Right sided endocarditis
- Atrial fibrillation

2. Non-thrombotic

- Fat embolism following bone trauma or a fracture
- Amniotic fluid embolism following delivery and caesarean section
- Septic (infective endocarditis)
- Tumour embolism (choriocarcinoma, renal cell carcinoma)
- Parasitic eggs (schistosomiasis)
- Air embolism (pulmonary barotrauma in divers and during neurosurgery from central venous catheter

the legs (Fig. 5.1C) and 10–15% from pelvic veins, calf vein thrombi rarely embolise. They propagate proximally to popliteal and iliofemoral veins and then embolise. The mechanism of thrombus formation in the veins is similar to thrombus formation anywhere, and involves three factors, i.e. *stasis of blood, hypercoagulability of the blood and abnormalities of the vessel wall*.

Pulmonary embolism and DVT are two manifestations of same disease.

The *clinical risk factors* that predispose to DVT and embolism are:

1. Surgery, trauma (*in-plaster injuries* or fracture of lower limb bones)

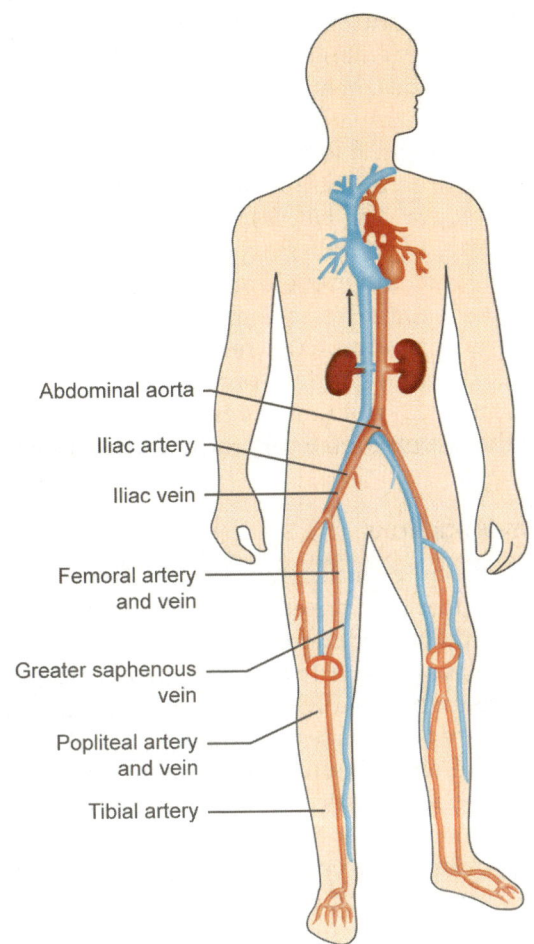

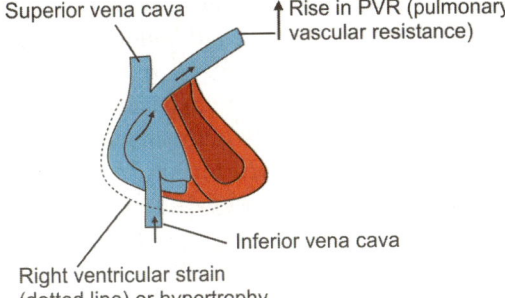

B. Haemodynamic consequences of pulmonary embolism

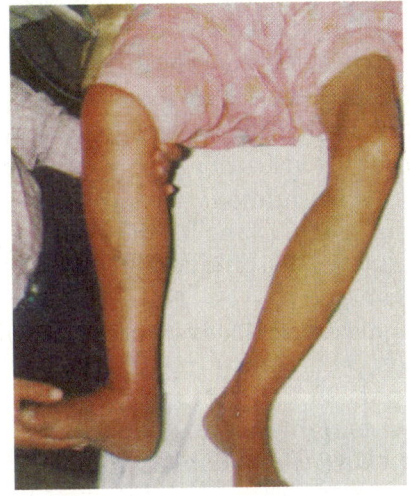

C. Deep vein thrombosis (DVT) of right leg. Note the swelling of the leg and positive Homan's sign (the sign is now-a-days not elicited). The patient presented with pain chest and haemoptysis. CT angiogram confirmed the diagnosis of pulmonary embolism

A. Veins of lower limbs and site of venous thrombosis and passage of embolism

Fig. 5.1A to C: Patient with DVT and pulmonary embolism

2. Prolonged immobilisation (stroke, or intensive care unit patients)
3. Oral contraceptives, hormonal replacement therapy, pregnancy, postpartum
4. Cancer and cancer chemotherapy
5. Varicosity of the veins
6. Chronic kidney disease, arterial hypertension, blood transfutions
7. Congestive heart failure (stasis of blood), COPD with cor pulmonale
8. Physical inactivity, e.g. obesity and smoking
9. Hypercoagulability (deficiency of protein C and S, antithrombin) prothrombin gene mutation, antiphospholipid antibodies, polycythemia
10. Inherited gene defect (resistance to activated protein C, and factor V Leiden mutation)
11. Long-hour air travel, air pollution.

Pathophysiological Consequences (Fig. 5.1B)

When deep vein thrombi detach from the site of formation they travel through vena cava, right atrium and ventricle to lodge in the pulmonary vasculature constituting *pulmonary embolism* (PE). The consequences are:

1. **Increased pulmonary vascular resistance** due to vascular obstruction and vasoconstriction due to neurohumoral factors.
2. **Impaired gas exchange due to:**
   - Increased physiological alveolar dead space from vascular obstruction leading to wasted ventilation. There will be large areas of the lungs which are ventilated but not perfused.
   - Hypoxaemia from alveolar hypoventilation in the non-obstructed lung and right to left shunting .
   - Loss of gas exchange surface.
3. **Increased airway resistance** due to reflex bronchoconstriction promotes wheezing.
4. **Reduced pulmonary compliance** due to lung oedema, lung haemorrhage and loss of surfactants, produces increased work of breathing.
5. **Right ventricular dysfunction:** As pulmonary vasculature resistance increases, it puts strain on the right ventricle and causes right ventricular dilatation (*acute cor pulmonole*) and myocardial ischaemia. Consequently the interventricular septum bulges into normal left ventricle reducing left ventricular cavity and its filling (*Bernheim effect*). Underfilling of left ventricle may lead to fall in left ventricular output causing hypotension and global myocardial ischaemia. Eventually, circulatory collapse and death can occur.

Clinical Features

The clinical picture is highly variable from *asymptomatic disease* to *catastrophic acute illness*. The massive pulmonary *embolism produces features of* **acute cor pulmonale**; while multiple microembolisation leads to features of **chronic cor pulmonale**. The triad of a pulmonary infarct is *haemoptysis, pleuritic chest pain* and *wheeze* that occurs due to embolisation of small peripheral blood vessels near the pleura. The clinical features (symptoms and signs) of pulmonary embolism are given in Table 5.2.

Dyspnoea, syncope, hypotension or shock indicate massive embolisation; while pleuritic pain, cough, haemoptysis, wheeze indicate a small embolisation located distally near the pleura. The *physical signs* depend on the severity of embolism, type of vessel/vessels involved and development of an infarct. Massive (large vessel) embolisation produces acute cor pulmonale, recurrent or medium vessel embolisation produce chronic cor pulmonale while small vessel embolisation is either asymptomatic or produces a pulmonary intarct.

Investigations

1. **Blood examination:** It may show leucocytosis and raised ESR if patient develops a pulmonary infarct.
2. **Chest X-ray:** It may be normal (12% of patients in PIOPED study had normal X-ray even in severe embolism). However, the most frequent radiological findings are atelectasis, elevated hemidiaphragm, enlargement of cardiac shadow, enlarged pulmonary conus, pleural effusion and consolidation.
   - Avascular lung zone (*Westermark's sign*), wedge-shaped opacity above hemidiaphragm (*Hampton's hump*) and an enlarged right descending pulmonary artery (*Palla's sign*).

> **Note:** All these signs are non-specific. The chest X-ray is done to exclude the other possibilities.

3. **The ECG:** The 12 lead ECG may be normal (70–80% of cases just show sinus tachycardia) in mild to moderate cases. In severe cases, the ECG changes represent P pulmonoles acute right ventricular strain (T wave inversion in $V_1 - V_4$) or myocardial ischaemia (ST segment depression indeed I and II) or both. Right axis deviation and clockwise rotation is common. The $S_I Q_{III}$, T_{III} syndrome in which there is S wave in lead I and Q wave in lead III with T

Table 5.2 Clinical features of pulmonary embolism

Size of vessel involved	Clinical syndrome	Haemodynaimc consequences	Symptoms	Signs
• Massive (large vessel) embolisation	Acute cor pulmonale (primary pulmonary hypertension)	• >50% ↓ in PV bed • ↑↑ PVR • ↑↑ RV afterload • RV failure • ↓ CO and shock	• Acute dyspnoea • Tachypnoea • Tachycardia • Sweating • Haemoptysis • Chest pain • Syncope	• Hypotension or shock • Raised JVP • Cyanosis • Loud P_2 with wide splitting • An ejection systolic murmur at P_2 area • Signs of RV hypertrophy, S_4
• Multiple or recurrent embolism (chronic pulmonary embolism)	Primary pulmonary hypertension or chronic cor pulmonale	• >50% ↓ in PV bed • ↑ PVR • ↑ RV afterload • RV dysfunction • No shock	• Dyspnoea • Fatigue • Weakness • Syncope	• Raised JVP • Cyanosis • Oedema • Hepatomegaly • Loud P_2 with narrow splitting • Parasternal heave and RV hypertrophy
• Small or medium sized vessels embolisation	Pulmonary infarct(s) or asymptomatic	• <50 in PV bed • PVR—normal • No RV dysfunction • No shock	• Pleuritic chest pain • Haemoptysis • Wheeze • Jaundice, mild, occasional • Fever	• Pleural rub • Tachycardia • Either signs of pleural effusion or atelectasis • Crackles (rales)

↓: decrease; ↑: increase; ↑↑: marked increase; RV: right ventricle; PVR: pulmonary vascular resistance; PV: pulmonary vascular bed and, CO : cardiac output

inversion, if present is highly suggestive of acute pulmonary embolism.

Transient development of incomplete RBBB is indicative of acute pulmonary embolism. Recurrent episodes of arrhythmias, e.g. sinus tachycardia, atrial flutter or fibrillation may also occur.

> **Tip:** ECG changes are transient in nature, hence, appearance and disappearance of above mentioned changes on serial ECGs is highly diagnostic. It must be born in mind that normal ECG does not rule out pulmonary embolism.

4. **Arterial blood gas (ABG) abnormalities:** It shows hypoxaemia with respiratory alkalosis.
5. **Echocardiagram:** The two-dimensional echocardiography is particularly helpful as it may reveal right ventricular dilatation/dysfunction, hypokinesia, septal flattening and tricuspid regurgitation. These echocardiographic findings in patients with DVT are virtually pathognomonic.

Transthoracic echocardiography is particularly helpful in critically ill patients as it may show a clot in right heart or the main pulmonary arteries.

6. **Plasma D-dimers:** D-dimer; a specific degradation product of fibrin is released into circulation after fibrinolysis of the clot. Its elevated levels in blood (ELISA method) suggest active thrombosis. It has not much diagnostic value as it may be raised in other conditions such as myocardial infarction, pneumonia, heart failure, cancer, etc. On the other hand, it is an excellent tool to exclude the pulmonary embolism, i.e. low levels of D-dimers (<500 mg/ml) exclude pulmonary embolism, hence, is most useful initial screening investigation (Fig. 5.3). Serum troponin I and T, plasma brain or B-type natriuretic peptide (BNP) are higher and correlate with adverse outcome. They are not useful in making the diagnosis.

7. **Non-invasive tests for deep vein thrombosis:** Any objective evidence confirming DVT (Doppler ultrasound, impedances plethysmography, contrast venography, contrast MRI, etc.) definitely raises the possibility of thromboembolism in an appropriate setting (echocardiographic evidence of right ventricular dysfunction, dilatation, etc.).

8. **CT pulmonary angiography:** It is accepted as a gold standard for the diagnosis of pulmonary embolism. Contrast material is injected in the main pulmonary artery which provides direct visualisation of *intraluminal filling defects or abrupt cut-off the vessel* caused by pulmonary embolism. It is hazardous in patients with pulmonary hypertension, right heart failure or respiratory failure. It is strongly indicated in establishing the diagnosis of life-threatening embolism where thrombolytic therapy or mechanical intervention or surgery are being considered.

   MRI: It has sensitivity and specificity equivalent to contrast venography in diagnosis of DVT. An intraluminal filling defect in more than one projection is virtually diagnostic of PE.

9. **Radioisotopic ventilation perfusion (V/Q) scan:** It is second line diagnostic test. It includes two scans done simultaneously, i.e. lung perfusion scan (^{99m}technetium) and ventilation scan (by radioactive ^{133}Xenon). Lung perfusion scan is a simple procedure in which particles of macroaggregated albumin labelled with ^{99m}technetium are injected intravenously. The under perfused area(s) of the lung is shown as *'cold area/spot'* or *'avascular zone'* in the scan.

   A perfusion scan can demonstrate area/areas of hypoperfusion but cannot identify the cause of perfusion defect.

A perfusion defect/defects can occur with any parenchymal or pleural lesion such as COPD, asthma, atelectasis, pneumonia and pleural effusion.

A normal perfusion scan in a patient with suspected pulmonary embolism virtually excludes it.

In a ventilation scan, radioactive ^{133}Xenon or krypton is inhaled and exhaled by the patient, while the gamma camera records its distribution throughout the alveolar gas exchange units. The test is based on the assumption that ventilation is preserved in areas of reduced perfusion due to pulmonary embolism and is abnormal when perfusion defects are due to pulmonary disease. The sensitivity and specificity of V/Q scans were established in general representative US Population by Prospective Investigation of Pulmonary Embolism Diagnosis (PIOPED) study and is used as a criteria for interpretation of V/Q scan (i.e. *high probable, intermediate* and *low probable*).

A **high probable scan** is defined as two or more segmental perfusion defect with normal ventilation, indicates pulmonary embolism. A **low probability scan** and a strong clinical impression that pulmonary embolism is unlikely make the possibility of pulmonary embolism remote.

10. **Spiral contrast chest CT:** It is a principal imaging test for diagnosis. This approach is best suited for identifying emboli that are situated in the proximal pulmonary vasculature but may not pick up emboli in distal vascular bed.

Helical CT pulmonary angiography is now a-days investigation of choice than V/Q scan in PE.

Diagnosis

Well's diagnostic scoring system for DVT and clinical prediction rule for PE is depicted in Box 1.

The recommendations for the diagnosis on V/Q scan are depicted in Figs 5.2 and 5.3.

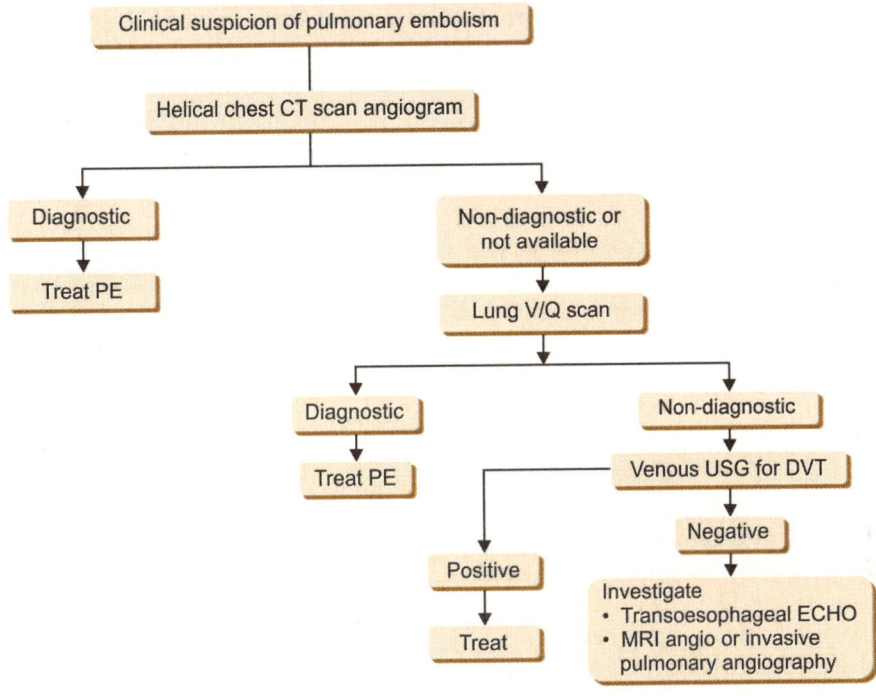

Fig. 5.2: Algorithm for diagnosis of clinically suspected cases of pulmonary thromboembolism

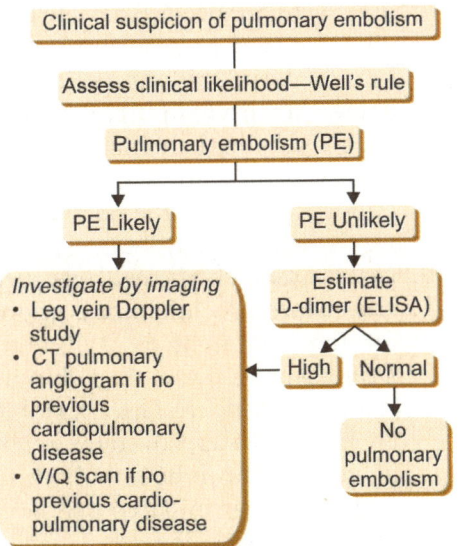

Fig. 5.3: Initial screening of the patients with suspicion of pulmonary embolism (PE)

Box 1 Well's diagnostic scoring system	
Feature	*Points*
• Clinical symptoms/signs of DVT	3.0
• An alternative diagnosis is less likely, i.e. other conditions have been excluded	3.0
• Heart rate >100/min	1.5
• Immobilisation or surgery during past 4 weeks	1.5
• Previous episode of DVT/pulmonary embolism	1.5
• Hemoptysis	1.0
• Malignancy (on treatment/treated in past 6 months)	1.0

Note: Total score is 12.5. If score is ≤4.0, then clinical diagnosis is less likely.

Management

Massive pulmonary thromboembolism is a life-threatening emergency, carries a mortality of 43–80% in first 2 hours following the event, hence, appropriate preventive measures in high-risk patients are most useful. However, once massive pulmonary thromboembolism has occurred, immediate recognition and institution of treatment are mandatory. Diagnosis mainly rests on the clinical suspicion together with contrast chest CT and V/Q scan (as discussed in algorithm Fig. 5.2). The steps of management are:

1. **Initial supportive measures:** Opiates may be necessary to relieve pain and distress but should be used with caution in hypotensive patients. Resuscitation by external cardiac massage may be sometimes successful in moribund patient by dislodging and breaking up a large central thrombus. Other measures include:

   i. *Oxygen administration* through mask
   ii. *Fluid therapy* for hypotensive and shocked patients. It should be given cautiously.
   iii. *Vasoactive drugs* such as norepinephrine and dobutamine to raise the BP in hypotensive or shocked patients. Diuretics and I.V. vasodilators should be avoided during acute setting.

2. **Prompt anticoagulation:** If the patient remains haemodynamically stable with or without supportive treatment, anticoagulation with heparin should be given to all patients with a high clinical suspicion of pulmonary embolism whilst confirmatory test results are awaited. Heparin accelerates the action of antithrombin III to inactivate thrombin, factor Xa and factor IX, prevents the further formation and extension of thrombosis and permits endogenous fibrinolysis to dissolve some of the clots. The standard regimen of heparin followed by 6 months of oral warfarin results in an 80–90% reduction in risk of PE. Heparin without oral anticoagulation is the treatment used throughout pregnancy to manage pulmonary embolism in high-risk pregnant patients. Heparin is used in the dose which prolongs the activated PTT or INR to 1.5 to 2 times over control.

   Different modes of anticoagulation are:

   i. *Aggressive unfractionated heparin therapy:* Heparin is started in the dose of 5000–7500 units as a bolus dose, followed by 1000 U/hr as an infusion monitoring the PTT.

   ii. *Short course of heparin* (5 days) and simultaneous administration of warfarin. The dose is adjusted to maintain the INR at 1.5 to 3 times that of control. Early discharge of the patient from hospital is possible with this treatment.

   > **Note:** International normalisation ratio (INR) is the PT ratio that would be obtained if the WHO standard thromboplastin was used in performing a given PT test. An INR of 2.0 to 3 is equal to a PT ratio of 1.3 to 1.5 approx. **Warfarin monitoring should ideally be done with INR.**

   iii. *A low molecular heparin,* i.e. enoxaparin (1 mg/kg bid) or tinzaprin (175 U/kg OD) with normal kidney function or fondaparinux given subcutaneously in a weight adjusted dosage is equally effective as unfractionated heparin in the treatment of pulmonary thromboembolism.

   iv. *Warfarin:* This vitamin K antagonist oral anticoagulant needs 5 days to become effective, therefore, during first 5 days both heparin and oral anticoagulant should be used simultaneously then followed by oral anticoagulant alone. Dose is 5 mg daily. The major risk of anticoagulation is haemorrhage, with warfarin, it is about 3%.

   v. *Newer noval oral anticoagulants: Rivaroxaba*—a factor Xa inhibitor is approved for the treatment of DVT and PE, *Debigartan*—a direct thrombin inhibitor and *endixaban* a factor Xa inhibitor are likely to be approved for treatment of venous thromboembolism (DVT and PE) after an initial course of parenteral anticoagulation.

   Duration of anticoagulation for DVT is about 3 months and for DVT and PE ia about 3 to 6 months. For patients with cancer and venous thromboembolism it is given indefinitely till the patient is cancer free.

3. **Thrombolysis:** Patient with an acute massive pulmonary embolism with haemodynamically compromised state, i.e. evidence of right ventricular dysfunction on ECHO or of hypotension, should be considered for urgent thrombolytic therapy when the diagnosis is confirmed. Streptokinase is given as a loading dose of 250,000 I.V. over 20 to 30 minutes, after pretreatment with 100 mg of I.V. hydrocortisone. This is followed by continuous I.V. infusion of streptokinase 100,00. I.V. per hour for 24 hours. The lysis can be confirmed by measuring either PTT, FT, TT, fibrin split products or whole blood euglobin lysis time. Treatment with urokinase (a loading dose of 4400 ID/kg over 10 minutes followed by 4400 IU/kg/hr for 12 to 24 hours) is equally effective. Before initiation of thrombolytic therapy, heparin is administered. Alteplase (human tissue plasminogen activator-tPA is preferred thrombolytic (fibrinolytic) agent. It is more expensive but less likely to lead systemic side-effects and hypotension. A dose of 100 mg I.V. infusion administered over 2 hours is sufficient. Heparin should be given subsequently. The contraindications for thrombolytic therapy are intracranial disease, recent surgery and trauma

Box 2	Acute management of pulmonary embolism

Risk stratification

Normotension plus normal RV	Normotension plus RV dysfunction	Hypotension
Secondary prevention • Anticoagulation • IVC filters	Individualize therapy	Primary/aggressive therapy • Anticoagulation plus thrombolysis • Embolectomy/surgery

uncontrolled hypertension, bleeding diathesis and recent or past history of GI bleed or stroke and chronic liver disease.

Surgery

The advent of thrombolytic treatment has reduced the need for surgical procedures (*embolectomy, percutaneous transvenous catheter fragmentation* and *distal dissipation of proximal pulmonary embolism*). However, contraindications to thrombolytic therapy or refractory hypotension despite thrombolytic therapy have kept embolectomy a viable option.

Table 5.3	Prophylaxis of DVT and pulmonary thromboembolism
Risk factors	*Preventive measures/treatments*
1. **High to moderate risk general surgery patients**	• Low dose heparin, **or** • Low molecular weight heparin (LMWH) **plus** • Intermittent pneumatic compression devices. These devices apply pressure to calf, enhance venous return and fibrinolytic activity
2. **Neurosurgery, urosurgery, major knee surgery**	• Intermittent pneumatic compression **plus** graduated compression stocking
3. **Effective hip surgery, surgery for fracture hip**	• Low molecular weight heparin, or low dose heparin • Adjusted dose warfarin to keep PT at upper half of normal control value (INR 2.5)
4. **Very high-risk general surgery patients**	• Low molecular weight heparin or low dose heparin started preoperatively
5. **Medical patients with clinical risk factors for venous thromboembolism**	• Intermittent pneumatic compression • Low molecular weight heparin or low dose heparin

Surgical Methods (Caval Filters)

Patients with recurrent pulmonary embolism despite adequate anticoagulation or failure of anticoagulation control get benefit from the insertion of a filter placed in inferior vena cava (caval filter obstruction) below the origin of the renal vessels. Such filters are safe and effective in preventing embolisation.

Emotional support therapy: These patients though appear healthy and fit but are reluctant to continue life-long anticoagulants, hence, need support group therapy to remove their doubts.

Prophylaxis

The incidence of pulmonary embolism and deaths due to pulmonary embolism can be reduced by applying prophylactic strategies given in Table 5.3. Prevention of DVT in lower limbs will reduce the frequency of embolism. Patients with a high risk for developing pulmonary embolism should be given prophylactic therapy. Prophylactic therapy may be medical or surgical. The medical therapy in high risk patients is given in Table 5.3.

Pneumothorax

Definition

Pneumothorax is defined as the entry of air into the pleural space. The incidence is higher in males aged 15–30 years.

Classification

The pneumothorax is divided into two main categories, i.e. *spontaneous* and *traumatic* (Box 1). The *spontaneous pneumothorax* may be *primary* (underlying lung is healthy) or *secondary* (occurs as a complication of some lung disease).

The *traumatic pneumothorax* results either from a chest injury or from a clinical procedure (iatrogenic).

Causes

1. **Primary spontaneous pneumothorax:** It is caused by rupture of subpleural emphysematous blebs or a pleural bleb which may be congenital or acquired at pulmonary end of a pleural adhesion. Now, it has been established that 80% of patients with primary spontaneous pneumothorax have some emphysematous changes on CT scan. The *risk factors* identified for primary pneumothorax are:
   - Thin as well as tall body habitus in age groups of 10–30 years
   - Heavy smoking (>20 cigarettes/day).
   - Marfan's syndrome
   - Mitral valve prolapse
   - Going to high altitude
   - Bronchial anatomical abnormalities
2. **Secondary spontaneous pneumothorax:** It is most commonly seen in patients of COPD and pulmonary tuberculosis. Almost every lung disease may be associated with pneumothorax. *Pneumocystis carinii pneumonia* is an emerging cause of pneumothorax in patients of AIDS.

Box 1   Classification of pneumothorax

A. Spontaneous

i. *Primary:* There is no evidence of overt lung disease. Air enters into the pleural space either through rupture of a small subpleural emphysematous bulla or a pleural bleb at the pulmonary end of pleural adhesion.

ii. *Secondary:* There is an overt underlying lung disease, most commonly COPD or tuberculosis. It is also seen in bronchial asthma, pulmonary infarct, lung abscess, bronchogenic carcinoma and all forms of fibrotic and cystic lung lesions. In *tuberculosis* or *lung* abscess, there is *usually hydropneumothorax* because these lesions *lead to exudative pleural fluid.*

B. Traumatic

It occurs following chest trauma/injury or may result following thoracic surgery or biopsy called *iatrogenic*.

The other lung diseases associated with pneumothorax are:

- *Infections,* e.g. necrotising pneumonia, lung abscess. These commonly cause hydropneumothorax or pyopneumothorax.
- *Interstitial lung diseases*
- *Occupational lung disease,* e.g. silicosis, coal workers pneumoconiosis.
- *Malignancy lung,* e.g. bronchogenic carcinoma.
- *Miscellaneous rare causes* such as pulmonary infarct, asthma, cystic fibrosis, eosinophilic granuloma, post-irradiation, tuberous sclerosis, catamenial pneumothorax (endometriosis).

3. **Traumatic pneumothorax:** It results from:
   - Blunt injury to thorax or abdomen.
   - Penetrating thoracic injury.
   - Procedural (iatrogenic), e.g. pleural tap, pleural biopsy, bronchoscopy, lung biopsy, endoscopy and sclerotherapy, subclavian or internal jugular vein catheter placement and positive pressure mechanical ventilation.

Pathological Types (Fig. 6.1)

1. **Closed:** The rupture site closes and lung is deflated. The air in the pleural space is absorbed slowly and lung expands to its original position over few weeks. The mean pleural pressure is negative (less than atmospheric pressure).

2. **Open:** The rupture site does not close but forms a communication between the pleural cavity and the bronchus (*bronchopleural fistula*). The mean pleural pressure is atmospheric, hence, the lung cannot re-expand. Infection such as pyopneumothorax is a common complication of bronchopleural fistula. Open pneumothorax also can result from penetrating chest wall injury.

3. **Tension (valvular):** The communication between the pleura and the lung persists, and acts as a check valve (discussed on next page).

Clinical Features

Symptoms

Primary spontaneous pneumothorax develops suddenly without any provocation. Symptoms of pneumothorax depend on the amount of air in the pleural cavity. *A small pneumothorax* (<15% of a hemithorax) is usually asymptomatic and detected by chance on routine chest X-ray. Moderate amount of air in pleural space produces chest pain and dyspnoea. Chest pain is sharp, pleuritic and localised to the side of pneumothorax. Dyspnoea is proportional to the amount of pneumothorax.

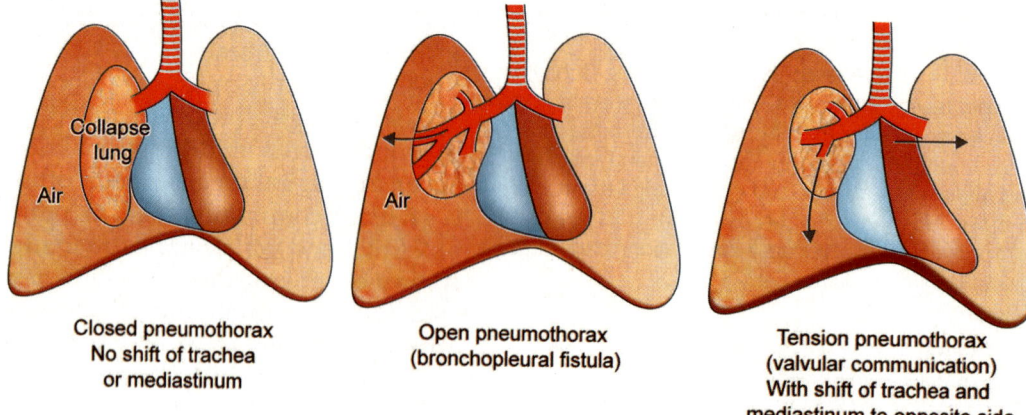

Closed pneumothorax
No shift of trachea
or mediastinum

Open pneumothorax
(bronchopleural fistula)

Tension pneumothorax
(valvular communication)
With shift of trachea and
mediastinum to opposite side

Fig. 6.1: Various types of pneumothorax

Secondary pneumothorax is usually more symptomatic because of pre-existing lung disease.

Signs

The *clinical signs* of pneumothorax are localised to the side involved. These are:

1. Fullness of intercostal spaces
2. Decreased movement of chest wall
3. Hyper-resonant percussion note
4. In closed and tension pneumothorax, breath sounds, vocal fremitus and vocal resonance are diminished due to collapsed lung.

    In open pneumothorax, an *amphoric bronchial breathing* with increased vocal fremitus and vocal resonance and presence of whispering pectoriloquy if a large bronchopleural fistula develops.

5. If associated with infection, e.g. open pneumothorax (commonly associated with infection) or pneumothorax due to tuberculosis there will be accumulation of fluid or pus in the pleural cavity (*hydro- or pyopneumothorax*), then there will be physical signs like horizontal shifting level of dullness and succussion splash, and in addition there will be signs of toxaemia.

6. *Recurrent spontaneous pneumothorax occurs* in patients with emphysema due to rupture of bullae and these invariably occur on the same side.

7. Very rarely, one may get bilateral small spontaneous pneumothorax; it may be difficult to diagnose such a case clinically as there will be hyper-resonant note and diminished breath sounds on both the sides and there will be no shift of trachea. All these signs are also present in emphysema from which it will be differentiated only on X-ray chest.

Tension Pneumothorax (Medical Emergency)

As the name suggests, the air in pleural cavity (pneumothorax) is under tension, i.e. mean pleural pressure is positive, hence, causes compression collapse of the lung. It is a medical emergency. It develops due to persistent air leak into the pleural cavity by a communication which opens during inspiration allowing the air to enter, and closes during expiration, preventing the air to escape, thus, acts as check valve. In this way, air accumulates with each successive breath and causes rise in intrapleural pressure thereby shifting the mediastinum to the opposite side and puts pressure on the great vessels. There is decreased venous return to the heart and cardiac output falls leading to *hypotension* (*cardiac tamponade*) and *cyanosis*.

It can occur in the setting of penetrating trauma, lung infection, cardiopulmonary resuscitation or positive-pressure mechanical ventilation. The **clinical features** include:

- Patients may present with acute onset of dyspnoea and cough or there may be sudden increase in symptoms in a patient of pneumothorax.
- Prominent chest (hyperinflated chest) with diminished or absent movement on the side involved.
- Trachea and mediastinum are shifted to the opposite side due to push of air pressure.
- Decreased or absent breath sounds on the side affected. Occasionally, there may amphoric breathing at a localised place.
- Tachypnoea, tachycardia, hypotension, cyanosis and pulsus paradoxus are usually present.

Diagnosis

The diagnosis is made on physical signs.

Investigations

I. **Chest X-ray:** Air in the pleural cavity gives hypertranslucent area devoid of lung markings in the periphery with a thin pleural line indicating the outer border of the collapsed lung (Fig. 6.2). In a doubtful case of small pneumothorax, a lateral decubitus or an end-expiratory film may help to delineate the free air in the pleural cavity. The diagnosis of pneumothorax on a film taken in supine position is more difficult and may be suggested by '*deep sulcus sign*', i.e. the presence of rim of air on the superior border of the diaphragm, making the diaphragmatic outline very sharp on the affected side.

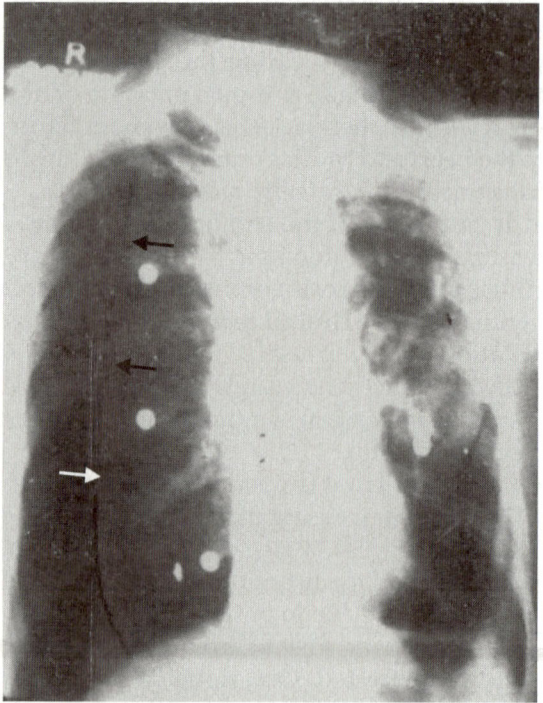

Fig. 6.2: Pneumothorax. X-ray chest (PA view) shows hyperinflated right lung with hyperlucency in the periphery devoid of markings. The underlying lung is collapsed indicated by a thin line (darkened) indicated by arrows

The amount of air can be calculated by the following formula on chest X-ray:

$$\text{Pneumothorax} (\%) = \frac{(d_L)^3}{(d_T)^3} \times 100$$

It is represented as percentage (%) of hemithorax volume occupied by air, roughly derived by measuring the average diameter of the collapsed lung (d_L) and hemithorax (d_T).

Tension pneumothorax on chest X-ray produces shift of the trachea and mediastinum to the opposite side, may not be shifted in small or closed pneumothorax or

bronchopleural fistula. Lung on the affected side is markedly collapsed and pasted along the hilum; but may not collapse if it is already diseased and fibrosed and fixed. Similarly, mediastinum may not be shifted and yet the hemodynamic compromise of tension pneumothorax may be evident.

In addition to pneumothorax, the chest X-ray may show signs of underlying disease (COPD or tuberculosis) hydro-pneumothorax.

Differential Diagnosis

It has to be differentiated from a large emphysematous bulla, which at times, may be difficult. The distinguishing feature is the outline or pleural margins of the collapse or deflated lung, but if pneumothorax is also loculated, then CT scan is helpful for differentiation.

Management

Aims

- To remove the air from the pleural space and to allow the lung to expand.
- To prevent recurrence.

Steps of Treatment

Patient should be treated for cough and chest pain.

A. *Removing air from pleural space:*

   i. *Conservative approach:* A small pneumothorax (<15%) is usually asymptomatic and should be left as such for spontaneous re-absorption and resolution with reexpansion of the lung which may take 4 weeks. This process can be hastened by supplemental oxygen inhalation at high concentration.

   ii. *Aspiration of air:* Tension pneumothorax and any pneumothorax which is >20% and symptomatic patient needs to be aspirated by the methods described below:

     1. *Simple needle aspiration:* Simple needle (16/18G) or a drainage catheter (I.V cannula) is used for

aspiration. A small pneumothorax can easily be drained with a 50 cc syringe and a three-way valve attached to it. Air comes out continuously as air bubbles in water, confirms the diagnosis. Air is drained till no air comes out and then *catheter is* left *in situ* for 4 to 6 hours keeping it well closed. Repeat chest X-ray is taken and compared with original one. If X-ray chest shows no recurrence or a small amount of air (<20%), catheter is removed. If recurrence is seen, then intercostal tube drainage is required.

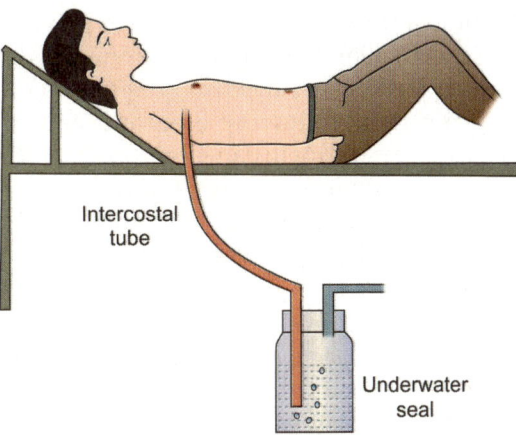

Fig. 6.3: Intercostal tube drainage of pneumothorax

2. *Intercostal tube drainage (ICTD):* It is required for all patients with moderate to large pneumothorax who fail on simple needle aspiration or who present with *tension* or *large pneumothorax*. Even a small pneumothorax can cause severe respiratory distress/failure in patients with underlying chronic lung disease, hence, all such patients require intercostal tube drainage (*tube thoracostomy*) and in-hospital observation.

If required, an intercostal drain should be inserted in the third or fourth intercostal space in mid-axillary line following blunt dissection through the parietal pleura. The tube is advanced in the apical direction and connected to underwater seal (Fig. 6.3). Once the lung expands, chest X-ray should be repeated to exclude the recurrence before removing the tube. Clamping of the tube before removal is potentially dangerous, should not be attempted. The drain should be removed 24 hours after the lung has fully reinflated and bubbling stopped. If bubbling in the underwater seal stops prior to full reinflation of the lung, then the tube is either blocked, kinked or displaced.

3. All patients should receive supplement O_2 to accelerate air reabsorption.

Note: Tension pneumothorax needs immediate relief of tension. It can be accomplished by just simply inserting the needle (16G) into the second intercostal space and removing 2–2.5 litres of air or till the patient gets relief in dyspnoea even without any underwater seal. The needle is left in place till the insertion of intercostal tube drainage.

4. Patients should not fly or dive for 3 months after full expansion of the lung. They should stop smoking to reduce the risk of a further attack. Future exposure to high altitude should be avoided.

B. **Prevention of spontaneous pneumothorax:** About 25% patients with primary pneumothorax have recurrence during the first year. Risks for further recurrences are still higher reaching up to 80% after the third episode. The recurrence rate in secondary pneumothorax is low.

Indications of thoracoscopy and *open throacotomy* include recurrences of spontaneous pneumothorax or bilateral pneumothorax or failure of tube drainage for the first episode. *Surgery* permits resection of the blebs and pleurodesis can be attempted.

Due to seriousness of this condition, pleurodesis (chemical or surgical) is recommended in all such patients with primary spontaneous pneumothorax following a second episode (even if ipsilateral) or in patients following their first pneumothorax where there is persistent air leak (>7 days). Surgical pleurodesis is recommended in all patients with secondary pneumothorax.

In *chemical pleurodesis*, the drug of choice is injectable *tetracycline, doxycycline* or *minocycline* which is instilled into pleural space in doses of 20 to 25 mg/kg. Alternative is *talc insufflation*. Currently, pleurodesis is limited due to non-availability of these drugs in our country, hence, surgical pleurodesis is done wherever indicated. This can be achieved by *pleural abrasion*, or *parietal pleurectomy* at thoracotomy or thoracoscopy.

A *small chest tube* attached to a *Heimlich valve* has been proposed for the treatment of *pneumocystis pneumonia with pneumothorax*. Patients who plan to continue activities that increase the risk of complications (e.g. flying or diving) should also undergo preventive treatment after the first episode of spontaneous pneumothorax.

Re-expansion Pulmonary Oedema

This is a rare complication that can occur with sudden withdrawal of air or fluid from the pleural space. This is unilateral pulmonary oedema that occurs more frequently if the lung has remained collapsed for longer period and if negative pressure is applied for drainage. The pathogenesis is not well understood. Loss of surfactants from the collapsed lung is the presumed hypothesis. Unilateral pulmonary oedema can lead to variable degree of hypoxia and cardiovascular compromise, and rarely, can be fatal. It is recognised by sudden onset of cough and dyspnoea soon after or during thoracocentesis or ICTD. Chest X-ray shows unilateral pulmonary oedema.

Treatment is supportive once it occurs. It can be prevented by slow removal of air/fluid, avoidance of negative pressure during drainage and monitoring of intrapleural pressure during such procedures.

Asphyxia

Definition

Clinically asphyxia refers to an airway obstruction leading to less or non-delivery of atmospheric O_2 to the lungs resulting in CO_2 retention. Asphyxia can be *mechanical* (obstruction extrinsic to airways) or *nonmechanical* (obstruction intrinsic to airways).

Causes

I. **Mechanical**
  - Covering of face (e.g. plastic bag)
  - Gag or pad smothering (closing of the external respiratory orifice by hand or by other means such as closing of nose and mouth with cloth, pad, etc.)
  - Gagging
  - Food or foreign body obstruction (choking)
  - Throttling (compression of the neck manually)
  - Hanging and strangulation
  - Drowning
  - Traumatic asphyxia

II. **Nonmechanical:** Suffocation may occur from diseases such as:
  - Diphtheria, infectious mononucleosis, *H. influenzae* in children
  - Rupture of aortic aneurysm in air passages
  - Haemoptysis in pulmonary tuberculosis
  - Erosion of bronchus by a tubercular gland
  - Laryngeal oedema due to any cause (e.g. steam inhalation, ingestion of irritant substances, drug allergies and poisons)
  - Retropharyngeal abscess
  - Laryngeal or bronchial growths
  - Nonpenetrating injury to front of the neck

FOREIGN BODY AIRWAY OBSTRUCTION (CHOKING)

Choking is a form of asphyxia caused by an obstruction within air passages.

Choking is almost always accidental. It results from the objects being lodged in the throat, is commonly seen in the children, elderly persons, psychiatric patients and in the infirms particularly where the ability to swallow or masticate is severely impaired.

Causes

1. It commonly occurs during a meal when the food is accidentally inhaled especially when victim is laughing or crying.
2. Vomitus may be inhaled by a person under the influence of liquor, during anaesthesia or an epileptic fit.

3. Infants usually regurgitate clotted milk after a meal and this may fall into the larynx.
4. Choking may occur due to inhalation of blood from facial injury, dislodged teeth, impaction of solid object, i.e. piece of meat, fruitstone, corn, button, coin, tag and rubber teat, gauge piece.
5. *Cafe coronary* (obstruction by a bolus of food or meat results in heart attack).

The choking or obstruction may be partial or complete. In complete obstruction, the victim becomes severely asphyxiated and may die suddenly or may develop severe brain damage or complication if obstruction is not relieved immediately.

If obstruction is partial, the resultant hypoxia may result in complications involving various organs.

Clinical Manifestations

The clinical feature varies according to severity of obstruction.

I. In partial obstruction due to a foreign body, the patient may struggle with the obstruction and tries to *'cough it out' or tries to swallow or 'wash it down with water'*: The victim is responsive and can cough forcibly. If air entry is poor, then signs of poor air exchange will appear such as weak ineffective cough, high-pitched noise while inspiration (stridor), increased respiratory difficulty and cyanosis.

II. With complete airway obstruction, the patient may clutch the neck with the thumb and fingers (universal distress sign for choking, Fig. 7.1) and following signs may appear:
   • Inability to speak, breath and cough.
   • Pallor followed by cyanosis.
   • Loss of consciousness and collapse.

If obstruction is not relieved immediately patient may develop cardiac arrest and die.

Diagnosis

The diagnosis is based on the circumstances and the clinical features. To find out the cause

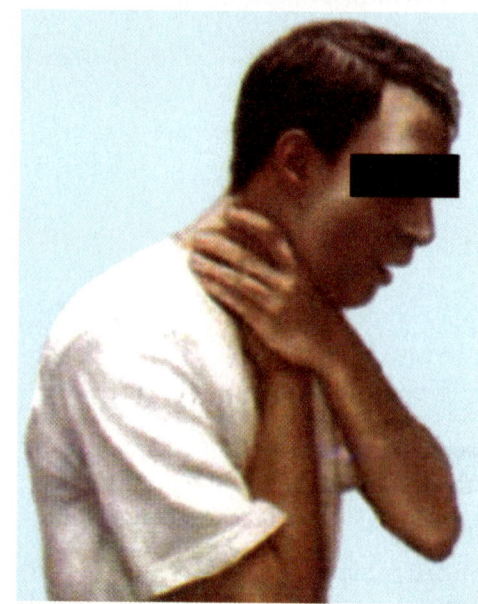

Fig. 7.1: Asphyxia due to foreign body airway obstruction

of obstruction, ask the following points in the history:
• Age of the patient.
• History of epilepsy, recent surgery or anaesthesia or psychiatric illness.
• History of recent intake of food or milk. If the obstructing agent is a fragment of food, the victim will be invariably the infant/child and the mother will tell the history of milk feed.
• Any history of trauma or facial injury.

Examination

• Examine the patient for signs of injury, loosening or missing of any teeth or wearing of artificial denture especially in old persons.
• Examine the mouth for sticking of food or any other material that can choke the throat.
• **Vital signs:** Examine the pulse, BP, temperature and respiratory rate. Look for cyanosis.

Management

The basic aim of management is to relieve the obstruction either by expelling the foreign body by artificial coughing (Heimlich's

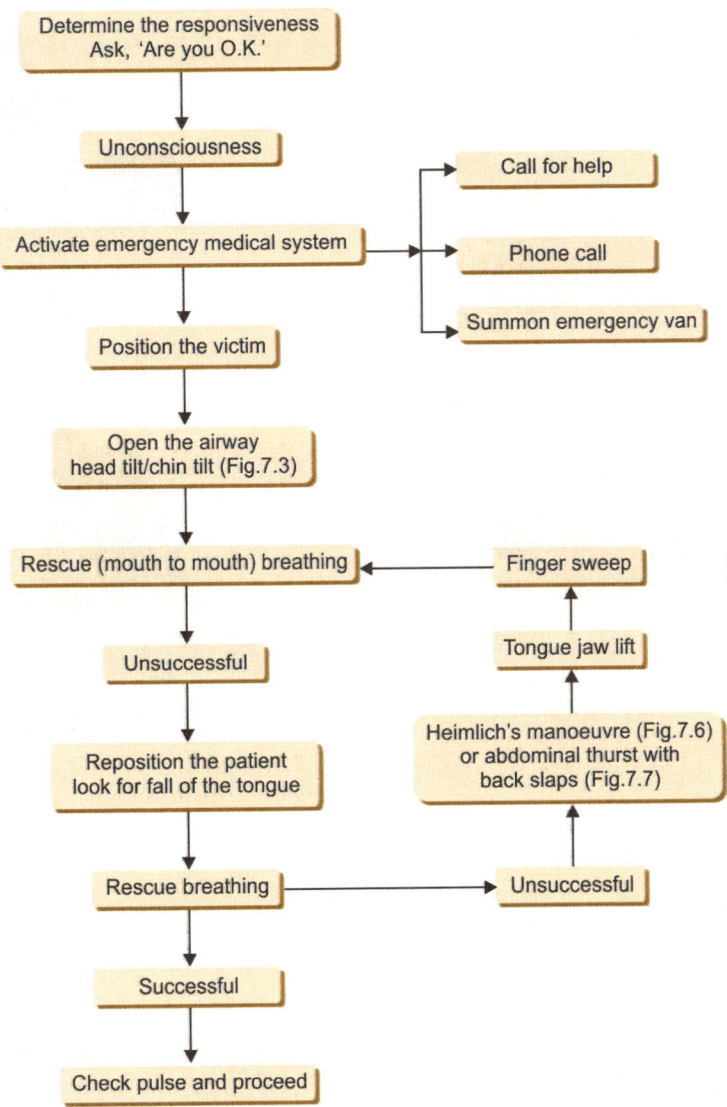

Fig. 7.2: Action plan for foreign body airway obstruction

manoeuvre or subdiaphragmatic abdominal thrusts) or its removal by sweeping the middle and index finger into the mouth cavity or with forceps. The plan of action in suspected foreign body airway obstruction is depicted in Fig. 7.2.

AIRWAY

Clearing the airway is a critical step in preparation of the victim for cardiac resuscitation. If tilting the head and lifting the chin (Fig. 7.3) do not clear the airway, then it seems that a foreign body might be obstructing the airway. First try to remove it by sweeping the fingers in the mouth. If desired result is not achieved, give five firm blows between the scapulae (Fig. 7.4), this may dislodge a foreign body by compressing the air that remains in the lungs, thereby producing an upward thrust of force behind the obstructing material and dislodging it and leading to its subsequent expulsion.

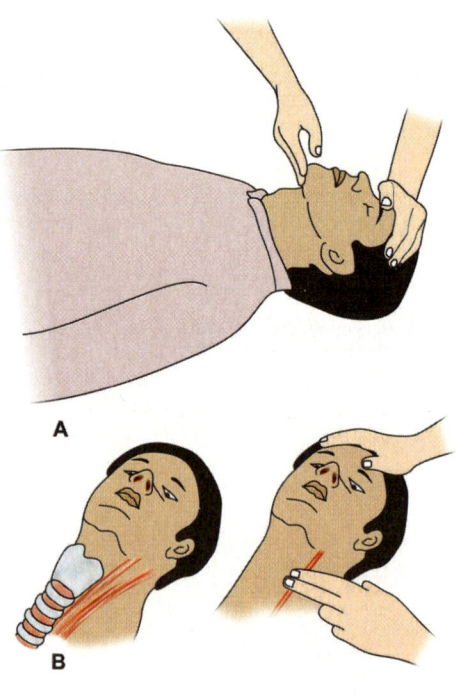

Fig. 7.3A and B: (A) Head tilt and chin lift, and (B) checking the pulse

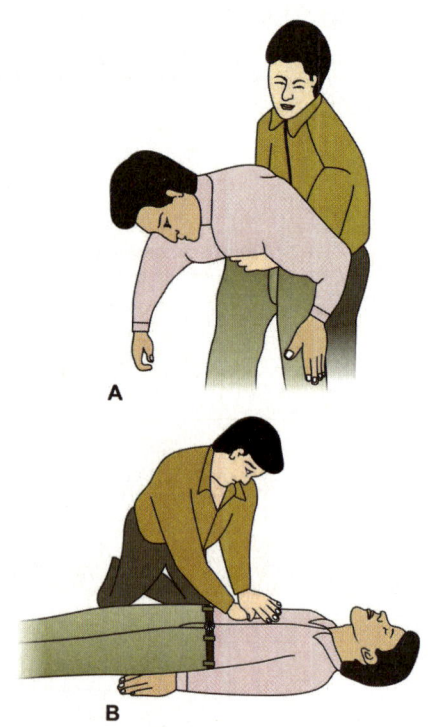

Fig. 7.5A and B: Abdominal thrust: (A) Conscious patient, and (B) in unconscious patient

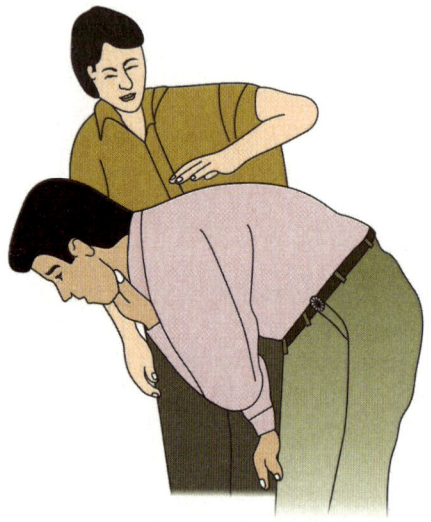

Fig. 7.4: Discharge the back blows to dislodge a foreign body

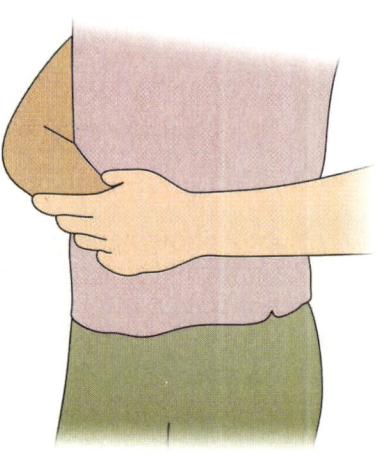

Fig. 7.6: Abdominal thrusts in conscious patient

If both the fingers sweep and back blows are not able to clear the airway, then try five abdominal thrust (Fig. 7.5A). If person is unconscious, then kneel over the victim, make a fist of one of your hand (place one hand over the other) and place it immediately below the victim's xiphisternum (Fig. 7.5B) and discharge the thrusts.

In conscious patient, one can use Heimlich's manoeuvre or discharge abdominal thrusts with back slaps as described in Fig. 7.6.

The Heimlich's Manoeuvre (Abdominal Thrust with back Slaps)

Grasp your fist with your other hand and push firmly and suddenly upward and backwards (Fig. 7.6). Discharge alternative abdominal thrust with back slaps (Fig. 7.7). The Heimlich's manoeuvre is not entirely benign. Rupture of abdominal viscera in the victim have been reported.

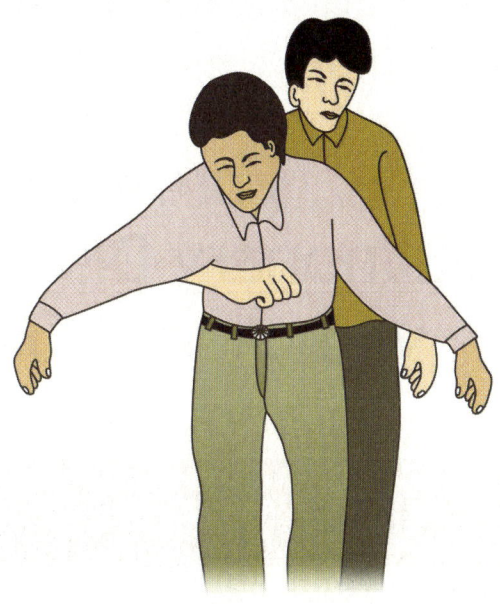

Fig. 7.7: Alternate abdominal thrust with back slaps

Chronic Obstructive Pulmonary Disease (COPD) with Acute Exacerbation

CHRONIC OBSTRUCTIVE PULMONARY DISEASE (COPD) WITH ACUTE EXACERBATION

Chronic Obstructive Pulmonary Disease has been defined by **GOLD (Global initiative for Chronic Obstructive lung disease)** as a disease state characterised by increased airflow resistance that is not fully reversible. Historically it includes, *emphysema*—a parenchymal lung disease characterised by destruction and dilatation of alveoli/air spaces and *chronic bronchitis*—a disease state in which cough occurs most of the day, 3 months in a year for two consecutive years. Bronchial asthma which is characterised by reversible resistance to airflow is not included in COPD. Similarly, chronic bronchitis without airflow obstruction is not included in it.

What Does Exacerbation of COPD Mean?

Exacerbations are defined as episodes of increased dyspnoea, cough and change in the amount and nature/character of the sputum with other signs of illness or infection such as fever, myalgia, sore throat and leucocytosis. Exacerbations are common during the natural course of COPD, the frequency of which increases as airflow resistance increases. Usually patients with moderate to severe COPD (Gold stages III and IV) have 2–3 episodes in a year.

With each exacerbation, there is worsening of pre-existing COPD.

The Precipitating Causes

1. **Infections:** Bacterial infections precipitate exacerbations of COPD in most of the cases while viral infection is present in one-third of patients.
2. **Thick, viscid secretion:** Thick viscid secretion produced by allergens may plug the smaller bronchi.
3. **Active or passive smoking (Fig. 8.1C):** It increases the airway resistance.
4. **Industrial pollutants/air pollutants** (dust and smoke) at workplace. It may also produce exacerbations.
5. **Physical or mental stress:** Though not proved, but still in few patients where no cause is found then this factor is blamed to be incriminating factor.
6. **Airway hyper-responsiveness:** Some patients of COPD like asthma exihibit airway hyper-responsiveness to external stimuli.

Pathophysiology

Airflow obstruction (both large and small airways), hyperinflation due to air-trapping resulting in large voluminous lungs and inadequate gas exchange leading to *hypoxemia* and *hypercapnia* are the most frequently encountered changes that constitute the clinical picture of COPD.

Persistent reduction in expiratory flow rates is hallmark of COPD. Increase in residual volume, ratio of residual volume to total lung capacity, uneven ventilation and ventilation-perfusion mismatch occur in COPD.

Changes in the large airways (bronchitis) produce cough and sputum while changes in the small airways and alveoli (gas exchange apparatus), are responsible for hypoxaemia and hypercapnia. In most cases of COPD, both bronchitis and emphysema are present but their relative contribution to obstruction vary from person to person.

Acute exacerbation factually means the super-imposition of acute bronchitis over and above the picture of COPD.

Clinical Presentations

1. **Symptoms of COPD:** *Cough*, *sputum* and *exertional dyspnoea* of long duration (>2 years) are the usual symptoms of COPD. These symptoms are gradual in onset and occur during exertion or activities. Activities performed below the arm level using the accessory respiratory muscles (walking on tread mill, pushing a wheel chair or just doing routine activities) are better tolerated than the activities involving the significant arm work above the shoulder level. As the disease advances, progressive dyspnoea on mild exertion occurs with increasing intrusion on the ability to perform vocational and avocational activities.

2. **Symptoms of acute exacerbation:** Acute worsening of symptoms of COPD with fever, tachycardia, tachypnoea, difficulty in speech, appearance or progression of cyanosis indicate acute exacerbation. These symptoms develop due to resting hypoxaemia and patients complain of giddiness, headache, light headedness and vertigo.

3. **Physical signs**

During acute exacerbation, the patient may be cyanosed and respiration is fast and shallow (Fig. 8.1). They usually have *purse-lip breathing* and sit in particular position (*propped up*). *Clubbing* is usually not present. Pulse rate is fast. There are decreased movements of the chest due to hyperinflated lungs and there is indrawing of the ribs during inspiration (*Hoover's sign*). There is evidence of increased mucus secretion due to superimposed infection leading to fever, rales and end-inspiratory and expiratory crackles. *Signs of emphysema* (barrel shaped chest, obliteration of cardiac and liver dullness, decreased respiratory excursion of the diaphragm) are present. The breathing is vesicular with prolonged expiration but the intensity of the breath sounds is diminished. *Papilloedema* may be present.

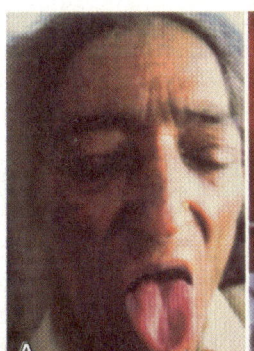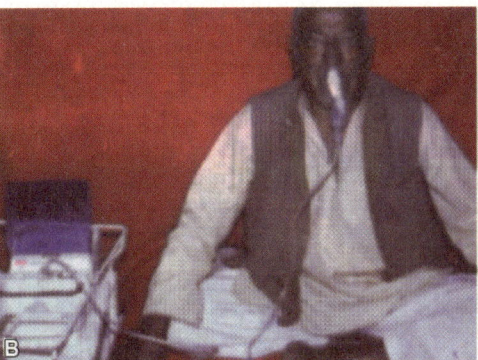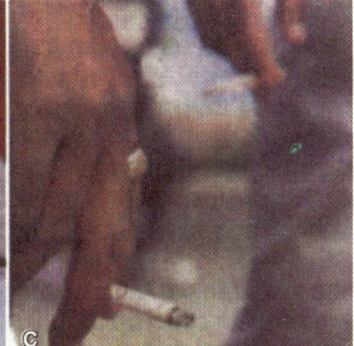

Fig. 8.1A to C: Chronic obstructive pulmonary disease with acute exacerbation. (A) Cyanosis in a patient with COPD, (B) nebulised β-adrenoreceptor agonist therapy, and (C) smoking—a precipitant factor

Investigations

1. **Blood count:** There may be leucocytosis indicating infection. There may be increase in haematocrit (PCV).

2. **Pulmonary function test:** Due to airflow obstruction, there is reduction in FEV_1/FVC ratio depending on severity of the disease (GOLD criteria). There is increase in total lung capacity, residual volume and functional residual capacity. Due to emphysema, diffusing capacity is reduced and there is alteration in blood gas analysis, i.e. decrease in PO_2 and increase in PCO_2. Arterial blood gas analysis demonstrate resting or exertional hypoxaemia and hypercapnia. Arterial pH allows the classification of respiratory failure defined as $PCO_2 > 45$ mmHg into acute or chronic.

Acute alteration in blood gas analysis is a common finding in a patient of COPD with acute exacerbation.

3. **Radiology:** The chest X-ray (PA view) will reveal the usual findings of COPD (e.g. hypertranslucency with decreased vascular makings of the lungs, presence of bullae and low flat diaphragm). CT scan is the current definite test for establishing the presence and absence of emphysema but practically it is not useful for patients of COPD during acute exacerbation.

Management

Aims

- To assess the severity of illness as well as an exacerbation.

Acute onset of fever, increasing breathlessness even on minimal activities, changes in colour or quantity of sputum, tachypnoea, tachycardia, cyanosis, use of accessory muscles and associated nausea, vomiting, myalgia, diarrhoea, chills, mental confusion suggest an exacerbation and these patients should be hospitalized for institution of treatment. These patients are unable to speak complete sentences, take frequent rests to complete them.

- To identify the precipitant and plan strategies to reduce frequency of exacerbations.
- To institute appropriate therapy.

1. *Initial assessment of patients:* A detailed history and physical examination should be included in initial assessment of patient illness. Chest examination with focal findings of decreased air entry and large airway obstruction should have chest x-ray and pulmonary function test for exacerbation. An attempt should be made to establish the severity of the exacerbation as well as severity of the pre-existing COPD. An exacerbation will destabilise the patient and may push the patient into *cor pulmonale* or *respiratory failure* if the disease is already advanced.

   The GOLD criteria for the severity of COPD are given in Table 8.1.

2. *Identification of the precipitant:* A variety of stimuli (precipitants) are known to exacerbate the symptoms of pre-existing COPD. The infection (bacterial and viral) is a common precipitant, should be found out by investigations. Smoking may also be a precipitant, hence, to be abandoned.

Table 8.1	GOLD criteria for severity of COPD		
Stage	*Severity*	*Symptoms*	*Pulmonary function tests*
0	At risk	Cough and sputum	Normal
I	Mild	With or without chronic cough or sputum	$FEV_1/FVC < 0.7$ and $FEV_1 > 80\%$ predicted
II	Moderate	-do-	$FEV_1/FVC < 0.7$ and FEV_1 between 50% and 80% predicted
III	Severe	-do-	$FEV_1/FVC < 0.7$ and FEV_1 between 30% and 50% predicted
IV	Very severe	-do-	$FEV_1/FVC < 0.7$ $FEV_1 < 30\%$ predicted with respiratory failure or signs of right heart failure

3. *Institution of treatment*

i. *Hospitalisation* and comfortable resting (prop up or sitting) position.

ii. *Controlled O_2 therapy:* Start with 24% controlled O_2 therapy through flow mask and increase it slowly to relieve hypoxaemia (to keep arterial O_2 saturations $\geq 90°$). However, COPD studies have demonstrated the O_2 therapy does not reduce minute ventilation during acute exacerbation but may result in slight increase in PCO_2. This alteration in PCO_2 must not deter O_2 therapy.

iii. *Inhaled bronchodilators:* These patients are treated initially either with an inhaled [β-agonist (salbutamol / terbutaline] with the addition of an anticholinergic agent either separately or together, or by nebulised therapy or meter-dose inhaler. The frequency of administration depends on the severity of exacerbation.

iv. *I.V. infusion theophylline:* The addition of theophylline or aminophylline in the drip (250 to 500 mg in 5% dextrose) may be considered; if above therapy is not effective, the serum levels of theophylline should be monitored.

v. *Antibiotics:* It is customary to treat patients with moderate to severe infection with a course of antibiotics even in the absence of an evidence of infection (leucocytosis) or identification of specific pathogen. Most common pathogens implicated during exacerbations include *S. pneumoniae, H.influenzae, M.catarrhalis, Mycoplasma pneumoniae* or *Chlamydia pneumoniae,* hence, initially a broad-spectrum penicillin with clavulanic acid (amoxiclav) is started and later on patient be shifted to appropriate antibiotic after culture and sensitivity of the sputum. The therapy is continued for >10 days. Most physicians treat an exacerbation with empirical antibiotic therapy in the absence of evidence of infection.

vi. *Corticosteroids:* Oral glucocorticoid therapy used in hospitalised patients has demonstrated beneficial effects in reducing the hospital stay, hasten the recovery and reduction in incidence of subsequent exacerbations. Based on these findings GOLD guidelines recommend 30–40 mg of oral steroid, i.e. prednisolone or its equivalent for 10–14 days.

The acute side effects of steroids include moon facies, hyperglycaemia and precipitation of diabetes, hypertension must be monitored.

vii. *Assisted ventilation:* Mechanical ventilatory support (invasive vs. noninvasive) is indicated to combat severe hypoxaemia in patients with COPD and exacerbation with impending respiratory failure ($PaCO_2$ >45 mmHg). The initiation of noninvasive positive-pressure ventilation (NIPPV) if not contraindicated in patients with respiratory failure ($PaCO_2$ >45 mmHg) results in significant improvement in mortality rate, need for intubation and reduction in hospital stay.

Invasive (conventional) mechanical ventilation via endotracheal tube is indicated in patients with life-threatening hypoxaemia and hypercapnia, acidosis, obtunded consciousness and cardiovascular instability. This therapy helps to improve oxygenation, clearance of air passages by suction and thus reduces mortality and morbidity.

viii. *Influenza vaccine:* The influenza vaccine has been shown to reduce exacerbation rates in patients with COPD.

Type II
Acute Respiratory Failure

RESPIRATORY FAILURE

Definition

The primary function of the lungs is to supply the body with adequate O_2 and to remove CO_2. Normally the respiratory system maintains partial pressure of oxygen (PaO_2 >95 mmHg) and CO_2 ($PaCO_2$ 36–45 mmHg) with a narrow margin of variation. When the respiratory system can no longer function to keep the gas exchange within normal range, respiratory failure is said to be present. The condition is suspected on the clinical ground, but confirmation is done by arterial blood gas analysis. For all practical purposes, PaO_2 less than 60 mmHg or $PaCO_2$ more than 50 mmHg indicates respiratory failure.

Classification (Fig. 9.1)

In respiratory failure, hypoxaemia (low PaO_2) is always present but partial pressure of CO_2 in the blood varies from low, normal to high. The retention of CO_2 in blood more than normal is called *hypercapnia*. Depending on the arterial blood gas analysis, respiratory failure is divided into *hypoxaemic (type I)* and *hypercapnic (type II)*.

HYPOXAEMIC (TYPE I) RESPIRATORY FAILURE

Acute type I respiratory failure has also been discussed as ARDS.

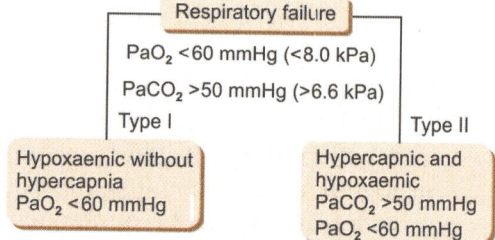

Fig. 9.1: Classification of respiratory failure based on arterial blood gas analysis

HYPERCAPNIC (TYPE II) RESPIRATORY FAILURE

It is defined as the failure of the lungs to maintain an adequate alveolar ventilation resulting in rise in $PaCO_2$ >50 mmHg. There is always hypoxaemia as well as hypercapnia.

A. *Acute:* This is called asphyxia. There is hypercapnia with acidosis. (This has been discussed as separate emergency).

B. *Chronic:* There is slow and insidious rise in CO_2 in the blood.

C. *Acute on chronic type* of respiratory failure (acute exacerbation of stable type II respiratory failure). This will be discussed here.

The **pathophysiological mechanisms** involved are:

1. *Alveolar hypoventilation* due to impaired CNS respiratory drive (drugs, brain stem injury, hypothyroidism etc.), impaired strength with failure of neuromuscular

function in the respiratory system (myasthenia, GB syndrome, motor neuron disease) and respiratory muscle weakness (fatigue, myopathy, electrolyte disturbance).

2. *Severe low ventilation/perfusion (V/Q) mismatch* (i.e. pulmonary embolism, respiratory diseases)
3. *Increased CO_2 production.*

The **causes** of type II respiratory failure are given in Box 1.

TYPE III RESPIRATORY FAILURE (PERI-OPERATIVE RESPIRATORY FAILURE)

This occurs due to lung atelactasis after general anaesthesia due to decrease in functional residual capacity.

TYPE IV RESPIRATORY FAILURE

This occurs in patients with shock due to hypoperfusion of respiratory muscles. Pulmonary oedema, lactic acidosis, anaemia lead to this type of failure in shocked patients. This is due to fatigue of the respiratory muscles due to excess of CO_2 in the muscles.

TYPE II RESPIRATORY FAILURE

Diagnosis

The diagnosis is based on the clinical features (listed in Box 2). The symptoms and signs of hypoxia and hypercapnia are non-specific and overlapping.

Dyspnoea is the presenting feature irrespective of the type of respiratory failure. The confirmation of the diagnosis is done by arterial blood gas analysis which also judges the type and severity of respiratory failure.

Once the diagnosis of respiratory failure is confirmed, the cause of respiratory failure should be established by history, detailed physical examination and specific investigations.

- A history of wheezing, cough, mucoid expectoration, shortness of breath and seasonal variations indicate asthma as the cause.
- History of cough with or without expectoration on most of the days for consecutive 3 months in a year for two consecutive years in a person indicates COPD (chronic bronchitis).
- A short history of fever, pain chest with rusty sputum indicates pneumonia.
- A history of exertional dyspnoea and dry cough indicates an interstitial lung disease.
- A history of sudden onset of dyspnoea and chest discomfort indicates pneumothorax.

Box 1	Causes of type II respiratory failure

I. Respiratory
- Severe acute asthma
- Pulmonary embolism
- An inhaled foreign body
- Laryngeal oedema
- Multiple fractured ribs (flail chest)
- Chronic bronchitis (COPD)
- Terminally ill patients
- Any progressive respiratory disease
- Kyphoscoliosis (severe chest deformity)
- Obesity (Pickwickian syndrome)
- Sleep-apnoea syndrome

II. Extrarespiratory
- Drug overdose (narcotics)
- Brainstem infarction
- GB syndrome
- Metabolic alkalosis
- Infections
- Respiratory muscles paralysis
- Myxoedema
- Heart failure
- Myasthenia gravis and Eaton-Lambert syndrome
- Retention of secretions (sputum retention syndrome)
- Ribs fracture, flail chest

Box 2	Symptoms and signs of type II respiratory failure

Hypoxia	*Hypercapnia*
• Dyspnoea	• Disorientation, delirium
• Mental confusion	• Somnolence
• Agitation anxiety	• CO_2 narcosis
• Tachypnoea	• Flapping tremors
• Tachycardia	• Headache, dyspnoea
• Restlessness	• Papilloedema
• Cyanosis	• Bounding pulses
• Hypertension	
• Cardiac arrhythmia	

- A detailed neurological examination may reveal neuropathy, myopathy or CNS disease as the underlying cause.

Management

The most common cause of type II respiratory failure is COPD. In this condition, CO_2 is retained slowly and is potential for acidaemia being corrected by renal conservation of bicarbonate which results in normal plasma pH. The *status quo* is usually maintained until there is a further respiratory insult in the form of infection, retention of secretions, bronchospasm, chest injury (ribs fracture), drug overdose (CNS depression) or pneumothorax which precipitates an episode of acute respiratory failure (Box 1).

The principal aims of treatment are:

- To achieve a safe PaO_2 (>7.0 kPa) without inducing extremes of $PaCO_2$ or pH by respirative support.
- Controlled O_2 therapy. Start with 24% controlled flow mask and increase it slowly to achieve $PaO_2 \geq 7$ kPa.
- Pharyngeal suction and physiotherapy.
- To identify and treat the precipitating cause. These patients of type II respiratory failure may not be overtly distressed despite being critically ill (Fig. 9.2).
- Antibiotics for treatment of infection.
- Nebulised bronchodilators.

Although relief of hypoxaemia is the first priority in management of acute type II respiratory failure, the hypercapnia and respiratory acidosis also must be addressed. Therefore, in initial assessment (Box 3), it is important to evaluate the conscious level of the patient, his/her ability to respond to commands and ability to cough effectively. This will give an idea whether patient needs intubation and tracheal suction or mechanical support.

If the hypercapnia with physical signs of CO_2 nacrosis (confusion, flapping tremors, bounding pulses, etc.) is secondary to depressed CNS drive due to sedatives overdose or poisoning, the patient should be intubated and put on mechanical ventilation straightway.

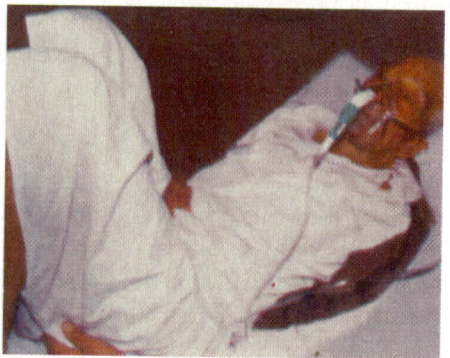

Fig. 9.2: A patient of type II respiratory failure with venture mask for O_2 therapy. The patient is not much distressed in spite of being critically ill

Box 3 Initial assessment
• Consciousness level (response to command, ability to cough)
• Signs of CO_2 narcosis (confusion, warm extremities, flapping tremors, bounding pulses, etc.)
• Signs of airway obstruction, e.g. wheeze, intercostal indrawing, pursed lips, tracheal tug
• Signs of right heart failure or cor pulmonale, e.g. raised JVP, oedema, hepatomegaly, ascites, etc.
• Signs of precipitating events or underlying cause (Box 1).
• Arterial blood gas analysis for severity of hypoxaemia, hypercapnia and acidosis.
• Chest X-ray for underlying disease or precipitating factor.

Prompt intervention may occasionally be necessary for some precipitating conditions, e.g. intercostal tube drainage for pneumothorax or injection of local anaesthetic for fractured ribs and torn muscles. Such interventions can result in dramatic improvement of respiratory functions.

Ventilatory Support

Ventilatory support consists of maintaining patency of the airway and ensuring adequate alveolar ventilation. Mechanical ventilation may be provided via face mask (noninvasive) or through tracheal intubation.

1. *Noninvasive positive-pressure ventilation:* NPPV delivered via a full face mask or nasal mask has become first-line therapy in COPD patients with hypercapnic

respiratory failure who can protect and maintain the patency of their airway, handle their own secretions, and tolerate the mask apparatus. Several studies have demonstrated the effectiveness of this therapy in reducing intubation rates and ICU stays in patients with ventilatory failure. A bilevel positive pressure ventilation mode is preferred for most patients.

2. *Tracheal intubation:* Indications for tracheal intubation include: (1) hypoxemia despite supplemental oxygen, (2) upper airway obstruction, (3) impaired airway protection, (4) inability to clear secretions, (5) respiratory acidosis, (6) progressive general fatigue, tachypnea, use of accessory respiratory muscles, or mental status deterioration, and (7) apnea. In general, orotracheal intubation is preferred to nasotracheal intubation in urgent or emergency situations because it is easier, faster, and less traumatic commonly only tracheal tubes with high-volume, low-pressure air-filled cafts should be used. Cuff inflations pressure should be kept below 20 mmHg if possible to minimize tracheal mucosal injury.

3. *Mechanical ventilation:* Indications for mechanical ventilation include (a) apnea, (b) acute hypercapnia that is not quickly reversed by appropriate specific therapy, (c) severe hypoxemia, and (d) progressive patient fatigue despite appropriate treatment.

Several modes of positive-pressure ventilation are available. Controlled mechanical ventilation (CMV; also known as assist-control or A-C) and synchronized intermittent mandatory ventilation (SIMV) are ventilatory modes in which the ventilator delivers a minimum number of breaths of a specified tidal volume each minute. In both CMV and SIMV, the patient may trigger the ventilator to deliver additional breaths. In CMV, the ventilator responds to breaths initiated by the patient above the set rate by delivering additional full tidal volume breaths. In SIMV, additional breaths are not supported by the ventilator unless the pressure support mode is added. Numerous alternative modes of mechanical ventilation now exist, the most popular being pressure support ventilation (PSV), pressure control ventilation (PCV), and CPAP. *Complications* of mechanical ventilation include migration of the tip of the endotracheal tube, bronchotrauma, respiratory alkalosis, hypotension and pneumonia.

- **If $PaCO_2$ continues to rise** or patient cannot achieve a safe PaO_2 without severe hypercapnia and acidosis, respiratory stimulant (e.g. doxapram 1.5 to 5 mg/min IV infusion) or mechanical ventilation (NIPPV or invasive) may be required. **In case of COPD with acute exacerbation**, if the patient is alert and the pH is >7.25, patient can be managed on noninvasive intermittent positive pressure ventilation (NIPPV) therapy through nasal or venture masks. **If patient is visibly fatigued** and has pH <7.25, then early mechanical ventilation will be ideal.

Monitoring for;

- Level of consciousness
- CVP
- Arterial bloodgases
- Pulse oximetry
- ECG, TLC, DLC.
- Urine output
- Pulse, BP, temperature, respiration
- Urea, creatinine, electrolytes

Treatment of Type III Respiratory Failure

- Frequent change in posture prevents atelectasis during postoperative period.
- Chest physiotherapy.
- Upright posture.
- Encourage coughing in postoperative period.
- Control of pain.
- Noninvasive positive pressure ventilation (NPPV).

Treatment of Type I.V. Respiratory Failure

- Treatment of shock.
- Maintenance of vitals.
- Intubation and mechanical ventilation.

Acute Empyema Thoracis

ACUTE EMPYEMA THORACIS

Definition

Empyema thoracis is defined as collection of pus in the pleural cavity or grossly purulent effusion (Fig. 10.1). The most common cause of empyema is the *bacterial pneumonia*. About 30–40% hospitalised cases of bacterial pneumonia have an associated pleural effusion. A small percentage (10%) of these parapneumonic effusions require drainage for their resolution and are called *complicated parapneumonic effusion*. Therefore, recently, the term empyema has been broadened to include all these cases of complicated parapneumonic effusions. The characteristic feature of these effusions is *exudative pleural effusion* which contains significant number of WBCs (but less than empyema) and contains organisms as demonstrated by Gram's stain and/or culture.

> *Parapneumonic effusions are exudative pleural effusion with low WBC count as compared to empyema but contain organisms as demonstrated on Gram stain and/or culture, are included in the designated term '**empyema**' which was previously used for frank pus in the pleural space.*

Pathology

In acute empyema, there is accumulation of large amount of pleural fluid with many polymorphs, bacteria and cellular debris. Fibrin gets deposited on both the layers of pleura (visceral and parietal) and there is tendency towards loculation. Later, as the empyema becomes chronic, fibroblasts grow from both the layers into the exudate resulting in adhesions of both the surfaces of pleura and form an inelastic membrane called *thickened pleura* or *pleural peel* (Fig. 10.2).

Causes

The empyema results from infection of pleura (parapneumonic effusion as a result of pneumonia, lung abscess and bronchiectasis) from the infection of lungs (liver abscess

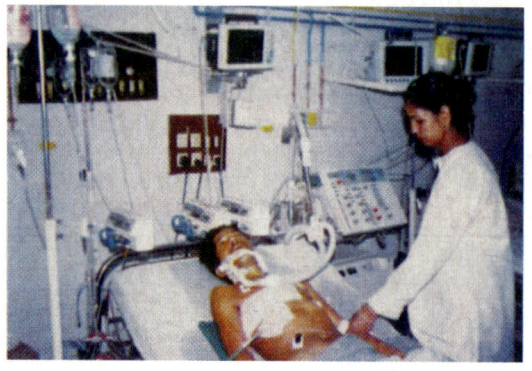

Fig. 10.1: Empyema thoracis. Intercostal tube drainage by self-retaining catheter in a patient with empyema thoracis

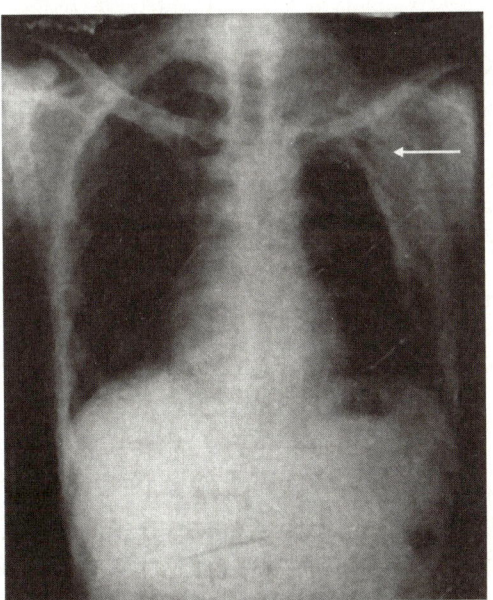

Fig. 10.2: Chronic empyema thoracis, X-ray chest shows thickened pleura on the left side (←). The shifted mediastinum has not returned to its original position

Table 10.1 Causes of empyema thoracis

1. **Diseases of lung:** Infection travels from the lung to pleura
   • Lung abscess   • Bronchiectasis
   • Pneumonia   • Tuberculosis
   • Fungal infection • Bronchopleural fistula

2. **Diseases of abdominal viscera** (infection travels from abdominal viscera to pleura)
   • Liver abscess (unruptured or ruptured)
   • Subphrenic abscess
   • Perforated peptic ulcer

3. **Diseases of mediastinum:** There may be infective focus in the mediastinum from which it travels to pleura
   • Cold abscess
   • Oesophageal perforation
   • Osteomyelitis, e.g. vertebrae, sternum

4. Trauma with superadded infection
   • Chest wall injuries (gunshot wound, stab wound)
   • Postoperative

5. **Iatrogenic:** Infection introduced during procedure   • Chest aspiration   • Liver biopsy
6. **Blood-borne infection**   • Septicaemia

perforated peptic ulcer, subdiaphragmatic abscess), abdominal viscera or mediastinum. It may also result from blood-borne infection (*septicaemia*) or iatrogenic infection (*following procedures*). There may be secondary pleural infection following chest injuries or post-operative. The causes are given in Table 10.1.

Pathogenic Organisms

1. Gram-positive aerobic organisms, e.g. *S. aureus, S. pneumoniae, S. pyogenes.*
2. Gram-negative aerobic organisms, e.g. *E. coli, B. proteus, H. influenza, Klebsiella, Pseudomonas* and *Enterobacter* species.
3. Anaerobic bacteria, e.g. *bacteroides, Fusobacterium, peptostreptococci.*
4. *M. tuberculosis.*
5. Parasites—*E. histolytica, T. echinococcus.*
6. Fungi, e.g—*Aspergillus, Cryptococcus, Blastocomycosis,* etc.

Predisposing Conditions

The common **predisposing conditions** include; *cardiopulmonary disorders, diabetes, alcoholism, drug abuse, malnutrition, presence of neoplasm, neurological disorders* and *immunocompromised state* (e.g. HIV, use of corticosteroids or cytotoxic drugs). Mortality is high in immunocompromised patients.

Clinical Features

The empyema can occur in any age group but commoner in elderly and debilitated persons.

Patients with aerobic infections (parapneumonic pleural effusion) present with acute onset of fever with chills, cough with purulent expectoration (bronchopleural fistula), dyspnoea and chest discomfort. In these patients, empyema develops as a complication of necrotising pneumonia and pleural effusion. Patients with anaerobic infections present with subacute illness with non-specific symptom and signs such as weight loss, leucocytosis, mild anaemia and history/evidence of predisposing factor for aspiration from oral cavity. Tubercular empyema presents with low grade fever of weeks and months duration with weakness and cough.

Physical Signs

Physical examination reveals signs of toxaemia (*fever, tachypnoea, tachycardia*) and pleural effusion during acute phase. Presence of tenderness on percussion with some oedema of chest wall provides a clue to empyema. *Clubbing of fingers* and *toes* is usually seen. Rarely, empyema may track into subcutaneous tissue of chest wall and presents as a localised swelling with positive cough impulse. This is termed as *empyema necessitans* and is mostly seen with actinomycotic infections.

Chronic cases with pleural thickening (thickened pleura Fig. 10.2) and loculation of pus will show significant deformity with retraction of chest on the same side of empyema and even scoliosis. The signs will be dull percussion note with diminished breath sounds. Extensive pleural calcification may occur. Tubercular empyema is often chronic and present with thickened pleura.

Investigations

The possibility of a parapneumonic effusion and empyema should be considered in each and every case of pneumonia if patients develop signs of toxic pleural effusion. Investigations to be done include:

1. **Leucocyte count:** There is leucocytosis with raised ESR in acute empyema.

2. **Chest X-ray:** All the three views (PA, lateral and decubitus) of chest X-ray are helpful. The X-ray picture of empyema initially is same as pleural effusion (Fig. 10.3A). Later on loculation of empyema which occurs posterolaterally is better seen on a lateral film. An air and fluid level if present, indicates *pyopneumothorax* which may be due to *bronchopleural fistula*. A large lung abscess with thin walls may have to be differentiated from a loculated pyopneumothorax.

3. **Ultrasonography:** It is most helpful investigations and guides the site of aspiration of loculated empyema. Fibrin strands and loculations (pockets) of empyema may

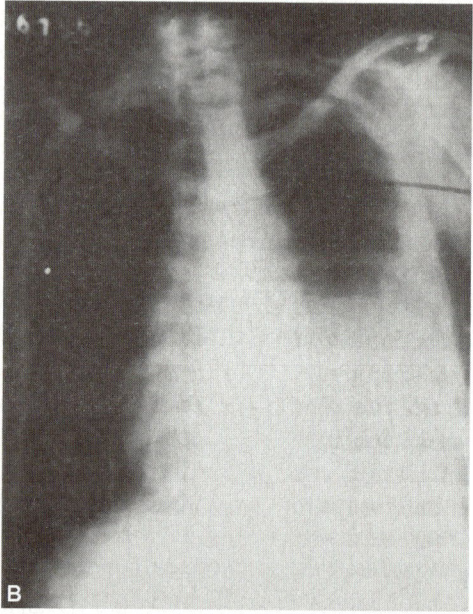

Fig. 10.3A and B: Empyema thoracis. Chest X-rays are displayed showing (A) empyema thoracis before needle aspiration, and (B) after needle aspiration and removal of 400 ml of pus

be seen on USG and may be aspirated under ultrasound guidance to confirm the diagnosis. All loculations should be aspirated as character of pleural fluid may vary from one loculation to other.

4. **CT scan:** It is most useful to distinguish pleural fluid loculations from peripheral parenchymal infiltrates, pleural thickening or lung abscess. It is particularly useful in identifying multiple small loculations.

5. **Aspiration of pus (thoracentesis, Fig. 10.1):** Initial aspiration of pus (thoracentesis) should be therapeutic cum diagnostic. The fluid (pus) aspirated should be examined for colour (anchovy souce pus in ruptured amoebic liver abscess), turbidity (thick pus is pyogenic) and odour (foul putrid smell is due to anaerobic infections) and discharge of sulphur granules (actinomycosis). Alquots are sent for cytology and biochemical analysis (i.e. glucose, proteins, pH, LDH, amylase level and TLC and DLC). Acidic effusion tends to loculate rapidly than alkaline.

Pleural fluid should be subjected to *Gram staining* and *culture for pyogenic organisms* and AFB. The pleural fluid pH is usually less than 7.2, the LDH level is more than 1000 IU/L and glucose content is <60 mg/dl. Low pH and glucose of parapneumonic pleural effusion indicates impending empyema.

Complications

1. Thickening of pleura with calcification (Fig. 10.2).
2. Empyema necessitans and chronic discharging sinus.
3. Bronchopleural fistula.
4. Fibrosis with bronchiectasis in the underlying lung.
5. Metastatic infection, e.g. brain abscess, meningitis, suppurative pericarditis.
6. Amyloidosis.
7. Gross deformity of thoracic cage.
8. Septicaemia.

Management

Aims

• To achieve expansion of lung by early drainage of pus and chest physiotherapy.
• To sterilize the pleural space to control septicaemia or systemic infection with appropriate antibiotic therapy.

1. *Antibiotic therapy based on culture and sensitivity:* In *gram-negative infection*, a 3rd generation cephalosporins along with an aminoglycoside is used. In *community-acquired infection*, β-lactam (oral cefpodoxime, cefuroxime, amoxycillin and clavulanic acid combination) *plus* an oral macrolide may be used. If *staphylococcal infection* is suspected, then targocid or vancomycin is preferred. *For anaerobes*, a combination of clindamycin or metronidazole and amoxycillin plus clavulanic acid is used.

   In the absence of culture and sensitivity report, a combination of penicillin (amoxycillin), an aminoglycoside (gentamicin, amikacin) and metronidazole may be used to cover both aerobic and anaerobic infections. In severe infections, systemic antibiotics in standard doses should be used. The duration of treatment is 6 weeks. Empyema due to tuberculosis or other organisms such as *Entamoeba histolytica* and *Actinomyces* should be treated accordingly.

2. *Drainage of the pus or empyema fluid:* The aim is to evacuate the pus rapidly to allow the underlying lung to re-expand. Drainage of pus may be *closed* or *open*. The *closed drainage* may be either intermittent via a wide-bore needle aspirations (*thoracentesis*) or continuous intercostal tube drainage.

   A. *Intermittent needle aspiration (thoracentesis):* The first needle aspiration is indicated in all cases of empyema to classify the nature of fluid (pus). During initial aspiration, the fluid or pus should be removed as much as possible and sent for diagnostic evaluation, hence, it is therapeutic **cum** diagnostic aspiration. If fluid recurs, serial thoracenteses (aspirations) are to be done provided patient is clinically better and there is no formation of loculations. Before each aspiration, chest X-ray is to be repeated (Figs 10.3A and B) or USG done to decide the site of aspiration. After each aspiration, fluid should be sent for cytology and biochemistry along with Gramstain and culture. During aspiration, a three-way cannula should be used to prevent air entry into pleural cavity. If response to antibiotic treatment is good, then fluid will become more serous (thin) at each aspiration and will become sterile after 3–4 aspirations. Chest X-ray repeated after each aspiration will demonstrate lung expansion (Fig. 10.3B) provided there is no underlying cause for non-expansion (underlying lung disease).

During aspiration, if patient develops, respiratory distress, pain and tachycardia, aspiration should be stopped immediately as uncommonly pleural shock and air embolism can occur.

Failure to needle aspiration: Needle aspiration will fail if:
1. Wrong site is selected.
2. Needle is too narrow and syringe is small sized.
3. Thick clot and fibrin tags block the aspirating needle, which should be made thin with use of fibrinolytic agents or proteolytic enzyme (hylase).

B. *Closed intercostal tube drainage (tube thoracotomy drainage):* The decision to institute chest tube drainage are:
   • The presence of thick pus in the pleural space which is difficult to aspirate through needle.
   • Organisms isolated on Gram stain or on culture of fluid.
   • Glucose level of the fluid is <60 mg/dl.

• Pleural fluid pH <7.2 or 0.15 units lower than the arterial pH. This is because acidic pleural fluid is likely to loculate rapidly, at times, within hours.
• Marked elevated WBC count in the pleural fluid.
• Bronchopleural fistula.
• Failure of serial thoracentesis.
• Bilateral acute empyema.
• Severe toxaemia.

The chest tube, traditionally, a large bore (28 to 32 French) catheter or any self-retaining catheter is put in the most dependent part of the empyema cavity and connected to underwater seal (Fig. 10.1). Recently, it has been advocated that in complicated parapneumonic effusions, smaller catheters (8 to 16 French) can be used percutaneously, especially for satellite pleural pockets formed due to pleural adhesions. These are easier to put and less painful but require ultrasonic guidance.

Success of tube drainage: If drainage is successful, then there will be clinical and radiological improvement within 24 hours.

Duration of drainage: Chest tube should be left in place until the volume of pleural drainage is less than 50 ml/24 hours for 2 consecutive days and the drainage fluid becomes clearly yellow.

Failure of tube drainage: It occurs if:
• Tube is in wrong place.
• Multiple loculations.
• Bronchopleural fistula.
• Failure of the pleural cavity to collapse and obliterate due to thickened pleura (pleural peel).
• Undiagnosed or unsuspected tuberculosis. A CT scan will be helpful to distinguish these possibilities.

Note: If the purulent drainage continues through the chest tube for more than a week in spite of proper method of drainage and after proper selection of an antibiotic, then instillation of a thrombolytic agent may be attempted to break the loculations and adhesion.

Use of Intrapleural Thrombolytic Agents

These agents have a role to break the loculations in multiloculated empyema. Intrapleural instillation of a fibrinolytic agent, i.e. streptokinase (usual dose is 250,000 U in 100 ml saline) or urokinase (100,000 U diluted in 100 ml of saline) or tissue plasminogen activator 10 mg through a chest tube is helpful if drainage stops because of loculations and opacities on chest X-ray persist. After each instillation, the chest tube is clamped for 2 hours to allow the thrombolytic agents to attack the fibrin membranes responsible for loculations. Thrombolytic agents can be daily instilled for up to 14 days. This is a costly treatment. The intrapleural injection of thrombolytic agents does not affect the systemic coagulation system as these do not diffuse through the pleura.

Contraindications of Thrombolytic Therapy

- Presence of bronchopleural fistula.
- Recent trauma.
- Recent bronchial suturing.

Surgical Interventions/Procedures

If the closed chest tube drainage and thrombolytic agents are unsuccessful, then surgical intervention either by rib resection, thoracoscopy with breakdown of adhesions, decortication, lung resection, thoracoplasty may be required. These are aggressive approaches of drainage of pus.

Rib resection is indicated when closed chest tube drainage has not helped the patient because now the drainage is gravity dependent or fibrin clots block the tube. Complete cure may take 6 to 8 weeks by tube drainage following rib resection. It will also fail if pus is too thick or a bronchopleural fistula has developed or pockets of pus become loculated and inaccessible. This will require major surgical interventions, such as;

A. **Thoracoscopy with manual breakdown of adhesions and chest tube drainage:** In this, chest tube is positioned optimally with the help of thoracoscope. In addition, pleural surface can be inspected to determine the necessity for decortication. If this procedure is successful, lung expands and drainage stops and after 2 to 3 days, the tube can be removed.

B. **Decortication:** It is procedure of choice if:
1. The fluid is too thick to drain.
2. There is an evidence of pleural adhesions.
3. The lung is not expanding on serial chest X-rays.
    In this procedure, all the fibrous tissue is removed from the visceral pleura, and all pus is evacuated from the pleural space.

Decortication is not possible in heavily thickened pleura which is usually seen in tuberculosis.

C. **Lung resection:** If the underlying lung is diseased, or the lung does not expand after decortication and there are chances of reactivation of the disease such as tuberculosis; in such patients, pleuropneumonectomy or pleurolobectomy is indicated.

D. **Open drainage:** If patient is not fit for major surgical procedures described above and empyema has become completely walled off, then open drainage by flap procedure (Floesser flap) can be done. In this procedure, the pleural space is exposed to the surface, i.e. to atmospheric pressure, hence, there is danger of developing pneumothorax if the empyema cavity is not walled off, therefore, it should not be done too early. Open drainage should be continued till the pleural cavity is completely evacuated and obliterated. It requires regular irrigation of the cavity with antibiotics and antiseptic dressings. The cavity will become obliterated within few months.

Pulmonary Hypertension and Cor Pulmonale

Definition

Pulmonary hypertension refers to increase in pulmonary systolic pressure >30 mmHg or mean pulmonary pressure greater than 20 mmHg due to increase in pulmonary vascular resistance. **Cor pulmonale** commonly referred to a pulmonary heart disease is defined as altered right ventricular structure (RV hypertropy/dilatation) and/or function secondary to pulmonary hypertension caused by diseases of lung parenchyma, pulmonary vasculature or thoracic cage abnormalities.

ETIOPATHOGENESIS

Cor pulmonale develops in response to pulmonary hypertension which may be *primary* or *secondary*. Normally pulmonary arterial pressure is <15 mmHg which is increased in setting of parenchymal lung diseases, primary pulmonary vascular disease, chronic hypoxia due to any cause and changes in pulmonary vascular bed (remodelling, vasoconstriction or destruction). As a result of above mechanisms, pulmonary arterial pressure and RV afterload increase, resulting in cor pulmonale.

The cor pulmonale secondarily leads to alteration in cardiac output as well as salt and water retention. Anatomically RV is thin walled, compliant chamber can withstand volume overload than pressure overload. The sustained pressure overload due to pulmonary hypertension leads to RV failure. **Acute cor pulmonale** is RV hypertophy or dilatation due to acute rise in pulmonary arterial pressure as a result of primary pulmonary vascular disease or due to multiple pulmonary thromboembolism.

Acute decompensation in patients with chronic cor pulmonale is uncommon, results in florid signs of right-sided failure with worsening dyspnoea and cough called **acute exacerbation of cor pulmonale**.

The acute precipitants are:
- Atmosphere pollutants (smoke, dust)
- Respiratory infection (pneumonia
- Hypoxia due to any cause
- Acidemia (exacerbation of COPD)
- Acute pulmonary embolism
- Arrhythmias
- Hypervolaemia (salt intake)

Causes

The causes are:
I. **Diseases of lung parenchyma**
- COPD (emphysema, bronchitis)
- Cystic fibrosis
- Pulmonary fibrosis (primary or secondary)
- Sarcoidosis
- Bronchiectasis
- Hypoventilation syndrome, i.e. idiopathic, obesity related (Pickwickian)

II. **Pulmonary vascular diseases**

- Primary pulmonary arterial hypertension.
- Thromboembolic pulmonary hypertension
- Venoocclusive disease
- Parasitic, e.g., schistosomiasis

III. **Chest wall disorders**

- Kyphoscoliosis

IV. **Neuromuscular disorders**

- Poliomyelitis
- Myasthenia gravi

Clinical Features

The symptoms and signs of cor pulmonale are related to:

1. **Symptoms of COPD,** e.g. cough, sputum, dyspnoea, chest discomfort, headache etc.
2. **Symptoms of right heart involvement**/failure, e.g. abdominal pain, swelling legs ascites.

Physical Signs

- **Patient is orthopnoic,** sits with elbows supported on a table and legs dangling by the side of the bed.
- **Purse-lip breating** (Fig. 11.1) and cyanosis (lips, tongue and buccal cavity) will be present in patients with COPD with acute exacerbation.

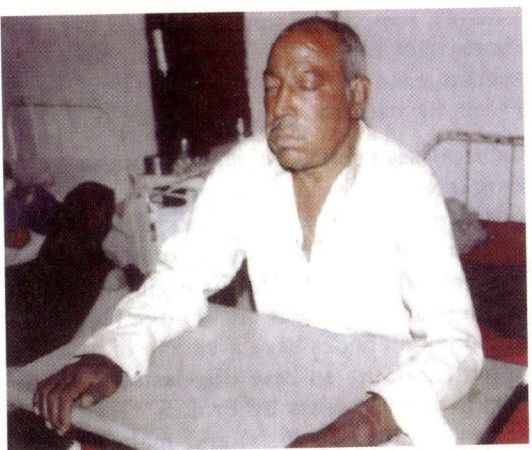

Fig 11.1: Purse-lip breathing in COPD. Note the sprouting of the lips during inspiration

- Periorbital oedema.
- **Neck veins:** Distended with raised JVP and 'VY' collapse due to tricuspid regurgitation.
- Peripheral oedema.

Systemic Signs

- Respiratory system may show **signs of COPD** (barrel-shaped chest, restricted chest movements and expansion, hyper-resonant note and vesicular breathing with prolonged expiration, muffled breath sounds).
- **Signs of RV hypertrophy or failure**, e.g. parasternal heave, loud P2, midsystalic and early diastolic (*Grahm-steel*) murmur and pansystolic or holosystolic murmur of tricuspid regurgitation (*Carvallo's sign*) may be present.
- **Abdominal examination:** Abdomen may be distended with tender hepatomegaly. Hepatojugular reflex may be present. Ascites may also be present.

Diagnosis

Diagnosis is suspected on the clinical findings and confirmed by following investigations.

- Blood count may show leucocytosis of the acute exacerbation is due to infection. The hematocrit may be raised indicative of secondary polycythaemia.

Chest X-rays (PA and lateral views): This will show enlargement of main pulmonary artery and hilar vessels. Heart may be enlarged. In addition there may be changes of basic disease causing cor pulmonale such as COPD.

ECG: There will be right axis deviation, p-pulmonale and right ventricular hypertrophy. An arrhythmia may be present.

Echocardiogram: 2D-echocardiography will demonstrate right ventricular hypertrophy or dilatation. Doppler echocardiography can be used to assess pulmonary arterial pressure.

Pulmonary function tests: Spirometry and lung volumes can identify obstructive or restrictive lung defects indicative of pulmonary lung diseases.

Arterial blood gases: They may demonstrate hypoxia and hypercapnia.

Spiral CT scans of chest are useful for diagnosing thromboemboli. High resolution CT scan is needed to diagnose interstitial lung disease.

Sophisticated investigations such as ventilation perfusion scan or MRI of heart are usually not required unless specifically indicated.

Brain natriuretic peptide (BNP) levels: Serum BNP levels are raised due to right ventricular dysfunction. They are dramatically elevated in acute cor pulmonale (pulmonary thromboembolism).

Emergency

Management

1. Patient is rested in supine comfortable position. Advised to avoid smoking.

2. *O$_2$ therapy:* O$_2$ therapy to be given intermittently.

3. *Salt restriction and diuretics:* Salt restriction is advised to avoid fluid retention and RV volume overload. Intravenons diuretics (fursemide) are given to relieve fluid overload.

4. *Bronchodilators:* They are given intravenously to relieve bronchospasm due to acute exacerbation to improve oxygenation.

5. Carbonic-anhydrase inhibitor, e.g. acutazolamide to be given to relieve hypercapnia.

6. Antibiotics to treat superadded infection causing acute exacerbation.

7. *Reduction of afterload* by angiotensin converting enzyme inhibitor in patients with left heart failure causing right heart failure.

8. Treatment of the basic cause.

Emergencies in Gastroenterology and Hepatology

- ○ Acute Vomiting
- ○ Acute Diarrhoea
- ○ Upper Gastrointestinal Bleed (Haematemesis)
- ○ Lower Gastrointestinal Bleed (Bleeding Per Rectum)
- ○ Acute Pancreatitis
- ○ Amoebic Liver Abscess
- ○ Hepatic Encephalopathy (Acute and Chronic Liver Failure)
- ○ Biliary Colic

Acute Vomiting

Definition

Vomiting refers to forceful expulsion of gastric contents through the mouth by sustained contractions of abdominal muscles. *Nausea* refers to feeling of an imminent desire to vomit. Nausea often precedes or accompanies vomiting. *Retching* refers to laboured rhythmic contractions of respiratory and abdominal muscles. It also frequently precedes or accompanies vomiting (Fig. 12.1).

Reflex Pathway of Vomiting

1. **Central control:** Vomiting is controlled by two centres located in the medulla, i.e.

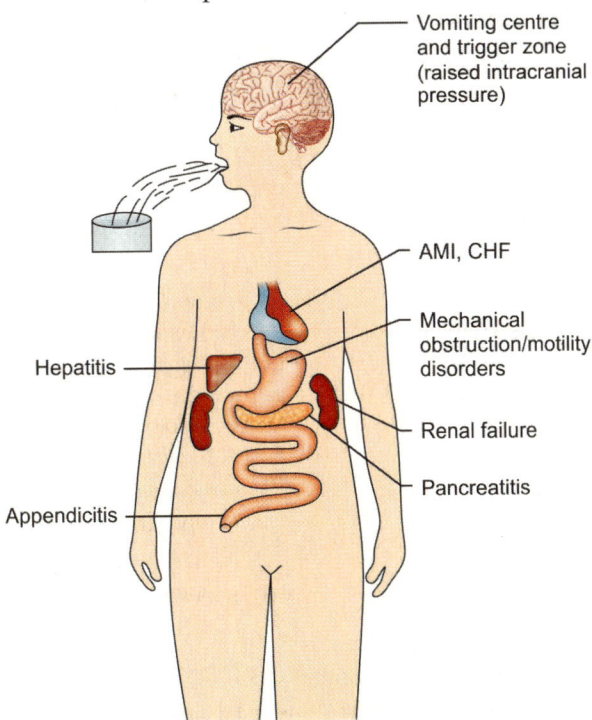

Fig. 12.1: Possible causes of vomiting

Vomiting centre and trigger zone (raised intracranial pressure)

AMI, CHF

Mechanical obstruction/motility disorders

Renal failure

Pancreatitis

Hepatitis

Appendicitis

vomiting centre in lateral reticular formation and *chemoreceptor trigger zone* in the floor of fourth ventricle.

2. **Afferent pathway:** The vomiting centre receives afferent impulses from the GI tract, from the brainstem and cortical centres especially labyrinthine apparatus and from the chemoreceptor trigger zone. The chemoreceptor trigger zone by itself is incapable of mediating the act of vomiting. The activation of this zone results in efferent impulses to the medullary vomiting centre, which in turn initiates the vomiting.

3. **The efferent pathway:** The important efferent pathways in vomiting are phrenic nerves (to the diaphragm), spinal nerves (to intercostal and abdominal muscles) and visceral efferent fibers in the vagus nerve (to the larynx, pharynx, oesophagus and stomach). The causes of vomiting are given in Table 12.1.

Clinical Consequences of Vomiting

1. Repeated vomiting, if forceful may lead to pressure rupture of oesophagus *(Boerhaave's syndrome)*.
2. It may cause a linear mucosal tear at or near the cardioesophageal junction leading to haematemesis *(Mallory-Weiss syndrome)*.
3. Prolonged vomiting may lead to fluid loss (dehydration), loss of HC1 (metabolic alkalosis), loss of K^+ (hypokalaemia) and loss of nutrients (malnutrition).
4. Vomiting in an unconscious patient or in patient with depressed consciousness may result in aspiration pneumonia.

Clinical Evaluation

History

The history is an important step in clinical evaluation of a case with vomiting because temporal relationship of vomiting to eating may be helpful in diagnosis as detailed below:

• Vomiting without abdominal pain is usually caused by food poisoning, infective gastro-enteritis, drugs or systemic illness.

Table 12.1 Causes of vomiting

1. Gastrointestinal

  i. *Mechanical obstruction*
    • Gastric outlet obstruction following peptic ulcer or malignancy
    • Small intestinal obstruction, e.g. volvolus, adhesions, malignancy

  ii. *Motility disorders*
    • Gastroparesis due to diabetes, drugs, post-vagotomy and idiopathic

  iii. *Inflammation*
    • Bacterial food poisoning
    • Appendicitis
    • Acute pancreatitis

  iv. *Gastrointestinal irritants*
    • Alcohol
    • Drugs, e.g. NSAIDs, oral antibiotics

2. Hepatobiliary
  • Hepatitis A and B
  • Portal hypertension
  • Acute cholecystitis
  • Gallstones

3. CNS disorders

  i. *Vestibular causes*
    • Labyrinthitis
    • Meniere's disease
    • Motion sickness

  ii. *Raised intracranial pressure*
    • CNS tumours
    • Subdural/subarachnoid haemorrhage
    • Hydrocephalus, meningitis, encephalitis

  iii. *Migraine*

4. Cardiovascular
  • Acute MI, congestive heart failure

5. Renal
  • Renal failure

6. Endocrinal
  • Diabetes mellitus
  • Hypo- and hyperthyroidism
  • Thyrotoxic crisis, adrenal crisis

7. Systemic causes
  • Infection
  • Pregnancy

8. Psychogenic

9. Radiation therapy

10. Bulimia
  • Psychiatric disorders

11. Postoperative

• Early morning vomiting without retching is seen in pregnancy and uraemia. Alcoholic gastritis produces retching with early morning vomiting.

- Vomiting occurring during or immediate after eating may indicate psychogenic vomiting or pylorospasm/pyloric obstruction.
- Vomiting occurring after 4 to 6 hours of eating with expulsion of large quantities of gastric contents, is seen in pyloric obstruction or gastroparesis or cardia achalasia.
- A projectile vomiting suggests raised intracranial pressure.
- Persistent vomiting suggests pregnancy, gastric outlet obstruction, gastroparesis and psychiatric illness.
- A long history of vomiting with little or no weight loss indicates psychogenic basis.
- Associated symptoms such as tinnitus, vertigo indicate vestibular involvement (*Meniere's disease*).
- Relief of abdominal pain with vomiting is typical of peptic ulcer.
- A large amount of gastric contents in vomiting indicates gastric outlet obstruction or *Zollinger-Ellison syndrome*.
- The presence of blood in the gastric contents usually denotes bleeding from the oesophagus, stomach or duodenum.
- Fever indicates inflammation or infection of oesophagus or stomach as the cause of vomiting.
- History of drug intake may indicate drug-induced vomiting.

Physical Examination

Every effort should be made to find out the cause of vomiting and also to assess the status of hydration.

1. **Status of hydration** is assessed by pulse, BP, skin turgor, moistness of mucous membrane and other vital signs.
2. **Abdominal examination** provides clues to the diagnosis and the cause of vomiting:
   - Abdominal distension with sluggish bowel sounds on auscultation indicates either an appendicitis or cholecystitis.
   - Abdominal distension with tenderness and visible peristalsis suggest acute intestinal obstruction, while succession

splash upon abrupt lateral movement of the patient suggests gastroparesis or pyloric obstruction.
   - Abdominal distension with board-like rigidity, tenderness may suggest peritonitis.
   - Presence of jaundice, hepatomegaly and subcostal tenderness (thumping sign) indicates hepatobiliary disease.
   - Altered sensorium, signs of meningeal irritation, focal neurological deficit, seizures, papilloedema indicate intracranial pathology with raised intracranial tension.
   - Nystagmus, ear discharge, deafness suggest either otogenic or cerebellar disease.

Diagnostic Investigations

A battery of tests to cover all the causes of vomiting, is given below out of which one has to select investigations depending on the presumptive cause.

- Complete blood count for iron deficiency anaemia.
- Urine analysis.
- Renal profile, e.g. blood urea, creatinine for azotemia.
- Serum electrolytes, e.g. K^+ for hypokalemia or metasolic alkalosis.
- Hepatic profile, e.g. serum bilirubin, hepatic enzymes.
- Serum amylase for pancreatic disease.
- USG of abdomen for liver and pancreatic disease.
- CSF analysis and CT scan of the head for any neurological cause.
- Pregnancy test should be done in all potentially pregnant women.
- Serum drug levels of certain drugs.
- Supine and erect X-ray to be done in a case suspected of intestinal obstruction or perforation.
- Upper GI endoscopy for peptic ulcer and/or gastric outlet obstruction/gastroparesis.
- EKG for myocardial infarction.

Table 12.2 Antiemetic drugs

Agent	Dose and route	Indications	Side effects
1. Antihistaminics and anticholinergics			
Diphenhydramine	25–50 mg, 4 to 6 hourly orally **or** parenterally	• Vomiting due to motion sickness, pregnancy, inner ear disease, uraemia and postoperative vomiting	• Sedation, dizziness, dry mouth, blurred vision, epigastric discomfort, constipation, urinary retention
Meclizine	25–50 mg orally/day		
Promethazine	25 mg 4–6 hours/orally **or** parenterally		
Scopolamine	1.5 mg/3rd day patch		
2. Dopamine receptors inhibitors			
• Phenothiazine (prochlor-perazine)	5–10 mg oral/IM/IV every 4–6 hourly 25 mg suppository every 6 hourly	All types of vomiting except motion sickness and labrinthine disease	Hypotension, extrapyramidal side-effects, akathisia; drowsiness, anxiety, sedation
• Promethazine	12.5–25 mg 6–8 hourly oral **or** IV 25 mg suppository	• Gastroparesis	
• Metoclopramide	10–20 mg **or** 0.5 mg/kg IV 6 hourly 10–20 mg orally 6–8 hourly	All types of vomiting	Extrapyramidal side effects, mood and sleep disturbance
• Domperidone	20–40 mg orally 3–4 times a day	-do-	Hyperprolactinemia
3. Sedative			
• Lorazepam	1 to 2 mg every 4–6 hours/orally **or** IV	• Added to metoclopramide or steroids to control vomiting in cancer patients	Sedation
4. Serotonin (5HT$_3$ receptors antagonists)			
• Dolasetran	100 mg **or** 1.8 mg/kg/IV once daily **or** 200 mg oral daily	• Chemotherapy and radiation induced vomiting in combination with corticosteroids	• Mild headache, diarrhoea or constipation, transient rise in transaminases
• Ondansetron	4–8 mg or 0.15 mg/kg infusion **or** 8 mg twice daily orally	• Postoperative nausea and vomiting	-do-
• Granisetron	10 µg/kg infusion **or** 1–2 mg once daily	• Chemotherapy or radiation induced vomiting	-do-
5. Corticosteroids			
• Dexamethasone	4 mg I.V. once 4–8 mg oral once	They are combined with metoclopramide to control vomiting due to cancer chemotherapy or postoperative vomiting	Side effects are of corticolsteroids
• Methylprednisolone	40–100 mg IV		
6. Antibiotic			
• Erythromycin	125 mg q 6 hours orally	Gastroparesis	• Abdominal cramps, bloating, nausea

Contd.

Table 12.2 Antiemetic drugs (Contd.)

Agent	Dose and route	Indications	Side effects
7. Neurokinin receptor antagonists			
• Aprepitant	125 mg once before chemotherapy then 80 mg on day 1 and 2 of chemotherpay	Chemotherapy induced vomiting	
• Fosaprepitant	115 mg once 30 minutes before chemotherapy	Prevention of vomiting during chemotherapy	

Management

1. The initial step of management is to find out the cause and treat/correct it appropriately. Electrolyte imbalance, gastric outlet obstruction, systemic infections, metabolic disorders, e.g. diabetes, uraemia and CNS disorders must be identified and treated accordingly.
2. Most cases of vomiting are mild and self-limited, require no specific treatment.
3. Patients with severe vomiting should be hospitalised and intravenous fluids started to prevent or correct dehydration. Electrolyte balance is corrected by infusing saline and potassium supplementation to correct metabolic alkalosis and hypokalaemia.

   Control the sugar for diabetic ketoacidosis and gastroparesis.
4. Gastric decompression by Ryle's tube aspiration may be needed for gastric outlet obstruction, gastroparesis and acute intestinal obstruction, etc.
5. **Drug therapy:** Antiemetic drugs vary in their usefulness, hence, choice of drug depends on the availability and extent of control of emesis. The antiemetics are given in Table 12.2 with their action, indications and side effects.

Antihistaminergic and *anticholinergic* act on labrinthine pathways, hence, are useful for motion sickness and inner ear disorders.

Dopamine antagonists are used for all types of vomiting (medication, toxic and metabolic causes) while *prokinetics* (domperidone, metoclopromide, erythromycin) are effective against gastroparesis.

Intestinal pseudoobstruction respond to *octreotide*.

Substance P antagonists are being tried for control of vomiting in patients receiving cancer chemotherapy. Initial trials show promising results with no side effects.

Vomiting due to chemotherapy in cancer patients is a special problem and can pose as an emergency as these patients go into dehydration easily. The drugs used to control vomiting in such cases include a combination of *metoclopramide, steroids* and *serotonin receptor antagonists*, e.g. *dolasetran*. The neurokinin receptor antagonists are used in combination with 5-HT$_3$ antagonists or steroids or both in cancer patients for prevention of vomiting.

Few clinical trials conducted on nausea and vomiting during pregnancy found *meclizine, prochlorperazine* and *antiserotonergic* (*ondansetron*) useful but limited success.

Acute Diarrhoea

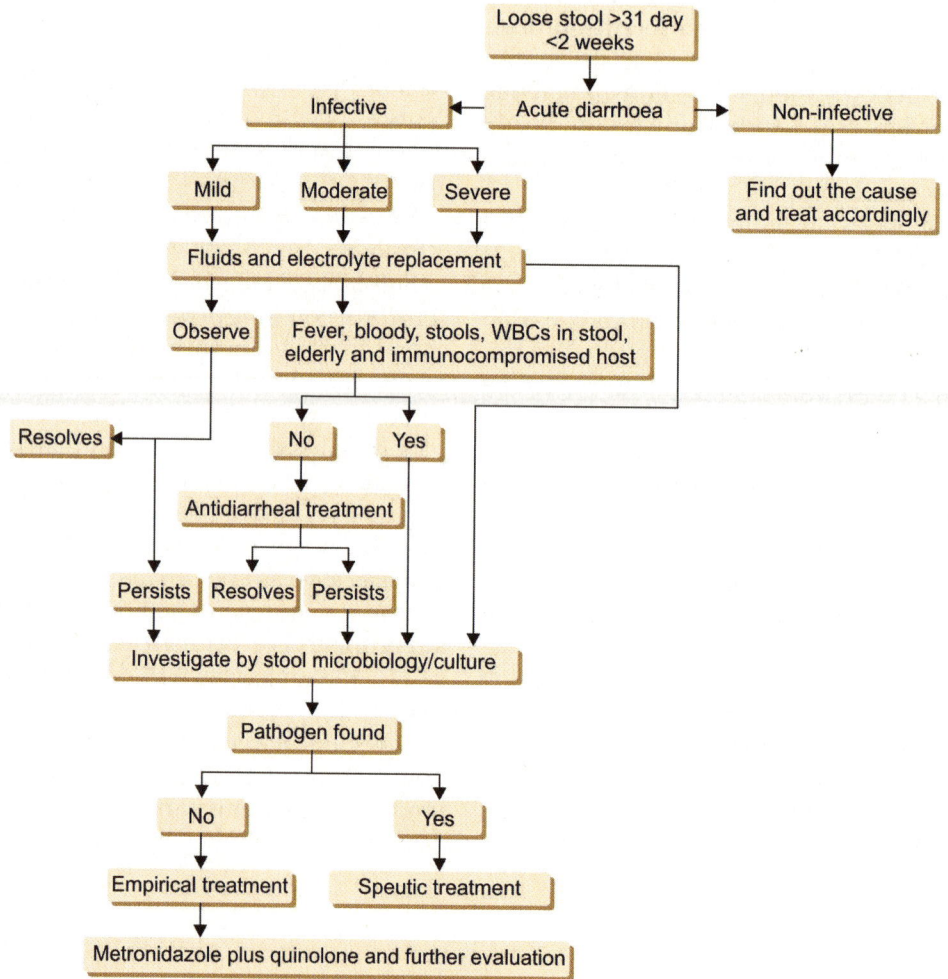

Fig. 13.1: Algorithm for management of acute diarrhoea

ACUTE DIARRHOEA

Definition

Normal stool content is <200 g/day and stool is well formed. Normal bowel frequency varies from three times a week to three times a day.

Diarrhoea is defined as an increase in daily stool content >200 g/day associated with increased loose stool frequency (>3/day). In diarrhoea, stool is usually liquid due to increase in water content. Diarrhoea is said to be *acute* if its duration is less than 2 weeks.

Diarrhoea must be distinguished from *pseudodiarrhoea* or hyperdefecation characterised by increased frequency of defecation without increase in stool weight above normal, often associated with rectal urgency or tenesmus or a feeling of incomplete evacuation indicates irritable bowel syndrome or proctitis and *faecal incontinence* is involuntary discharge of rectal contents and is most often caused by neuromuscular disorders or anorectal problems.

Spurious or *overflow diarrhoea* is due to rectal faecal impaction.

Causes

The acute diarrhoea can be classified depending on the *aetiology, site of involvement* (small bowel vs large bowel) or *pathophysiology* (i.e. whether secretory, osmotic, exudative or disordered motility) and *type of involvement*. Based on the aetiology and site of involvement, classification of acute diarrhoea is classified as inflammatory and non-inflammatory (Table 13.1). Contaminated food articles (water, milk, meat) or contact with farm animals are common reservoir of infection.

More than 90% of cases of acute diarrhoea are caused by infectious agents while 10% are due to non-infections causes (drugs, toxins, ischemia, food allergy or intolerance).

Clinical Features

Patients with acute infectious diarrhoea present with nausea, vomiting (common with toxins

Table 13.1 Causes of acute diarrhoea

I. Infective (90% cases)

- *Virus* e.g. rota, norovirus, cytomegalovirus, viral hepatitis.
- *Bacterial* e.g.
  - Enterotoxin-induced i.e. *S. aureus, B. cereus, C. perfringens, E. coli, V. cholera*
  - Cytotoxin induced (EHEC), i.e. *E. coli*, toxic shock syndrome
  - Mucosal invasion, i.e. *Shigella, Salmonella, Compylobacter, Yersinia,* Traveller's diarrhoea
- *Parasitic*
  - *Giardia, E. histolytica,* Cryptosporium, Cyclophora

II. Non-infective (10%)

- Drugs, e.g. laxative, digitalis, ampicillin
- Ischaemic colitis
- Pseudomembraneous colitis
- Diverticulitis, graft versus host disease
- Toxin induced, i.e. organophosphorus, insecticide, amanita and mushroom and seafood.
- Food allergy/intolerance

or toxigenic infection), abdominal pain which is mild, diffuse, crampy due to stimulation of peristalsis by hypervoluminous stool content, fever (e.g. infections) and loose watery, malabsorptive (bulky) or bloody stool depending on the specific pathogen. Profuse rice water stool suggests cholera.

The presence of systemic symptoms may provide important clues to the basic underlying cause, e.g. both *shigellosis* and *E. coli* (enterohaemorrhagic strain may be accompanied by haemolytic-uraemic syndrome particularly in very young and old persons. *Yersinia* infection and occasionally other enteric bacterial infections may be accompanied by *Reiter's syndrome* (arthritis, uveitis, urethritis), thyroiditis, pericarditis and glomerulonephritis. Tenesmus (painful rectal spasms) is a feature of proctitis due to *Shigella* or amebiasis.

The signs of dehydration may be present depending the severity of diarrhoea (Box 1). The clinical features of small bowel and large bowel diarrhoea are given in Table 13.2. It is important from the aetiological and therapeutic point of view.

Box 1 Symptom and signs of acute diarrhoea	
Symptoms	*Signs of dehydration may be present*
• Nausea, vomiting • Abdominal pain • Fever • Watery loose stools • Blood in the stool • Excessive thirst	• Patient irritable • Weak pulse, low BP • Depressed fontanelle • Dry pinched facies • Sunken eyeballs • Dryness of mouth, tongue, mucous membrane • Loss of skin turgor

Investigations

1. *Stool examination* for leucocytes, ova, parasites, blood and pus cells, etc.
2. *Stool for faecal lactiferin:* It is a sensitive marker of fecal leucocytes, indicates inflammatory diarrhoea. It is estimated by ELISA and latex agglutination test.
3. *Stool immunoassay* for bacterial toxins (*c. difficile*), viral antigen (rota virus) and protozoal antigens (*Giardia, E. histolytica*)
4. *Stool culture* for isolation of the infective agent, i.e. enterohaemorrhagic and other types of *E. coli*, Vibrio species and Versinia.
5. *Complete haemogram.*
6. *Blood biochemistry*, e.g. urea, creatinine, electrolytes.
7. *Blood culture.*
8. *Sigmoidoscopy* with biopsies and *upper endoscopy with duodenal aspirates* and biopsy if indicated.
9. *Abdominal X-ray,* or *CT scan.*

Clinical Evaluation and Management

Acute non-infectious-diarrhoea (Fig. 13.1) is usually mild and self-limited, responds well to rehydration therapy.

Acute infectious bacterial diarrhoea (Fig. 13.1) needs evaluation for hydration status, mental status and presence or absence of tenesmus stool should be sent for ova, parasite, blood, faecal leucocytes or lactoferrin determination.

The mainstay of treatment of acute diarrhoea is rest and prevention and treatment of

dehydration by fluid replacement. Hospitalisation is required for severe dehydration and altered mental status.

1. **Correction of fluid and electrolyte deficit:** Most deaths in acute diarrhoea result from fluid and electrolyte deficit, hence, must be corrected by fluid and electrolyte replacement. Intravenous fluid therapy may be necessary in severely dehydrated individuals, especially the infants and elderly. The key to effective management of diarrhoea is early replacement of fluid losses starting from home with available fluid administration early in the illness to prevent dehydration. As long as renal function is preserved, profound disturbances of electrolytes and pH do not occur.

   Depending on the degree of dehydration, the oral rehydration solutions (ORS) used in the treatment of cholera can also be considered in patients of acute diarrhoea.

   A. *Mild-dehydration* (i.e. irritability, dry mouth, increased thirst and weak pulse). Mild dehydration is treated

Table 13.2 Characteristics of small bowel (inflammatory vs large bowel diarrhoea (non-inflammatory)		
Characteristic	*Small bowel (inflammatory)*	*Large bowel (non-inflammatory)*
Pathogens	• *V. cholerae* • *E. coli* • *Rota virus* • *Norwalk virus* • *Giardia*	• *Shigella* • *E. coli* • *Campylobacter* • *E. histolytica*
Stool content	Large (profuse)	Small
Consistency of stool	Loose, watery	Viscus, mucoid
Presence of blood	Rare	Common
Presence of faecal leucocytes or faecal lactoferin	Rare	Common
Pain	Central (periumbilical)	Quadrantic (commonly left lower abdominal)
Proctoscopy	Normal	Abnormal

by home-available solution (plan A of WHO) such as coconut water, lemon sugar beverage (shikanjvi), weak tea, rice, water, etc. The fluid should be given as much as the patient can tolerate orally. This fluid therapy may be given in small sips or with teaspoon. If situation does not come under control, then home made oral rehydration solution (mixing of 6–8 TSF of sugar, one TSF of salt with or without lemon squeeze in one litre of water) should be started.

B. *Moderate dehydration* (dry tongue, depressed fontanella, irritability, reduced urine output, feeble pulse, excessive thirst, loss of skin turgor and postural drop in BP), requires WHO recommended ORS (i.e. glucose 20 g, NaCl 3.5 g, trisodium citrate 2.9 g and KCl 1.5 g or $NaHCO_3$ 2.5 g dissolved in one litre of safe drinking water). It is administered in small sips or with a teaspoon freely as much as person can tolerate without vomiting. It should be continued till dehydration is corrected.

> *ORS provides 90 mEq/L of Na^+, 20 mEq/L of K^+; 80 mEq/L of Cl^+ and 30 mEq/L of HCO_3^- which is usually sufficient for all types of diarrhoea at all ages.*

C. *Severe dehydration* with signs of acute peripheral circulatory failure, e.g. hypotension, oliguria, tachycardia, confusion and shock requires intravenous fluid replacement starting with Ringer's lactate or glucose saline solution at a rate of 20 ml/kg/hr in the next 2 hours. An adult should receive about 2 L of fluids within 2–3 hours.

A child who starts passing urine within 2 hours should receive 40 ml/kg of Ringer's lactate solution I.V. over next 2 hours as well. Concurrently, oral rehydration therapy should also be started as described above.

Oral rehydration therapy should be continued till losses have been corrected and patient is on maintenance requirement of fluids.

2. **Antibiotics:** Empirical antibiotic therapy in bacterial diarrhoea is controversial and generally not required in patients with mild or resolving disease but should be considered in patients with *shigellosis, traveller's diarrhoea, pseudomembranous colitis, cholera, food poisoning*, and *immunocompromised patients*, etc. Empiric treatment with fluoroquinolones (e.g. ciprofloxocin 500 mg, ofloxacin 400 mg twice daily is recommended in patients with non-hospital acquired diarrhoea with fever, tenesmus or blood stools. The treatment is revised after culture and sensitivity report. Only 5–10% of patients with diarrhoea require specific antibiotic therapy; the choice of which depends on the causative agent (Box 2).

3. **Antidiarrhoeal drugs:** Most of these drugs have little beneficial effect and can have potential side effects. These are not recommended in children. Loperamide and bismuth subsalicylate (2 tablets or 30 ml orally 4 times daily) have been shown to be

Box 2	Antibiotic treatment of acute diarrhoea
Organism	*Choice of antibiotic*
Shigella and E. coli	Quinolones (norfloxacin 400 mg bid or ciprofloxacin 500 mg bid for 5 days)
Traveller's diarrhoea	Rifaximin, a nonabsorbable oral antibiotic 200 mg tid for 3 days
Cholera (*Vibrio cholerae*)	Tetracycline (see the treatment of cholera)
C. difficile	Vancomycin orally (250–500 mg qid for 7–10 days)
Campylobacter	Erythromycin 250–500 mg qid for 5 days or azithromycin 500 mg OD × 5 days
Yersinia	Tetracycline 1–2 g/day for 7 days
Giardia	Metronidazole 200–400 mg tid for 7 days
E. histolytica	Metronidazole (400–800 mg tid for 5–7 days) or tinidazole 600 mg bid for 5–7 days or ornidazole 500 mg bid.

safe in patients with traveller's diarrhoea who have neither fever nor blood or pus in the stool. Loperamide is also a widely used drug for social convenience to decrease the frequency of stools in profuse diarrhoea. It is given as 4 mg initially followed by 2 mg after passage of each loose stool till either diarrhoea stops or maximum of 16 mg/24 hr. Anticholinergics (e.g. diphenoxylate are contraindicated.

4. **Symptomatic treatment of vomiting and distention of abdomen:** Occasional vomiting does not require treatment except the adjustment of oral rehydration therapy. Persistent vomiting may require antiemetic therapy.

   Abdominal distention due to hypokalaemia may be treated by withholding oral feeding and its replacement with parenteral fluids with potassium supplementation.

5. **Monitoring:** Patient with acute diarrhoea should be monitored for vitals, electrolytes, pH, urea and creatinine.

Upper Gastrointestinal Bleed (Haematemesis)

Definition

Bleeding occurring from upper gastrointestinal tract up to the ligament of *Treitz* is called upper GI (UGI) bleed. It is most common gastrointestinal emergency presenting.

Causes

The causes according to frequency are given in the Box 1 and Fig. 14.1 with therapeutic treatment.

Clinical Presentations

Patients with upper GI bleed invariably present with haematemesis (blood in the vomit) which may be red with clots when bleeding is profuse, or malena (black, tarry stool) in case of less severe bleeding.

Blood loss of less than 500 ml is rarely associated with systemic signs. A postural fall in systolic BP >10 mm usually indicates a 20% or more reduction in blood volume. There may be *syncope, dizziness, tachycardia, tachypnoea* due to hypotension resulting from intravascular volume depletion. Shock frequently ensues when blood loss is 25% to 40% of blood volume. Patients may occasionally experience vasovagal reaction with bradycardia. There may be symptoms and signs of anaemia if there has been a chronic blood loss due to repeated bleeding.

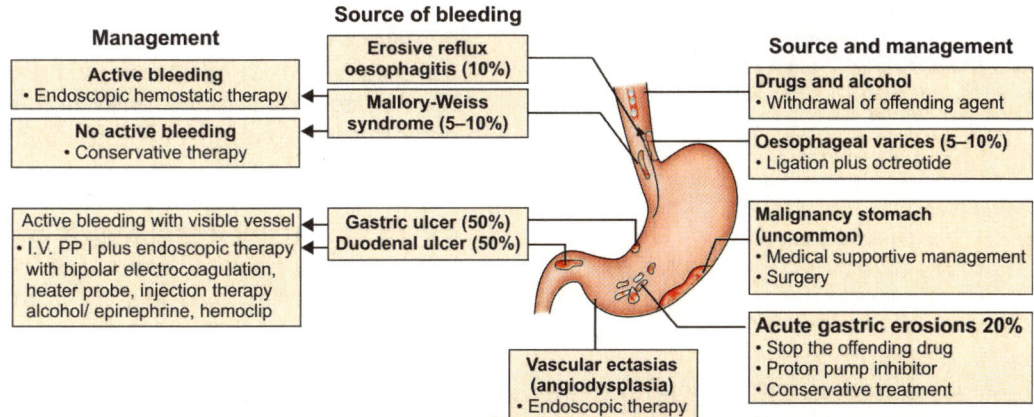

Fig. 14.1: Possible source(s) of acute upper GI bleed and their management

Initial Clinical Evaluation and Assessment

1. A history or symptoms suggestive of peptic ulcer disease, liver disease (portal hypertension), intake of NSAIDs (erosive gastropathy), bleeding from other sites (patient on anticoagulants), cutaneous malformations (telangiectatic lesion of Osler-Rendu-Weber disease) point towards the possible cause of UGI bleed. History of retching preceding haematemesis suggests Mallory-Weiss tear (Box 1).

2. Clinical examination also yields important informations. Stigmata of alcoholic liver disease (spider angiomata, gynaecomastia, jaundice, ascites, testicular atrophy, hepatosplenomegaly) suggest portal hypertension with bleeding from the varices (oesophageal or gastric).

Diagnosis and Management

A. Initial steps of management

I. Initial resuscitation and stabilisation

- Measurement of heart rate and BP
- Procure I.V. line using at least two larger bore cannula.
- Blood should be sent for complete blood count, prothrombin time (PT) with INR (international normalisation ratio), blood for urea, creatinine, glucose, liver enzymes, bilirubin and grouping and cross-matching.

- *Restoration of airway and O_2 administration:* Blood and blood clots should be removed from the mouth cavity to have patent and clear airway. Administer oxygen by facemask, if necessary.

- *Restoration of intravascular volume:* Intravenous fluids and blood may be administered to replace lost volume. Patients with shock and patients with haemoglobin less than 7 g% should receive blood transfusions. Always maintain two I.V. lines in patients with shock. Saline or Ringer's lactate solution should be infused to stabilise the vital signs. The haemoglobin should be kept above 9 g%. Periodic monitoring of PCV, haemoglobin and CVP (to avoid overtransfusion) is mandatory.

- *Vasopressors* are generally avoided because shock is hypovolaemic, needs fluid/blood replacement as early as possible.

- *Coagulopathy* is corrected by administration of platelets, fresh frozen plasma or whole blood and vitamin K. If INR is prolonged >1.8.

II. **Nasogastric tube insertion:** When there is history of haematemesis or malena, a nasogastric tube should be passed to empty the stomach and to determine whether the bleeding is proximal to the ligament of Treitz.

   If the initial nasogastric aspirate is clear, current active bleeding is unlikely and the tube may be removed. If ***blood or 'coffee ground'*** material is aspirated from the nasogastric tube. Patient is prepared for urgent upper GI endoscopy. Erythromycin (250 mg) administration 30 minutes prior to endoscopy to promote gastric emptying and improves quality of endoscopy.

III. **Gastric lavage:** Efforts to stop or slow bleeding by gastric lavage is of no benefit

---

Box.1   Causes of acute upper GI bleed frequency-wise

1. Peptic ulcer (35–50%) associated with NSAIDs and *H. pylori*.
2. Acute gastric erosion (about 20%), e.g. NSAIDs, alcohol induced, stress-induced ulceration
3. Oesophageal varices (5–10%), i.e. liver disease, portal hypertension.
4. Erosive oesophagitis (5–10%) usually associated with hiatus hernia.
5. Mallory-Weiss tear (5%), i.e. laceration of gastro-esophageal junction
6. Vascular (angiomatous) malformations (5%)
7. Cancer of oesophagus or stomach (2%)
8. Aortic graft (aorto-duodenal fistula—0.2%)
9. Miscellaneous (rare), i.e. bleeding disorders, corrosive injury, post-sclerotherapy or ligation ulcers.

and exposes the patient to an increased risk of aspiration.

IV. **Upper GI endoscopy:** It is the most preferred method of examination to find out the cause of upper GI bleeding.

Endoscopy should be done once the patient is hemodynamically stable. A diagnosis will be achieved in 80% of cases. Lesions located in certain blind areas may be missed on endoscopy such as fundus of the stomach, high lesser curvature and just inside the rim of pyloric opening. Oesophageal varices may not be apparent soon after UGI bleed. In case of multiple lesions, endoscopy can pinpoint the lesion responsible for bleed due to collapse. In torrential bleeding, endoscopic visualisation is impossible. Upper GI endoscopy also provides information about the risk of rebleed in patients with peptic ulcer. Patients who are found to have major endoscopic stigmata of recent haemorrhage in peptic ulcer (i.e. active spurting haemorrhage, a visible vessel) have 50–80% chances of rebleed. Similarly, varices, which are large and have stigmata of recent bleed, are likely to rebleed.

V. **Urgent angiography:** Selective mesenteric angiography usually localises the site of bleeding in about 75% of cases where endoscopy fails to reveal the bleeding lesion.

VI. **Acid inhibitory therapy:** Intravenous proton-pump inhibitors (esomeprazole or pantoprazole 80 mg bolus followed by 8 mg per hour continuous infusion for 72 hours) are given before endoscopy. It is a standard practice. The oral proton pump inhibitor are continued later on.

- *Monitoring:* Patients are monitored carefully for heart rate, BP, CVP and urine output.

VII. **Ultrasound of abdomen:** It can provide evidence of portal hypertension especially when the patient is unfit for endoscopy.

B. Specific therapy for underlying lesions

a. Peptic ulcer

i. *Therapeutic upper GI endoscopy:* Endoscopic haemostasis should be attempted as soon as patient is fit for endoscopy. It is safe and effective procedure, decreases the rate of rebleeding, duration of hospital stay, need for blood transfusions and also the mortality rates. The methods employed are:

- Injection sclerotherapy (with epinephrine, absolute alcohol, poridocanol, etc.).
- Laser photocoagulation (it is costly, not affordable, is available in specialised centres).
- Electrocoagulation.
- Heater probe.
- Use of hemoclips.

The efficacy of all the methods is almost similar but injection sclerotherapy is commonly employed because it is safe, effective and economical.

ii. *Acid suppression therapy* with I.V. proton pump inhibitor, is continued to reduce the risk of rebleed in patients with peptic ulcer. High dose oral esomeprazole 80 mg or lansprazole 60 mg twice a day for 5 days is given.

iii. *Surgery:* An urgent surgical operation is undertaken when:

- Endoscopic haemostasis fails to stop active bleeding.
- Rebleeding occurs on one occasion in an elderly or frail patient, or twice in younger patients.
- Significant number of blood transfusions (>5 units in 24 hours) are needed.

The choice of operation depends on the site and diagnosis of bleeding lesion,

iv. *Angiography and arterial embolisation:* Patients with persistent massive haemorrhage, who are not fit for surgery or endoscopic therapy, can be considered for arterial angiography (selective catheterisation of the bleeding artery) and then either a continuous infusion of vasopressin or intra-arterial embolisation may be attempted.

iv. *Prevention of rebleed:* It is done by acid suppression and eradication of *H. pylori.* Stop NSAIDs if found to be the cause.

b. **Acute variceal bleed**

i. *Endoscopic haemostasia:* The endoscopic measures used to control acute variceal bleeding include *sclerotherapy* and *banding.* Both sclerotherapy and variceal band ligation are methods of choice and are effective in up to 90% of cases. In experienced hands, they are safe and effective. Sclerotherapy carries a higher risk of complications such as oesophageal ulceration, perforation and stricture; whereas variceal ligation is equally effective and has low rate of complications. Variceal ligation is repeated until obliteration of all the varices is completed.

ii. *Reduction of portal venous pressure by vasopressin, or somatostatin/octreotide:*

• *Vasopressin* can be given as 20 units in 100 ml of 5% dextrose as I.V. infusion over a period of 10 minutes or may be given as continuous I.V. infusion. Though therapy lowers portal venous pressure but is highly risky and should not be used in patients of IHD, hypertension or other vascular diseases.

• *Somatostatin/octreotide:* Intravenous use of somatostatin (250 µg as a bolus dose followed by an infusion of 250 µg/hour) or octreotide (50 µg I.V. as a bolus dose followed by I.V. infusion of 50 µg/hour) is comparable to endoscopic treatment. The treatment is safe with minimal side-effects.

Combined treatment with octreotide and endoscopic therapy is superior to either. The therapy is continued for 3–5 days if varices are confirmed on endoscopy, if not confirmed, therapy is discontinued immediately.

Terlipressin 1–2 mg I.V. every 4 hourly is another alternative.

iii. *Balloon tamponade (variceal decompression):* It is quite effective in controlling the bleeding from oesophageal or gastric varices. Several tubes are available *(Sengs-taken-Blakemore tube, Minnesota tube, Linton tube)* for decompression. Use of balloon tamponade is associated with high risk of complications, some of which may be fatal, hence, this procedure should be reserved if therapeutic endoscopy and pharmacotherapy are either not available or cannot be instituted immediately.

iv. *Portosystemic shunt surgery:* It can be done if endoscopic and pharmacotherapy fail to stop the variceal bleeding. The success of surgery depends on the status of liver functions and the surgical expertise.

v. *Transjugular intrahepatic portosystemic shunt (TIPS):* It has been used increasingly in the recent past for control of bleeding from the gastric/oesophageal varices not responding to other therapeutic procedures. A metal stent is placed between hepatic vein and the portal vein (portosystemic shunt) to reduce the portal vein pressure by decompressing the portal vein. This is an alternative to surgery.

vi. *Other pharmacological therapies*

• Antibiotic prophylaxis either with oral or I.V. fluoroquinolones or I.V. third generation cephalosporin (ceftriazone 1 g/day for 5–7 days) reduces the risk of severe infection.

- *Vitamin K:* Cirrhotic patients with an abnormal PT (prothrombin time) should be given vitamin K (10 mg daily till desired PT is achieved).
- *Lactulose:* Encephalopathy may complicate an episode of GI bleeding in cirrhotic patients, hence, lactulose should be given in doses described under management of hepatic encephalopathy (read hepatic encephalopathy).

C. Erosive gastritis (acute gastric erosion)

Steps of management include:

i. Stop NSAIDs promptly if these are the cause
ii. Judicious use of antacids or I.V. proton pump inhibitor (pantaprazole IV) or mucosal protective agents.
iii. Treatment of associated stress and organ dysfunction.

D. Mallory-Weiss tear

i. Most patients stop bleeding spontaneously.
ii. Endoscopic haemostasis (injection sclerotherapy) and angiographic therapy with embolisation may be tried and has been found effective.

E. Stress ulceration

It is a frequent cause of GI bleeding in seriously ill patients admitted in ICU with head injuries, fulminant hepatic failure, multiple organ system failure, shock, etc. Prophylactic therapy in such patients with I.V. H_2 antagonists, proton-pump inhibitors (PPIs) or high doses of antacids orally or through Ryle's tube are very effective in preventing stress ulceration and bleed.

F. Angiodysplasias

These lesions are frequently multiple and may be present in other parts of the body. Gastric mucosal bleeding in this condition is treated by endoscopic means as discussed earlier.

Lower Gastrointestinal Bleed (Bleeding per Rectum)

LOWER GASTROINTESTINAL BLEED

Definition

Lower gastrointestinal bleeding is defined as bleed distal to ligament of *Treitz* or duodeno-jejunal flexure. It may present with fresh red blood in stool (hematochezia), maroon blood or occult blood. It must be remembered that melana (black tarry stool) is a sign of upper GI bleed, but rarely can occur in lower GI bleed such as bleeding lesion of right side of colon.

Causes

The causes of lower GI bleed are diagrammatically represented in Fig. 15.1 and summarised in Box 1.

Box 1	Causes of lower GI bleed	
Severe/acute	*Moderate chronic/subacute*
• Diverticular disease in old age	• Anorectal disease (e.g. fissure, haemorrhoids, Fig. 15.2)
• Ischaemic colitis	• Inflammatory bowel disease (e.g. Crohn's disease, ulcerative colitis)
• Angiodysplasias or AV malformations	• Infections (e.g. bacillary dysentery, tuberculosis, HIV colopathy, etc).
• Meckel's diverticulum	• Large polyps
	• Carcinoma colon/rectum
	• Angiodysplasia
	• Radiation enteritis, solitary rectal ulcer
	• Idiopathic (20%)

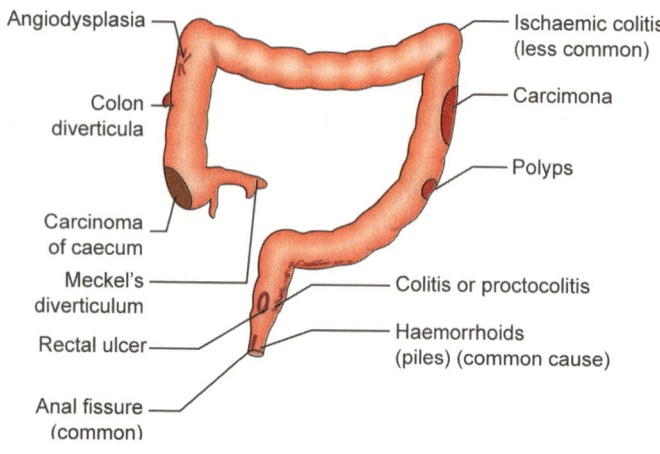

Angiodysplasia

Colon diverticula

Carcinoma of caecum

Meckel's diverticulum

Rectal ulcer

Anal fissure (common)

Ischaemic colitis (less common)

Carcimona

Polyps

Colitis or proctocolitis

Haemorrhoids (piles) (common cause)

Fig. 15.1: Causes of lower GI bleed diagrammatic representation

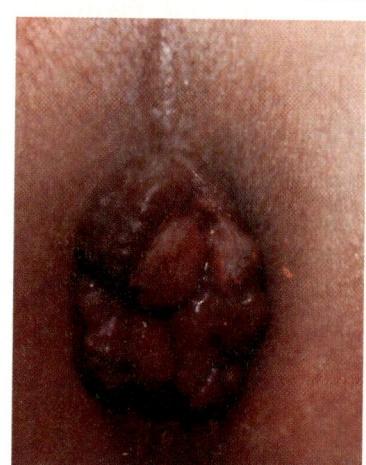

Fig. 15.2: Bleeding piles

Clinical Presentations/Features

The clinical features depend on the site, type and severity of the bleeding from lower GI tract. The clinical features with their important causes are given in Table 15.1. The causes of acute, subacute and chronic lower GI bleed are given in Box 1. Patients with profuse bleeding have underlying enteric or nonspecific ulcers, arteriovenous malformations (angiodysplasias) in elderly (>55 years) and diverticular disease (erosion of an artery within mouth of a diverticulum) in the young. Ischaemic or inflammatory bowel disease or tumour results in subacute or chronic blood loss with diarrhoea and pain.

Diagnosis and Differential Diagnosis

The colour of the stool helps distinguish upper from lower GI tract bleeding. *Brown stool* mixed with blood predicts anorectal or rectosigmoid region as source. *Bright red stool* suggests colonic cause, while *maroon colour* indicates bleeding from right colon. *Black stools* indicates either upper GI bleed or bleeding from small intestine.

Differential diagnosis of lower GI bleed has been presented in Table 15.1. The diagnosis is confirmed on investigations.

Investigative Evaluation (Fig. 15.3)

1. **Anoproctoscopy:** It is done to detect underlying lesions (e.g. haemorrhoids, rectal ulcer or cancer, proctitis etc.).

2. **Colonoscopy:** It is the investigation of choice in all patients with lower GI bleeding unless massive bleeding precludes this procedure. It is done both for diagnostic (visual examination of the lesion, biopsy) and therapeutic purposes (an application of sclerotherapy/heater probe/thermal ablation). Colonoscopy can detect many lesions that are often missed on barium enema studies. Colonoscopy also helps in localisation of the lesion (right or left colon) and to determine its possible aetiology (characteristic vascular spots in angiodysplasia).

3. **Angiography:** Angiography is a tool in expert hands to localise the lesion. Angiography may also disclose lesions like angiodysplasia (vascular spots as reminiscent of spider naevi) and diverticulosis even when active bleeding has stopped. During this procedure, vasopressin can be given intra-arterially. *Gelfoam* or *steel coils* can be injected into a bleeding vessel to stop the bleeding. This procedure is available only at specialised centres is indicated in patients with massive lower GI bleed and hematochezia.

Nuclear bleeding scan (technetium labelled RBC scanning): It is useful to detect lesions with low rates of bleeding

Table 15.1: Clinical features with their possible causes in lower GI bleed	
Features	*Possible cause(s)*
• Bleeding occurring as drops of red blood or small ooz at the end of defecation into the toilet bowel or pan associated with constipation.	Haemorrhoids (piles)
• Bleeding per rectum with pain and tenesmus	Fissure, proctitis
• Painless frequent bleeding occurring in a child	Polyposis, Meckel's diverticulum
• Painless rectal large volume bleeding with constipation	Diverticular disease
• Blood mixed with mucus diarrhoea and pain	Inflammatory bowel disease
• Bleed with a palpable abdominal lump, obstruction, weight loss, change in bowel habits, old age	Malignancy colon
• Perianal skin lesions	Crohn's disease
• Occult GI bleed (blood or blood products are present in the stool but cannot be seen) with anaemia	Colorectal cancer particularly carcinoma of right side of colon or of caecum

but can be normal in up to 30% of cases with bleeding from colonic site. Tc^{99m} pertechnetate scans are useful to detect ectopic gastric epithelium in Meckel's diverticulum in children and adolescents. In the presence of massive GI bleed (an emergency), angiography is preferred over scan. Accordingly angiograms are performed in patients with positive scan.

5. **Small intestine push enteroscopy or capsule imaging:** In minority of cases, small intestine bleeding may present as lower GI bleed. It is very difficult to evaluate this source of bleeding by upper endoscopy and colonoscopy. Therefore, the small intestine is investigated in patients with unexplained recurrent hemorrhage of obscure origin.

6. **Upper GI endoscopy:** It should be done if no lesion is found on investigations in lower GI bleed. About 5 to 10% of patients with bleeding per rectum may have a lesion found on upper GI endoscopy. It is advisable to perform upper GI endoscopy in each and every case of lower GI bleed to rule out upper GI lesion even when nasogastric aspirate is negative for blood.

Management

1. **General treatment:** The primary consideration in the case of bleeding patient is:
   - To maintain intravascular volume by fluids and blood transfusions.
   - Resuscitation of shock and to maintain haemodynamic stability. These measures have already been discussed in management of upper GI bleed.

2. **Specific treatment:** It depends on the cause (Box 2). Specific treatment can be (i) endoscopic (e.g. polypectomy, injection

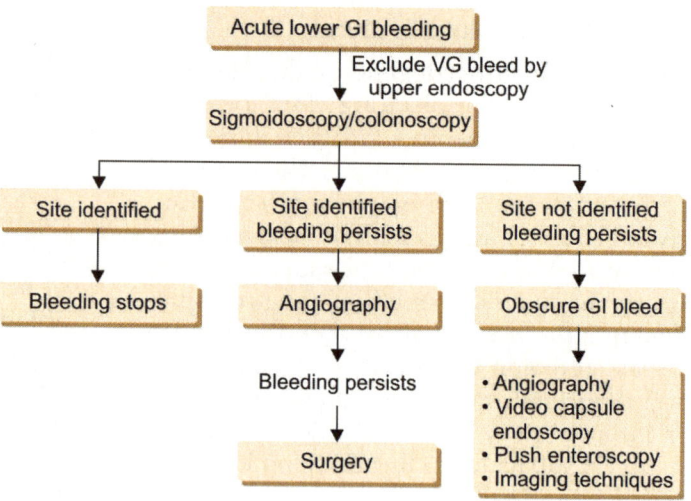

Fig. 15.3: Algorithm for evaluation of lower GI bleed

sclerotherapy, laser/thermal ablation), (ii) angiographic (arterial embolisation) or (iii) pharmacological (vasopressin, somatostatin in case of UGI bleed). Surgery is indicated for inaccessible lesions on colonoscopy, e.g. small bowel tumours or when source of bleeding remains unknown. In case of non-localisation of lesion on angiography with continued bleeding, hemicolectomy/colectomy may be performed as a life-saving measure.

Box 2	Treatment of commonly encountered lesions in lower GI bleeding
Lesion	*Treatment*
Haemorrhoids/piles	Injection sclerotherapy/banding/laser photocoagulation
Polyp(s)	Polypectomy
Amoebic colitis	Metronidazole/tinidazole
Bacillary dysentery	Appropriate antibiotics
Typhoid ulcers	Ciprofloxacin or ceftriaxone; if conservative treatment fails, then surgery
Malignancy	Endoscopic hemostasis, surgery
Nonspecific/ulcerative colitis	Steroids/5-ASA enemas
Angiodysplasias	Laser/heater probe/surgery
Rectocolonic varices	Somatostatin/surgery

Acute Pancreatitis

ACUTE PANCREATITIS

Definition

Acute pancreatitis is defined as an acute inflammation of the pancreas with variable involvement of regional tissues and remote organ system. It results from premature activation of zymogen granules which activate and release pancreatic enzymes (proteases), vasoactive substances and toxic material that digest the pancreas and the surrounding tissues leading to local and systemic complications.

Classification

The currently used terminology based on Atlanta system of classification is given in Table 16.1. The revised Atlanta classification of severity of acute pancreatitis uses the following three catagories:

1. **Mild disease** is the absence of organ failure, local or systemic complications.
2. **Moderate disease** is the presence of transient (<48 hours) organ failure or complications or both.
3. **Severe disease** is presence of persistent organ failure or complications or both.

Pathogenesis and Pathophysiology

The most accepted pathogenesis of pancreatitis is its autodigestion by its enzymes. It occurs as a result of:

1. Oedema or obstruction of the *ampulla of Vater*, reflux of bile into pancreatic ducts, and direct injury to acinar cells by premature activation of zymogen granules. A number of factors, e.g. toxins, viral infection, ischaemia, anoxia, direct trauma activate these proenzymes.
2. Release of activated proteolytic enzymes, e.g. proteases and cytokines.
3. Autodigestion (inflammation) of the pancreas and surrounding tissue by activities

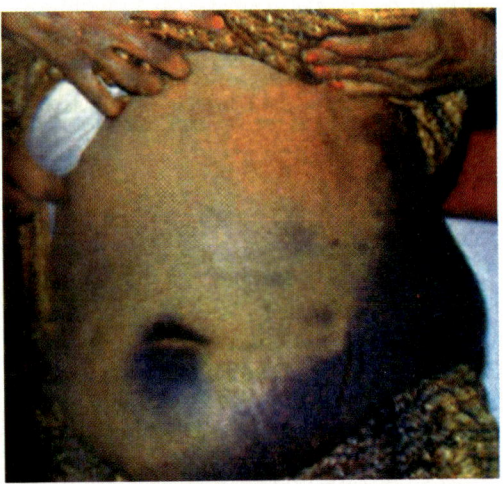

Fig. 16.1: Acute pancreatitis. A patient of pancreatitis showing haemorrhagic manifestations, e.g. brownish discolouration in periumbilical region (Cullen's sign) and in the flanks (Grey-Turner sign). Both the signs indicate acute necrotising haemorrhagic pancreatitis

Table 16.1 Revised Atlanta definitions of morphological features of acute pancreatitis

1. *Severe acute pancreatitis (necrotising pancreatitis):* Inflammation associated with pancreatic, parenchymal necrosis and/or peripancreatic necrosis.
2. *Mild acute pancreatitis (interstitial pancreatitis):* Acute inflammation of the pancreatic parenchyma and peripancreatic tissue. Uneventful recovery takes place within 3–5 days without organ dysfunction.
3. *Acute pancreatic fluid collections:* Occurs in acute interstitial pancreatitis without peripancreatic necrosis. Areas of paripancreatic fluid collection are detected on CT scan.
4. *Acute pseudocyst:* Collection of pancreatic juice and inflammatory exudates in lesser omentum enclosed by a wall of fibrous or granulation tissue. The entity occurs >4 weeks after on set of pancreatitis.
5. *Pancreatic necrosis:* Widespread focal areas of non-viable parenchyma (necrosis) and fluid collection involving the parenchyma and peripancreatic tissue; occurs only in the setting of acute necrotising pancreatitis.
6. *Pancreatic abscess:* Collection of pus within pancreas.
7. *Pancreatic ascites:* Exudative fluid in peritoneal cavity rich in amylase and lipase.

enzymes, i.e. trypsin leads to proteolysis, oedema, haemmorrhage and vascular damage and parenchymal necrosis, systemic inflammatory response syndrome (SIRS). ARDS and multiple organ failure are its distant effects.

The normal pancreas has only a poorly developed capsule, hence, adjacent structures including the common bile duct, duodenum, splenic vein and transverse colon are commonly involved in the inflammatory process. The severity of pancreatitis depends on the balance between proteolytic enzymes injury and anti-proteolytic defense.

Causes

The gallstones, alcohol, post-ERCP (endoscopic retrograde cholangiopancreatography) and idiopathic constitute 90% of cases of pancreatitis. Rest 10% are due to many other conditions given in Box 1. The causes of recurrent acute pancreatitis are given in Box 2. Rarely acute pancreatitis may be a presenting manifestation of a pancreatic or ampullary neoplams.

Clinical Features

Symptoms

1. *Abrupt epigastric pain*, which is severe and commonly radiates to the back is the presenting symptom. Radiation of pain to the left upper quadrant or periumbilical region is also seen. Pain may be dull or boring in character and is deep-seated.

Box 1 Causes of acute pancreatitis

Common (90%)	*Uncommon/rare*
• Gallstones	• *Infections*, e.g. viral (mumps, cytomegalovirus coxsackie), bacterial (salmonella) fungal and parasitic (round worm)
• Alcohol abuse	
• Idiopathic (microlithiasis)	
• Abdominal trauma (blunt)	• *Drugs* (azathioprine, thiazides, isoniazid, leflunamide tomoxifen valproate, dapsone, pentamidine, didanosine, sitagliftin, etc.
• Hyperlipidaemia, hypercalcaemia	
• Post-ERCP	• Perforating peptic ulcer
	• *End-stage renal disease*, peritoneal dialysis
• Post-surgical (abdominal/extra-abdominal)	• *Congenital anomaly* (pancreas divisium)
	• Pancreatic outflow obstruction
	• Severe hypothermia, shock, bites, etc.
	• *Organ transplantation* (kidney, liver), cardiopulmonary bypass
	• Vasculitis

Box 2 Causes of acute pancreatitis

- Drugs
- Pancreas divisum
- Sphincter of Oddi dysfunction
- Idiopathic
- Hypertriglyceridemia
- Pancreatic cancer
- Cystic fibrosis

The patient may feel relief of pain by sitting forward with bent-knees against the chest or lying on one side with knees flexed. There may history of alcohol intake or heavy meal preceding the attack

2. *Associated nausea and vomiting.* Weakness, sweating and anxiety are present during severe attack.
3. Distension of abdomen due to gastric and intestinal hypomotility and peritonitis.
4. Symptoms of other organ systems involvement, e.g. dyspnoea, GI bleed.

Signs

1. In severe cases, the patient looks acutely *ill, anxious, restless* with *low grade fever* (38–39°C) and *tachycardia*. Later, they become *hypoxic*, develop *hypovolaemic shock (hypotension)* and *oliguria* due to retroperitoneal sequetation of fluid.
2. *Abdominal signs* are absent initially, but develop gradually. These are:
   • *Abdominal tenderness, guarding* and *rigidity* due to peritoneal involvement.
   • *Abdominal distension* and *absent bowel sounds* due to development of paralytic ileus.
   • *Mild jaundice* may be seen. This is due to compression of intrapancreatic portion of common bile duct by inflammatory exudate.
   • *Erythematous skin nodules* due to subcutaneus fat necrosis may be present.
   • *Grey-Turner's sign* [brown discolouration of the flanks—Fig. 16.1] may be seen in acute necrotising haemorrhagic pancreatitis.
   • *Cullen's sign* [bluish-brown discolouration of the periumbilical region (Fig. 16.1)] is also seen in haemorrhagic pancreatitis due to blood dissecting along the tissue planes giving this discolouration,
3. *Chest signs:* Chest examination may reveal rales, atelectasis, pleural effusion, commonly on the left, is usually small, haemorrhagic and has high amylase content. Sometimes, there may be pneumonitis or development of ARDS (hypoxic respiratory failure).
4. *A palpable mass* two or more weeks after the onset may represent inflammatory mass/ necrosis or pseudocyst. Ascites may be present if pancreatitis is complicated.

Diagnosis

Diagnosis initially rests on the clinical picture. Acute pancreatitis should be suspected in any patient with severe upper abdominal pain or unexplained hypovolaemic shock. Ultimately, diagnosis is made on the basis of symptoms, signs, compatible biochemical and radiological investigations and exclusion of the other causes.

Investigations

i. **Serum enzymes (amylase, lipase, etc.) levels:** A number of enzymes i.e. amylase, lipase, elastase, phospholipase A etc. are elevated during acute pancreatitis, hence, their estimation form an important diagnostic clue.

   Serum *amylase* is elevated in 90% of cases, starts rising within few hours and persists for 3 to 5 days. It is not specific for pancreatitis because many extrapancreatic conditions (e.g. perforated bowel, intestinal obstruction, mesenteric infarction, peritonitis, acute appendicitis, renal failure, diabetic ketoacidosis, salpingids, diagnostic and therapeutic GI tract procedures, etc.) can raise it 2 to 3 times than normal. Therefore, higher levels more than 3 times than normal are suggestive of pancreatitis in a patient with upper abdominal pain. Persistence of high levels beyond first week indicates presence of extensive necrosis or pseudocyst formation. Separation of serum amylase into pancreatic and salivary fractions is more diagnostic than total amylase.

   Serum lipase levels are raised by 2 to 3 times than normal in about 90% cases of acute pancreatitis. Its elevation is more specific than serum amylase. Its estimation is helpful in conditions where hyperamylasemia is due to non-pancreatic causes. Therefore, combined measurement of serum amylase and lipase increases the sensitivity as well as specificity to about 90% in acute pancreatitis.

> *An elevated serum amylase or lipase at least 3 times than normal in a patient with recent onset of upper abdominal pain with or without shock is diagnostic of acute pancreatitis.*

ii. **Inflammatory markers:** Certain inflammatory markers such as IL-6 released by macrophages increase during acute pancreatitis. An elevated C-reactive protein >150 mg/L indicates severe disease but is not specific for pancreatitis. However, these markers have prognostic rather than diagnostic value in follow-up of cases.

iii. **Blood tests:** There may be leucocytosis (15,000–20,000 cells/mm^3) and hematocrit may be high (>44%). Blood urea is raised due to pre-renal azotemia.

iv. **Liver function tests:** Raised serum bilirubin, alkaline phosphatase and aminotransferases may occur.

v. **Serum calcium:** Hypocalcaemia may be seen in 25% of cases of severe pancreatitis. It results from sequestration of Ca^{++} in saponification of fats, increased glucagon and calcitonin levels. It is associated with bad prognosis.

vi. **Blood lipids:** There may be hypertriglyceridemia.

vii. **Blood sugar:** There may be hyperglycaemia.

viii. Methemoglobinemia may be seen in haemorrhagic pancreatitis due to entry of haematin into the circulation.

ix. **Blood gas analysis:** There may be hypoxia (arterial PO$_2$≤60 mmHg) which may herald the onset of ARDS.

x. **ECG:** ST-T wave abnormalities simulating myocardial ischaemia may be seen.

xi. **Other tests,** e.g. urinary trypsinogen-2, trypsinogen activation peptide and carboxypeptidase B are now becoming available.

Imaging Studies

i. **Radiology:** The radiological findings which may be seen on plain X-ray abdomen and X-ray chest are given in Box 3.

X-ray abdomen is also useful to rule out other causes of acute abdominal pain such as ruptured viscus and bowel infarction.

ii. **Abdominal ultrasound:** It is recommended in the emergency ward as an initial diagnostic modality and is very useful in diagnosis and management of acute pancreatitis and its local complications. It is useful in detection of gallstones, helps in identification of pseudocyst and ascites. In the early stage, it may show the swollen gland with periglandular fluid collections.

Endoscopic USG is useful in identifying occult biliary disease (sledge or a small stone) or microlithiasis, is indicated in suspected pancreatitis (severe pain) in person's over the age of 40 years.

iii. **CT scan/MRI scan:** CT scan shows swollen, oedematous gland with obliteration of peripancreatic fat. Pseudocyst formation

Box 3   Radiological findings in acute pancreatitis
Plain X-ray abdomen
• Ill defined tissue planes, dilated bowel loops and hazy renal and psoas shadows
• Isolated small bowel dilated loops near the pancreas due to isolated ileus (sentinal loop)
• *Colon cut-off sign:* It is a nonspecific finding. There is spasm in the transverse colon with absence of colonic gas beyond it
• Hazziness due to ascites
• Extraluminal gas bubbles indicating pancreatic abscess
X-ray chest (PA view)
• Raised domes of diaphragm
• Pleural effusion (left)
• Atelectasis
• Pneumonitis
• Cardiomegaly or CHF
• Interstitial fluffy shadows

may also be seen. MRI has no added advantages over CT scan, to be done if CT scan cannot be done. A contrast enhanced CT scan provides valuable information or the estimation of the presence and extent of pancreatic necrosis (severity).

iv. **ERCP or MRCP:** ERCP is indicated in pancreatitis associated with cholangitis or jaundice. MRCP or endoscopic USG should be considered especially after repeated attacks of acute pancreatitis. In selected cases aspiration of bile for crystal analysis may confirm microlithiasis. Sphincter of Oddi manometery may be done in recurrent pancreatitis.

Diagnosis and Differential Diagnosis

The diagnosis is established by two of the following three criteria:

1. Typical abdominal pain in the epigastrium radiating to the back.
2. Three fold or more elevation of serum amylase and/or lipase.
3. Confirmatory findings of acute pancreatitis on cross-sectional abdominal imaging (USG, CT sacn).

  Differential diagnosis includes the following conditions, i.e.

1. Perforated peptic ulcer
2. Acute cholecystitis and biliary colic
3. Acute intestinal obstruction
4. Inferior myocardial infarction
5. Mesentery vascular occlusion
6. Dissecting aortic aneurysm
7. Diabetic ketoacidosis
8. Vascalitis

Complications

They are both local and systemic:

I. **Local**
   • Pancreatic necrosis
   • Pancreatic fluid collection, e.g. abscess, pseudocyst
   • Pancreatic ascites
   • Involvement of adjoining organs and vessels
   • Obstructive jaundice

II. **Systemic**
   • *Pulmonary,* e.g. pleural effusion, pneumonitis, ARDS, atelectasis and mediastinal abscess.
   • *Renal,* e.g. oliguria, azotemia, ATN (acute tubular necrosis) and renal artery/vein thrombosis.
   • *Cardiovascular,* e.g. hypotension, pericardial effusion and sudden death.
   • *Haematological,* e.g. disseminated intravascular coagulation.
   • *GI haemorrhage,* e.g. peptic ulcer disease, hemorrhagic pancreatic necrosis, portal vein, thrombosis.
   • *Metabolic,* e.g hyperglycemia, hypertriglyceridemia, hypocalcemia and encephalopathy.
   • *CNS*—psychosis, fat emboli.

Urgent Management

There is no specific therapy which can arrest or interrupt the process of autodigestion, hence, the treatment is mainly supportive and symptomatic. Patient with mild disease may be treated in emergency ward, severe disease requires management in ICU with monitoring.

Steps of Treatment

• To establish the diagnosis and to assess its severity (Ranson's criteria, Box 4).
• Early institution of treatment whether disease is mild or severe. Mild disease resolves spontaneously within few days.
• Resuscitation of shock or maintenance of intravascular volume.
• Relief of pain.
• Detection and treatment of complications.
• Nutritional support and rest to the gland.
• Treatment of underlying cause, if found, specifically gallstones.

A. Mild pancreatitis

About 80-90% of cases of acute pancreatitis are self limited. Mild pancreatitis is treated by:

i. *Relief of pain* by meperidine hydrochloride (100–150 mg IM) or I.V. morphine, though not a preferred analgesic due to provocation of spasm of sphincter of Oddi but has been found useful alternative.

ii. *Nutrition and fluid replacement:* The fluid deficit must be corrected immediately by I.V. fluids (normal saline), if patient has vomiting so as to correct hypotension. The fluid therapy must be monitored by pulse, BP, skin turgor and urine output. Oral intake of fluids and food can be resumed when the patient is free of pain and bowel sounds are present. Clear liquids are given first followed by gradual advancement to low fat diet.

iii. *Rest to the gland:* Patient is kept on nil orally (NPO). A nasogastric aspiration should be done to keep the stomach empty in an attempt to prevent gastric acid from entering into the duodenum and stimulating the pancreatic secretions. There is no use of administering H_2 receptors antagonists or proton-pump inhibitor in order to reduce pancreatic secretions.

iv. *Antibiotics:* Prophylactic use of antibiotics in mild pancreatitis is not recommended.

v. *Nutrition:* Parenteral nutrition is not needed in mild disease, however if patient has vomiting and distension, parenteral feed for few days may be given. Once patient has improved and there is no pain and bowel sounds have returned oral feeds may be started. Clear fluids are given initially followed by gradual replacement with low fat diet according to tolerance of the patient may be given.

Treatment of the cause: Treatment of underlying cause:

- Following recovery from acute biliary pancreatitis, laparoscopic chalecystectomy is performed to reduce the rate of recurrent pancreatitits.
- In pancreatitis associated with pancreas divisum, insertion of a stent in the minor papilla may reduce subsequent attacks.
- For sphincter of Oddi dysfunction, biliary sphincterotomy alone is effective.

B. Severe pancreatitis (Boxes 4 and 5)

Patients with severe pancreatitis are best managed in ICU. Despite good management, mortality is 10–15%. Management includes:

i. *Relief of pain* by analgesic.

ii. *Nasogastric aspiration* to keep the stomach empty and to provide rest to the gland.

iii. *Parenteral fluids:* Intravenous fluid, e.g. Ringer's lactate or normal saline 500–1000 ml/hr for several hours followed by 250–300 ml/hr to maintain intravascular volume and urine output 0.5 ml/kg/hr. Pressor agents (dopamine) may be used to treat hypotension. Serial bedside monitoring is required every 6–8 hours to assess vital signs and oxygenation.

A decrease in haematocrit and BUN during first 24 hours is strong evidence that sufficient fluids are administered.

iv. *Parenteral nutrition:* After 3–4 days of I.V. fluids, if pain continues, there are a number of options to provide continuous nutrition including total parenteral nutrition with intralipids. Lipid infusion does not stimulate pancreatic secretions but it can produce hyperlipidaemia that can trigger further pancreatitis. As soon as pain is relieved, enteral feeding may be started with a low fat diet.

v. *Antibiotics:* Antibiotic therapy is indicated in severe pancreatitis with or without complications. Antibiotics having good diffusion capacity into pancreas, (e.g. imipenem, ofloxacin, metronidazole, and mezlocillin) may be started in severe pancreatitis. Those with necrotising pancreatitis should preferably receive imipenem 500 mg I.V. every 12 hourly for 7–10 days.

vi. Infusion of fresh frozen plasma or serum albumin may be necessary for coagulopathy or hypoalbuminemia.

vii. *Severe hypocalcaemia* is corrected by giving 10 ml of calcium gluconate I.V. slowly.

viii. *Patient with ARDS or respiratory distress* require O_2 therapy and respiratory support, i.e. intubation and mechanical ventilation with positive end-expiratory pressure.

Box 4	Clinical Criteria for severity of acute pancreatitis

Ranson's criteria	*Glasgow criteria*
1. At admission (three or more indicate severe disease)	
• Age >55 years	• Age >55 years
• TLC >16000/mm³	• PO, < 8 kPa
• Blood sugar >200 mg %	• WBC >15 107L
• LDH>350 IU/L	• Albumin <32 g/L (3.2 g%)
• Aspartate amino transferase 7250 units	• Serum calcium <2 mmol/L (corrected)
• Base deficit >4 mEq/L	
• Fluid sequestration >6 L	
2. Initial 48 hours (development of the following indicates worse prognosis)	
• Haematocrit decrease by >10%	• Glucose >10 mmol/L
• BUN increase by >5 mg%	• Urea >16 mmol/L (after rehydration)
• Serum calcium < 8 mg%	• ALT >200 U/L
• PaO$_2$ < 60 mmHg AST	• LDH >800 U/L

Box 5	CECT severity index (scoring system) in acute pancreatitis

Finding	*Points*
A. Degree of pancreatic necrosis	
• No necrosis	0
• Necrosis of one-third of pancreas	2
• Necrosis of 1/2 (one half) of pancreas	4
• Necrosis more than one-half of pancreas	6
B. CT grade of acute pancreatitis	
• Normal pancreas	0
• Pancreatic enlargement alone	1
• Inflammation of pancreas and peripancreatic fat	2
• One peripancreatic fluid collection	3
• Two or more fluid collections	4
Severity index = CT grade + necrosis score (0–10)	

Note:

1. Complications and mortality rates are negligible when severity index is 1 or 2; and low when score is 3 to 6.
2. High morbidity (92%) and significant mortality (17%) is reported when the severity score is >7.

ix. *Renal failure* is treated on the same lines as acute renal failure (read acute renal failure).

x. Patients who present with cholangitis or jaundice in association with acute severe pancreatitis should undergo urgent ERCP to diagnose and treat gallstones. Otherwise. ERCP has to be done once acute phase is over.

xi. Patients with diabetes and hyperlipidaemia (>1000 mg/dl) should receive insulin, heparin or plasmapheresis initially followed by control of diabetes, lipid lowering agents, weightloss and avoidance of drugs that raise lipids.

xii. Recently somatostatin, octreotide and the antiprotease gabexate mesylate have been found to reduce the risk of pancreatitis after ERCP. Placement of stent across the pancreatitis duct has also been shown to reduce post-ERCP pancreatitis.

Management of Complications

Patients who have developed *necrotising pancreatitis* (fever, leucocytosis), require urgent surgical debridement of the pancreas, followed by percutaneous aspiration. The aspirated material is stained with Gram's stain and sent for culture. This may be associated with left sided pleural effusion which should be aspirated.

Pancreatic abscess is treated by antibiotics and fine needle aspiration. Surgical drainage is required when percutaneous drainage of pus is not helpful.

Pancreatic pseudocysts are treated by drainage into the stomach or duodenum. This is usually done after at least 6 weeks, once a pseudocapsule is formed, using open surgery or endoscopic method.

Pancreatic ascites is exudative (protein > 2.5 g/L) and has high serum amylase levels (>1000 U/dl). Medical treatment includes nasogastric aspiration, total parenteral nutrition and octreotide therapy. As it occurs due to leakage from the cyst or duct, hence, surgery may be needed to correct this leakage.

Amoebic Liver Abscess

AMOEBIC LIVER ABSCESS

Definition

Amoebic liver abscess is an inflammatory pus collection within the liver caused by *Entamoeba histolytica*. It is the most common form of liver abscess encountered in clinical practice as an emergency. It is endemic in India, and is the most common presentation of extraintestinal invasive amoebiasis.

Pathogenesis

Liver abscess is always preceded by amoebic intestinal involvement which may be symptomatic or asymptomatic. Trophozoites invade the veins in the intestine by lysis of the wall and reach the liver through portal circulation (Fig. 17.1). Pathogenic strains are resistant to complement-mediated lysis—a property which makes them survive in the bloodstream. In contrast, *nonpathogenic* strains are rapidly

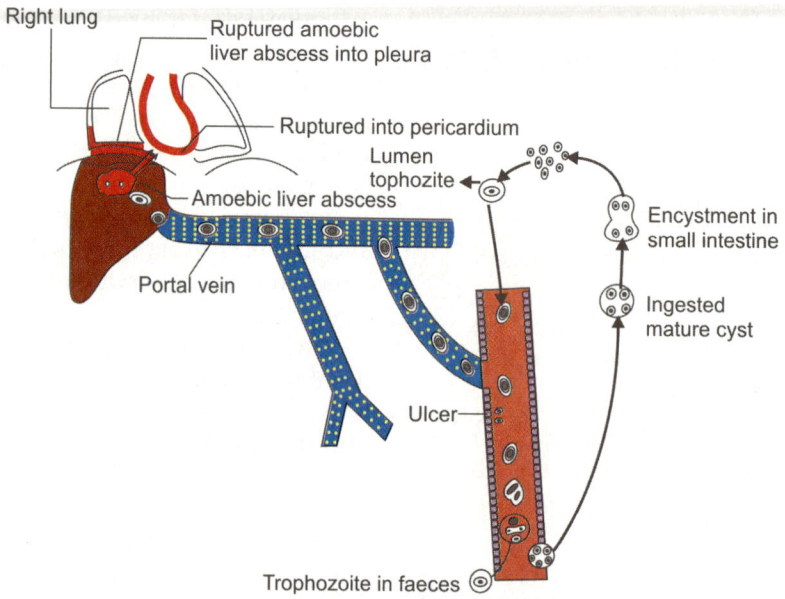

Fig. 17.1: Amoebic liver abscess-pathogenesis and its rupture into pleural space

lysed by complement and are thus restricted to the bowel lumen. The active trophozoites in the liver incite inflammatory reaction consisting predominantly of neutrophils. Later, the neutrophils are lysed by contact with amoebae and release of neutrophil toxin that may contribute to necrosis of hepatocytes. The liver parenchyma is replaced by necrotic material that is surrounded by a thin margin of congested liver tissue, i.e. there is formation of liver abscess demarcated by inflammed congested liver tissue. The oozing of blood from the vessel into necrotic tissue makes the liver abscess—a classical anchovy paste—called *anchovy sauce like pus* but the colour of fluid is variable with treatment and is composed of bacteriologically sterile granular debris with few or no pus cells. Trophozoites, if seen, tend to be found only near the walls of the abscess.

Clinical Features

Amoebic liver abscess can occur with colitis but more commonly presents without history of prior intestinal symptoms.

Of traveller's who develop amoebic liver abscess after leaving an endemic area, 95% do so within 4–5 months. Young patients with abscess are more likely to present in the acute phase with prominent symptoms of less than 10 days duration. The *presenting symptom is fever with right upper quadrant pain* which may be dull or pleuritic in nature and radiates to shoulders. **Point tenderness** over the liver and right sided pleural effusion (sympathetic effusion) is common. Although the parasites reach the liver from the intestine, concomitant diarrhoea is common. In older patients, unexplained weight loss, anorexia without fever or pain may be seen as a presenting complaint.

Hepatomegaly with intercostal tenderness (*thumping sign*) is a characteristic finding but may be absent in deep or centrally located lesion. *Jaundice* is not a common finding but a large abscess can cause compression of bile ducts and produce obstructive jaundice at a later stage.

Abscesses are most commonly single and in the right lobe of the liver, and they are more common in men.

Persistent or increase in local signs of inflammation on the skin suggest impending rupture. *Complications* occur due to rupture of the abscess into subdiaphragmatic, pleural, pericardial, intraperitoneal or intrabiliary space or into the lung. Compression of inferior vena cava (IVC) or hepatic veins may cause an outflow obstruction producing portal hypertension (*Budd-Chiari syndrome*).

> *Fever, tender hepatomegaly with intercostal tenderness of less than 10 days duration in a young person suggest an amoebic liver abscess*

Since 10–15% of patients present only with fever, therefore, amoebic liver abscess should be considered in the differential diagnosis of pyrexia of unknown origin (PUO).

Diagnosis

The diagnosis of amoebic liver abscess is made on history of fever, right hypochondrial pain with tender hepatomegaly. It is confirmed on ultrasound and other tests.

Investigations

1. **Stool examination** for trophozoites is usually negative. At least 3 stool specimens should be evaluated after concentration and staining.
2. **WBC count** may show leucocytosis (>10,000 cells/mm^3). There may be anaemia.
3. **Ultrasonography of liver:** It is useful non-invasive test to identify an abscess as a hypoechoic cyst or cavity with irregular shaggy walls. The abscess is more common in right than left lobe on its posterosuperior surface (Fig. 17.2). Multiple abscesses are likely to be pyogenic. Satellite lesions (microabscess) may be present around the main lesion. However, multiple lesions spread all over the liver in amoebic liver abscess should make one to suspect an

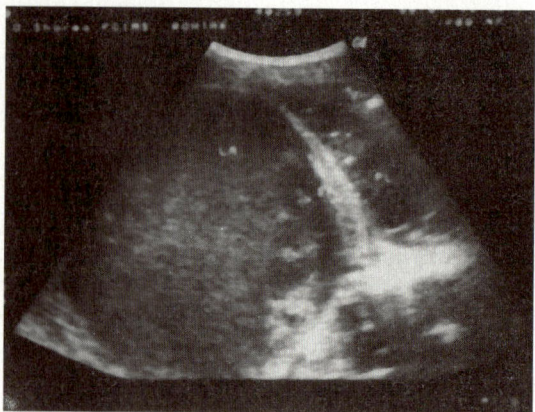

Fig. 17.2: USG showing a large amoebic liver abscess in right lobe

immunocompromised state which should be investigated. The USG findings change with the duration of the illness from a solid lesion, abscess-in-evolution to abscess formation. It is made clear that size usually increases with treatment and does not warrant aspiration unless associated with no response to treatment or impending rupture.

4. **CT scan/MRI:** These investigations do not have any advantage over USG which is gold standard for diagnosis of an amoebic liver abscess.

5. **Serological tests:** Indirect haemagglutination (IHA) and ELISA tests for amoebiasis have been the most extensively employed confirmatory tests and are almost always positive except very early in infection. Low titres are not diagnostic of recent infection. Titres >1:1024 are diagnostic of amoebic liver abscess. A negative IHA for amoebic liver abscess should be repeated after one week and if found again negative, it rules out amoebic abscess and warrants further investigations to look for other aetiologies like pyogenic abscess, primary or secondary hepatocellular carcinoma or an infected cyst. A commercially available amoebic antigen test (*Tech Lab II*) claimed to have sensitivity of >90% in amoebic colitis, can be used in serum with sensitivity

of 40%. It should be done before start of treatment.

6. When diagnosis is uncertain and there is high possibility of the abscess to be pyogenic, *a diagnostic aspiration* may be done. Demonstration of trophozoites in the aspirated fluid is not easy and their absence does not help in the differentiation of amoebic from pyogenic abscess. Aspiration for Gram staining and culture will help when diagnosis is in doubt.

7. **Other routine tests** such as liver function tests are normal. However with large liver abscess, the alkaline phosphatase, bilirubin and amino-transferases may be elevated slightly.

8. **Fluoroscopy** may show limitation of movement of right dome of the diaphragm.

9. **X-ray chest (PA views):** It is done to detect the complications such as pleural or pericardial effusion. Right dome of the diaphragm may be raised in amoebic liver abscess.

Treatment

1. **Relief of pain and fever** with analgesics.
2. **Drug treatment:** Single drug therapy with *metronidazole* (800 mg tid or 40 mg/kg/day) is treatment of choice for amoebic liver abscess. *Metronidazole* can be used introvenously, *Tinidazole*, (2 g daily orally for 3 days), *secnidazole* and *ornidazole* are other nitromidazole derivatives found to be effective in amoebic liver abscess. The **second line** alternative therapeutic drugs, i.e. dehydroemetine (1 mg/kg deep IM) and chloroquine 500 mg bid for 2 days and then 500 mg daily for 3 weeks should be reserved for nonresponders. South African and other studies done on liver abscesses have recommended an addition of luminal agent (diloxanide furoate 500 mg orally 3 times a day for 10 days) to metronidazole to eradicate cysts and prevent further transmission even if there is no evidence or past history of invasive amoebiasis.

Response to antiamoebic therapy is seen usually within 48–72 hours with prompt resolution of fever, pain, toxaemia, tender hepatomegaly; and therapy must be continued for 10 days. Relapses after adequate therapy are uncommon when a luminicidal agent has been added. Routine administration of antibiotics is not indicated as superadded bacterial infection is not common.

3. **Aspiration of the abscess (Fig. 17.3):** Routine aspiration of the abscess is not indicated because it has been shown clearly that aspiration does not change the course of the disease as compared to medical therapy alone. Most of the patients respond to medical therapy. Aspiration is indicated in certain situations given in Box 1. Its distinction from pyogenic abscess is not easy. Patients with pyogenic liver abscess typically are older and have history of underlying bowel disease or

Box 1 Indications for aspiration of amoebic liver abscess
• No response to medical treatment within 5 days
• Impending rupture. Thin rim (<1 cm) between abscess wall and liver capsule on aUSG.
• Abscess in the left lobe of the liver. It is aspirated to prevent rupture.
• Abscess size >10 cm. Aspiration may accelerate healing
• When distinction between pyogenic and amoebic liver abscess is uncertain.

recent surgery. There will be symptoms and sign of toxaemia. In pyogenic abscess sometimes, repeated aspiration of the amoebic liver abscess may lead to its conversion into pyogenic abscess, hence, repeated aspirations are to be avoided. Serial ultrasonographic follow up should be done to detect resolution of the abscess, which takes 3–6 months.

4. **Catheter drainage:** Along with medical therapy, aspiration with catheter may be required to treat abscess with complications (e.g. rupture).

5. **Surgical exploration** may become necessary in certain situations like bowel perforation or rupture into the pericardium.

Treatment of Complications (Box 2)

Box 2 Treatment of complications
Complication and treatment
1. Pleuropulmonary amoebiasis, i.e. amoebic sterile effusion. It is treated with drainage and medical therapy.
2. Hepatobronchial fistula (rupture of abscess into the lung). Treatment is drainage and antiamoebic therapy.
3. Rupture of abscess into peritoneum (peritonitis): Percutaneous catheter drainage with antiamoebic therapy is best option.
4. Rupture of abscess into pericardium (pericardial effusion): Percardiocentesis and medical therapy should be instituted.

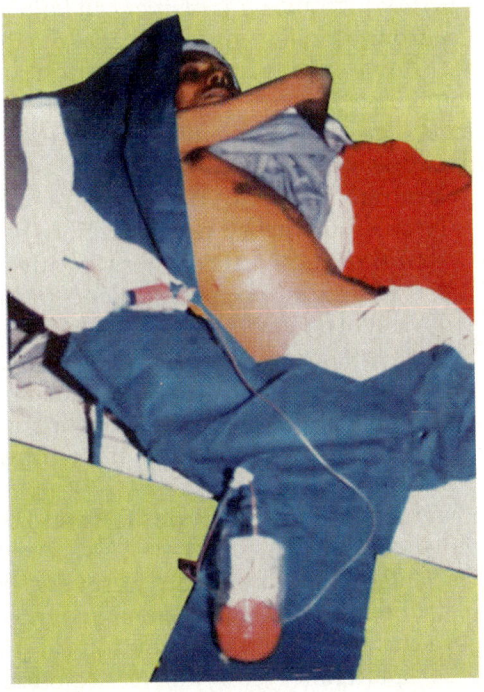

Fig. 17.3: Drainage of amoebic liver abscess

Hepatic Encephalopathy (Acute and Chronic Liver Failure)

HEPATIC ENCEPHALOPATHY

Definitions

Acute hepatic encephalopathy is a clinical syndrome of neuropsychiatric manifestations developing within a period of 8 weeks in a patient with acute fulminant hepatitis as a result of massive acute hepatocellular necrosis without any evidence of previous liver disease. **Chronic hepatic encephalopathy** develops between 8 weeks and 6 months after the onset of acute liver disease. **Acute on chronic liver failure refers** to acute deterioration of liver function in a person with pre-existing liver disease. This is due to entry of nitrogenous products and gut derived neurotoxins in the circulation and the brain. These nitrogenous products and neurotoxins normally originate in the intestine and are inactivated and metabolised in the liver. In hepatic failure, they bypass the diseased liver and reach the CNS through circulation leading to encephalopathy (Figs 18.1 and 18.2).

ACUTE HEPATIC ENCEPHALOPATHY

Causes (Acute Fulminant Hepatitis)

It is primarily seen in acute fulminant due to any cause. Hepatitis B accounts for more than 50% of cases; one-third of which are associated with hepatitis D virus (HDV) infection. It is

a life-threatening syndrome. The causes are given in Box 1. *Acute on chronic hepatic encephalopathy* occurs in a setting of acute exacerbation of chronic liver disease, i.e. hepatitis or cirrhosis.

Clinical Features

It consists of:
  i. Cerebral features
 ii. Symptoms and signs of liver cell failure.

Gastrointestinal symptoms, renal dysfunction, haemorrhagic phenomenon and adrenal insufficiency complicate acute liver failure. The symptoms in acute encephalopathy appear suddenly.

1. **Cerebral features:** These include poor alertness, disturbed concentration, behavioural changes, drowsiness, confusion, disorientation, disturbed sleep pattern (day-night reversal), slurred speech (dysarthria), constructional apraxia (Fig. 18.1), convulsions, delirium and coma. These cerebral features are divided into 4 grades depending on severity of liver disease (Box 2).

2. **Features of hepatocellular failure:** These include:
   • *Jaundice:* It is moderate to severe. Bilirubin >20 mg% carries poor prognosis.
   • *Fetor hepaticus:* It is an ammonical smell in patient's breath due to excretion of methylmercaptans.

- *Flapping tremors:* A flap on extended hands is visible in grade II and III coma but is lost in grade I.V. coma.
- *Bleeding diathesis:* Coagulopathy (INR 1.5 or higher) is invariably present. In some patients, purpura or severe gastro-intestinal bleeding may occur due to lowered coagulation factors. Bleeding can occur from any site, may be evident in the form of epistaxis, black coloured gastric aspirate, purpura, ecchymosis or from a punctured site.
- *Liver span:* The liver span is reduced to <10 cm (normal >13 cm) due to shrinkage.
- *Neurological manifestations,* e.g. hypertonia, decerebration may develop but are less common. Cerebral

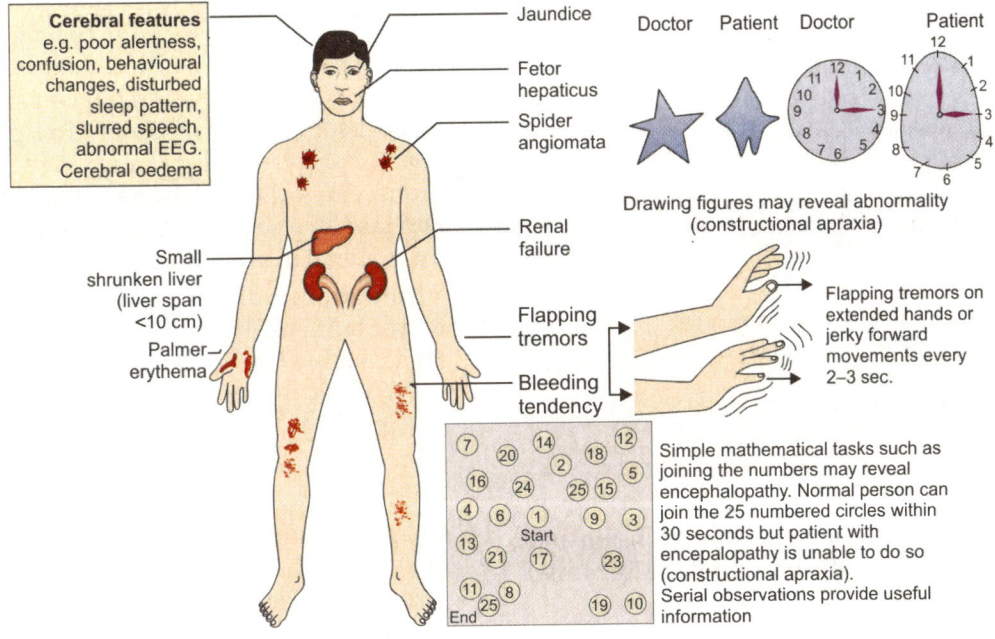

Fig. 18.1: Clinical spectrum of acute hepatic encephalopathy

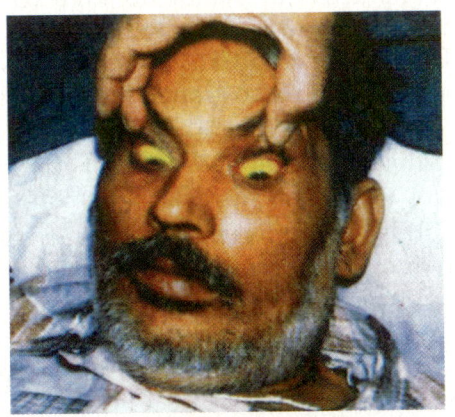

Fig. 18.2: A patient of hepatic coma. There was severe jaundice and unconsciousness

Box 1   Causes of hepatic encephalopathy

1. *Infection:* Viral hepatitis (B and D), yellow fever leptospirosis.
2. *Hepatotoxic drugs:* Anaesthetics (halothane), NSAIDs, acetaminophen overdose, antitubercular drugs, antiepileptics, etc.
3. *Vascular:* Hepatic vein thrombosis (*Budd-Chiari syndrome*), veno-occlusive disease.
4. *Poisons:* Carbon tetrachloride, poisonous fungi (*amanita phalloides*), phosphorous.
5. *Miscellaneous:* Wilson's disease, Reye's syndrome, fatty liver of pregnancy, autoimmune hepatitis, etc.
6. A *chronic hepatitis* or *cirrhosis* due to any cause (alcoholism is the common cause).

Box 2	Staging and clinical features of hepatitis encephalopathy		
Stage	Cerebral features	Asterixis (tremors)	EEG
Grade 0 (sub-clinical or minimal	Only minimal change in memory concen-tration and intellec-tual function. Unfit to drive.	–	Normal
I (mild)	Confusion, mood changes, slurred speech, disordered sleep	+/–	Triphasic slow (5 cycles/ sec waves
II (mode-rate)	Lethargy, drowsy but arousable, confusion, behavioural distur-bances	+	–do–
III (severe)	Marked confusion, incoherent speech, sleepy but arousable	+	–do–
IV (coma)	Coma, initially res-ponsive to noxious stimuli, later non-responsive	–	Delta waves

(+) : present; (–) : absent

oedema, intracranial hypertension and brainstem compression are terminal events.

Note: Patient may develop *acute on chronic hepa-tic encephalopathy* in patient with pre-existing liver disease such as cirrhosis. In such cases, features of chronic liver disease (clubbing, white nails, spider naevi, palmer erythema, gynaecomastia, testicular atrophy, parotid enlargement and symptoms and signs of portal hypertension) will be present.

Tip: Recent onset of encephalopathic features in a patient of hepatitis (within 8 weeks of onset) with small strunken liver on clinical examination (reduced liver span) as well as on USG suggest acute hepatic encephalopathy in a young person without any evidence of pre-existing liver disease.

Diagnosis

It is purely clinical, supported by investiga-tions.

Investigations

1. **Complete haemogram** may reveal anaemia (mostly macrocytic) and leucocy-tosis.

2. **Serum bilirubin** is slightly raised. Both conjugated and unconjugated fractions are increased. Serum bilirubin >20 mg% is a bad prognostic sign.

3. **Serum transaminases:** They are raised initially in hepatitis, may fall progres-sively with progression of the disease, hence, fall of SGOT/SGPT in acute hepatic coma is not a healthy sign but constitutes a bad prognostic parameter. The parac-etamol toxicity leads to much higher rise in enzymes (50–100 times). The **serum amylase** levels are elevated at least 3 times due to renal dysfunction.

4. **Virological studies:** This includes estima-tion of IgM anti-HBc, IgM anti-HAV, anti-HEV, HCV, CMV, herpes simplex and EBV.

5. **Serology:** Serum autoantibodies, ANA, anti-mitochondrial antibodies indicate autoimmune hepatitis.

6. **Coagulation profile:** Prothrombin time (PT) and PTT, INR are prolonged in severe form of the disease. PT >50 sec is also a bad prognostic sign in acute hepatic coma.

7. **EEG:** It is done to grade the hepatic coma. A characteristic symmetric high voltage triphasic slow waves pattern (2–5/sec) on EEG seen in grade I to III while delta wave activity appears in grade I.V. coma.

8. **Serum ammonia** levels are high and correlate with the development of enceph-alopathy and intracranial hypertension.

9. **Ultrasonography (USG)** of the liver shows reduced liver size (usually <10 cm) with normal echotexture.

10. **Toxicology screen of blood and urine.** Ceruloplasmin, serum and urinary copper may be done.

11. **Elevated serum troponin-1 levels** due to subclinical myocardial injury.

Management

Patient should be treated in intensive care unit under the direct supervision of specialists. Early diagnosis and early institution of therapy is essential to prevent its further progression.

Steps of Treatment

General emergency measures

- Patient should be isolated.
- Barrier nursing care.
- All medical personnel and attendants looking after the patient must be vaccinated against hepatitis B.
- A large bore central venous line should be put in for fluids, CVP measurements, drug administration and sample collection.
- A nasogastric tube and condom urinary drainage or catheter are also put. Maintain intake and output chart. Measure urine output.
- Monitor pulse, BP, temperature, respiration, size of pupils, ocular fundus, plantar response and grade of coma. Liver size on percussion or ultrasound be monitored periodically.
- Check the blood counts, urine, LFT, coagulation profile, blood urea, creatinine, arterial blood gases, electrolytes and blood sugar almost every day/alternate day.
- The cause of acute hepatic encephalopathy if known should be treated simultaneously. Infections surveillance by culture of blood, urine, cannula sites, sputum, chest X-ray and TLC and DLC must be done.

Specific measures

Intravascular volume by fluid administration is to preserved, large volume of hypotonic fluids should be avoided.

1. *Sedation:* No sedation is to be given until the patient is violent or irritable. However, if necessary, a small dose of phenobarbitone or 10 mg I.V. oxazepam may be given. Phenothiazines being hepatotoxic should not be used either as an antiemetic or as a sedative.

2. *Nutrition:* Restriction of proteins is advised. To preserve muscle mass and immune function, external administration of protein 1–1.5 g/kg/day is advised with careful monitoring of NH_3 level. Hypoglycaemia is an important cause of death, hence, 10–20% glucose drip is given continuously with potassium supplements. In early stages of coma, glucose can be given through nasogastric tube. Blood glucose is to be monitored frequently with a glucometer and should be kept above 100 mg%. Oral feeds including proteins are to be substituted once the patient starts recovering.

3. *Sterilisation of the gut and its emptying:*
   - Sterilisation of gut by a nonabsorbable antibiotic rifaximin (550 mg orally twice daily) has been very effective in treating encephalopathy. It is a preferred treatment. Metronidazole 250 mg orally thrice daily has shown benefit.
   - Increase the nitrogen content of stool by changing the bacterial flora with lactulose (30–60 ml through nasogastric tube after every 2–3 hours) till one or two loose stools are passed. Lactilol 30 g powder per day is also effective.
   - Repeated bowel/colonic wash to evacuate the bowel (colon) off its contents so as to reduce the ammonia formation from breakdown of proteins by coliform bacteria.

     Rectal use of lactulose (300 ml in 700 ml of saline or sorbitol as a retention enema for 30–60 minutes is indicated when patient is not able to take lactulose orally. Enema can be repeated every 4–6 hours. Continued use of lactulose after an acute episode reduces the frequences of further episodes.

     Bowel cleansing with polyethylene glycol is effective in acute overt hepatic encepholopathy.

4. *Treatment of infection:* Sputum, urine, intravenous catheter tip/site and blood culture

should be obtained periodically. Antibiotic should be given at the evidence of infection.

5. *Treatment of bleeding:* Patients may develop mucocutaneous bleeding, GI bleed or frank DIC. Often the haemorrhage is fatal. Bleeding is treated with fresh blood / packed RBCs infusion, fresh frozen plasma and vitamin K intravenously. Intravenous H_2 blockers (ranitidine) or proton pump inhibitors can be given through naso-gastric tube for prophylaxis of stress gastropathy. Prothrombin time, BT, CT and platelet count are done daily. Active suction through nasogastric tube should be avoided as it can produce gastric erosions.

6. *Treatment of renal failure:* Progressive azotaemia is a dangerous situation in acute hepatic encephalopathy, can be worsened by haemorrhage and sepsis. It should be corrected by volume repletion and monitored by CVP. Nitrogenous matter is removed by gastric lavage. Renal failure is managed by haemodialysis or venous haemofiltration.

7. *Cerebral oedema:* It is the most important cause of death. The diagnostic clues to cerebral oedema include; poorly reacting pupils, fluctuating BP, hypertonia and decerebrate posture. It is treated by rapid infusion of mannitol (20%) at a dose of 100 ml and can be repeated after 4–6 hours if patient passes adequate amount of urine. In the absence of diuresis, mannitol can produce hyponatraemia and water retention.

   Extradural sensors may be placed to monitor intracranial pressure and maintain it below 20 mmHg and the cerebral perfusion pressure above 70 mmHg.

   Hypothermia (temperature 32–34°C) may be used alternatively to reduce cerebral oedema.

8. *Liver transplantation:* If available, is the treatment of choice in patients with grade III–IV coma.

9. *Other recent therapies:* Acetyl-cysteine in paracetamol overdoses and role of prostaglandin E1 intravenously; penicillin and silymarin infusion for amanita (mush-room) poisoning, appear to be effective. Flumazenil—a benzodiazepine antagonist may have a role in hepatic encephalopathy precipitated by use of benzodiazepine (diazepam, lorazepam). Nucleoside analogs are recommended for patients with hepatitis B encephalopathy. *Plasmapheresis* combined with D-penicillamine has been used in fulminant Wilson's disease.

Complications of Acute Hepatic Failure

- Hypoglycaemia, hypokalemia, hypocal-caemia, hypomagnesaemia, metabolic acidosis.
- Cerebral oedema.
- Hypothermia.
- Hypotension.
- Respiratory failure.
- Pancreatitis.
- Progressive azotemia (renal failure).
- Bleeding tendencies.
- Sepsis.

ACUTE ON CHRONIC HEPATIC ENCEPHALOPATHY (ACUTE LIVER FAILURE)

Definition

This is a syndrome of mental and neurological features that occur acutely in patients with long-standing cirrhosis with or without portal hypertension. It results from failure of the liver to detoxity noxious agents of gut origin because of hepatocellular dysfunction and portosys-temic shunting. It is intermittent and reversible in nature if treated early and properly. Rarely irreversible CNS changes occur producing paraplegia, Parkinsonism and epileptic fits.

Precipitating and Pathogenic Factors

Chronic hepatic disease, i.e. cirrhosis due to any cause is the underlying cause of chronic hepatic encephalopathy which is precipitated acutely by certain precipitating factors, i.e.

1. High protein diet.

2. Infections (hepatic and systemic).

3. Trauma.

4. Surgery (portosystemic shunts).

5. GI bleed.

6. Hypokalaemia induced by diuretics

7. Constipation.

8. Rapid removal of ascitic fluid.

9. Uraemia (spontaneous or diuretic-induced).

10. Drugs, e.g. sedative, hypnotics, antidepressants.

Gut derived neurotoxins that are not removed by the liver because of portosystemic shunting and decreased hepatic mass, get into the brain and cause hepatic encephalopathy.

Ammonia is an identifiable and measurable toxin in hepatic encephalopathy. Cerebral oedema, reduced cerebral oxygen consumption, increased levels of oxygen reactive species, nitrous oxide and high levels of mercaptans and false neurotransmitters are other contributory factors.

Clinical Features

The clinical features of acute on chronic or chronic hepatic in cephalopathy are more or less same except the patients of chronic hepatic encephalopathy have stigmata of chronic liver disease, i.e. hepatitis or cirrhosis.

1. **Feature of encephalopathy,** e.g. day-night sleep reversal, drowsiness, confusion, asterixis, constructional apraxia dysarthria, tremors, delirium and coma.

2. **Stigmata of cirrhosis of liver and liver cell failure:** These include:
   - *Mild to moderate jaundice* due to hepatic decompensation.
   - *Ascites, pitting oedema pleural effusion:* They are due to combined effect of portal hypertension and liver cell failure.
   - *Skin changes,* e.g. palmar erythema, spider angiomata, cyanosis (AV shunting in the lungs). Pigmentation and Dupuytren's contractures, clubbing of fingers, white nails, etc.

- *Endocrinal changes,* e.g. loss of axillary and pubic hair, loss of libido.
  - *Men:* Gynaecomastia, impotence, testicular atrophy.
  - *Women:* Menstrual irregularity, ammenorrhoea, breast atrophy.
- *Haematological,* e.g. anaemia, pancytopenia (hypersplenism), bruises, purpura, menorrhagia (coagulopathy due to Vitamin K deficient factors). Glossitis and cheilosis occur due to vitamin deficiency.
- *Symptoms and sign of portal hypertension* e.g. caput medusae (collaterals around the umbilicus), variceal bleed (haemetemesis), rectal varices, fetor hepaticus and splenomegaly.
- *Alcoholic stigmatas:* Loss of axillary and pubic hair, gynaecomastia, red nasal tip and ear lobule, parotid enlargement, muscle weakness and wasting may be present in alcoholic cirrhosis. These are called alcoholic stigmatas.
- *Pyrexia:* Fever may be a presenting feature in up to 35% of patients and suggest alcoholic hepatitis, spontaneous bacterial peritonitis or intercurrent infection as the cause.
- *Bone changes* i.e. osteoporosis or osteopenia may be present due to chronic liver disease.

Differences between clinical features of acute versus chronic hepatic encephalopathies are given in Table 18.1.

Diagnosis

It is based on the clinical features (liver disease with mental features asterixis and investigations).

Investigations

They have been discussed in acute hepatic encephalopathy. In addition, the following investigations may be done:

Blood examination: Anaemia mostly macrocytic is due to bleeding, folate deficiency and

Table 18.1 Difference between clinical features of Acute versus chronic hepatic encephalopathy

Acute hepatic encephalopathy	Chronic hepatic encephalopathy
• Acute onset	• Slow chronic onset
• Acute fulminant hepatitis is the common cause	• Chronic hepatitis or cirrhosis is the commonest cause.
• No precipitating factors	• It is precipitated by certain factors
• Ascites and portal hypertension absent	• Ascites and portal hypertension present
• Liver span is reduced	• Liver span is normal or increased
• Prognosis is bad	• Prognosis is better

haemolysis. Pancytopenia indicates hypersplenism.

Prolongation of PT and PTTK may be due to reduced levels of clotting factors.

Raised liver enzymes, bilirubin and low serum albumin indicate decompensated cirrhosis.

1. **Ascitic fluid examination for biochemistry and cytology:** The fluid is transudate in cirrhosis of the liver with encephalopathy. An ascitic fluid with total leucocyte count >500 cells/mm^3 or >250 polymorphonuclear leucocytes suggests spontaneous bacterial peritonitis which is treated with antibiotics (amoxycillin and gentamicin or cefotaxime).

2. **USG of liver** will show evidence of chronic liver disease (disturbed shape, size and echotexture), presence of ascites, splenomegaly, increased portal vein diameter (>14 mm).

3. The role of neuroimaging studies (e.g. cerebral PET, magnetic resonance spectroscopy) in the diagnosis of hepatic encephalopathy is evolving.

Treatment

It is same as discussed under the heading of acute hepatic encephalopathy. In addition to it, the management include:

1. **Treatment of ascites** by salt and dietary proteins restriction and diuretics (potassium sparing or a combination of loop diuretic with potassium sparing). Hypokalemia must be avoided. Ascites should not be tapped routinely except for diagnostic purpose. If ascites is tense and causing respiratory embarrassment, then it should be tapped keeping in mind that sudden withdrawal of large amount of fluid can precipitate coma. Ascitic fluid can be shunted by a *Leveen shunt* to the central veins in patients, who fail to respond to medical treatment.

2. **Sterilisation the gut** (read acute hepatic encephalopathy. It is done by lactulose (oral or enema) and use of oral rifaximin 550 mg twice daily.

3. **Gastrointestinal bleeding** should be controlled and blood purged from the GI tract by oral magnesium citrate or lactulose every 3–4 hourly orally or by nasogastric tube until stool is free of blood.

    Fresh blood packed RBCs infusion, frozen plasma and vitamin K may be employed to control bleeding. I.V. proton pump inhibitors are useful.

4. **Cerebral edema:** It is reduced by I.V. mannitol (100 ml to be given every 4 to 6 hourly.

5. **Sedation:** For agitation, oxazepam 10–30 mg is given by mouth or through Ryle's tube.

6. **Zinc deficiency** if present may be corrected by oral zinc sulphate 600 mg/day in divided doses.

7. **Role of L-ornithine and L-cartitine (LOLA):** Sodium benzoate 5 g twice daily, ornithine aspartate 9 g orally thrice a day and L-acyl carnitine 4 g orally daily may lower blood ammonia levels but there is limited experience with these drugs.

8. **Flumazenil:** It is a benzodiazepine antagonist, is effective in severe hepatic encephalopathy.

9. Role of prebiotic and probiotic is under investigation.

10. Treatment of complication

- *Hepatorenal syndrome (type 1 and 2):* It is rare in acute hepatic encephalopathy. It occurs in chronic or acute on chronic hepatic encephalopathy. Type 1 hepatorenal syndrome (HRS) is characterized by progressive impairment of renal function and associated with poor outcome; type 2 HRS is characterized by stable renal function with slow reduction is GFR, hence, carries slight better prognosis. Treatment is midodrine, an α-agonist alongwith octreotide and I.V. albumin. The best therapy for HRS is liver transplantation.

- Fulminant septicaemia.
- *Spontaneous bacterial peritonitis (SBP):* In patients with variceal bleed, the frequency of SBP is significantly increased. It is treated with appropriate antibiotic cefotaxime 2 g 12 hourly. Alternatively ceftriaxone and amoxicillin clavulanic acid are used. Furthermore, in patients who have had an episode(s) of SBP and recovered once weekly administration of an antibiotic is recommended. Albumin infusion may be given to raise serum albumin.

Biliary Colic

Definition

It is an acute intermittent abdominal colic resulting from an obstruction in the biliary tract leading to increased intraluminal pressure and acute distension of biliary system (Fig. 19.1) followed by intermittent repeated biliary contractions to overcome this obstruction. Intermittent biliary contractions are responsible for pain. Infection usually supervenes producing acute cholangitis and/or acute cholecystitis and then the two conditions, i.e. obstruction and infection co-exist.

Pathogenesis

Two important factors in pathogenesis of acute biliary colic are obstruction with superadded or concomitant infection. Obstruction leads to dilatation of the biliary system proximal to obstruction resulting in rise in intraluminal pressure followed by or concomitant infection of the stagnant bile (Fig. 19.2). Infection or acute cholangitis causing acute biliary colic can occur in the absence of obstruction. Portal vein is the most significant pathway of bacterial colonisation of biliary system. Another route is invasion of biliary system directly from the gut through the sphincter of oddi or through the biliary enteric communications.

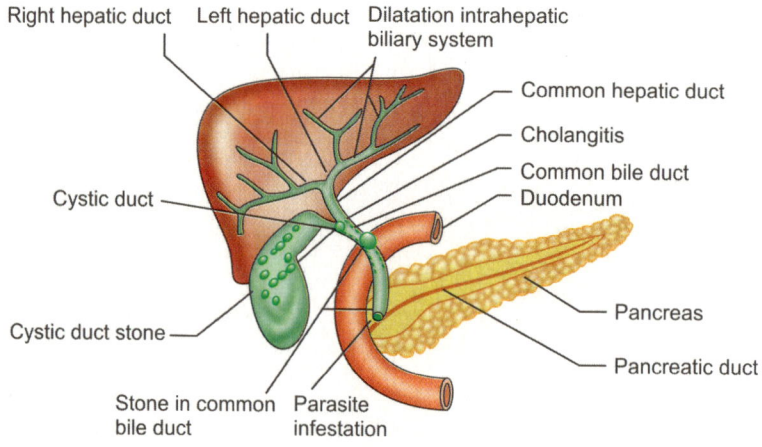

Fig. 19.1: Functional anatomy of biliary tract and aetiology of biliary colic

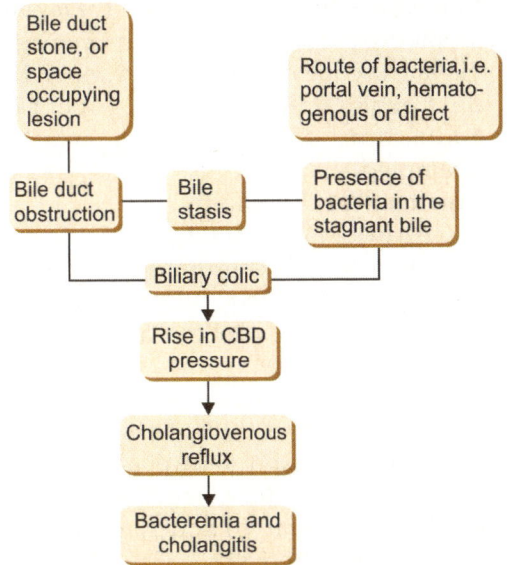

Fig. 19.2: Pathogenesis of billary colic and cholangitis

The fever and chills accompanying acute biliary colic indicate acute cholangitis due to bacteremia. As a result of obstruction, there may be regurgitation of bacteria from the bile into hepatic venous system and is directly proportional to biliary pressure.

Causes of Biliary Colic

1. Choledocholithiasis (70–75%).
2. Biliary stricture.
3. Malignant obstruction of biliary tract.
4. Parasitic infection (ascariasis, clonorchis sinensis).
5. Ductal compression by lymphadenopathy.
6. Primary sclerosing cholangitis.
7. Congenital anomalies of bile ducts such as choledochal cyst.
8. Chronic pancreatitis.

Clinical Features

1. **Acute abdominal pain,** colicky in nature, intermittent or continuous, is felt in the epigastrium or right upper quadrant of abdomen. It may radiate to interscapular region, right scapula or shoulder. There is no guarding or rigidity of abdomen.

Hepatomegaly and tenderness in right hypochondrium may be present in the calculous biliary obstruction.

2. **Pyrexia and chills:** Moderate pyrexia is not uncommon. The Charcot's triad (fever with chills and rigors, jaundice and right upper quadrantic pain) indicates obstructive cholangitis, is found in 70% of cases. The addition of altered mental status and hypotension (*Reynold's pentad*) indicates acute suppurative cholangitis.

3. **Jaundice:** There may be intermittent jaundice, i.e. during an attack of pain, slight jaundice may appear and when present, is helpful in diagnosis of biliary obstruction. In some cases, frank jaundice (obstructive) develops.

4. **Vomiting** *nearly always accompany pain, at times, may be severe.*

Diagnosis and Investigations

The diagnosis of acute cholangitis (Tokyo guidelines 2006) is established by (i) the Charcot triad, (ii) two elements of Charcot plus laboratory evidence of inflammation, i.e. leucocytosis, elevated CRP, raised liver enzyme and imaging evidence of biliary system dilatation.

- **Plain X-ray abdomen** will demonstrate stones in less than 20% of cases.
- **USG** is the method of choice to diagnose gallstones, cystic duct stone and stone in the common bile duct.
- **Endoscopic USG and helical CT** confirms the bile duct stones.
- **MRI cholangiography** is becoming increasingly available which can demonstrate gall-stones, bile duct stones and their complications such as cholangitis.
- **ERCP** (endoscopic retrograde cholangiopancreatography) can be used to diagnose obstruction and its cause, and to remove bile duct stones and to place stent. If ERCP fails, percutaneous transhepatic cholangiography may be undertaken to determine the accurate cause, location and extent of obstruction.
- **Routine investigation** such as *total leucocyte count (TLC)* and *differential leucocyte count*

(DLC) may reveal leucocytosis with neutrophilia if there is an evidence of infection, i.e. cholecystitis, cholangitis, etc. *Serum bilirubin* may be raised slightly with *raised alkaline phosphatase and transaminases* (>1000 U/L). Not uncommonly serum amylase levels are high due to secondary pancreatitis. *Hypoprothrombinemia* may result due to prolonged cholestasis and responds to parenteral vitamin K. *Blood culture* is usually sterile, but if there is an evidence of infection, it may yield the causative organism.

Treatment

1. **Relief of pain:** Several analgesics can be used to control pain but pethidine I.M. or pentazocine I.M. are commonly employed. Morphine is best avoided as it increases intrabiliary pressure.

2. **Treatment of bile duct stones:** Urgent ERCP with sphincterotomy and stone extraction is generally indicated for bile duct stones complicated by acute cholangitis and it is followed by laparoscopic cholecystectomy within 72 hours. Before ERCP, liver function tests, i.e. enzymes and PTI must be done and PT should be restored to normal by parenteral vitamin K. An alternative approach is laparoscopic cholecystectomy and bile duct exploration.

Choledocholithiasis discovered at laparoscopic cholecystectomy may be managed via laproscope or, if necessary, open bile duct exploration or by post-operative endoscopic sphincterotomy may be attempted.

3. **Treatment of cholangitis**
   - Ciprofloxacin 500 mg I.V. every 12 hourly plus metronidazole 500 mg every 6–8 hourly is most effective regimen. The ciprofloxacin penetrates well into the bile.
   - Alternative regimens include I.V. ampicillin and sulbactam 3 g every 6 hourly; cefoxitin 1–2 g every 6 hourly.

or

Ampicillin 2 g every 6 hourly plus gentamicin 80 mg every 8 hourly.

For severe or hospital acquired acute cholangitis: The antibiotic regimen includes I.V. piperacillin and tazobactum (3.375 g every 6 hourly), ticarcillin and clavulanate 3.1 g every 6 hourly or ceftriaxone and metronidazole combination.

Meropenam is used in high risk patients with antibiotic-resistant pathogens.

If medical therapy fails, decompression by a biliary stent or nasobiliary catheter can be done. After decompression, antibiotics are continued for another 3 days.

Emergency Related to Infections

- Septic Shock
- Dengue Fever
- Typhoid Fever and its Complications
- Rabies
- Tetanus
- Myonecrosis (Gas Gangrene) and Toxic Shock Syndrome
- Cholera
- Bacterial Food Poisoning
- Acute Dysentery (Amoebic *vs* Shigellosis)
- Cerebral Malaria
- Pyrexia of Unknown Origin (PUO)

Septic Shock

SEPTIC SHOCK (Fig. 20.1)

Definitions Used in Relation to Septic Patients

1. **Sepsis or systemic inflammatory response syndrome (SIRS):** In a patient with proven or suspected microbial infection, the presence of two of the following 4 symptoms and signs constitutes sepsis or SIRS.
   - Oral temperature of >38°C or <36°C.
   - Respiratory rate >24/min or $PaCO_2 < 32$ mmHg.

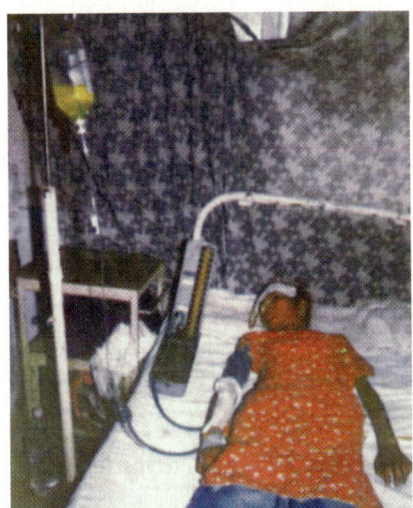

Fig. 20.1: A patient of gram-negative septic shock being treated in a hospital

- Heart rate >90/min
- Leucocyte count >12,000/μl or <4000/μl or >10% band forms.

2. **Septicaemia:** Systemic illness produced as a result of spread of microbial infection or entry of their toxins into the bloodstream.

3. **Bacteraemia:** Presence of viable bacteria in the blood as evidenced by positive blood culture.

4. **Hypotension:** Systolic blood pressure <90 mmHg or 40 mm fall of systolic BP from the baseline in a patient without any other reason for hypotension.

5. **Septic shock:** It is defined as sepsis with hypotension (SBP < 90 mmHg or fall of SBP by >40 mm below the patient's normal BP) for at least one hour despite adequate fluid replacement, blood lactate level more than 2 mmol/L and need for vasopressors to maintain SBP >90 mmHg.

6. **Refractory shock:** Shock is said to be refractory if it lasts for >1 hour and does not respond to fluid or pressor agents.

7. **Severe sepsis (sepsis syndrome):** It is defined as shock with one or more signs of organ dysfunction, i.e.
   i. SBP ≤ 90 mmHg or mean arterial BP ≤ 70 mmHg
   ii. Urine output < 0.5 ml/kg/hr for 1 hour despite fluid replacement

iii. $PaO_2/FiO_2 \leq 250$
iv. Platelet count < 80,000/μl or 50% fall in the count from highest value recorded over past 3 days,
v. Metabolic acidosis (pH < 7.30 and base deficit > 5.0 mEq/L).
vi. PCWP ≥12 mmHg or CVP < 8 mmHg after adequate fluid resuscitation.

8. **Multiple-organ dysfunction syndrome (MODS):** It is defined as dysfunction or failure of more than two organs/systems requiring intervention to maintain homeostasis.

Causes

Septic shock can result from gram-positive and gram-negative organisms and due to fungal sepsis. The most common cause is gram-negative sepsis (Fig. 20.1), and common organisms involved are *E. coli, Salmonella, Klebsiella, Pseudomonas* and *Enterobacter*. The gram-positive organisms involved are *Staphylococcus* and *Meningococcus* (Fig. 20.2) and fungus involved is *Candida* species. The portal of entry is via blood, GI tract, genitourinary tract, respiratory tract and the skin. The causes involved increased incidence of severe infection are given in Box 1.

The conditions that predispose to sepsis are given in Table 20.1.

Box 1	Sites of infection causing septic shock
Common	*Less common*
• Intravenous lines (particularly central)	• Heart valves (prostheses)
• Respiratory tract (nosocomial infection)	• Meninges (pyogenic meningitis)
• Abdomen (intra-abdominal organ infection, e.g. abscess, necrotic gut, pancreatitis, cholecystitis, etc.).	• Joints and bones (septic arthritis, osteomyelitis)
	• Nasal sinuses, ears, retropharyngeal space infection
• Urinary tract (e.g. infection)	• Genitourinary tract (e.g postpartum)
	• Gastrointestinal tract (e.g. infection)

Table 20.1 Predisposing conditions/factors to sepsis or septic shock

1. **Immunocompromised state**, e.g. diabetes mellitus, AIDS, cytotoxic and steroids use.
2. *Malignancies*, e.g. leukaemia, lymphoma
3. Cirrhosis of the liver (portosystemic infection)
4. Extensive burns
5. Neutropenia
6. Implants, prostheses, intravenous drug abuse
7. Antibiotic abuse
8. Invasive procedures
9. Malnutrition
10. Rupture of hollow viscus

The patient may be admitted with infection from home *(community acquired)* or develop it after hospitalisation *(nosocomial)*. The risk factors for hospital-acquired infections are:

1. Mechanical ventilation
2. Trauma
3. Catheters (intravenous or urinary) or tubes (nasogastric)
4. Prolonged hospital stay
5. Stress ulcer on prophylaxis with H_2-antagonists

Diagnosis and Clinical Features

The diagnosis of septic shock rests on clinical evidence of an infection in the setting of persistent hypotension, organ hypofunction, lactic acidosis, oliguria and altered mental status despite resuscitation. The septic response

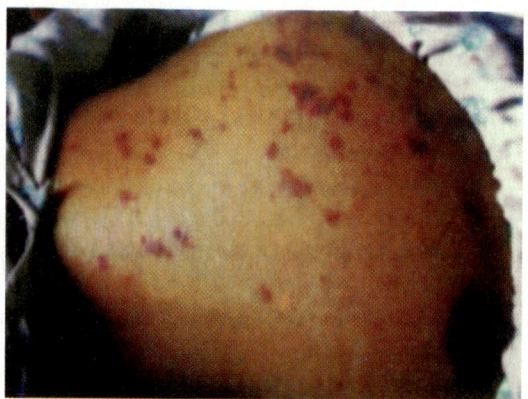

Fig. 20.2: Meningococcaemia with septic shock in an adult. Note the palpable purpuric rash over the abdomen and limbs (not shown)

can be quite variable especially in patients at extremes of age, those on immunosuppressive therapy (e.g. steroids, cytotoxic drugs), in patients with indwelling catheters or with co existing illness such as diabetes, malnutrition, cancer or transplantation. The clinical features are given in Table 20.2.

Majority of patients either present in stage I (warm shock) or stage II (cold stage). Both the stages can reverse with treatment. The patient may not recover with treatment, may develop third stage of multiple-organ dysfunction syndrome involving the lungs, heart, kidneys, brain, liver, etc.

Investigations

Investigations are given in Box 2. Repeated blood culture must be done from different sites to confirm the diagnosis. At least two blood samples should be obtained from two different venepuncture sites, in case of catheter one sample to be taken from tip of the catheter. DNA in peripheral blood or tissue samples by PCR may give definite diagnosis of microbes. Buffy coat smear of PBF is useful to detect meningococcemia.

Box 2 Investigations for a patient with septic shock
• Leucocytosis or leuco-penia, neutrophilia with toxic granules • Rise in serum bilirubin and hepatic enzymes • Metabolic acidosis (lactic acidosis) • Arterial blood gas analysis reveals hypoxia	• Thrombocytopenia • Features suggestive of DIC (prolonged thrombin time, low fibrinogen level, presence of D-dimers) • Proteinuria • Chest X-ray may show, underlying pneumonia, diffuse infiltrates of ARDS, volume overload • ECG may show tachycardia, non-specific ECG changes • USG and CT scan of chest/abdomen to exclude pelvic or other soft tissue pus collection.

Table 20.2 Pathophysiology and clinical features of septic shock

Pathophysiology	Symptoms and signs
Stage I (warm shock)	
• There is vasodilatation, opening of arteriove-nous shunts and increase in cardiac output	• The skin is flushed and warm with perspiration (diaphoresis) • Impaired consciousness, irritability and mental confusion • Tachypnoea and tachycardia • Blood pressure is normal or may be decreased • Urine output is normal or slightly decreased
Stage II (cold shock)	
• This is stage of vasoconstriction and leakage of circulating volume into interstitial spaces with decrease in cardiac output	• Cold, clammy skin and cold extremities • Severe hypotension BP < 80 mmHg • Weak, thready pulses tachycardia, tachypnoea and oliguria • Restlessness, listlessness, confusion, disorientation, stupor, coma • Arrhythmias
Stage III (multi-organ failure)	
• There is poor tissue perfusion, microthemobi in leaking capillaries, disseminated intravascular coagulation, metabolic acidosis, circulatory collapse, respiratory and renal failure	• Cold extremities • Weak, thready pulse with severe hypotension, arrhythmias • Oliguria or anuria • Shallow respiration (acidotic breathing), worsening hypox-aemia, tachypnoea, etc. • Disorientation, stupor and coma • Bleeding tendencies

Management

Aims

1. To find out the underlying cause and to treat it properly.
2. To treat local and/or systemic infection.
3. To sustain life by basic life support with an assessment of airway, breathing and circulation and haemodynamic and ventilatory support.
4. Symptomatic treatment of pain, fever, etc.
5. Other measures.

I. General considerations

- Initial assessment by pulse, fever, BP for severity of shock.
- Procure I.V. line and collect blood samples for blood count, sugar, electrolytes, ABG analysis, coagulation profile, lactate levels, typing and cross-matching and cultures.
- Foley's catheter may be put to measure use urine output.
- ECG may be done for arrhythmias.
- Haemodynamic monitoring, e.g. CVP.

II. Specific therapy

1. *To remove the source of infection wherever possible:* It includes *surgical drainage of abscesses, debridement of necrotic tissue,* to relieve obstruction of hollow viscus or to exclude pelvic or soft tissue pus collection by CT scan.
2. *Antimicrobial therapy:* The indwelling I.V. catheter should be removed; culture should be taken from the tip and a new catheter should be inserted at a different site. The best way to treat septic shock is to initiate empiricial antibiotic therapy as soon as possible.

   Samples of blood and from other relevant sites should be taken for culture. The choice of initial therapy is based on the knowledge of the likely organisms at specific sites of local infections and predisposing factors operating in the patient and the location (community or a hospital). Pending culture reports, it is reasonable to start an antibiotic which is effective against both *gram-positive* and *gram-negative* organisms such as a combination of third generation cephalosporin (cefotaxime 2 g I.V. 6 hourly or ceftriaxone 2 g I.V. 12 hourly) and a aminoglycoside (amikacin 1 g bid); if anaerobes are being suspected then add penicillin, metronidazole or clindamycin. If methicillin resistant *S. aureus* (MRSA) is suspected, then add vancomycin. For respiratory infections, a macrolide is added. Similarly a quinoline (ciprofloxacin) may be added for urogenital sepsis. Empirical antifungal therapy should be considered if the septic patient.

   When culture results become available, then antibiotic regimen be simplified using specific antibiotic effective against specific organism. Most patients require antibiotic therapy for 1 week, but can be extended depending on the underlying cause/disease. Antibiotic therapy is to be given intravenously in shocked patients.

III. Supportive therapy

A. *Resuscitation of shock (hemodynamic support)*

   i. *Fluids therapy:* Patients of septic shock are dehydrated due to capillary leak, hence, need a large amount of volume replacement by fluids. Both crystalloids and colloids can be administered. Initially 1–2 L of saline is infused over a period of 1–2 hours, followed by infusion of fluids to maintain systolic BP >90 mm and cardiac index >4 L/min/m². Caution must be exercised with large volume resuscitation with unwarmed fluids because this can induce hypothermia and hypothermia-induced coagulopathy, warming of fluids before administration can avoid this complication. If these guidelines are not met by fluid replacement, then vasoactive agents are indicated.

ii. *Corticosteroids:* Adrenal insufficiency, glucocorticoid receptor resistance should be considered if severe refractory hypotension is present in patients with sepsis. Recent trials have recommended low dose supplemental hydrocortisone 50 mg I.V. after every 6 hours.

iii. *Vasopressor agents:* Patients with low mean arterial pressure, low cardiac output and low or normal pulmonary capillary wedge pressure need inotropic support with dopamine (2–$10\,\mu g/kg/min$).

• *Vasopressin (antidiuretic hormone-ADH):* Infusion of low dose vasopressin (0.01–0.04 units/min) adjunct to catecholamine may be safe and effective in refractory septic shock.

> *Fluid therapy is to be monitored by CVP (to be kept at 8–12 cm H_2O) and PCWP (to be kept 12 to 16 mmHg) and urine output (to be kept above 30 ml/hr).*

B. **Respiratory support (ventilatory support)**
Oxygenation: Ventilatory support is needed in about 85% of patients with progressive hypoxaemia, hypercapnia, neurological deterioration and respiratory muscle failure. Intubation is often undertaken for adequate oxygenation. If respiratory drive and muscle power is adequate, then adequate tidal volumes (4–$6\,ml/kg$) can be delivered by pressure support; and PEEP is only indicated in few patients. Arterial O_2 saturation of 90% is adequate. Blood transfusion is indicated to improve oxygenation if haemoglobin level is $<7\,g/dl$.

C. *Metabolic support*
i. *Correction of metabolic (lactic) acidosis:* Mild acidosis does not require therapy. Severe acidosis is corrected by bicarbonate administration if arterial pH is <7.2. Electrolytes need constant monitoring and appropriate management.

ii. *Coagulopathy or DIC:* For severe DIC with major bleeding, transfusion of fresh frozen plasma and platelets is indicated.

iii. *Nutritional supplementation* is needed to reduce the hypercatabolism. Nutrition is provided by enteral feeding or parenteral feeding.

iv. *Renal failure:* Acute renal failure due to sepsis require treatment with antibiotics, vasoactive substances and fluid therapy. Most of the patients improve and only a few of them may need dialytic support.

D. **Other measures:** To reduce the mortality due to septic shock, two types of drugs, i.e. anti-endotoxin agents (monoclonal antibodies to endotoxin, human neutrophil protein, a polymyxin B-dextran conjugate, etc.) and antimediators agents (anticytokines drugs, PAF antagonists, bradykinin antagonists and ibuprofen) are being investigated but still not been found successful.

Recently recombinant activated protein C (aPC)—an anticoagulant agent has been cleaved by US food and Drug Administration (PDA) to be used specifically in patients with septic shock who are >18 years of age and who meet the APACHE II score ≥ 25 and have a low risk of haemorrhage related side effects. Dose of continuous infusion is $24\,\mu g/kg/hr$ for 96 hours, clotting parameters should be monitored as haemorrhage is serious complication of this therapy.

E. **General measures** include good nursing care, prevention of nosocomial infection, *good enteral nutrition*, prevention of stress ulcer and GI bleed by *H$_2$-blockers* (I.V. ranitidine), care of skin and prevention of *deep vein thrombosis by heparin* in patients who do not have active bleeding or coagulopathy. They contribute significantly to reduce the mortality. Intensive glucose monitoring and control (blood sugar to be kept around 150 mg/dl) during first 3 days of sepsis is essential, if need be, insulin may be given and blood sugar monitored.

Complications

1. *ARDS or shock lung:* ARDS develops in 20 to 25% cases of septic shock.

2. *Renal failure:* Oliguric and nonoliguric renal failure can develop.

3. *Coagulopathy or DIC.*

4. *Nutritional deficiencies.*

The treatment of these complications has already been discussed in the management.

Dengue Fever

DENGUE FEVER AND RELATED EMERGENCIES

Dengue Fever

It is a mosquito-borne virus infection character-ized by febrile illness (*classic dengue*), bleeding manifestations (*dengue haemorrhagic fever*) and shock (*dengue shock syndrome*).

The disease is transmitted from human to human by bite of a female mosquito *(Aedes aegypti)* and is caused by one of the distinct 4 types of *flavi viruses (dengue virus 1 to 4)*. The disease occurs in endemic and epidemic forms. In India, many outbreaks have been reported, but recent one occurred in the capital (Delhi) in 1996.

The incubation period is 3 to 7 days. The viraemia begins 24 hours before the fever and subsides with the end of fever. The virus disse-minates to the regional lymph nodes, then through the lymphatics throughout the body (Fig. 21.1).

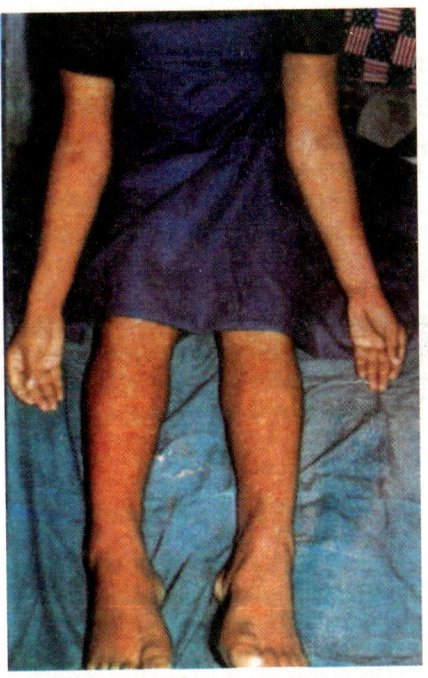

Fig. 21.1: Rash of classic dengue fever

Clinical Characteristics

Three distinct entities of dengue fever have been described depending on the severity of infection and whether infection is primary or secondary.
 1. *Classical dengue fever.* The clinical features of classical dengue are given in Box 1.

 2. *Dengue haemorrhagic fever* (DHF).
 3. *Dengue shock syndrome* (DSS).
 The secondary infection may be more severe due to circulating antibodies. Sequential infection by any 2 out of 4 sero types of dengue virus may lead to severe dengue leading DHF and DSS in *hyperendemic* areas. Chronic infection by this virus is unknown. The features of classical dengue are described in Box 1.

Box 1　Clinical features of classical dengue

Symptoms	Signs
• After incubation period of 4–7 days there is sudden onset of fever, headache, retro-orbital pain, back pain with severe myalgia for which a common term 'break-bone fever' is used. In children, there is associated cough, sore throat, nausea, vomiting and abdominal pain. • Macular erythematous rash (Fig. 21.1) which blanches on pressure may be seen on trunk within 24 hours of fever. There may be flushed facies with scleral injection (redness of eyes). At the time of defervescence on days 3–5—this maculopapular (see Fig. 21.1) rash beginning on the trunk and spreading to the extremities and the face. This fades over next few days. The illness lasts for a week. • Epistaxis, petechiae and purpura are often noted in uncomplicated dengue.	• Pharyngeal congestion • Scleral congestion/injection • Suffused facies • Abdominal tenderness • Lymphadenopathy • A positive tourniquet test for capillary fragility • >10 petechiae over 2.5 cm² area • Cutaneous hyperaesthesia.

Treatment

The treatment of classic dengue fever is entirely symptomatic with analgesics for relief of pain and fever. Patient is advised rest during the stage of fever. Transfusion of blood or blood products is indicated in case of severe bleeding. The disease is self-limiting.

SEVERE DENGUE: DENGUE HAEMOR-RHAGIC FEVER (DHF) AND DENGUE SHOCK SYNDROME (DSS)

Dengue haemorrhagic fever is characterized by all manifestations of classical dengue fever, thrombocytopenia, vascular instability and increased permeability resulting in leakage of intravascular fluid to interstitial space (haemoconcentration) and local haemorrhage (*positive tourniquet test*, spontaneous petechiae and/or purpura) or frank haemorrhage (epistaxis, gum bleeding, bleeding into GI tract, i.e. malena and menometrorrhagia) have been described. The haemorrhage is inconstant and is thought to be a combined effect of vascular damage and thrombocytopenia.

As the plasma leakage increases, patient may become restless, irritable and develops hypotension and shock (cold extremities) called *dengue shock syndrome (DSS).* In severe cases, frank shock is present with low pulse pressure (<20 mmHg), cyanosis, hepato-megaly, pleural effusion and ascites. In some cases, severe ecchymosis and GI bleeding may be seen.

Diagnosis

The diagnosis is purely clinical and the full blown picture of dengue haemorrhagic fever is easy to recognise. The grading of DHF (WHO) is given in Box 2. The **laboratory findings** that support the diagnosis include *leucopenia, thrombocytopenia* and *raised serum aminotrans-ferases*. The *diagnosis* is helped by *antibody detection* (IgM, IgG ELISA) or paired serology during recovery or by antigen or the specific viral protein NS1 detection (ELISA or RT-PCR) during acute phase. Virus can also be isolated from the blood by virus culture.

Management

Early recognition is necessary because of the need for virus-specific therapy and supportive measures. The treatment include:

1. **Judicious fluid therapy:** All patients do not require admission. Patients with mild circulatory collapse or hypoten-sion require fluid replacement by mouth and close monitoring of the vital signs. Patients presenting with circulatory collapse (*hypovolaemia, cold extremities, pallor, oliguria*) and *falling platelet count* require hospitalisation for fluid replace-ment. Intravenous fluids (5% dextrose in

Box 2	WHO classification of dengue and its related syndrome			
Grade	*Platelet nadir (per ml)*	*Plasma leakage*	*Circulatory collapse*	*Others*
Classical dengue	Variable	Absent	Absent	• Tourniquet test variable
Dengue haemorrhage fever				
Grade I	< lac	Present	Absent	• Tourniquet test positive
Grade II	< lac	Present		• Tourniquet test positive and frank haemorrhage
Dengue shock syndrome	<1 lac	Present	Pulse pressure <20 mmHg	• Tourniquet test positive
Grade III				• Haemorrhage may be present
Grade IV	<lac	Present	Blood pressure unrecordable	• Tourniquet test variable
				• Haemorrhage may be present

half normal saline or Ringer's lactate) are given in the beginning. If no improvement occurs, or in severe cases, a plasma expander may be given as rapidly as possible to produce volume expansion. Fluids are to be continued till patient comes out of shock and vital parameters improve.

2. **Pressor agents:** Pressor agents along with fluid therapy may be used to resuscitate shock in severe cases. Blood pressure is to be maintained above 90 mmHg.

3. **Oxygen therapy** should be used to improve oxygenation.

4. **Blood transfusion** is given in the presence of massive bleeding with falling haematocrit.

5. **Coagulopathy or thrombocytopenia** may need cryoprecipitate and platelets transfusion. Platelet transfusions may be considered for severe thrombicytopenia (count <10,000/ mcL) or when there is evidence of bleeding. IVIG Anti-Rho globulin have been found effective in thrombocytopenia.

6. **Corticosteroids** are of not much help.

7. **Antiviral therapy** has also not been found useful.

Prevention and Control

• Avoidance and eradication of mosquito vectors.
• During an epidemic, fumigation of insecticide by road vehicles or air crafts in the area affected.
• Removal of breeding sites/containers.
• Avoid the use of stored water and try to use piped water.
• No effective vaccine available. At least two live attenuated vaccines have been evaluated in clinical trials but results are not encouraging. The Dengvaxia made by Sanofi Pasteur is approved for use in Mexico for persons aged 9–45 years.

Differential Diagnosis

Other conditions that produce haemorrhagic fever are:

1. Lassa fever
2. Yellow fever
3. Meningoccocaemia
4. Kyasanur Forest disease
5. Rift Valley fever
6. Rickettsioses
7. Haemorrhagic fever with renal syndrome

Typhoid Fever and its Complications

TYPHOID FEVER AND ITS COMPLICATIONS

Typhoid fever is an acute systemic illness caused by infection due to *S. typhi* and *S. paratyphi*. The disease is acquired by oro-faecal route through faecal contamination of food, water, drinks and other eatables. The reservoir of infection include patients suffering or convalescing from typhoid or chronic carriers of typhoid (food handlers). Health care workers (doctors, paramedical staff, laboratory technician) acquire enteric fever after exposure to infected patients or during processing of clinical specimens and cultures.

Typhoid fever is characterized by fever, malaise, abdominal pain, rash, splenomegaly and leucopenia (Box 1). The untreated patients may develop complications during second and third week due to toxaemia and septicaemia. In some cases, it may be fatal.

Clinical Features

The incubation period is 5–14 days. The onset is usually insidious. The clinical manifestations are variable from mild illness to acute systemic illness which may last for 6–8 weeks

Box 1 Clinical symptoms and signs of typhoid fever
1. During first week (first 5–7 days)
• Remittent fever (38.5–40.5°C), headache, body-ache, malaise, constipation, leucopenia, relative bradycardia.
2. Between first and second week
• Rose spots (pink papules over trunk which fade on pressure), coated tongue splenomegaly, bronchitis, abdominal pain, abdominal distension, epistaxis and diarrhoea. The fever reaches its maximum (*step ladder rise*) and persists. The patient looks ill and more toxic.
3. Beyond second week
• If everything is well and treatment is effective, patient recovers. In severe infection, the patient may develop complications (discussed below). The temperature may remain slightly above normal in the convalescence period.
• Relapse occurs in 5–10% cases after 7–14 days of defervescence. It is milder than the initial attack.

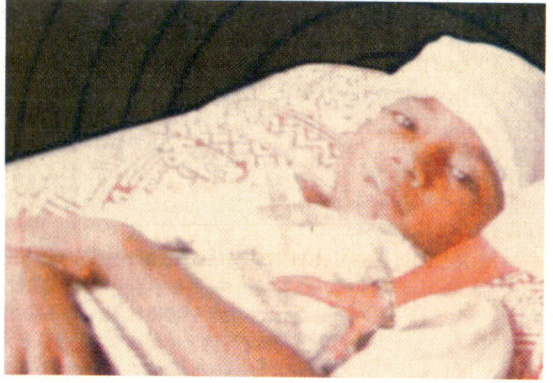

Fig. 22.1: A patient of uncomplicated typhoid fever being treated in the hospital

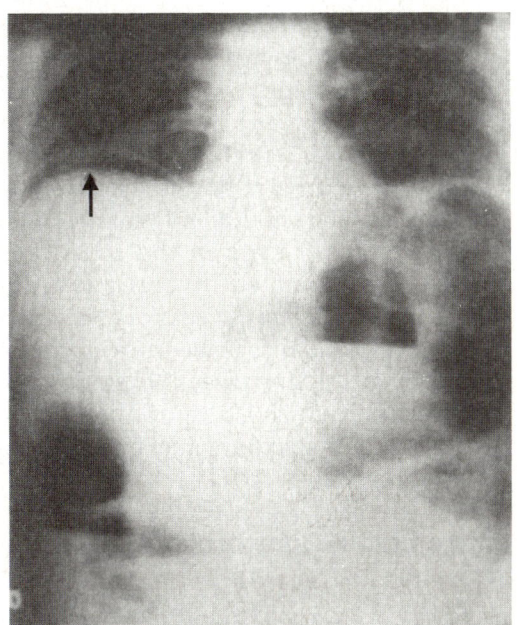

Fig. 22.2: Enteric perforation. Note the air under right dome of diaphragm

if untreated. The symptoms and signs of typhoid fever are summarised in Fig. 22.1 and Box 1.

Complications

1. **Gastrointestinal,** e.g. intestinal perforation (Fig. 22.2), or acute paralytic ileus, intestinal haemorrhage, pancreatitis.
2. **Hepatobiliary,** e.g. hepatitis, necrotising cholecystitis, hepatic abscess.
3. **Cardiovascular** e.g. myocarditis, endocarditis pericarditis.
4. **Hematological,** e.g. aplasia of bone marrow, pancytopenia, DIC, haemolytic anaemia.
5. **Renal,** e.g. nephritis, haemolytic uraemic syndrome, urinary retention.
6. **Respiratory,** e.g. bronchitis, pneumonia.
7. **Bone and joints,** e.g. osteomyelitis.
8. **Neurological,** e.g. enteric encephalopathy, encephalitis, brain abscess, meningitis, peripheral neuropathy, G.B. syndrome, coma vigil (muttering delirium).
9. **Miscellaneous,** e.g. parotitis, splenic abscess.

Diagnosis

The diagnosis is suggested by the clinical features; whereas the definite diagnosis still depends on the isolation of the organism from culture blood or bone marrow, rose spots, stool culture, the overall yield of culture is disappointingly low about 90% in first week, falls to less than 50% in untreated patient during third week. Yield can be approximately 100% when both blood and bone marrow culture are done in patients not receiving antibiotics. Stool culture may be positive in 75% cases during third week, while it is negative during first week. The culture of intestinal (duodenal) secretions aspirated through Ryle's tube gives better results than stool culture.

Serological diagnosis is made by **Widal test** which is less reliable than culture. In the absence of immunisation, a higher titre of agglutinins on Widal test (1:300) is suggestive but not diagnostic. A four-fold rise in antibody titre between paired sera samples is highly suggestive. *Rapid tests (typhi dot test)* to detect antibodies to outer membrane proteins or antigen are available in developing countries (India) but have lower positive predictive value than culture.

DNA probe have been developed for identifying *S. typhi* from culture isolates and from blood. Recently a PCR based test using 2 pairs of oligo nucleotide from a fragment of *S. typhi* flagellum gene (Hl-d) was found to be 93% sensitive and 100% specific on clinical trials, but still is not commercially available. Another test—PCR based on the nucleotides sequencing using Vi antigen (VaB region) has been developed. In addition there may be leucopenia or neutropenia is about 50% cases.

Treatment

With the emergence of chloramphenicol resistant strains, it no longer remains the drug of choice now-a-days. Fluoroquinolones and third generation cephalosporins are antibiotic of choice due to development of multi-drug resistance.

1. For treatment of drug susceptible typhoid fever 4-fluoroquinolones such as ciprofloxacin 500–750 mg bid or levofloxacin 500 mg orally once daily or gatifloxacin 400 mg once a day are sufficient to treat uncomplicated typhoid fever. Parenteral preparations (e.g. ciprofloxacin 200 mg I.V. bid) are used in typhoid with complications.

   When there is decreased susceptibility to ciprofloxacin such as in Asia, high doses of ciprofloxacin for prolonged period (10–14 days) or the third generation cephalosporins such as ceftriaxone and cefoperazone are used in dosage of 1 g twice a day I.V. or 50 mg/kg/day for 7 to 10 days or at least 3 days after defervescence. *Azithromycin* (1 g/day orally for 5 days) is also effective. In pregnancy, the third generation cephalosporin is preferred drug over fluoroquinolone. Alternatively ampicillin 6–12 g/daily for adults or 100 mg/kg for children in divided doses is also useful. If sensitivity to chloramphenicol is present then it is given 2–4 g/day.

   Ceftriaxone, cefofataxime, and oral cefixime are effective for treatment of muti-drug resistant (MDR) typhoid fever. Oral azithromycin (1 g/day) is equally effective for both susceptible and multi-drug resistant typhoid.

2. Antipyretics are used orally or I.V. for fever and pain. Hydrotherapy for high grade fever is indicated (Fig. 22.1).

3. Patient is advised to take oral liquids and semi-solid diet so as to avoid fluid loss/deficit due to fever during defervescence. I.V. fluids are to be given if there is state of dehydration.

4. Relapse and primary attack are similarly treated.

5. **High doses steroids:** In one Indonesian study, it has been reported that high doses of corticosteroids in typhoid fever with CNS manifestations and/or evidence of DIC if given along with antibiotic therapy, reduces the mortality rate.

Dexamethasone 3 mg/kg I.V. as a bolus followed by 1 mg/kg I.V. every 6 hours for 24–48 hours should be considered in such a typhoid state.

6. **Treatment of carriers:** A person is said to be carrier if he/she excretes the organisms in the stool after 1 year following illness. Carrier state in the absence of gallstones is treated by oral ampicillin 100 mg/kg/day for 6 weeks or cotriamoxazole 960 mg/day for 4 weeks or ciprofloxacin 750 mg bid for 4 weeks to sterilise the gallbladder which is responsible for this state. Cholecystectomy may be necessary in some cases.

Management of Complications

Enteric Encephalopathy

It is a toxic complication, occurs commonly during second or third week of typhoid fever, is characterized by fever with an altered state of consciousness ranging from disorientation to coma and has a mortality rate exceeding 40%.

Treatment

It includes:

1. Care of semiconscious or unconscious state.

2. Intravenous fluids to treat dehydration and to maintain proper hydration and blood pressure so as to prevent other complications. Vitals are to be monitored.

3. Intravenous antibiotics specially third generation cephalosporin, e.g. ceftriaxone 2 g I.V. 12 hourly for 2–3 days then 1 g after every 12 hours over few days is highly effective.

4. High dose corticosteroids: High dose corticosteroids has been recommended in this complication. Dose and duration of therapy has already been discussed.

5. If patient recovers, he/she has to be treated with one of the drugs used to treat carrier state. This is given for 4 weeks to sterilise

the gallbladder and to prevent relapse and to eradicate the organisms to prevent carrier state.

Intestinal Haemorrhage

It is characterized by bleeding per rectum in a patient of typhoid during second and third week, followed by development of anaemia. The patient is pale, dehydrated and has toxic look. There is tachypnoea and tachycardia. There may be hypotension or shock depending on the loss of blood.

Management

- Resuscitation of shock by fluids and vasopressor.
- Endoscopy, coeliac axis angiography, radio-isotopic scanning to localise the site of bleeding.
- Supportive therapy by intravenous fluids and antibiotics.
- Blood or blood products transfusion.
- Surgical intestinal resection may be required occasionally.
- Monitoring of vital parameters.

Rabies

RABIES

It is an acute *viral* infection of the brain (Fig. 23.1) caused by RNA virus of rhabdoviridae family and affects all the mammals. It is transmitted by the infected secretions, commonly the saliva containing the virus through the bite of infected animal (Fig. 23.1). In most areas of the world, the dog is the most important vector for rabies virus transmission to humans (Fig. 23.2). However, other animals such as wolf, mongoose, vampire bat and cats may also be important vectors. Several cases of human-to-human transmission of rabies through corneal transplantation have been reported, otherwise human rabies (human bite) is exceedingly rare.

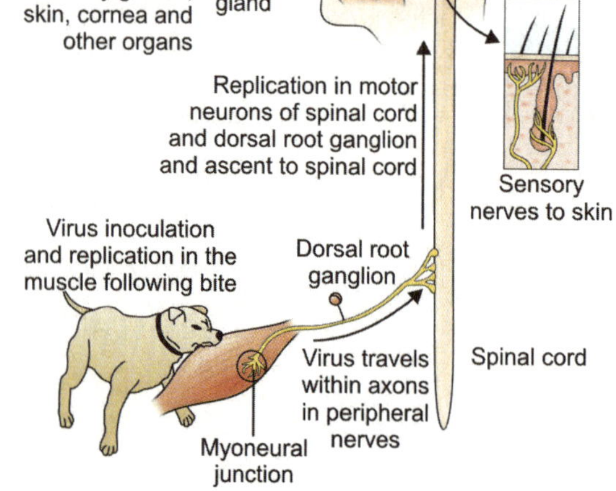

Infection of brain neurons with neuronal dysfunction

Brain

Centrifugal spread along nerves to salivary glands, skin, cornea and other organs

Salivary gland

Replication in motor neurons of spinal cord and dorsal root ganglion and ascent to spinal cord

Sensory nerves to skin

Virus inoculation and replication in the muscle following bite

Dorsal root ganglion

Spinal cord

Virus travels within axons in peripheral nerves

Myoneural junction

Fig. 23.1: Schematic representation of pathogenic pathway following inoculation of rabies virus by an animal bite

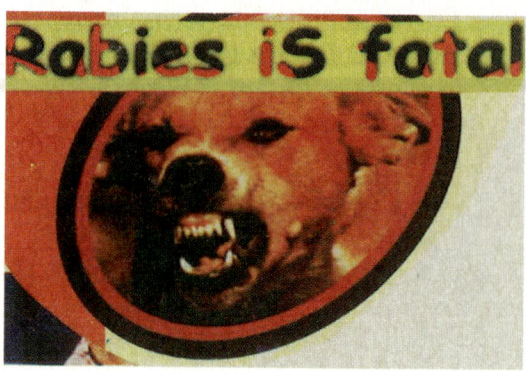

Fig. 23.2: Rabies—a fatal disese is caused commonly by rabid dog bite

Pathogenesis

The incubation period of rabies is between 20–90 days but is extended up to 1 year in rare cases. Following inoculation of virus by dog bite, the virus binds to neuromuscular junction and multiplies in the muscles. Then it spreads centrifugally along the peripheral nerves to the spinal cord and brain. Once the virus enters CNS, it rapidly disseminates to other regions of the CNS along neuroanatomic connections. Neurons are mainly attacked by the virus. After CNS infection becomes established it spreads centrifugally along the sensory and autonomic nerves to salivary glands, eye, skin and other organs (Fig. 23.1).

Clinical Features

These are given in Box 1.

Diagnosis

The diagnosis of rabies is generally made on clinical ground supported by investigations.

1. **Serum neutralising antibodies** to rabies virus are diagnostic in an unimmunised patient. The presence of rabies virus—specific antibodies in CSF suggest rabies encephalitis regardless of immunisation status.

2. **RT-PCR Amplification to detect rabies virus RNA** is highly sensitive and specific. This technique can detect virus in fresh saliva sample, skin, CSF and brain tissue.

3. **Direct fluorescent antibody testing** is highly sensitive and specific. In skin biopsy rabies virus antigen can be detected in cutaneous nerves at the base of hair follicles.

4. **MRI** shows nonenhancing ill defined hyperdense changes in brainstem, hypothalamus and subcortical regions.

5. **Confirmation** is done by classical *Negri bodies* at postmortem examination of brain.

Management

1. **Once the disease is established, therapy is symptomatic:**
   - The patient should be nursed in a quiet, isolated, darkened room with all facilities.

Box 1 Clinical featues of rabies (hydrophobia)		
Prodromal symptoms	*Encephalitic symptoms*	*Brainstem dysfunctions*
Non-specific prodromal symptoms include fever, headache, malaise, myalgia, GI symptoms, pain, pruritus, paraesthesias and/or fasciculations around the site of inoculation of virus indicate multiplication of virus in dorsal root ganglia of sensory nerve supplying the area.	(A) **Furious rabies (80%):** It is characterised by episodes of CNS hyperexcitability followed by periods of complete lucidity that become shorter as the disease progresses. The features are: • Agitation, excitation, enhanced motor activity • Confusion, hallucinations, bizaree thoughts • Fear of water (hydrophobia), muscles spasms meningismus, opisthotonus • Seizures and focal paralysis • Hyperesthesia with excessive sensitivity to bright light, noise, touch and even gentle breeze is common • *Temperature is elevated* • Autonomic symptoms and signs, e.g. dilated irregular pupils, lacrimation, salivation, postural hypotension and cardiac arrhythmias • Change in the voice (vocal cord paralysis) • Evidence of UMN paralysis, e.g. exaggerated reflexes with plantar extensor is the rule (B) **Dumb rabies or paralytic rabies (20%).** It presents with a symmetric ascending paralysis resembling Guillain-Barré syndrome. Cardinal features of encephalitic rabies, i.e. hydrophobia, hyperexcitability and aerophobia are lacking. Sphincter involvement is common. It lasts for 2–10 days.	• Cranial nerve palsies • Hydrophobia (Fig. 23.3) • Priaprism and spontaneous ejaculation • Unconsciousness or coma • Death

Box 2   Algorithm for post-rabies prophylaxis

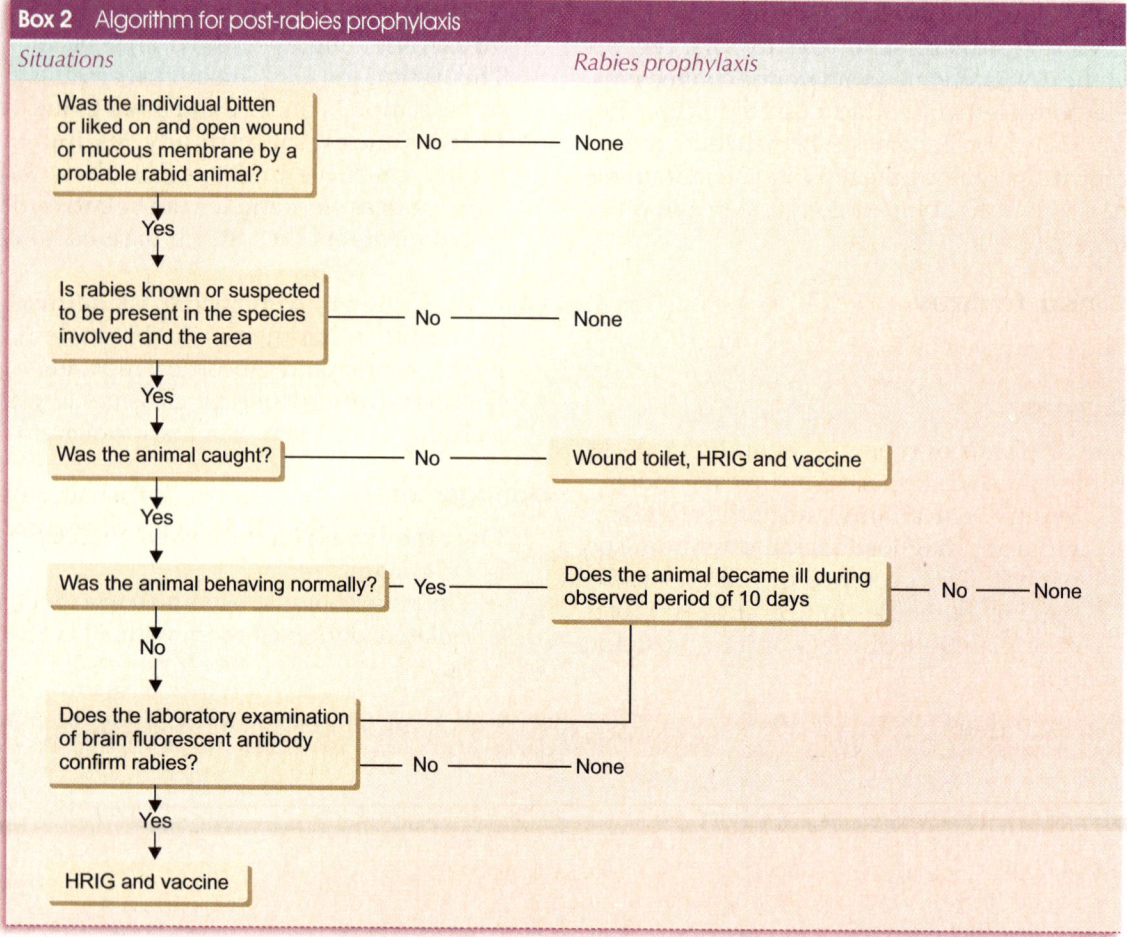

Situations   Rabies prophylaxis

- Nutritional, respiratory and cardiovascular support to be provided.
- To reduce psychomotor excitation, morphine, diazepam and chlorpromazine should be used liberally in such patients.
- Maintain water and salt balance because dehydration results due to aversion to drinking water and excessive perspiration. Intravenous fluids are to be administered liberally.
- Prednisolone and mannitol may be given in patients with raised intracranial pressure.

2. **Prevention of rabies:**

   A. *Post-exposure prophylaxis (see the algorithms in Box 2):* Dramatic clinical

features and fatal outcome in rabies make the prevention of rabies essential. The steps of prophylaxis include:
- To decide whether post-exposure prophylaxis is warranted.
- If animal remains healthy during observed period, no need for prophylaxis.
- If animal develops signs of rabies (abnormal behaviour), it should be euthanised immediately, the head should be transported to laboratory under refrigeration, rabies virus should be sought by direct fluorescent antibody (DFA) test and virus should be isolated by culture/mouse inoculation. In high risk exposures

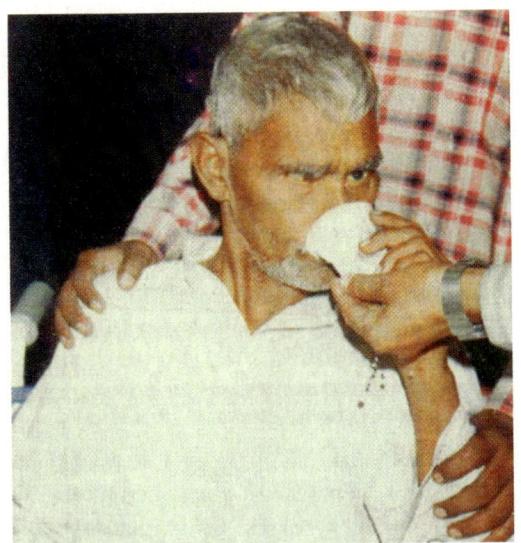

Fig. 23.3: A patient of rabies depicting hydrophobia. Note the severe phobic reaction following just holding of a glass of water by the observer while the patient is supported by his attendant. Patient ultimately died after 24 hours

and in areas where canine rabies is endemic, post-exposure prophylaxis should be initiated. If laboratory test is negative, immunisation should be discontinued. If animal escapes after exposure, prophylaxis must be instituted.

- Local treatment of the wound
- Immunisation (active and passive).

i. *Local treatment of the wound:* It consists of:
  - Wound toilet with soap and water: The wound is scrubbed with soap and flushed with water so as to remove the saliva from the wound.
  - *Chemical cleansing of the wound:* After removal of soap with water, chemical cleansing is done by any quaternary ammonium compound (1–4% benzalkonium chloride or 1% cetrimonium bromide) to inactivate the rabies virus.
  - Tetanus toxoid and antibiotics should be administered.
  - Wound must not be stitched.

ii. *Passive immunisation with antirabies serum of either equine or human origin:* The antirabies serum provides passive immunity in the form of ready-made antibodies against rabies virus. Human rabies immunoglobulin (HRIG) is preferred because equine antiserum may cause serum sickness.
  Dose: Total dose of HRIG is 20 units/kg, and equine antiserum is 40 units/kg. Half the dose is infiltrated around the wound and remaining half is given by deep intramuscular injection into the gluteal region. The antirabies serum needs sensitivity test; while HRIG does not require any prior sensitivity testing.
  Warning: When a person is re-exposed to rabies virus after administration of antirabies vaccines, antirabies strum should not be injected.

iii. *Active immunisation with antirabies vaccine:* In the developed world, human diploid cell vaccine (HDCV) is recommended which is least antigenic and systemic (1–4%) and local reactions (15–20%) are uncommon.

In the developing world, several other rabies vaccines have seen licenced and used extensively. These include vaccines made in chick embryonic cells, vero-cells and duct embryonic cells. These preparations are safe but immunogenic and are effective for post-exposure prophylaxis. In India, HDCV is not available. Other tissue culture vaccines are; primary chick-embryo cell vaccine (PCECV) and purified vero-cells rabies vaccine (PVRV). The dose schedule of vaccine recommended by WHO is given in Box 3.

Pre-exposure Prophylaxis

Some individuals who are at high risk of contact with rabies virus due to their profession such as veterinarians, laboratory research workers

> **Box 3** Dose schedule of vaccine in post-exposure prophylaxis (WHO schedule)
>
> • Four doses of the vaccine available are given intramuscularly, preferably in the deltoid region, the first dose is administered as soon as possible after exposure (Day 0) and should be accompanied by injection of HRIG. The other 3 doses are to be given within 14 days on the following schedule—days 3, 7 and 14. Day 0 indicates the day of vaccination started and the day of the bite. Pregnancy is no contraindication.
> • The fifth injection at 90th day has also been recommended by WHO in those persons who are either immunodeficient or are on steroid therapy and/or at the extremes of ages.
> • Period of immunity conferred is 3–5 years.
> • Adverse effects with tissue culture vaccines are minimal such as sore arm, headache, nausea, fever, localised oedema at the site of injection. Symptomatic treatment is advised to the patient.

and animal handlers should receive pre-exposure prophylaxis with three doses of rabies vaccine on days 0, 7 and 21 or 30. Neutralising antibody titre is to be checked after vaccination.

Depending on the level of risk, serological testing to be done at 2 to 6 years intervals. If titres of neutralising antibody falls below 1:5, booster doses should be given.

Post-exposure prophylaxis in individuals who have received pre-exposure prophylaxis consists of initial two injections on days 0 and 3. HRIG is not given. The indication for postexposure vaccination with or without rabies immune globulin depends on the type of contact with rabid animal (Box 4).

> **Box 4** Types of contacts and treatment
>
> Category I: Just feeding animal licks the skin. No treatment is required.
> Category II: Nibbling of uncovered skin, minor scratches or abrasions without bleeding, licks on broken skin. Immediate vaccination is done.
> Category III: Single or multiple transdermal bites or scratches, contamination of mucus membrane with saliva during licking; exposure to bat bite or scratches, vaccination plus HRIG plus flushing of all bites and scratches.

Tetanus

It is a disorder of neuromuscular excitability caused by an exotoxin (e.g. *tetanospasmin*) elaborated by *Clostridium tetani,* characterised by rigidity and powerful muscle spasms. It manifests clinically in many forms, i.e. *generalised, neonatal, cephalic* and *localised.* It is a vaccine preventable disease.

Aetiopathogenesis

C. tetani—a causative organism of tetanus, is a motile, gram-positive, spore forming obligatory anaerobic organism found in the soil and the environment. It is a normal commensal of animals and human GI tract and is excreted in the stool/excreta. The organism is heat-resistant but sensitive to penicillin and metronidazole. The spores can resist boiling and disinfectants, survive for many years in adverse circumstances.

The organism attacks the wound finding suitable anaerobic environment with low redox potential (low oxidation-reduction potential). The development of tetanus depends on the immune status of the individual. The tetanus occurs sporadically in non-immunised or partially immunized persons mostly through the contaminated wound having local anaerobic conditions. It is common in ruralites than urbanites, and during summer months. It is common in neonates and children in under developed countries where a comprehensive immunisation policy is not followed. It is common in extremes of ages.

The majority of cases occurs after an acute injury with abrasion, laceration or punctured wound. The portal of entry is contaminated wounds containing the spores of *C. tetani* but sometimes entry cannot be identified as injury may be trivial or goes undetected. Following contamination, if local environment of the wound is anaerobic (low oxidation-reduction potential), the spores germinate and produce exotoxin.

Skin abrasions/ulceration, abscesses, gangrene are the wounds commonly predisposed to tetanus. The predisposing conditions include: burn, surgery, abortion, childbirth, drug abuse and tattooing presence of a foreign body in the wound.

The exotoxin (*tetanospasmin*) released from the wound, enters locally through the peripheral motor neurons to axons and travels to the nerve cell bodies in the brainstem and spinal cord. The length of the nerve determines the time of ascent and explains why the disease first manifests in the muscles supplied by short cranial nerves in cephalic tetanus.

The *tetanospasmin*—a zinc metalloprotease cleaves synaptobrevin—a protein essential for neurotransmission. Thus tetanospasmin interferes or blocks the release of inhibitory neurotransmitter-GABA at myoneural junction or synapse. Therefore:

- *In tetanus,* central inhibition is abolished resulting in free play of alpha (α) and gamma (γ) neurones producing typical rigidity.
- The loss of central inhibition also affects the autonomic nervous system resulting in sympathetic overactivity.
- With lessened inhibition, the agonists and antagonists contract simultaneously resulting in spasms.

In **cephalic or local tetanus**, the muscles supplied by involved local nerves are paralysed initially followed by rigidity of the affected muscle following central inhibition

In **tetanus neonatorum**, the portal of entry is infected umbilical cord stump.

Clinical Features

The features of adult generalised tetanus in nonimmunised or partially immunised status of an individual, are given in Box 1.

Neonatal tetanus: It develops in children born to mothers who have been either not immunised or inadequately immunised during pregnancy. It follows infection of umbilical cord stump by unsterilised means. The onset is common during first 2 weeks of life. It occurs in generalised form, proves fatal if left untreated. Poor sucking, failure to thrive, grimacing and irritability followed by rigidity and spasms are its diagnostic features. Mortality is high.

Loal tetanus: It is characterised by rigidity and spasms restricted to the muscles around the wound, is thus a limited form of tetanus, hence, carries excellent prognosis.

Cephalic tetanus: It is an uncommon form and follows injury of face or head and neck region or the ear. The incubation period is short. The *trismus* (*lock jaw*) and dysfunction of one of the cranial nerve mostly the seventh nerve are its common manifestations. Generalised tetanus may or may not develop. The mortality is high due to early and severe involvement of brainstem.

Box 1   Clinical features of general tetanus

1. *Incubation period* is about 7 days (varies from 5 days to 15 weeks).
2. The initial symptom may be pain and tingling at the site of inoculation followed by rigidity.
3. *Hypertonia and rigidity of muscles:* Hypertonia of muscles of face [*risus sardonicus—grinning expression of face* (Fig. 24.1)], jaw (*lock jaw* or *trismus*), neck, shoulder, chest pain and stiffness, abdomen (abdominal rigidity) and back (*opisthotonus—arched back*). These painful spasms occur spontaneously or are induced by noise, light and handling of the patient.
4. *Visceral manifestations:* Painful strong spasms of muscles of respiration and glottis may result in cyanosis and respiratory obstruction or failure. Oesophageal and urethral spasms result in dysphagia and urinary retention. The patient may be febrile due to strong muscular contractions. Deep tendon reflexes may be increased. Strong spasms produce tendon avulsion and crush fractures.
5. *Autonomic symptoms:* These include labile (fluctuating) or sustained hypertension, tachycardia, arrhythmias, fever, sweating, etc. and may require β blockade if become severe.

Investigations

There is no single test which can confirm tetanus including culture of the organism from the wound; however, recovery of the organisms from the wound in the symptomatic patients of tetanus is highly suggestive. Other tests are:

i. Leucocyte count may be elevated.

ii. **Other tests such as EMG** may show continuous motor units discharges and shortening or absence of silent interval (normally, these intervals, are seen).

iii. **ECG:** It may be done frequently in patients with autonomic dysfunction.

iv. **Muscle enzymes:** The creatine phosphokinase (CPK), aldolases may be high during acute phase.

v. Serum anti-toxin levels ≥ 0.1 IU/ml are deemed protective, do not support the diagnosis.

vi. PCR has been used for detection of toxin but its sensitivity is unknown.

Management

Aims

  i. To eliminate the source of toxin (care of the wound).

  ii. To neutralise unbound toxin.

 iii. To prevent muscle spasms.

 iv. To maintain patent airway by tracheostomy.

  v. Ventilatory support if needed.

Treatment

1. **General measures:**

  a. *Good nursing* care is the single most important measure to reduce mortality significantly. The patient should be nursed in a dark, quiet, well ventilated isolated room.

  b. *Proper hydration and nutrition:* Initially or in case of diarrhoea, nutrition is given in the form of intravenous fluids. Calories expenditure is high in a patient with tetanus, hence more than 2500 kcal and 70 g proteins are needed daily, may be given through nasogastric tube for long-term management.

  c. *Wound debridement:* Cleansing of the wound and its debridement is necessary to eliminate the anaerobic environment of the wound so as to eliminate the source of the toxin.

  d. *Care of the unconscious patient:* Meticulous care of the skin to prevent bed sores, proper urinary drainage, maintenance of vitals is necessary.

  e. *Patent airway or tracheostomy (Fig. 24.1):* It is always required in the presence of laryngeal spasms or excessive secretions. Tracheostomy should be done electively and as early as possible. Frequent suction of the secretions is mandatory to prevent aspiration and to maintain patent airway.

2. **The role of antibiotic:** Metronidazole 500 mg I.V. 6 hourly or 1g 12 hourly for 7 days is preferred drug due to its potent anaerobicidal action. The penicillin is

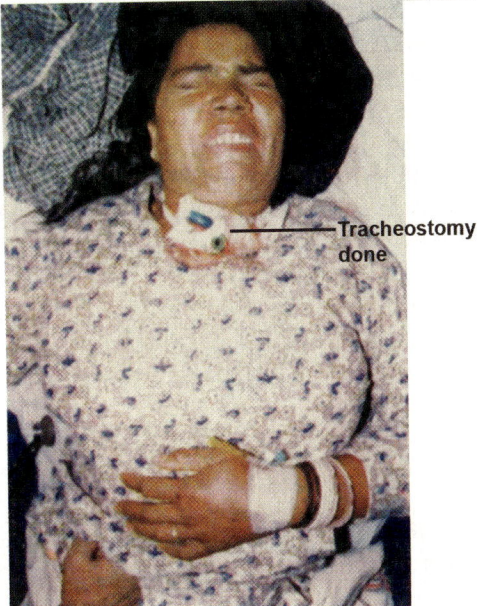

Tracheostomy done

Fig. 24.1: Risus sardonicus in a patient with tetanus. A 40-year-old woman developed tetanus following injury. Note the grimacing or grinning appearance of the face due to facial muscle spasms

alternate drug of choice in doses of 10–12 million units I.V. daily for 10 days or a single injection of benzathine penicillin 2.4×10^6 units provides bactericidal concentrations for a period of 2 weeks. Tetracyclines, clindamycin and erythromycin are other alternative antibiotics.

3. **Antitoxin:** The antitoxin (ATS-antitetanus serum) is given as 10,000 IU intravenously after testing the sensitivity to neutralise the circulatory as well as unbound tetanus toxin in the wound. Local infiltration of the wound is obsolete now-a-days.

  Human tetanus immunoglobulin (TIG) 500 units should be given I.M. within 24 hours of presentation then up to 3000 units in divided doses; however, 1500 IU is considered as optimal dose now-a-days. The intrathecal administered of TIG has no role but found useful in one of the trials.

4. **Control of muscle spasms:** Diazepam—a benzodiazepine derivative and GABA agonist is the drug of choice. Continuous

I.V. infusion of 100–200 mg daily may be needed initially to control the painful spasms, then dose is reduced to maintenance dose. Lorazepam and midazolam are other alternatives. Barbiturates and phenothiazines are second-line agents. The spasms that are unresponsive to medication or that threaten ventilation are best treated with mechanical ventilation and therapeutic muscular *paralysis by neuromuscular blockade*, e.g. *curarisation*. Alternative agent is propofol but is expensive. I.V. magnesium sulphate has been used as muscle relaxant. Baclofen and dantrolene may be used with the hope that their use will shorten the period of paralysis.

5. **Control of autonomic symptoms when and if they arise:** A hemodynamic monitoring is needed for autonomic dysfunction. β-blockers (esmolol), clonidine and verapamil are used in case of sympathetic overactivity to control hypertension and prevent arrhythmias. Bradycardia or bradyarrhythmias may require pacemaker insertion. Hypotension responds to volume expansion and pressor agents. The heavy sedation and parenteral $MgSO_4$ are used for autonomic stability.

6. **Vaccine:** Active immunisation with full course of toxoid is given before discharge of the patient from the hospital. It is necessary in view of the fact that patients of tetanus do not generate sufficient antitoxin in the blood after recovery.

7. **Treatment of intercurrent infection** by appropriate antibiotic.

Prophylaxis

Tetanus is preventable by good wound care and active immunisation. For primary immunisation in adults Td (tetanus and diptheria toxoids vaccine) is administered as two doses 4–6 weeks apart with a third dose 6–12 months later. For one of the doses Tdap (tetanus toxoid, low dose diphtheria toxoid and acellular pertussis vaccine) should be substituted for Td. Booster doses are given at 10 years or at the time of injury. A single dose of Tdap is preferred to Td prophylaxis if the patient has been previously vaccinated with Tdap.

Passive immunisation with TIG (tetanus immune globulin 250 units) is given intramuscularly to non-immunized persons and for those whose immune status is uncertain, active immunisation with tetanus toxoid is begun simultaneously.

Complications

1. **Pulmonary infection** occurs due to:
   - Aspiration of infected secretions.
   - Depressed cough and swallow reflex.
   - Impaired ventilation and mucociliary defense mechanisms following tracheostomy.

2. **Autonomic dysfunctions** such as hypertension, tachy and bradyarrhythmias and hypotension. They require monitoring and proper treatment.

3. **Vertebral fractures of the dorsal spine** during violent and severe spasms.

4. **Myositis ossificans** due to deposition of calcium in the ligaments around the joints (knee, elbow) can occasionally occur.

5. **Decubitus ulcer/pressure sores occur due to:**
   - Prolonged immobilisation.
   - Skin contamination with urine and faeces.

Myonecrosis (Gas Gangrene) and Toxic Shock Syndrome

MYONECROSIS (GAS GANGRENE)

Myonecrosis (gas gangrene) is produced from invasion of healthy muscle from adjacent traumatised muscle or soft tissue infected by anaerobes especially clostridial group of organism. About 80% cases are caused by *C. perfringens;* while remainders are due to *C. novyi, C. septicum* and *C. histolyticum. C. sordellii* as the causative organism in toxic shock syndrome during pregnancy and medically-induced abortion. The finding of gas in the muscle, soft tissue or uterus (Fig. 25.1A) is not pathognomonic of clostridial infection as other bacteria particularly anaerobes, mixed with aerobes can also produce gas.

Aetiopathogenesis

Gas gangrene is a serious complication seen in devitalised and devascularised muscle(s) following trauma, repeated injections, surgery or amputation. The causative organisms are present in the soil and in the Gl tract of animals and humans. The development of gas gangrene requires an anaerobic environment and contamination of wound with spores or vegetative organisms. The presence of necrotic tissue, foreign bodies or ischaemia in a wound reduce locally available oxygen (low oxidation-reduction potential) and permit the organism to grow and produce toxin.

The **predisposing factors** for traumatic gas gangrene include crush injury, open fractures of bones that are contaminated with soil or bits of clothing containing bacterial spores. In the traumatic gas gangrene organisms introduced in the injured tissue proliferate and produce toxins alpha (α) and theta (θ) called *perfrinolysin*.

The concerned toxins spread through tissue and expand them in aerobic area. The alpha (α) toxins of *C. perfringens* result in the destruction

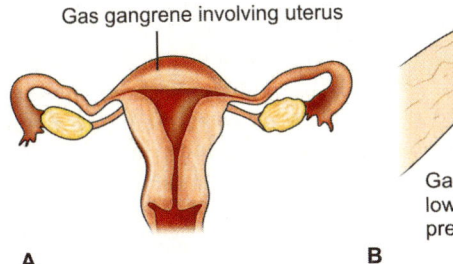

Gas gangrene involving uterus

A

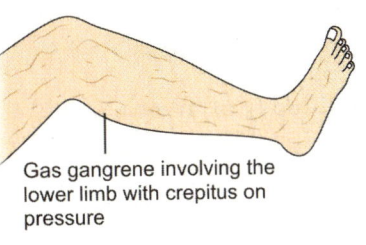

Gas gangrene involving the lower limb with crepitus on pressure

B

Fig. 25.1A and B: Gas gangrene (myonecrosis). A. Uterus and B. lower limb

of muscles fibres by disrupting the phospho-lipid in cell membranes. *Collagenases* and *hyaluronidases* destroy the partitions of connective tissue and enable the infection to spread, through muscles. In less virulent infection, local fasciitis rather than myositis may result. Cardiovascular collapse and end-organ failure occur late in the course of gas gangrene and are largely attributed to the effects of these toxins.

Toxic shock syndrome is due to infection caused by *C. sordellii,* can develop after gynaecological procedures, childbirth or abortion.

Clinical Features

The clinical features are summarised in Box 1. Gas gangrene is a true emergency because it is accompanied by bacteremia, hypotension and multiple organ failure, hence requires immediate surgical debridement.

Investigations

- There may be *leucocytosis, haemolytic anaemia, thrombocytopenia* (DIC) due to toxaemia or toxic shock syndrome.
- **Muscle enzymes:** There may be raised creatine phosphokinase (CK).
- **Radiograph of the involved area** may show collection of gas with ill-defined soft tissue shadow.
- **USG and CT scan** may confirm badly damage muscle and presence of gas.
- **Isolation of the organism from scrapping from** uterus, smears from the wound or cervical discharge by Gram's staining. **Blood culture** for isolation of the organism to be placed in anaerobic media.
- **Frozen section biopsy of muscle** confirms the diagnosis.

Diagnosis

The diagnosis of gas gangrene is primarily on the clinical findings with demonstration of gas in the muscles, soft tissue or uterus and isolation of the organism from the site

involved (smears of wound exudates, uterine scrappings or cervical discharge) or from the blood cultures to be placed in selective media and incubated under anaerobic conditions. The diagnosis is confirmed by frozen section biopsy of the muscle.

Management

1. **Eradication of source of infection:**
   a. *Surgery:* It includes debridement of local soft tissue infection, debridement of all the involved muscles in abdominal myonecrosis or surgical removal of the source of infection such as

---

Box 1 Clinical features of clostridial myonecrosis

- *Incubation period* is short, i.e. less than 3 days, frequently less than 24 hours.
- *Precipitating or incriminating factors* include: Deep muscle trauma (*lacerated wound*), surgery or intramuscular injection which creates an anaerobic environment for growth of clostridia.
- *The initial symptom* is *pain* of sudden onset, severe, localised to the infected area and then may spread. This is followed by *local swelling, oedema* and *haemorrhagic exudation* from the wound. There is associated elevation of temperature and marked tachycardia. There may be *frothiness of the wound* on compression at this stage. The symptoms progress rapidly, i.e. swelling, oedema and toxaemia increase and a profuse serous discharge with sweetish smell appear. *Gram's stain* of the wound may reveal— Gram-positive rods with few inflammatory cells. At this stage, there is an evidence of suppuration, and gas in the soft tissues (subcutaneous crepitance) (Fig. 25.1) as well as overwhelming toxaemia.
- *These patients preserve consciousness* in spite of hypotension, renal failure and body crepitance. They lapse into toxic delirium and coma in later phases. In untreated cases, skin becomes bronzed; bullae appear, become filled with dark red fluid and are accompanied by dark patches of cutaneous gangrene. Jaundice is rare, if present is associated with haemoglobinuria, haemoglobinaemia and septicaemia. DIC may be seen in severe infection.
- **Toxic shock syndrome** following childbirth or abortion is characterised by *pain, nausea, vomiting* and *diarrhoea*. Patient is usually afebrile, *systemic manifestations* include *oedema, effusion, hypotension* and *multiple organ failure*.

amputation of a limb or hysterectomy for uterine myonecrosis.

b. *Antibiotics:* Penicillin g (20 million units a day in adults) have been the drug of choice till now. Recently its role has become controversial because of increasing resistance to this drug. Clindamycin (600 mg every 6 hourly) and penicillin combination has been found to be superior than either of them alone. In case of penicillin allergy, other antibiotic (chloramphenicol, metronidazole, imipenem, doxycycline) should be used. Broad spectrum antibiotic with a aminoglycoside may be used for the aerobic (suppurative) gram-negative bacteria involved in mixed infections.

2. **Polyvalent gas gangrene antitoxin:** It is still recommended by some authorities but at present its role has become controversial because of questionable efficacy and risk of hypersensitivity to horse serum from which it is derived.

3. **Hyperbaric oxygen:** Its role has also become questionable because:

   i. Its efficacy is not proved but addition of hyperbaric O_2 to the therapeutic regimen provides additional benefit provided if surgery and antibiotic therapy precede oxygen therapy.

   ii. Expert surgical and medical management and control of complications are the most important factors in the treatment of gas gangrene.

Cholera

CHOLERA

Cholera is an acute diarrhoeal illness caused by *Vibrio cholerae* 01 or *V. cholerae* 0139. The two biotypes—classical and *E1 Tor* are major causes of cholera. Each biotype has two serotypes—*Ogawa* and *Inaba*. All are pathogenic strains. Transmission occurs through ingestion of food and drinks contaminated directly or indirectly with faeces or vomitus of an infected person (feco-oral route).

It is hypersecretory acute watery diarrhoea produced by the action of exotoxins elaborated by *V. cholerae* producing loss of water and electrolytes resulting in dehydration, acidosis, hyponatraemia, hypokalaemia and renal failure as a complication.

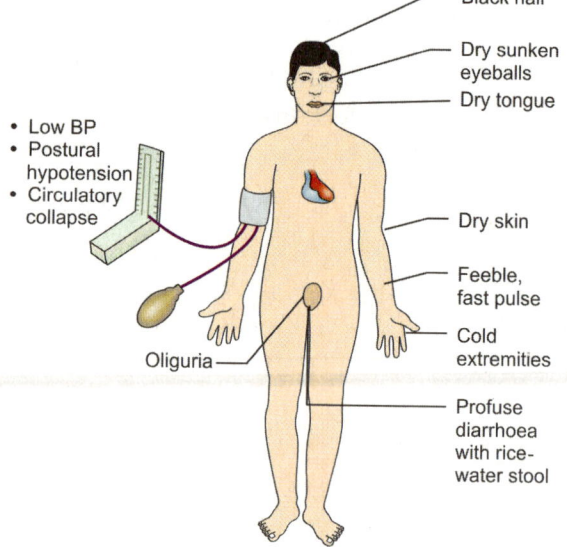

Fig. 26.1: Clinical features of cholera

Clinical Features (Fig. 26.1)

Cholera is a disease of children (most common during 1–5 years of age). The incubation period is few hours to 6 days.

Cholera occurs in epidemics under conditions of crowding, war and famine (e.g. refugee camps) and where sanitation is not proper. Infection occurs via oro-fecal route by contaminated water and food.

The disease may be mild or remains asymptomatic but typical cholera presents with severe diarrhoea without pain or colic followed by vomiting. Following the evacuation of normal

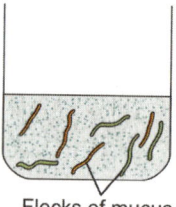

Fig. 26.2: Commode showing rice-water stools—flecks of mucus

gut faecal contents, typical 'rice-water' material (gray, turbid) is passed consisting of clear fluid with flecks of mucus floating in the watery stool (Fig. 26.2). Classical cholera produces significant loss of fluids (8–10 L) and electrolytes resulting in dehydration with muscle cramps. Later on, shock and oliguria (acute renal failure), develop but mental clarity is preserved. Improvement is rapid with proper treatment. Death occurs due to acute circulatory collapse in untreated patients. The clinical hallmarks of cholera are given in Box 1.

Box 1	Clinical hallmarks of cholera

- Rapid onset of symptoms
- Profuse watery diarrhoea (liquid stools) typical rice-water stool. There is loss of about 8–10 L of fluids
- Absence of fever
- Occasional vomiting
- Symptoms and signs of dehydration, hypovolaemic shock, acute renal failure, acidosis, hypokalaemia

Diagnosis

Diagnosis is easy during an epidemic and depends on clinical features. Confirmation is done by bacteriological culture of the stool for isolation, identification of agents— *V. cholerae* 01 and 0139 and antibiotic sensitivity. Stool specimens or rectal swabs must be taken for culture before antibiotic therapy. Agglutination of vibrios with specific sera can be demonstrated.

It is better to collect the specimen and place it immediately in the transport medium viz *Cary-Blair, Venkataraman Ramkrishnan fluid (V.R. fluid)*. If transport medium is not available, then blotting paper strips soaked in liquid stool may be preserved in sealed plastic bags.

Management

Management of cholera is similar to acute watery diarrhoea from other causes (read also acute diarrhoea as an emergency). The main aim of treatment is to maintain circulation by adequate replacement of fluids and electrolytes. It should be accomplished as early as possible to reduce the risk of hypovolaemic shock. The steps of treatment are:

1. **Assessment of dehydration** (e.g. restlessness, irritability, sunken eyeballs, dry tongue, excessive thirst, dry skin, weak pulse and low blood pressure).
2. **Rehydration therapy:** Rehydration is mainly oral by oral rehydration solution (ORS), but intravenous fluids therapy is necessary for severely dehydrated patients and for those with acidosis (pH < 7.2). Replacement of fluids by ORS is highly effective and saves countless lives of dehydrated patients.

The components of ORS are given in Box 2. The fluid therapy and its type depend on the degree of dehydration:

1. **Mildly dehydrated patients** need ORS (75 ml/kg in 4 hours). A simple home made ORS includes one TSF of table salt, 4 TSF of sugar and 1 liter of H_2O. Reassess after 4 hours and then further treatment depends on degree of dehydration. Hydration can be maintained by allowing liberal amount of fluids as much as he/she can take.
2. **Severely ill dehydrated patients** need I.V. Ringer's lactate and the diarrhoea treatment solution (NaCl 4.0 g, sodium acetate 6.5 g, KCl 1.0 g and glucose 9.0 g/L). If not available then normal saline (100 ml/kg I.V. in 3 hours and in 6 hours

Box 2	Oral rehydration solutions		
Content	WHO/* UNICEF	Cereal based ORS*	UK/Europe ORS**
Sodium (mmol/L)	90	90	35–60
Potassium (mmol/L)	20	20	20
Chloride (mmol/L)	80	80	37
Bicarbonate (mmol/L)	—	—	90–200
Glucose (mmol/L)	111	—	90–200
Citrate (mmol/L)	10	10	10
Rice (g/L)	—	50–80	—

* Used in cholera
** ORS currently recommended in children UK/Europe

in infants), 30% of fluid rapidly within half an hour followed by ORS as soon as the patient can drink orally. Rehydration can be maintained after correction of dehydration by adequate amount of fluids in adults; 100 ml of fluid after each stool in <2 years old; 200 ml after each loose stool in 2–9 years old.

- *Electrolytes to be monitored during treatment.*
- *Frequent assessment of dehydration to be done.*

The maintenance of hydration by replacement of ongoing fluid losses to be continued until diarrhoea stops.

3. **Antibiotics:** Antibiotics are generally not essential for most of the cases of cholera but should be used in severely dehydrated patients. They reduce the loss of amount of fluids and duration of diarrhoea and shorten the period of *V. cholera* excretion. Tetracycline (250–500 mg 6 hourly for 3 days or 2 g as a single dose) or doxycycline (300 mg as a single dose) or ciprofloxacin lg/day as single dose for 3 days are effective to eradicate the infection. Ampicillin, azithromycin (1 g as a single dose) and cotrimoxazole are also effective. Recently during an epidemic of cholera in Delhi (2000), the antimicrobial agents effective against both *V. cholerae* 01 and *V. cholerae* 0139 were nalidixic acid and furazolidine followed by cotrimoxazole. WHO recommends erythromycin as an alternative to tetracycline.

4. **Feeding:** Feeding should be continued to the extent possible. Normal diet should be instituted as soon as vomiting stops. Breast-feeding in infants should be continued uninterruptedly even during rehydration with ORS.

Prevention

- Strict personal hygiene (wash your hands after defecation and before preparing and eating food. Use soap for washing hands).
- Drink water from a safe source or use boiled water or disinfected water.
- Store drinking water in clean, covered and narrow mouthed container.
- Avoid raw and uncooked food. Cook food thoroughly and eat it while it is hot.
- Keep the flies away from food.
- Old parenteral cholera vaccines are of limited use because of low efficacy and short duration of protection. New generation cholera vaccines (WC/rBS and CVD 103-HgR) provide convincing protection. The WC/rBS vaccine is given orally in 2 doses, 10–14 days apart, confers 80–90% protection for 6 months. The *booster dose* is given after every 6 months to persons remaining in areas where cholera is a hazard. The level of protection is still about 50%, 3 years after immunisation in those who were >5 years of age at the time of vaccination. The vaccine is indicated in population believed to be at imminent risk (within a period of 6 months) of a cholera in an epidemic, but not to contain an epidemic once it has occurred. Vaccine WC/rBS is currently licenced in some countries but is not available in India as yet.
- Mass chemoprophylaxis, immunisation with conventional parenteral vaccines and cordon sanitaire are useful measures during an epidemic but all are ineffective in preventing and controlling the epidemic.

Bacterial Food Poisoning

BACTERIAL FOOD POISONING

Bacterial food poisoning or enterocolitis is an acute short-lived infection of the intestine due to a wide variety of organisms. It is characterized by fever, malaise, cramping abdominal pain, bloody diarrhoea and vomiting. Occasionally cholera like picture may be present. The incubation period of this illness is variable. It is self-limiting illness that lasts for 2–3 days.

Aetiology and Clinical Features

These are given in Box 1.

S. aureus is a common commensal in the anterior nares. Poor hygiene is the cause. Transmission occurs via the food handlers who do not keep up hygiene to the foodstuffs especially dairy products, cheese and cooked meat. Inappropriate storage of these eatables allows the growth of the organisms and production of one or more heat-stable exotoxins (Fig. 27.1).

Spores of C. perfringens are widespread in the gut of large animals and in soil. If contaminated meat products are incompletely cooked and stored in anaerobic conditions, spores germinate and viable organisms multiply. Sporulation is associated with production of enterotoxins. Botulism (food poisoning by C. botulinum) occurs due to ingestion of contaminated foodstuffs, commonly the canned meat, fish and preserved vegetables (Fig. 27.2).

Bacillus cereus causes food poisoning by ingestion of preformed toxins in the contaminated

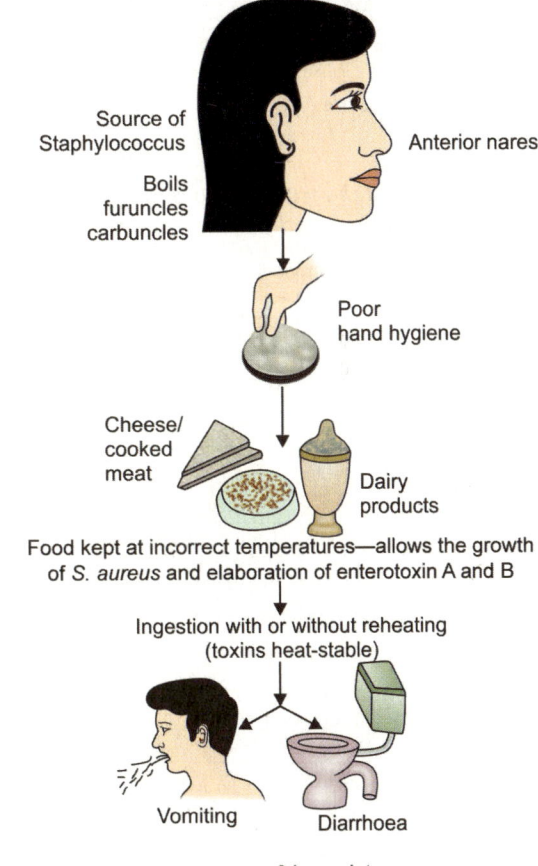

Source of Staphylococcus
Boils furuncles carbuncles

Anterior nares

Poor hand hygiene

Cheese/ cooked meat

Dairy products

Food kept at incorrect temperatures—allows the growth of S. aureus and elaboration of enterotoxin A and B

Ingestion with or without reheating (toxins heat-stable)

Vomiting

Diarrhoea

6 hours later

Fig. 27.1: Staphylococcal food poisoning

food (Fig. 27.3). Fried rice or freshly prepared vanilla sauces are frequent sources. The organisms grow and produce exotoxins during storage. The *'Chinese restaurant*

syndrome' is caused by this organism, characterised by rapid onset of vomiting within hours of food ingestion followed by some diarrhoea.

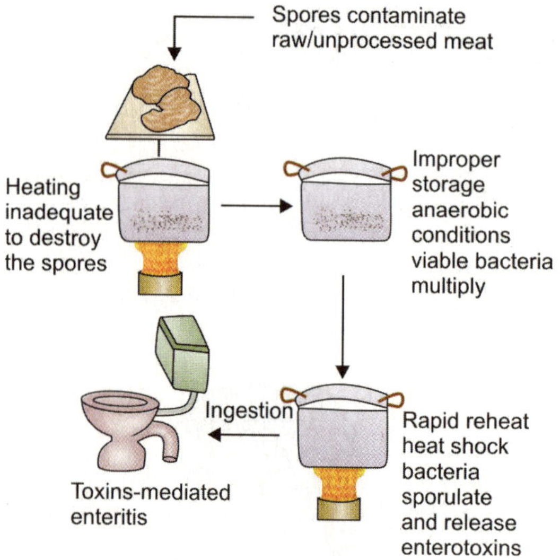

Management

It is an emergency. Patient needs replacement of fluids and electrolytes to prevent the development of peripheral circulatory failure. The steps of management include:

1. **Fluid and electrolytes:** The patient should be given fluids (ORS) to compensate the fluid loss in the stools and to correct dehydration which is commonly present in these cases. Patient with severe dehydration should receive I.V. fluids such as Ringer's lactate. The pulse, BP, temperature and urinary output should be monitored. The electrolytes should be monitored and corrected accordingly.

2. **Antibiotics:** Specific treatment of bacterial diarrhoea includes oxytetracycline (500 mg after every 6 hours) for shigellae

Fig. 27.2: *Clostridium perfringens* food poisoning

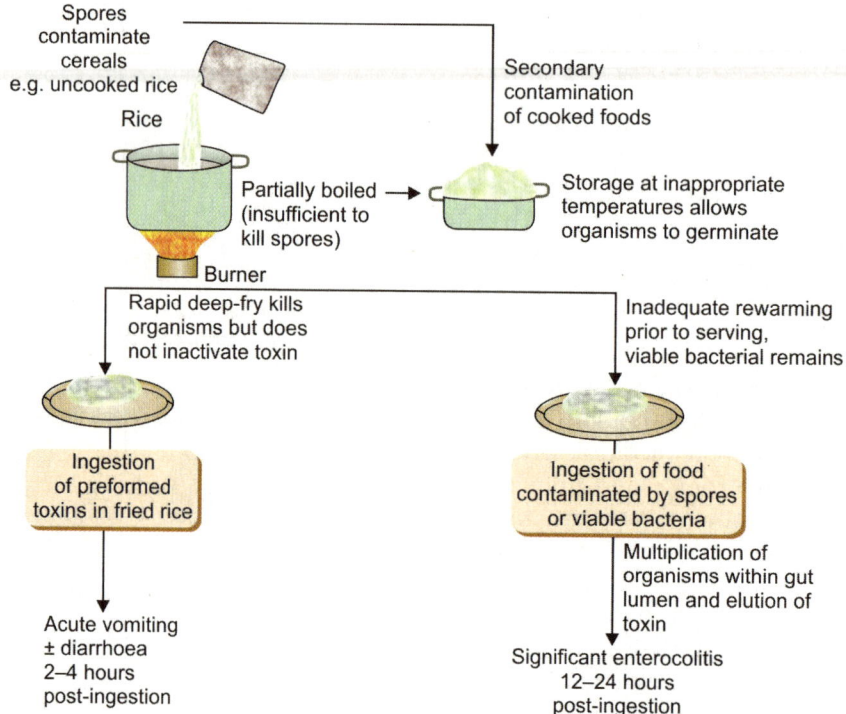

Fig. 27.3: *Bacillus cereus* (Chinese restaurant) bacterial food poisoning

Box 1 Bacterial causes of acute diarrhoea (food poisoning)

Pathogen	Source	Clinical features	Investigations	Treatment and recovery
Staphylococcus aureus (preformed toxin)	Contaminated food or other eatables	Incubation period 2–6 hours. Diarrhoea, vomiting, fever and dehydration are symptoms	Clinically vomitus or stool can be tested for toxin	Rapid within few hours with supportive care
Bacillus cereus (preformed toxin)	Spores in food (often rice) resistant to boiling	Incubation period is 1–6 hours. Diarrhoea, vomiting and dehydration occur	Clinical, stool and food can be tested for toxin	Rapid with supportive care
Clostridium perfringens	Spores in food (meat and poultry dish) survive boiling	Incubation period is 8–20 hours. Watery diarrhoea and abdominal cramps occur (toxin-induced enteritis). 'Point source' outbreaks, in which a number of cases become symptomatic following ingestion, classically occurs following school or canteen lunches where meat stews are served.	Culture the organisms in faeces and food	2–3 days with supportive care
Clostridium botulinum	Canned or bottled food. Spores survive cooking and germinate in anaerobic conditions	Incubation period is long (24–36 hours). Brief diarrhoea and gut paralysis due to neuromuscular block by neurotoxin. There is bulbar or ocular nerves palsies (difficulty in swallowing, blurred or double vision, proptosis)	Demonstration of toxins in food and stool. Stool and food can be cultured	Recovery within 10–14 days. Treatment requires clear airway, ventilation and I.V. polyvalent anti-toxin.
Shigella spp.	Contaminated food and water	Bloody diarrhoea/dysentery, cramps, tenesmus	Culture the organism in stool	Recovery within 2–5 days with fluoroquinolones
Salmonella enteritidis (phage type 4), sometimes S. typhimurium	Eggs, poultry, contaminated food and water, unpasteurised milk	Incubation period is 12–24 hours. Fever, vomiting and diarrhoea (+ blood) occur	Culture the organism in stool	Usually 2–5 days with antibiotic treatment, but may take 2 weeks
Campylobacter jejuni	Bowel of animals especially fowls; and cattle (Zoonotic infection). The most common source of infection is meat such as chicken or contaminated milk product	Incubation period is longest (1–3 days). Fever, pain abdomen and diarrhoea with or without blood occur. Campylobacter species have been linked to Guillain-Barré syndrome and reactive arthritis	Culture the organism in stool	Recovery within 3–5 days. Treatment includes azithromycin or fluoroquinolones for severe disease
Vibrio cholerae (enterotoxins)	Contaminated food, fish and eatables	Incubation period is few hours to few days. Profuse, painless, watery diarrhoea (rice-water stools), dehydration, hypotension or shock are its manifestations	Stool culture for organisms	Recovery is variable (may be fatal). Treatment includes I.V. fluids or ORS to replenish fluid and electrolytes.

Contd.

Box 1	Bacterial causes of acute diarrhoea (food poisoning) *(Contd.)*				
Pathogen	Source	Clinical features	Investigations	Treatment and recovery	
Enterohaemo-rrhagic or entero-toxigenic E. coli	Infected food and water. Incubation period 16–24 hours	Watery or bloody diarrhoea and abdominal cramps	Stool culture for organism	Tetracyclines and azithromycin shorten the duration of diarrhoea. 2–4 days. In travellers fluoroquinolones shorten disease Give activated charcoal to absorb toxin.	
Sea food poisoning (toxin produced by fishes)					
Shellfish poisoning (Saxitoxin blocks sodium conductance and neurotransmission in muscles		Consumption produces gastrointestinal symptoms (pain, vomiting, diarrhoea) within 30 minutes followed by respiratory paralysis		No specific antidote. Supportive therapy with fluids and electrolytes. Observe for paralysis	
Ciguatera fish poisoning (ciguatoxin)	Consumption of fish	Incubation period is 1–6 hours, G.I. symptoms are associated with paraesthesias of lips and extremities, distorted temperature sensation, myalgia, progressive flaccid paralysis	—	The gastrointestinal symptoms resolve rapidly but neuropathic features may persist for months	
Scomprotoxic fish poisoning (histamine and other chemicals)	Ingestion of fish-tuna bonito, skip jack and canned dark meat of sardines	Symptoms are immediate, allergic-like occur within minutes, include flushing, burning, sweating urticaria, pruritis, colic nausea, vomiting and diarrhoea, bronchospasm and hypotension	—	Symptoms resolve with treatment with H_2 blocker, anti-histamines and salbuta-mol; I.V. fluid replacement cures dehydration	

Note: Toxins found in fishes or shellfish can produce food poisoning (by ingestion)

infection and ciprofloxacin 500 mg bid or bismuth subsalicylate (2 tab after half an hour intervals up to 8 doses) for *E. coli*, Salmonella or other bacterial diarrhoea. Metronidazole 400–800 mg tid is effective against anaerobes.

Conventionally, it is better to start with ciprofloxacin *plus* metronidazole in such an acute situation so as to cover most of the causative organisms till a final report of stool culture is received. Parenteral antibiotic therapy is indicated if patient is not accepting orally. The treatment is continued for few days. Depending on the response, most of the patients show rapid recovery.

3. **Anticholinergic and antimotility:** Drugs have no role. However, loperamide has been used to reduce the frequency of stool. It is given 4 mg initially followed by 2 mg with each stock (maximum 8–12 mg) in *E. coli* induced food poisoning.

Acute Dysentery (Amoebic *vs* Shigellosis)

Acute dysentery is an acute inflammation of the large intestine characterised by diarrhoea with blood and mucus in the stool. Its causes are bacillary (*Shigella* spp., enterohaemorrhagic *E. coli* and *Vibrio parahaemolyticus*) or amoebic infection. It has to be differentiated from bloody diarrhoea which may be due to infections and noninfectious causes (read acute diarrhoea).

Clinical Features

Bacillary dysentery presents as acute illness with *diarrhoea, lower abdominal cramps* and *tenesmus*. Stools are mixed with blood and mucus. **Systemic symptoms**, i.e. *fever*, chills, malaise are present. Abdomen is tender. The clinical features between two types of dysentery are summarised in Box 1. Bacillary dysentery must be distinguished from *Salmonella enteracolitis* and from disease due to enterotoxigenic *E. coli*, campylobacter, and *Yersmia enterocolitica*.

Complications

Complications of shigellosis are summarised in Box 2.

Diagnosis

The diagnosis of acute dysentery is based on the clinical features and confirmation is done by stool examination (shows many leucocytes and RBCs) and stool culture to isolate the organism. Mixed infection (amoebic plus bacillary) is also

Box 1 Distinguishing features of two common types of dysentery	
Amoebic dysentery (Fig. 28.1)	Bacillary dysentery
Onset is subacute.	Onset is acute.
1. 4–8 motions (<10 motions/day)	8–12 motions (>10 motions/day)
2. Fairly large stools with streaks of dark blood and mucus seen on the surface	Small amount of stools mixed with fresh blood and mucus
3. Offensive (foul smelling) and acidic stools	Odourless, alkaline stools 'red current Jelly'
4. Stools are semisolid or viscid, stick to the container or latrine sheet	Liquid or semisolid stools do not stick to the container
5. Tenesmus is not usual	Tenesmus is usual
6. A lot of mucus, scanty pus and RBCs present. Charcot layden crystals present. Trophozoites with ingested RBCs may be present	Microscopically, stool contains numerous pus cells, RBCs and macrophages with ingested RBCs. No charcot layden crystals. Few bacteria visible
7. Tenderness over the whole colon (diffuse)	Tenderness over the left colon and caecum
8. Fever, weakness but usually no signs of dehydration	Fever with dehydration and weakness common

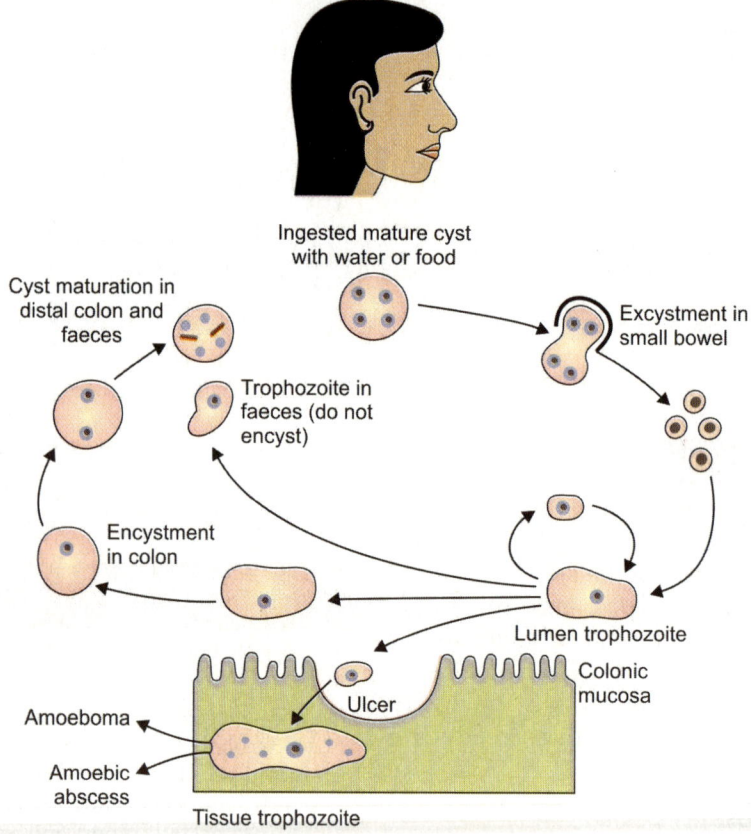

Cyst maturation in distal colon and faeces

Ingested mature cyst with water or food

Excystment in small bowel

Trophozoite in faeces (do not encyst)

Encystment in colon

Lumen trophozoite

Colonic mucosa

Amoeboma

Ulcer

Amoebic abscess

Tissue trophozoite

Fig. 27.1: Pathogenesis of amoebic dysentery with life cycle of *Entamoeba histolytica*

common which will have features of both types of dysentery, i.e. patient experiences acute bowel symptoms with more frequent stools, the passage of much blood and mucus. There may be fever with chills and rigors.

Sigmoidoscopy reveals an inflamed, engorged mucosa with punctate and sometimes large areas of ulceration.

Management

The bacillary dysentery has to be differentiated from amoebic dysentery from therapeutic point of view (Box 1). The stools are to be examined for trophozoites, pus cells, RBCs and culture be immediately sent. The steps of management include:

1. Assessment of dehydration should be done and oral rehydration therapy (WHO/UNICEF solution) may be started if dysentery is mild or moderate. In severe cases, intravenous fluids and electrolytes should be given to correct fluid and electrolyte deficit. The pulse, BP, urine output, temperature and electrolytes be monitored.

2. **Antimicrobial therapy:** Ciprofloxacin 750 mg bid for 7 days or levofloxacin 500 mg daily for 3 days is drug of choice in bacillary dysentery; ceftriaxone and azithromycin are alternatives. Amoebic dysentery needs metronidazole 800 mg 8 hourly for 5 days or tinidazole single dose of 2 g daily for 3 days. Diloxanide furoate 500 mg should be given orally 8 hourly for 10 days to eliminate the luminal cyst.

Box 2	Complications of shigellosis (acute bacillary dysentery)

A. Intestinal
- Toxic megacolon
- Intestinal perforations
- Rectal prolapse

B. Bacteraemia
- Rare

C. Metabolic/toxic
- Hypoglycemia
- Hyponatraemia and dehydration
- Toxic encephalopathy

D. Blood
- Haemolytic uraemia syndrome

E. Joint
- Reactive arthritis (Reiter's syndrome)

Parenteral antibiotics may be given if patient has associated vomiting or cannot take orally or has serious illness.

Before starting specific treatment and before the stool culture report, an empirical treatment with ciprofloxacin *plus* metronidazole or tinidazole is advised. The treatment is to be revised after report of stool culture.

3. **Antimotility drugs** should be avoided.

4. **Treatment of complications:**

   A. *Toxic megacolon*
   - Correct dehydration, anaemia and electrolyte.
   - Nasogastric aspiration.
   - Parenteral nutrition and antibiotics.
   - Surgery if above medical treatment fails.

   B. *Haemolytic uraemic syndrome*
   - Water and salt restriction (discontinue ORS).
   - Haemofiltration if needed.

Cerebral Malaria

CEREBRAL MALARIA

Cerebral malaria is defined as failure to respond appropriately to noxious stimuli and an unarousable coma (for more than 30 minutes after a generalised convulsion in adults). It is caused by *P. falciparum* parasitaemia.

It results from engorgement of cerebral capillaries and venules with parasitized and non-parasitized RBCs. As falciparum malaria attacks all stages of RBCs, hence, there is heavy parasitization, and red cells containing schizonts adhere to capillary (cyto-adherence) in brain and other organs leading to vascular occlusion making them anoxic or hypoxic. Rupture of schizonts liberates toxic and antigenic substances which trigger cytokines production which may cause further damage.

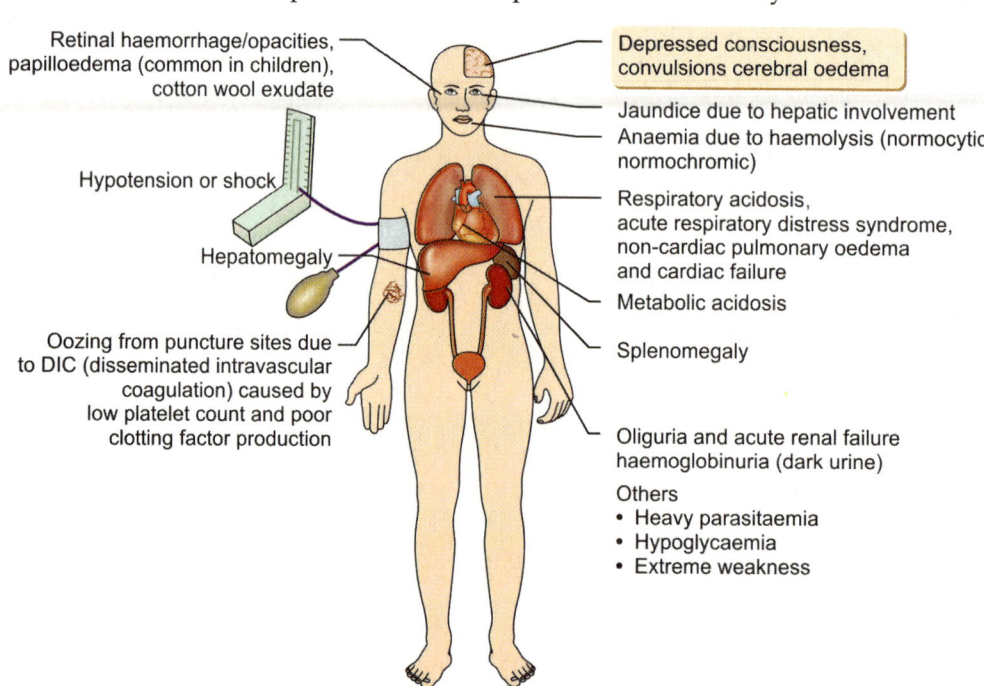

Retinal haemorrhage/opacities, papilloedema (common in children), cotton wool exudate

Hypotension or shock

Hepatomegaly

Oozing from puncture sites due to DIC (disseminated intravascular coagulation) caused by low platelet count and poor clotting factor production

Depressed consciousness, convulsions cerebral oedema

Jaundice due to hepatic involvement
Anaemia due to haemolysis (normocytic normochromic)

Respiratory acidosis, acute respiratory distress syndrome, non-cardiac pulmonary oedema and cardiac failure

Metabolic acidosis

Splenomegaly

Oliguria and acute renal failure haemoglobinuria (dark urine)

Others
• Heavy parasitaemia
• Hypoglycaemia
• Extreme weakness

Fig. 29.1: Organ involvement in cerebral malaria

High levels of cytokine 'tissue necrosis factor-TNF' upregulates the nitrous oxide synthetase activity. It is possible that large amounts of nitrous oxide produced locally due to sequestration of parasitized RBCs, diffuses across the wall of the affected cerebral vessels into the brain parenchyma where it interferes with the calcium influx mechanisms and synaptic transmission leading to coma.

Clinical Features (Fig. 29.1)

Cerebral malaria is the most severe form of *P. falciparum* malaria with high levels of parasitaemia. The WHO criteria for severe malaria are given in Box 1. About 1% patients with *P. falciparum* infection develop cerebral malaria or severe malaria.

Cerebral malaria is a diffuse encephalopathy in which focal neurological signs are unusual though reported in Indian series. Coma is a characteristic and ominous feature of falciparum malaria and carries high mortality rates (20% in adults and 15% in children). Therefore lesser degree of disturbance in consciousness barring coma should be taken seriously. The onset may be gradual or sudden following a convulsion. The following symptoms and signs occur in cerebral malaria:

1. **Symptoms:**
   - Fever, high grade, irregular.
   - Convulsions—generalised, common among children. Adults rarely have convulsions.
   - Disturbance in consciousness lapsing into coma.
   - Petechial haemorrhage in skin and mucous membrane occur rarely.
   - Haemetemesis presumably from stress ulcerations or acute gastric erosions can occur.
2. **Signs:**
   - Pulse rate is fast (tachycardia).
   - BP may be low (hypotension) to normal.
   - *Neurological manifestations* include *signs of meningism* (passive resistance to head flexion) but not of meningitis, *divergent eyeballs* and *pout reflex* are common.

Box 1   WHO criteria for severe falciparum malaria

- Cerebral malaria (unexplained unarousable coma)
- Severe anaemia (Hb <5 g/dl or haematocrit <15%)
- Renal failure (oliguria—urine output <400 ml/day or <12 ml/kg/day plus serum creatinine >3 mg/dl or 265 µmol/L)
- Noncardiogenic pulmonary oedema (ARDS, hypoxaemia, respiratory failure)
- Hypoglycaemia (whole blood glucose <40 mg/dl or 2.2 mmol/L)
- Circulatory collapse (systolic BP <70 mmHg with cold clammy extremities)
- Spontaneous bleeding, DIC (prolonged PT, PTT) and thrombocytopaenia
- Repeated generalised convulsions (>3 in 24 hours)
- Acidaemia (arterial pH <7.25) or acidosis (plasma bicarbonate <15 mmol/L)
- Haemoglobinuria (not drug induced)
- Jaundice (icterus or serum bilirubin >3 mg/dl)
- Hyperparasitaemia (>5% in nonimmune patients or >10,000/ml)

Other primitive reflexes are absent. Corneal reflexes are preserved except in deep coma. The pupils are normal and react to light. Motor system examination reveals variable muscle tone and deep tendon reflex are usually brisk and the plantar reflexes are usually extensor (UMN signs) but at times flexor. The superficial reflexes (abdominal and cremasteric) are absent. In advanced stages of the disease, there may be generalised hypertonia, opisthotonus and abnormal (flexor or extensor) posturing in the form of decerebrate or decorticate rigidity.

- *Associated other signs;* such as severe anaemia, hemolytic jaundice, acidotic breathing, bleeding due to DIC, tachypnoea and tachycardia (due to ARDS) and/or oliguria (due to acute renal failure).
- Hepatosplenomegaly.

Diagnosis and Investigations

Diagnosis of cerebral malaria depends on the clinical manifestations (already discussed), the severity of falciparum infection to be decided by WHO criteria and confirmation of the diagnosis is done by demonstration of asexual forms (ring stage in case of falciparum) of the parasite in thick and thin of peripheral blood.

Blood test: There may be anaemia, thrombocytopaenia, leucopaenia (pancytopaenia). The ESR, C-reactive protein levels are high. The PT and aPTTK may be prolonged. Blood urea and creatinine raised if ARF develops. There may be metabolic acidosis and electrolytes may be abnormal.

Giemsa stained smear: Single film is diagnostic in infected individual but in nonimmune individuals with low parasitaemia, smear should be repeated after 8–24 hours. The parasite load or degree of parasitaemia is seen in thin film as percentage of infected red cells in PBF. Immunochromatographic *'dipstick or card test'* tests for *P. falciparum* antigen in finger-prick blood samples are now available for detection of this infection. They should be used in parallel with blood film examination but are less sensitive than a carefully examined blood film. Other tests are done to detect complications. Hypoglycaemia is common.

Serological Tests

Serological tests such as PCR are not useful for diagnosis of acute infection because in immune populations PCR has limited value because of subclinical infection. It is more sensitive than microscopy and other tests. It is useful in identifying asymptomatic infections as control and eradication programs drive has no value in the diagnosis of acute illness.

Management

Severe malaria is a medical emergency and cerebral malaria is the common presentation and cause of death in adults. The management of severe malaria or cerebral malaria includes:
1. Early appropriate antimalarial therapy.
2. Active treatment of complications or severe manifestations.
3. Correction of fluid, electrolyte and acid-base disturbances.

4. Avoidance of harmful ancillary treatments.
5. Supportive measures and care of unconscious patient.
1. **Appropriate antimalarial therapy:** *Artesunate/artemether* is the drug of choice for falciparum infection everywhere.

As per WHO and in India and some other areas, the Chinese drugs derived from artemisinin (*artemether, artesunate*) have become first-line treatment for severe malaria as controlled trials in Asia have shown superior efficacy of parenteral artesunate over quinine. In quinine-resistant cases, the artesunate or artemether is drug of choice. Artesunate should be given as a loading dose of 2.4 mg/kg I.V. every 12 hourly for one day then daily for 3 days. Artemether dose is 3.2 mg/kg (loading dose) I.M. stat then 1.6 mg/kg I.M. daily. A rectal formulation of artesunate has been developed for patients in rural tropics who can not take oral medicines. Mefloquine should not be used for severe malaria as no parenteral formulation is available.

Quinine is as effective as artesunate, is being used worldwide due to less cost and easy availability. It is used alternatively if artesunate is promptly not available. Intravenous quinine in 10% dextrose is given as an infusion of 20 mg/kg over a period of 4 hours as a loading dose, followed by 10 mg/kg after every 8 hours till patient regains consciousness and starts accepting orally. Oral therapy (10 mg/kg after every 8 hours) to be given as soon as patient can take orally and be continued for total of 10 days including parenteral therapy. The loading dose should not be given if the patient has received quinine outside during the previous 24 hours. Tinnitus, nystagmus and ECG changes (prolonged QRS duration and QTc interval) should be looked for especially in the cardiac patients; and the dose of quinine reduced if these are present. Blood glucose should be monitored every 4–6 hours and 5–10%

Table 29.1 Management of complications/manifestations of falciparum infection

Lesion/Pathogenesis	Manifestations	Treatment
• **Coma** (cerebral malaria). Unarousable coma as a result of heavy parasitisation of cerebral vessels	• Coma persisting >30 minutes after generalised convulsion.	• Maintain patent airway • Exclude other causes of coma (e.g. hypoglycaemia, bacterial meningitis) • Nursing care in the side position • Care of skin, bowel, bladder • Monitor pulse and BP
• **Hypoglycaemia.** It occurs due to failure of hepatic gluconeogenesis and consumption of glucose by both the host and the parasite	• Plasma glucose <40 mg%	• Measure blood glucose • Give 25–50% glucose injection stat followed by 10% glucose infusion
• **Hyperpyrexia** (heavy parasitaemia with destruction of all types of RBCs releasing malarial toxins)	• Fever >41.5°C	• Parenteral antipyretic • Cold sponging, fanning etc.
• **Convulsions** (common in children, rare in adults, occurs due to heavy cerebral vessels parasitaemia)		• Parenteral diazepam or phenobarbitone • Maintain patent airway
• **Severe anaemia and thrombocytopenia** (due to destruction of RBCs and ineffective erythropoiesis)	• Hb<5 g% and PCV <15% with parasitaemia <10,000/ml	• Transfuse fresh whole blood, packed cells, platelet concentrates
• **Acute pulmonary oedema** (noncardiogenic) Pathogenesis unclear. The condition is aggrevated by vigerous administration of I.V. fluid.	• X-ray chest reveals bilateral hilar haze	• Prop up position • Give O_2, diuretics • Stop I.V. fluids • Intubate and add PEEP/CPAP in life-threatening hypoxaemia • Haemofiltration
• **Acute renal failure** (acute tubular necrosis). It is due to erythrocytes sequestration and agglutination interfering with the microcirculation of kidneys and its metabolism.	• Rise in blood urea and nitrogen	• Exclude pre-renal cause • Check fluid balance and urinary sodium • Give diuretics and dopamine if urine output falls • Peritoneal dialysis, haemofiltration or haemodialysis if available. Consider exchange transfusion for high parasitaemia (>5 to 10%)
• **Spontaneous bleeding and DIC** (coagulation abnormalities, thromboxytopaenia, DIC contributes to bleeding). Haematemesis is common.	• Bleeding from gums, nose, petechiae are evidences of DIC	• Transfuse fresh whole blood/cryoprecipitate/fresh frozen plasma and platelets if available • Injection vitamin K
• **Metabolic acidosis.** It occurs due to accumulation of organic acids, lactic acid. Renal impairment, hypoglycaemia contribute to it.	• Arterial pH <7.25. Bicarbonate <15 mmol/L Lactate level >5 mmol/L	• Exclude or treat hypoglycaemia, hypovolaemia and gram-negative septicaemia • Give O_2. Consider sodium bicarbonate for severe acidosis
• **Shock** (fluid loss, perspiration and gram-negative infection)	• BP <50 mmHg in children and <80 mmHg in adults.	• Consider gram-negative septicaemia • Take blood cultures • Give parenteral antibiotics

Contd.

Table 29.1 Management of complications/manifestations of falciparum infection (*Contd.*)

Lesion/Pathogenesis	Manifestations	Treatment
• Aspiration pneumonia (common due to aspiration during obtunded consciousness)	• X-ray chest may reveal opacity/ opacities	• Correct haemodynamic disturbances • Monitor pulse, BP, urine output • Take X-ray • Give parenteral antibiotics • Change posture • Physiotherapy • O$_2$ inhalation • Consider exchange transfusion
• Heavy parasitaemia, e.g >15% of circulating erythrocytes in a patient with malaria		

glucose coadministered to decrease the likelyhood of hypoglycaemia.

2. **Severe manifestations and complications on falciparum malaria** are to be actively treated as given in Table 29.1.

3. **Maintenance of fluid, electrolyte and acid-base balance:** Intravenous fluids are given to replace fluid loss. If hypotension or shock present, saline should be given. 25% dextrose to be given in case hypoglycaemia develops. *Blood transfusion* to correct severe hemolytic anaemia and *sodium bicarbonate* for metabolic acidosis may be needed. Blood sugar, pH and electrolytes are to be monitored. As soon as patient accepts fluid, oral therapy should be instituted.

4. **Avoidance of ancillary treatments** such as corticosteroid, decongestive therapy, low molecular dextran, heparin and adrenaline should be avoided as they have been proved of no value, and even may be harmful.

5. **Care of unconscious patient:** Place the patient on his/her side. Care of the skin, bowel and bladder should be taken. Frequent change of position, self-retaining catheter to measure urinary output and maintenance of pulse, BP and temperature chart should be undertaken.

Radical cure and chemoprophylaxis of malaria: Read antimalarial drugs.

Pyrexia of Unknown Origin (PUO)

PYREXIA OF UNKNOWN ORIGIN (PUO)

A clinical problem in practice is the patient who has pyrexia (fever) either intermittent or continuous that lasts for one week or more and in whom routine investigations fail to reveal the cause. PUO may be a manifestation of diseases of diverse origin (tuberculosis, endocarditis, gall bladder disease, HIV or opportunistic infections). The important causes of PUO are given in Box 2.

Categories of PUO

1. **Hospital associated PUO:** It refers to hospitalised patients of fever of 38.3° C or higher on several occasions in whom initial cultures are negative and the diagnosis remains unknown after 3 days of investigations.

2. **Neutropenic PUO:** It refers to fever of 38.3°C or higher on several occasions in neutropenic patients with less than 500 neutraphils/µL in whom initial cultures are negative and diagnosis remains uncertain after 3 days.

3. **HIV-associated fever:** It pertains to HIV-positive patients with fever of 31.5°C or higher who have been febrile for 4 weeks or more in whom the diagnosis remains uncertain after 3 days of investigations.

Box 1   Some important causes of PUO

1. Infection
- Pyogenic abscess (liver, kidney, brain, bone, subdiaphragmatic pelvis)
- Tuberculosis
- Urinary tract infection, bone infection
- Biliary tract infection (cholangitis)
- Subacute infective endocarditis
- CMV and EBV infection
- Q fever
- Typhoid
- Malaria
- Brucellosis
- Toxoplasmosis
- Leishmania
- Thyroiditis
- Thrombophlebitis

2. Malignancy
- Lymphomas (Hodgkin and non-Hodgkin)
- Leukaemia, multiple myeloma
- Solid tumours (renal, liver and pancreas)
- Atrial myxoma

3. Immunological
- Connective tissue and autoimmune disorders, e.g. rheumatoid arthritis, SLE, polyarthritis nodosa, Giant cell arteritis, polymyalgia rheumatica
- Drugs (drug fever)
- Sarcoidosis, Mediterranean fever
- Inflammatory bowel disease

4. Factitious
- Switching thermometers
- Injection of pyrogenic material

5. Undiagnosed PUO

4. **Fever after organ transplant** and **fever in the returning traveller** are of common concern.

Evaluation and Investigations

The evaluation of pyrexia of unknown origin is given in Box 2.

Age is a common denominator since infection is common cause of PUO in neonates, children and young adults, though no age is immune to infection. Cancer and connective tissue disorders are more common in elderly. Immunocompromised persons are susceptible to infectious diseases than nonimmunocompromised persons and often present with unusual spectrum of infection. In adults over 65 yrs of age giant cell arteritis, palymyalgia, rhumatica, temporal arteritis, sarcoidosis, RA account for 25–30% of all PUO.

Duration of fever: The cause of PUO changes dramatically in patients who have been febrile for 6 months or longer.

- Infection, cancer and autoimmune disorders combined account for only 20% cases of PUO. Granulomatins disease (hepatitis, Crohn's disease, ulcerative colitis and factitions fever) became important causes.
- 25% patients who admit fever for 6 months of longer actually have no fever or underlying disease. Instead, they experience normal circadian variations in temperature (0.5–1.0°C higher in the afternoon than in the morning).
- Patients who experience episodic or recurrent fever (who meet the criter for PUO but have fever-free periods of 2 weeks or longer) are similar to those with prolonged fever. Infection, malignancy and autoimmune disorder account for only 20–25% of such fever whereas various miscellaneous disease i.e. crohn's disease, familial mediterrannean fever, allergic alveolitis account for another 25%. About 50% cases still in this category remain undiagnosed but have benign course with eventual resolution of fever.

Box 2   Evaluation of PUO
1. Repeat the history, especially for:
• Contact with source of infection (tuberculosis) or animals (brucellosis) • Sexual contacts   • Travel outside the country • Occupation   • Drug intake • Recent surgery or dental treatment (abscess or endocarditis)
2. Repeat examination
• Heart examination for changing murmurs or new murmurs (endocarditis) • Spleen enlargement (typhoid, malaria, kala azar) • Lymph nodes (infectious mononucleosis, reticulosis, HIV, syphillis, tuberculosis)
3. Review the investigations and order them a fresh, if needed
• Re-examine the chest X-ray, if need be repeat it, if there is suspicion of minimal lesion • Biochemical results abnormal (liver involvement) • Haematological results abnormal (leukaemia, lymphoma, etc.) • Microbiological results abnormal (pyuria, e.g. tuberculosis, gonorrhoea, UTI) • Echocardiogram (endocarditis atrial myxoma)
4. Investigate the patient further if there is no clue on routine investigations
• Serological investigations (typhoid, brucella) • CT/MRI scanning (for abdominal/thorax lymph nodes, tumours). USG, upper GI studies • Tissue biopsies (histology and culture for tuberculosis, malignancy)
5. Empirical therapeutic trial as a last resort
• Antitubercular drugs (cryptic miliary tuberculosis) • Corticosteroids (connective tissue disease)

Immunological Status

1. In neutropenic pateints, fungal infections and occult bacterial infections are common causes of PUO.
2. In patients taking immunosuppressive medications, particularly organ transplant patients, CMV infections and fungal infections, nocardiosis *Pneumocystitis pneumiae* and mycobacterial infections are common causes.

A patient with PUO needs aggressive approach to reach at some diagnosis. A specifice diagnosis will influence management and result in curative treatment. It is always worthwhile to repeat the history and examination as new signs may have evolved since admission of the patient to the hospital. The drug therapy should be reassessed and, if possible, stopped.

Clinical Findings

- First of all it is imperative to document the presence of fever. This is done by observing the patient while the temperature is being taken to ascertain that fever is not factitious.
- Note the associated features that accompany fever, i.e. chills, tachycardia, perspiration and piloerection.
- Take a through history including family, occupational, social (sexual and drugs intake), dietary exposure (unpasteurised products, raw meat), exposure to animal, chemicals and travel history may give clues to the diagnosis.
- **Physical examination** include examination of heart, lungs, reticuloendothelial system (liver, spleen, lymph nodes) which can be repeated frequently along with history (Box 2)

Laboratory Tests

The addition to routine laboratory studies (*complete hemogram, urine, blood biochemistry*) *blood cultures* should always be obtained preferably when the patient has not taken antibiotics for several days and should be withheld for 2 weeks to detect slow growing organisms. Culture for special media are requested if *Legionella, bartonella* or *nutritionally deficient streptococi* are suspected pathogens. *'Screening tests'* with *immunologic* or *microbiologic serologies* should not be done. When a specific diagnosis is suggested then specific serological tests corresponding to the diagnosis should be performed for rise and fall in antibody titre.

In addition to blood cultures, other body fluids should be cultured such as *urine, sputum, CSF, stool, morning gastric aspirates* (for tuberculosis). **Direct smear of blood examination** may establish a diagnosis of malaria or relapsing fever. Frequent review of investigations should be dne and order them afresh, if needed (Box 2).

Imaging Studies

All patients with PUO should have a *chest X-ray*. Studies such as *sinus CT, upper GI studies* with *small bowel follow through, sigmoidoscopy, barium enaema* should be reserved for patients who have symptoms, signs or a history suggestive of involvement of these body regions. *CT Scan of abdomen* and *pelvis* is useful for looking at occult lesion access in the liver spleen and retroperitoneum. The role of *MRI* is limited. It is better than CT in diagnosis of CNS disorders and vasculitis. USG is useful to detect lesions of kidney, pancreas and biliary tract. *Echocardogram* should be done if one is suspecting endocarditis or atrial myxoma. The usefulness of *radionuclide studies* in diagnosis PUO is variable. *Indium labelled immunoglobulin* may prove to be useful in detecting infection and neoplasm and can be used in neutropenic patients.

Biopsy

Any abnormal finding should be aggresively evaluated. Headache requires **CSF examination** to rule-out and meningitis. **Skin biopsy** should be done for cutaneous lesions. **Enlarged lymph nodes** should be aspirated or biopsied for neoplams and sent for culture. **Bone marrow aspiration with biopsy** is useful for detecting mycobacterial infection especially in HIV patients.

MANAGEMENT OF PUO

The protocol for treatment is depicted in Table 30.1.

1. Record/monitor vital signs, urine output.
2. Use on antipyretic for fever.
3. Maintain nutrition and proper hydration.

Although it is tempting to begin an empiric course of antimicrobials covering both

Table 30.1 Protocol for treatment of pyrexia

1. At admission

Order the following investigations immediately before embarking on treatment.

- **Blood film** (thin and thick) for malaria; repeat, if negative
- **Total and differential leucocyte counts.**
- **Blood culture** (repeated thrice, if initial negative), if patient is on antibiotics, bone marrow culture is advised. *Culture of urine*, *throat swab* and *stool* if diarrhoea (cholera suspected).
- **Liver function tests.**
- **Urine** for blood, proteins, sugar and microscopic examination.
- **Store serum for serology.**
- Start treatment on clinical grounds in those conditions, where either there is no confirmatory test (e.g. tick typhus) or where delay is unjustified (malaria).

2. Over next three dyas

- Daily examine the patient and review the physical signs and investigations done.
- Treat the infection diagnosed.

3. After three days

- Reassess, if getting better; wait and watch, if not. Repeat the initial tests.

- Now consider *X-ray chest*, *ultrasound abdomen*.
- **Consider serology** for EB virus, HIV, dengue, rickettsia, toxoplasma, entamoeba, schistosomiasis on the basis of clinical and epidemiological situation.
- Now consider treatment on the clinical grounds alone if there is no clue on examination. If the patient is getting worse and clinical picture suggests typhoid, treat it accordingly.

4. After 10 days

- Consider for other *chronic infection* (e.g. tuberculosis, brucellosis, HIV, leishmaniasis)
- Consider *non-infectious cause of fever*
- Obtain a second opinion.

gram-positive, gram-negative and anaerobes organisms but it is rarely helpful and may delay the diagnosis if aetiology is infectious by reducing the sensitivity of blood cultures.

Empiric administration of corticosteroids should also be discouraged because they can suppress fever and excerbate many infectious disease.

Treatment should be diagnosis-specific once the diagnosis is made.

Emergencies in Cardiology

- Acute ST-Elevation Myocardial Infarction (STEMI)
- Cardiogenic Shock
- Shock or Acute Circulatory Failure
- Heart Failure (HF)
- Left Ventricular Failure (Acute Cardiogenic Pulmonary Oedema)
- Management of Tachyarrhythmias
- Management of Bradyarrhythmias and Stokes-Adams Attacks
- Acute Coronary Syndrome (ACS)
- Cardiac Tamponade
- Acute Chest Pain
- Cardiac Arrest and Sudden Cardiac Death
- Hypertensive Emergencies or Urgencies

Acute ST-Elevation Myocardial Infarction (STEMI)

ACUTE ST-ELEVATION MYOCARDIAL INFARCTION (STEMI)

Definition

Myocardial infarction is characterised by acute cardiac pain due to sudden and complete occlusion of a coronary artery due to thrombus. The thrombus is formed at the site of rupture of an atheromatous plaque in a coronary artery. Rarely AMI may also result from prolonged vasospasm, inadequate myocardial blood flow (e.g. hypotension) or excessive metabolic demand, embolic occlusion and vasculitis. Cocaine is a cause of infarction in young persons without risk factors. The present hospital mortality of AMI is 6.5% which is significantly decreased from prethrombolytic era. Spontaneous thrombolysis can occur but takes time, and by this time, the damage has already occurred, therefore, induced thrombolysis (revascularisation) is the mainstay of treatment nowadays. The myocardial infarction is more common in those having one or more risk factors enumerated in Box 1.

Clinical Features

The myocardial infarction is characterised by *typical anginal pain at rest* (Fig. 31.1) which is more severe and prolonged, radiates to left arm or to other sites and is associated with signs and symptoms of sympathetic overactivity

Box 1	Risk factors for AMI
• Age (old age)	• Smoking, alcohol
• Sex (males are more prone)	• Mental stress/ psychosocial factors
• Family history	• Obesity (abdominal, metabolic syndrome)
• Hypertension	
• Hypercholestrolaemia (hyperlipidemia)	• Polyunsaturated fatty acid deficiency
• Diabetes mellitus	• Sedentary habits/ physical inactivity
• Hyperfibrinogenaemia and hyperhomocysteinaemia	
• Low levels of antioxidant vitamins (too low consumption of fruits and vegetables)	
• Low levels of protein C and S	• Elevated high sensitivity CRP (hsCRP)

i.e. *sweating*, *feel weak* and *apprehensive*. They may have associated symptoms, e.g. *vomiting*, *dyspnoea* etc. About 25% of AMI may have atypical symptoms such as atypical chest pain, nausea, vomiting, dyspnoea, fatigue, exhaustion, etc. Myocardial infarction may also be painless, masquerade as the development or worsening of CHF, appearance of an arrhythmia (more common in anterior MI), an overwhelming sense of apprehension, profound exhaustion, acute indigestion, pericarditis, stroke or peripheral embolism.

The symptoms and signs are given in Box 2. About 50% of AMI patients die before they arrive at hospital. The cause of death is cardiac arrest due to ventricular fibrillation.

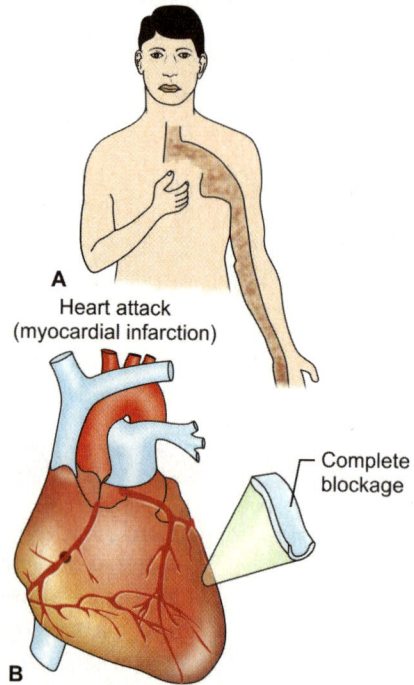

A
Heart attack
(myocardial infarction)

Complete
blockage

B

Fig. 31.1: (A) A patient of acute MI showing character of pain by thrusting the fist into anterior chest at the site of pain and radiation of pain to left arm and forearm, (B) coronary angiogram showing coronary occlusion (diagram)—a common cause of acute MI.

Diagnosis

It is very important to examine the patient of acute myocardial infarction before embarking on the treatment. The diagnosis of MI suspected clinically must be confirmed by ECG (Fig. 31.2). Cardiac markers (CPK-MB), troponin I and T, LV global or regional ischemia on echocardiography, imaging studies (MRI with gadolinium contrast enhancement Tc^{99m} pyrophosphate scintigraphy help in the diagnosis).

Management

It is divided under three heads:
1. Management of uncomplicated AMI:
   • Pre-hospital management.
   • In-hospital management.
2. Management of complications of AMI.
3. Secondary prevention of infarction.

Box 2	Myocardial infarction

A. Symptoms

i. Prolonged and severe retrosternal chest pain radiating to left arm, throat, shoulder, epigastrium and back. Most infarction pain occur at rest and early morning hours
ii. Anxiety, fear, apprehension of impending death. Patient move about in the bed seeking a position of comfort
iii. Nausea, vomiting, sweating, feeling of weakness
iv. Dyspnoea, orthopnoea, cough
v. Giddiness or syncope or collapse
vi. Painless infarction occurs in one-third patients especially in older women and diabetics

B. Signs

i. *Signs of sympathetic overactivity* usually present, e.g. pallor, perspiration, tachycardia
ii. *Signs of vagal stimulation* may be present as in inferior wall infarction, e.g. bradycardia
iii. *Signs of myocardial dysfunction* and/or left heart failure may be evident if complicated:
   • Cold extremities, hypotension or shock or fall in BP in patients with hypertension
   • Oliguria
   • Low volume pulse, low pulse pressure, an arrhythmia (e.g. UPCs)
   • Quiet first heart sound
   • Diffuse apical thrust. Mid-systolic murmur of papillary muscles dysfunction may be present
   • Fine crackles at the bases, respiratory distress, and S$_3$ gallop.
iv. *Signs of tissue damage*, e.g. fever, leucocytosis and raised ESR
v. *Heart examination*, e.g. pericardial rub may be present. Mid-systolic or pansystolic murmur due to mitral regurgitation or papillary muscle dysfunction are not uncommon. Soft heart sounds and atrial gallop (S$_4$) is common than ventricular gallop (S$_3$).

I. Management of Uncomplicated AMI (Fig. 31.3)

Pre-hospital management

Most out-of-hospital deaths from MI are due to development of arrhythmias (particularly ventricular fibrillation). Out of these, 50% occur in first one hour. Therefore, the major steps in management of suspected AMI in developed countries include:

  i. Recognition of the symptoms by the patient,
 ii. Rapid deployment of an equipped emergency ambulance to provide advanced cardiac life support.
iii. Expeditious transportation of the patient to a hospital.

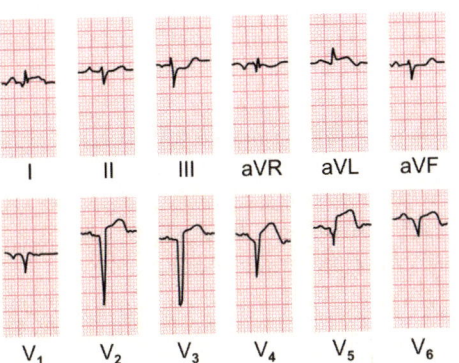

Fig. 31.2: Acute anterior myocardial infarction. The EGG showing ST-elevation, QS pattern from V2–V6 and leads I and aVL. T-wave is dragged up.

Pre-hospital treatment includes
 a. Routine measures.
 b. Aspirin.
 c. Nitrates.
 d. Thrombolysis.
 a. *Routine immediate measures include:*
   • High-flow O$_2$.
   • I.V. access.
   • ECG monitoring and a 12-lead ECG.
   • Nitroglycerine (0.3 mg) or isosorbide dinitrate (5 mg) sublingual to be given to relieve pain before morphine. The dose can be repeated at 5 minutes interval up to 3–4 doses. If no relief occurs after 15 minutes, patient should be hospitalised.
   • Analgesia (opiates) and an antiemetic—Adequate analgesia is essential not only to relieve severe distress, but also to lower adrenergic drive and thereby reduce pulmonary and systemic vascular resistance. Intravenous morphine 10 mg and an antiemetic (prochlorperazine 12.5 mg or cyclizine 50 mg) should be

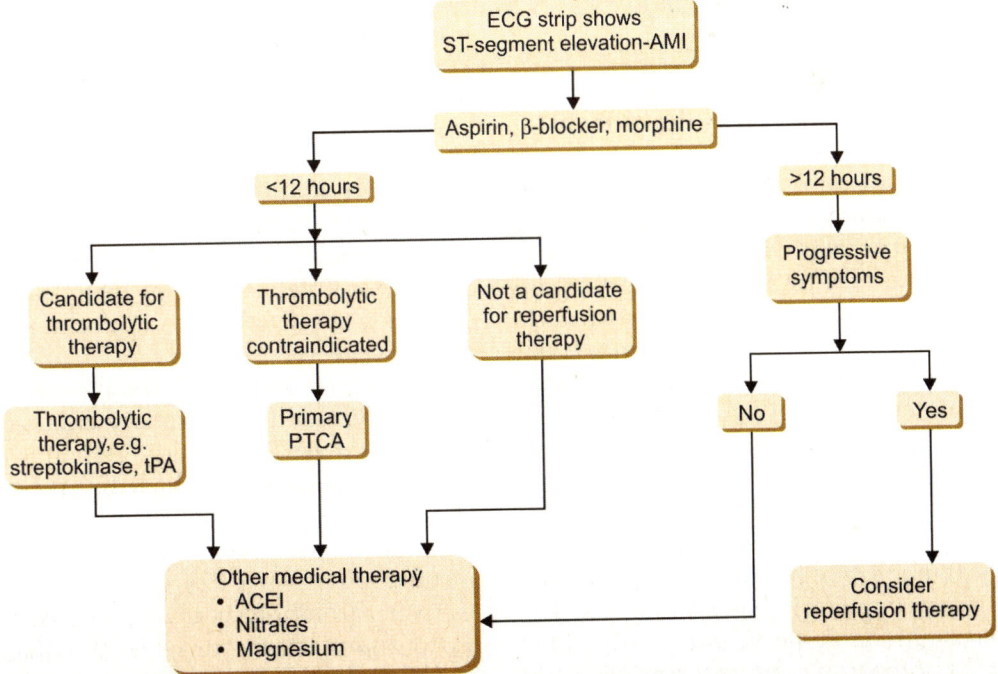

Fig. 31.3: Algorithm for management of ST segment elevation myocardial infarction (STEMI).

given stat through a cannula and to be titrated according to the response.

b. *Aspirin:* Oral administration of 75–310 mg of aspirin daily improves survival by 25% on its own, hence, is called *'poor man's,* streptokinase' and enhances the effect of thrombolytic therapy. The first tablet of 310 mg to be given in a soluble or chewable form and then daily dose should be continued indefinitely if there are no contraindications. Clopidogrel in combination with aspirin is more beneficial, should be given to all patients with STEMI. Prasugrel (P 2Y12 inhibitor) is considered to be superior to clopidogrel. It is given 60 mg orally on day first then 10 mg daily. It is contraindicated in patients with history of stroke or who are older than 75 years.

c. *Acute reperfusion by thrombolysis:* Earlier the thrombolysis, better the prognosis and the maximum benefit is achieved when it is given, within first 1–2 hours. So, if possible, thrombolysis can be done out-of-hospital in a well-equipped ambulance by the trained staff.

In-hospital Management

A. **Accidental and emergency department**

1. *Routine measures include* bed-rest, O_2 therapy, administration of analgesia and intravenous nitroglycerin if pain or ST-segment elevation persists. Before morphine is administered, sublingual nitroglycerin (0.3 mg) or isosorbide dinitrate (5 mg) can be given if not taken already. Up to 3–4 doses at an interval of 5 minutes can be given. Nitrates reduce myocardial O_2 demand (reduce preload) and increase myocardial O_2 uptake (by dilating the infarct-related artery or collateral vessels). If response occurs, nitroglycerin infusion (0.6–1.2 mg/hr) is given to relieve ongoing ischaemia diagnosed by persistent chest pain. Nitrates are avoided in hypotension and inferior or right ventricular infarction.

2. *Intravenous beta-blockers:* They are useful in the control of the pain of AMI by reducing myocardial O_2 demand and hence ischaemia. Most important, there is evidence that I.V. beta-blockers reduce in-hospital mortality. A commonly employed regimen is I.V. metoprolol 5 mg every 2 to 5 minutes or atenolol 5 mg given over 5 minutes for a total of 3 doses provided the patient has heart rate >60/min and BP >100 mmHg and P-R interval <0.24 seconds. 15 minutes after the last dose, an oral regimen consisting of 50 mg 6 hourly for 48 hours followed by 100 mg after every 12 hours may be started. However, the Chinese COMMIT/CCS-2 trial found no overall benefit to I.V. followed by oral metoprolol.

Avoid beta-blockers if there is heart failure, heart block or severe bradycardia.

Unlike beta-blockers, calcium channel blockers are of little help in AMI, rather they may be detrimental.

3. Aspirin (75–310 mg/day) and/or clopidogrel 75 mg/day if not given already. *Dual antiplatelet therapy:* In patients with an acute coronary syndrome, dual antiplatelet therapy is indicated for 1 year in all patients (including those with medical therapy and those patients undergoing revascularisation irrespective of stent type (drug eluting or bare metal stents) Dual antiplatelet therapy includes aspirin plus P 2Y12 inhibitor, e.g. clopidogrel, prasugreel).

4. *Primary percutaneous coronary intervention (PCI):* Immediate coronary angiography and primary PCI including stenting of the infarct related artery have been shown to be superior to thrombolysis if performed within 90 minutes called *'door-to-balloon'* time. Otherwise PCI is generally preferred over thrombolysis in opening occluded coronary arteries or when the diagnosis is in doubt or cardiogenic shock is present.

Bivalirudin, a direct thrombin inhibitor or glycoprotein IIb/IIIa inhibitors specifically abciximab have been shown to reduce major thrombotic events when added to heparin for patients undergoing PCI.

Facilitated PCI where a combination of fibrinolytic agent with or without glycoprotein IIb/IIIa inhibitor is given followed by PCI is not recommended. Patients treated with fibrinolytic therapy appear to have improved outcome if transferred for routine coronary angioplasty and PCI within 24 hours.

Thrombolysis or fibrinolysis: Coronary thrombolysis preferably done within 3 hours (door-to-needle time) helps to restore coronary patency, preserves left ventricular function and improves survival. Mortality related benefit is maximum if window period is less than 6 hours. Beyond a period of 12 hours, there is no rationale for administration of thrombolytic therapy. Between 6 and 12 hours it has been realised that it may be beneficial in those selected patients who have on-going chest pain and persistent ST-segment elevation of at least 1 mm in at least two contiguous leads on ECG.

> *The benefit of thrombolysis is more in anterior myocardial infarction, non-diabetic patients and younger subjects (< 55 years of age).*

The thrombolytic agents i.e. tissue plasminogen activator (tPA), streptokinase and anisoylated plasminogen streptokinase activator complex (APSAC) have been approved by PDA for intravenous use in acute MI. These drugs act by promoting the conversion of plasminogen to plasmin which lyse the fibrin clot (fibrinolysis). The principal goal is prompt restoration of coronary arterial patency (TIMI-grade 3 flow).

Streptokinase 1.5 million units (7,50,000 units over 20 minutes and 7,50,000 units over next 40 minutes in 100 ml of saline given as an IV infusion over a period of one hour, is a widely used regimen. It is cheap but antigenic and occasionally causes serious allergic reaction. The drug may cause hypotension, which can often be managed by stopping the infusion and restarting at a slower rate. Being antigenic, it induces antibodies which can render subsequent infusions of streptokinase ineffective, so it is advisable to use another non-antigenic agent if the patient requires further thrombolysis in future. The summary of thrombolytic therapy is given in Box 3.

Box 3	Streptokinase therapy

- *Maximum benefit* is achieved when administered within few hours (<6 hours) of infarction with ST-segment elevation in more than 2 leads without Q-waves.
- *Thrombolysis* is not beneficial in patients with ST-segment depression and even may be harmful.
- *Parameters of success of thrombolysis* include:
  - Relief of pain.
  - Significant reduction (>70%) or complete resolution of elevated ST-segment.
  - Transient arrhythmias, e.g. idioventricular rhythm.
  - Reinfarction or reocclusion is indicated by recurrence of pain and ST-elevation during hospital stay, is treated by readministration of a thrombolytic agent or immediate PCI.
- *The drawback and disadvantage of thrombolytic* therapy include stroke (1%), bleeding (7%) and re-infarction (5%), allergic reactions (<2%) and hypotension (<5%).

Note: It is less effective in opening occluded arteries and also less effective in reducing mortality than tenecteplase.

Alteplase (human tissue plasminogen activator or tPA) is a genetically engineered drug, which is not antigenic but is more expensive than streptokinase. It seldom causes hypotension. It results in 50% reduction in circulating fibrinogen.

Many ICU use tPA or tenectephase/reteplase if streptokinase is contraindicated but there is evidence that it produces better survival rates than streptokinase.

The standard regimen of tPA given over 90 minutes includes bolus dose of 15 mg, followed by 0.75 mg/kg but not exceeding 50 mg over 31 minutes and then 0.5 mg/kg but not exceeding 35 mg over 60 minutes.

Tenecteplase (TNK-t PA) and *Reteplase* (rPA) are fibrin specific and more effective than alteplase in restoring full reperfusion, i.e. TIMI grade 3 coronary blood flows. They are referred as bolus fibrinolytics since their administration does not require infusion.

- Tenecteplace is given as single weight adjusted bolus 0.5 mg/kg
- Reteplase is given as 10 units as bolus over 2 minutes, repeated after 31 minutes

The contraindications of thrombolytic therapy includes:

a. Active internal bleeding.
b. Previous subarachnoid or intracerebral bleed or stroke or CVA within one year.
c. Uncontrolled hypertension (BP >180/110 mmHg at presentation).
d. Recent surgery (within 1 month).
e. Recent trauma (within 2–4 weeks).
f. Suspicion of active peptic ulcer.
g. Pregnancy.
h. Bleeding diathesis.
i. Diabetic retinopathy.
j. Suspicion of aortic dissection.
k. Current use of anticoagulants (INR more than 2–3)

5. *Heparin and thrombolysis:* Administration of aspirin and heparin (4000 U Stat followed by 1000 U/hr), then adjusted to PTI) after thrombolysis with streptokinase or tenecteplase has an added advantage to prevent reinfarction. However, heparin should perhaps be continued for 24–48 hours, when tPA is given as a thrombolytic agent.

The low molecular heparin *enoxaparin* 310 mg I.V. bolus and 1 mg/kg every 12 hours can be used alternative to unfractionated heparin. *Fondaparine* 2.5 mg S.C. daily is also useful.

Prophylactic treatment with proton-pump inhibitors or antacids and an H_2-blocker is recommended in all patients with STEMI treated with intensive antithrombotic therapy.

B. **Management in coronary care units**

These units are routinely equipped with a system of continuous ECG monitoring of each patient and haemodynamic monitoring of selected patients. Facilities of advanced life support, pacemaker and pacing catheters and flow-directed balloon tipped catheters are also available in addition to staff trained in the management of various aspects of AMI.

Patients should be admitted to a coronary care unit (CCU) early in their illness so that they can derive maximum benefit during the critical phase of infarction. The duration of stay in coronary care unit depends on the need for intensive monitoring. Patients in whom AMI have been ruled out should be shifted out of coronary care units after 8–12 hours of observation. Similarly patients with confirmed infarction who are considered to be at low risk (no prior infarction and no persistent chest pain or no complication and haemodynamically stable) may be safely shifted out of CCU within 24–36 hours.

Note: Antiarrhythmic prophylaxis with lidocaine infusion is not recommended.

Steps of Management in CCU

- *General measures:* Record the pre-hospital treatment given. Coronary care monitoring should be instituted as early as possible.
  1. *Bed-rest* for first 12 hours is necessary in acute infarction. However, in the absence of complications, patient can resume an upright posture on bed within first 24 hours followed by sitting in a chair. Provided no complication occurs, patient can be made ambulatory in the room by the third day with

increasing duration and frequency of movements. By day 4 to 5 after infarction, patient should be increasing their ambulation progressively to a goal of 600 feet at least 3 times a day.

Low flow O_2 therapy (2–4 L/min) should be given if O_2 saturation is reduced.

2. *Diet:* Patient should receive either nothing or only clear fluids by mouth during first 6 to 12 hours. During first 4–5 days, a low caloric diet, low in sodium, high in K^+ and magnesium divided into multiple small frequent meals is advisable.

3. *Analgesia and sedation:* Morphine 4–8 mg should be given to relieve pain followed by small doses at frequent intervals. Most patients require sedation in CCU in order to withstand the period of enforced inactivity with tranquillity. Diazepam (5 mg) or lorazepam (0.5 to 2 mg 3 to 4 times a day is effective. Appropriate sleeping medication may be given at night to ensure to dream free sleep. It should be given for few days.

4. *Bowels:* Constipation is a problem and occurs due to prolonged rest and use of opiates. Most patients are not comfortable using a bed pan, which frequently results in straining during defecation. A bedside commode, a fibre-rich diet, routine use of stool softener or a laxative are recommended.

5. *Other drugs (pharmacotherapy):* Several drugs are important in routine treatment of AMI. They need to be started early but may not be required on an emergency basis.

   i. *Beta-blockers:* They reduce both short and long-term mortality, hence, to be started as early as possible after AMI if there is no contraindication (such as heart failure, left ventricular dysfunction, heart block, orthostatic hypotension or a history of asthma). They are also given after PCI and stenting.

   ii. *Angiotensin converting enzyme inhibitor (ACEI):* Now there is convincing evidence that ACEIs have additive advantages in reducing mortality in addition to those achieved with aspirin and beta-blockers. The mechanism of action is to reduce ventricular remodeling after infarction so as to reduce the subsequent risk of CHF. Hence, recent recommendation is to start ACEI therapy in all patients of AMI with EF <40% or with large infarction within 24–48 hours, continue it during hospital phase and reassess after 4–6 weeks later to decide whether or not to continue for long-term benefits.

   iii. *Calcium channel blockers:* Current practice is not to use calcium channel blockers routinely after AMI as they have been shown to increase mortality rates.

   iv. *Nitrates:* They are beneficial in limiting the infarct size and may be used for this reason in addition to aspirin and thrombolysis. They have been shown to have added advantage over aspirin and thrombolysis. They are, otherwise, indicated in the presence of angina and heart failure (to decrease preload).

   v. *Glucose-insulin-potassium, magnesium infusion:* Though some small studies have shown benefits, but it is difficult to justify the routine use unless a large trial shows conclusive benefit. However, ISIS-IV trial has shown no benefit of such therapy.

   vi. *Long term antithrombotic therapy* (heparin and anti-platelet agents) is continued for few days and then heparin is stopped. Patient is discharged on aspirin. Patient who have received a coronary stent should also received dual antiplatelet therapy (aspirin plus clopidogrel).

vii. *Rescue angioplasty:* For patients who fail to reperfuse (<50% resolution in ST elevation) should undergo rescue angioplasty. Similarly patients with recurrent ischemic pain should undergo catheterisation, and, if indicated, perform revascularisation.

II. Treatment of Complications of STEMI

Treatment of complications of STEMI is given in Table 31.1.

Table 31.1 Treatment of complications of STEMI

Complication	Corrective measures
I. Hypotension may result due to one or more causes	• Find out the cause and treat it accordingly. • Drugs like nitrates, beta blockers and ACEI should either be stopped or their dose is reduced. • I.V. fluids and inotropic support if required. • If hypotension is due to rhythm disturbances, then correct arrhythmia. • Cardiogenic shock due to CHF is most serious cause of hypotension and also a marker of poor prognosis. Treat it urgently (read cardiogenic shock as an emergency).
II. Arrhythmia and conduction disturbance	
i. VPCs	• Find out the cause and treat it accordingly. • VPCS may be asymptomatic but some forms of VPCs are markers of poor prognosis, hence, to be treated with either beta-blockers or amiodarone.
ii. VT	• Correction of aggravating factors such as ischaemia, electrolyte disturbance. • Antiarrhythmics like lidocaine (1 mg/kg bolus), amiodarone (150 mg over 10 minutes, may be repeated if needed followed by 360 mg over 6 hours and 540 mg over 18 hours). • DC shock (100–200J) • VT occurring after 48 hours of AMI need long-term amiodarone or AICD implantation, while occurring within 48 hours does not require such a measure.
iii. VF	• Primary VF (occurring within 24 hours) does not alter long-term prognosis but requires immediate defibrillation (300J) • Resistant VF may require bretylium or amiodarone followed by repeat cardioversion while CPR is being carried out • Late VF is associated with an adverse long-term outcome and may recur, hence, use of AICD is recommended in such cases.
iv. Complete heart block (occurs in 5 to 15% cases)	• Complete heart block with idioventricular rhythm originating from infranodal or bundle of His (escape rhythm >45/min) is common and may respond to atropine. If not responding to atropine, temporary pacing may be required. • When escape rhythm originates below the bundle of His (15–45/ min), it requires an immediate pacing. • If complete heart block is persistent and irreversible, then a permanent pacemaker is indicated.
v. Ventricular dysfunction	• Ventricular remodelling soon occurs after MI. • ACE I should be prescribed in patients with EF <40% regardless of whether or not CHF is present.
vi. Pump failure	• Monitor LV filling pressure (PCWP). • Fluid or diuretic therapy depending on the LV filling pressure. • Adjust the vasopressor/vasodilator therapy depending on PCWP.

The common arrhythmias in acute MI are give in Box 4.

III. Secondary Prophylaxis (Secondary Prevention of Infarction)

- Control of risk factors and life-style modifications.
- Drug therapy such as betablockers and aspirin to be continued for life or for 5–7 years of infarction. Nitrates can be used for long-term if there is angina, left ventricular dysfunction, thrombus or recurrent sustained VT/SVT or AF.
- Revascularisation either by PTCA and adjuvant techniques like stenting, atherectomy, laser and rotablation is required in selected cases. Coronary artery bypass surgery may be required in few selected patients depending on the findings of stress-testing and angiography (e.g. left main coronary artery disease).

Box 4 Common arrhythmias in AMI

Ventricular	Atrial
• Ventricular premature complexes (VPCs)	• Atrial tachycardia
	• Sinus tachycardia or PSVT
• Accelerated idioventricular rhythm	• Atrial fibrillation
• Ventricular tachycardia	• Sinus bradycardia, heart blocks especially in inferior wall infarction
• Ventricular fibrillation	

Cardiogenic Shock

CARDIOGENIC SHOCK

Definition

Cardiogenic shock is a state of acute circulatory failure resulting from severe depression of cardiac functions (*systolic and diastolic*) leading to tissue hypoperfusion and hypoxaemia, which may become irreversible if not promptly corrected.

Criteria of Cardiogenic Shock

1. *Systolic BP <90 Hg or >60 mm fall below baseline level.*
2. *Cardiac index* <2.2 L/min/m². It is calculated by cardiac output divided by body surface area. Normal cardiac index is 2.6–4.2 (L/min) m².
3. *Left ventricular filling pressure* or pulmonary capillary wedge pressure >18 mmHg; and pulmonary oedema is usually present.

Transthoracic echocardiography (TTE): It is a noninvasive technique, provides same informations as PCWP and CVP. It also differentiates hypovolaemic shock (LV filling pressure is low but contractility is preserved) from cardiogenic shock (LV filling pressure is high but contractility is low/decreases)

These haemodynamic parameters with clinical evidence of peripheral circulatory failure (e.g. altered mental state, cold clammy skin and oliguria with urine output <20 ml/hr) constitute clinical syndrome of Cardiogenic shock.

Causes

They are:
1. **Following myocardial infarction**
   i. Involvement of critical muscle mass (>40%) and /or refractory arrhythmias (80%).
   ii. *Mechanical complications of AMI*
      - Acute mitral regurgitation due to rupture of papillary muscle or chordae tendineae of 6–7%.
      - Acquired ventricular septal defect (3–4%).
      - LV free wall rupture/tamponade.
      - Ventricular aneurysm.
2. **Severe valvular lesions**
   - Severe aortic (stenosis/regurgitation) or mitral (stenosis/regurgitation) valve disease.
   - Left ventricular outflow tract obstruction
   - Obstructive cardiomyopathy.
3. **Extracardiac obstructive causes**
   - Pericardial effusion with tamponade (1–1.5% cases).
   - Massive pulmonary embolism.
   - Severe pulmonary hypertension (primary or Eisenmenger).
   - Severe restrictive cardiomyopathy.

4. **Inflammatory/infectious myocardial disease**
   - Severe myocarditis.
   - Acute endocarditis with myopathic or valvular involvement.
5. **Severe myocardial depression**
   - Septic shock.
   - Acidosis or alkalosis.
   - Hypoxia.
   - Drugs, e.g. beta-blockers, calcium channel blockers, anaesthetics and anti-arrhythmics.
   - Post-cardiac arrest, post-cardiotomy
6. **End stage of myocardial disease**
   - Dilated cardiomyopathy.
7. **Traumatic,** e.g. pericardial, myocardial or valvular injuries.

Clinical Features and their Pathogenesis (Fig. 32.1)

Irrespective of the cause of cardiogenic shock, it is characterised by a vicious circle of severe myocardial (systolic and diastolic) dysfunction (Fig. 32.1). **Systolic dysfunction** results in fall in cardiac output, BP and thereby coronary perfusion pressure falls. Hypotension, oliguria, confusion or altered mental state, tachypnoea, tachycardia and cold, clammy extremities are the manifestations of low output state or acute circulatory failure.

Diastolic dysfunction on the other side of cycle causes a rise in CVP, left ventricular end-diastolic pressure, rise in PCWP, pulmonary congestion and oedema, leading to hypoxia which further worsens the myocardial ischaemia. Breathlessness, orthopnoea, PND, cyanosis, cough, haemoptysis, hypoxia, perspiration and *inspiratory crackles* at the bases of the lungs, and S3 and S4 gallops are features of acute pulmonary oedema.

A systemic inflammatory response syndrome (SIRS) may accompany large infarctions and shock. Inflammatory cytokines and excess nitric oxide may contribute to genesis of cardiogenic shock. Severe acidosis (lactic acidosis) reduces the efficacy of catecholaminers and provoke arrhythmias.

A Swan-Ganz catheter can be used to measure the pulmonary artery wedge pressure which is >18 mmHg.

Untreated or refractory shock leads to multiple organ dysfunction, e.g. heart, brain, lungs, kidneys and liver.

Older patients mostly females, prior MI, diabetes and extensive anterior MI (EF <30%) are at increased risk of cardiogenic shock.

Diagnosis

It is based on the evidence of:
1. **Clinical features (Fig. 30.1):** The features of acute circulatory failure combined with features of the cause of cardiogenic shock occur. These patients have dyspnoea appear pale, apprehensive, diaphoretic, confused and agitated. Sensorium may be altered. The pulse is weak/feeble and rapid (tachycardia) or slow (bradycardia/brady-arrhythmia/heart blocks). The systolic BP is reduced (<90 mmHg) with narrow pulse pressure (< 30 mmHg). Tachypnoea and Cheyne-Stokes breathing and raised jugular venous pressure may be present.

   Cardiovascular findings may include a weak apical impulse, quiet precordium, feeble heart sounds and an S_3 gallop. Murmurs of severe MR and of septal/tendinal rupture may be audible. Rales are audible with wheezing in most of the patients. Oliguria is common.

2. **Haemodynamic parameters:** It includes BP <80 mm of Hg, cardiac index <1.8 L/min/m² and pulmonary capillary wedge pressure >18 mmHg. EF is usually <30% on TTE (Transthoracic echocardiography).

Differential Diagnosis

It is based on the cause of cardiogenic shock.
- **Acute MI** is diagnosed by cardiac pain, typical ECG changes and raised cardiac enzymes. Echocardiography will give

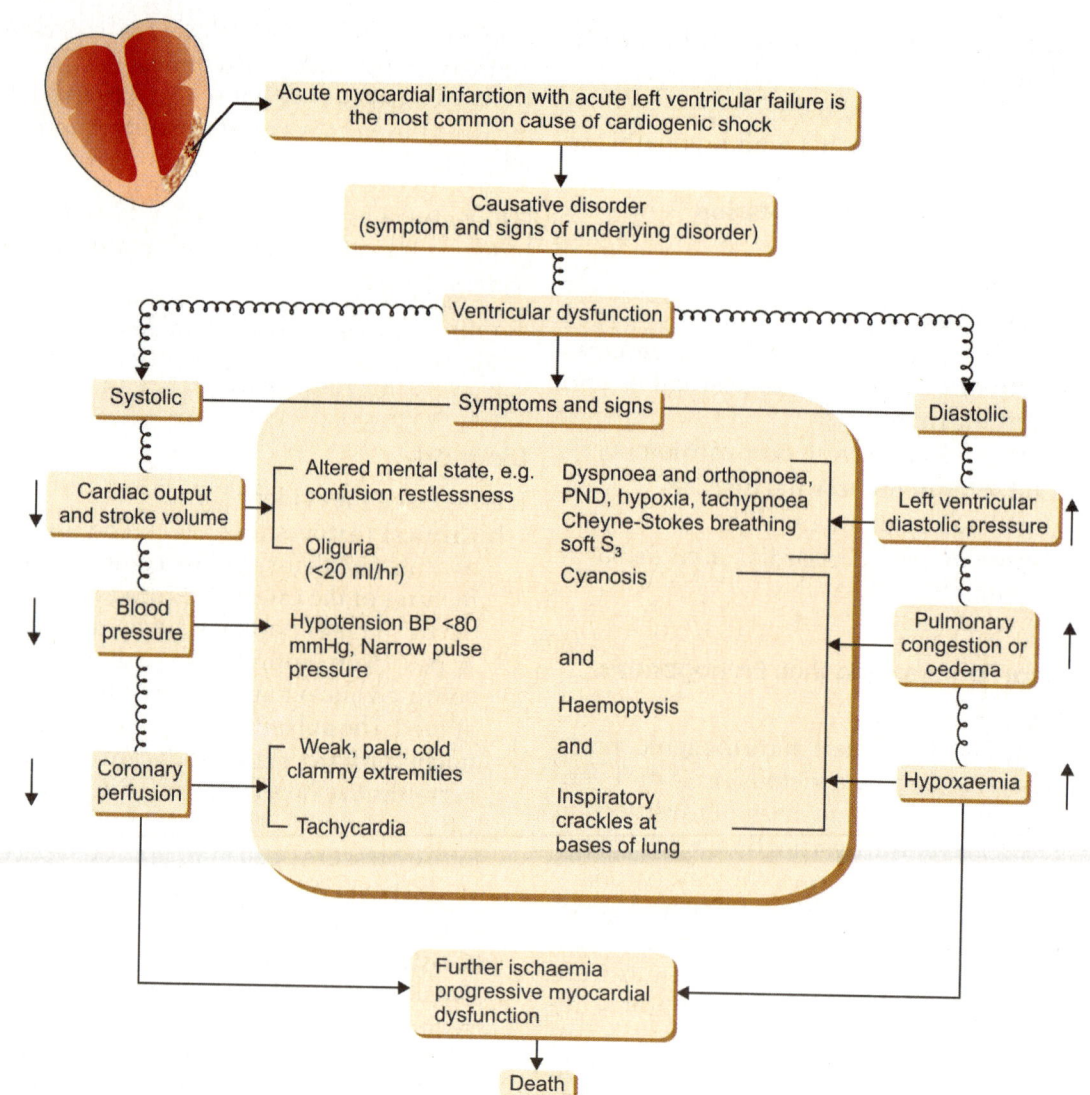

Fig. 32.1: Cardiogenic shock. The clinical features and their pathogenesis. The systolic dysfunction leads to fall in cardiac output, BP and coronary perfusion; while diastolic dysfunction causes pulmonary congestion and hypoxaemia.

estimate of extent of myocardial damage and is useful to detect mechanical complications such as acute MR and VSD.

- *Valvular heart lesions* are diagnosed by clinical features, echocardiography and cardiac catheterisation.
- *Cardiac tamponade* presents with raised JVP, pulsus paradoxus X-ray chest for

pericardial effusion and echocardiography.

- *Massive pulmonary embolism* with shock. Echocardiography may demonstrate a small vigorous left ventricle with dilated right ventricle. Sometimes a thrombus in right ventricular outflow tract may also be seen. Spiral CT confirms the diagnosis, which is nowadays preferred over ventilation perfusion scan and pulmonary angiography.

- *Myocarditis* is diagnosed by systemic illness supported by identification of the virus and endomyocardial biopsy can be used for confirmation.
- *Aortic dissection* presents with classical tearing or stabbing pain with pulse deficit, acute AR and neurological manifestations. Echocardiography confirms the diagnosis.

Investigations:

- *Routine blood tests* and *kidney function tests.*
- *ECG* and *cardiac enzymes* may point to myocardial infarction. Cardiac markers, i.e. troponins (I and T) are elevated.
- *X-ray chest* may show signs of pulmonary oedema. Heart size is usually enlarged with bilateral hilar haze.
- *Arterial blood gas analysis* may show hypoxaemia, metabolic acidosis, may be compensated by respiratory alkalosis.
- *Echocardiogram* will show depressed LV functions, and helps to find out the cause, e.g. left to right shunt (Doppler study) due to rupture of interventricular septum, pericardial effusion, aortic dissection, etc.
- *Measurement of pulmonary capillary wedge pressure (PCWP)* and *cardiac output* by pulmonary artery catheterisation to confirm the diagnosis and to optimize treatment (fluids and vaso-pressure).
- *Left heart catheterisation* and *coronary angiography to measure LV pressure and to define coronary anatomy.*

Management

The management is divided into:
- General principles of management of shock.
- Specific measures.

General Management

The major goals are:
i. To recognise the condition as early as possible and to correct the initial insult so as to maintain adequate tissue perfusion and preservation of vital functions.
ii. To find out and treat the underlying cause.

The steps of initial management include:
- Whenever possible, patient should be treated in ICU.
- ECG monitoring to assess heart rate and rhythm and for prompt diagnosis of arrhythmias.
- Monitoring of clinical parameters, i.e. heart rate, rhythm, BP, cerebral function, skin temperature and urine output.
- Measure blood gases and correct hypoxaemia (O_2 therapy).
- Consider intubation if $PaCO_2$ is >6.5 kPa, respiratory rate >25/min and impaired consciousness (glasgow coma scale < 7).
- Correct acidaemia with I.V. bicarbonate if pH < 7.20 and $PaCO_2$ <6 kPa.
- Correct hyperglycaemia, if present, with insulin.
- Measure CVP (off ventilator): If CVP < +6 mmHg from mid-axillary line, give volume challenge (250 ml of normal saline or colloid). If CVP >+6 mmHg or poor ventricular function, use 100 ml of fluid only as a challenge and consider the insertion of PA catheter to direct further treatment with fluids and vasoactive drugs and to monitor the response to treatment.

Specific Measures

They are directed depending on the cause:

A. Cardiogenic shock due to AMI

In addition to the usual treatment of acute AMI, initial therapy is aimed at maintaining adequate perfusion and left ventricular filling pressure.

1. *Relief of pain and anxiety:* Pain should be relieved with judicious use of morphine

or pethidine sulphate; but may be given cautiously as they may reduce BP.

2. *Oxygen inhalation and ventilatory support:* O₂ inhalation should be delivered through nasal catheters at a rate of 5–10 L/min to relieve hypoxaemia and maintain O₂ saturation beyond 90%. Ventilatory support may be needed if there is severe hypoxaemia leading to acute respiratory acidosis or there is failure to achieve adequate oxygenation with high flow system.

3. *Fluid therapy:* Hypovolaemia though uncommon, may be ruled out by assessing the pulmonary capillary wedge pressure (PCWP) which is normal or elevated in AMI with cardiogenic shock. The initial fluid therapy depending on the CVP has been described under general measure, i.e. if CVP < +6 mmHg, 250 ml of saline be given and if >+6 mm then 100 ml of fluid is given, the further fluid therapy is guided by monitoring of pulse, BP, urine output and CVP/PCWP. Maintenance fluid therapy is given daily under CVP monitoring to keep LV filling pressure adequate.

4. *Emergency reperfusion and revascularisation:* If patient is seen within first 4 to 8 hours of the onset of infarction, early reperfusion either by PTCA or CABG (coronary artery bypass graft) may reduce infarct size and improve LV function and thereby reduce the mortality rate in AMI (mortality was reduced in **SHOCK** trial). Thus, for hospitals without revascularisation facilities, a strategy of early TT and intra-aortic balloon pumping (IABP) followed by an early transfer for PTCA or CABG may be appropriate.

5. *Treatment of an arrhythmia:* Sustained VT in a patient with haemodynamic instability or VF, must be treated with DC shock and I.V. bolus lidocaine 1–2 mg/kg followed by an infusion at a rate of 1–2 mg/min.

6. *Vasoactive drugs:* A variety of intravenous vasoactive drugs may be used to augment arterial pressure and cardiac output in patients with cardiogenic shock. Inotropic drugs such as dopamine or dobutamine or combination improves haemodynamics (cardiac output and BP) in cardiogenic shock but does not improve hospital survival significantly.

- *Dopamine:* At moderate dose 2–5 µg/kg/min); it has both chronotropic (increase HR) and inotropic (increase contractility) effects as a consequence of beta-receptor stimulation. Intravenous dopamine is started at an infusion rate of 2–5 µg/kg/min and the dose is increased every 2 to 5 min to a maximum of 20–50 µg/kg/min.

- *Dobutamine:* It is a synthetic sympatho-mimetic amine with positive inotropic and minimal positive chronotropic effects and less peripheral vasocons-trictive action. It should not be used alone when vasoconstrictor effect is required. Therefore, it should not be used alone in cardiogenic shock to raise the BP, but be given simultaneously with dopamine infusion. The dose is 2–10 µg/kg/min.

- *Norepinephrine:* It is sympathomimetic amine, may be used to increase diastolic BP of 90 mmHg and to maintain coro-nary perfusion. Dose is 2–4 mg/min and titrated upwards as necessary.

- *Amrinone and milrinone* are phospho-diestrase inhibitors with both positive inotropic and vasodilator action. These drugs resemble dobutamine in their pharmacological action, but have a more potent vasodilator action. Both the drugs have longer half-live and can cause hypotension, so they are reserved for use when other agents have proven ineffective.

Other Mechanical Measures

- **Intra-aortic balloon pumping (IABP):** In cardiogenic shock, mechanical assistance with an intra-aortic balloon pumping capable of augmenting both diastolic pressure and cardiac output have been found useful in reducing the in-hospital mortality. This therapy is reserved for patients whose condition merits mechanical (surgical or angioplastic) intervention, i.e. in patients with acute mitral regurgitation or ventricular septal rupture. It is contraindicated in presence of aortic regurgitation or aortic dissection.

- Recently **venoarterial extracorporeal membrane oxygenation** (VA-ECMO, a pump in combination with oxygenator) device resulted in better haemodynamic support as compared to IABP.

- **Percutaneous cardiopulmonary bypass support:** It is used where intra-aortic balloon pumping is ineffective, for example, in patients with unstable rhythm, i.e. frequent VT/VF or those with severe LV dysfunction.

- **Hemopump** is a catheter mounted LV assist device which is capable of augmenting cardiac output and providing systemic perfusion without intrinsic LV function.

- **External ventricular assist device** such as pneumatically driven thoracic system can be used for intermediate terms (day or months) for support of either or both ventricles in refractory cases.

Treatment of complications of AMI:

1. *Intraventricular septum rupture:* Circulatory support by IABP and inotropic agents followed by surgical repair.
2. *Free wall rupture (pseudoaneurysm):* Pericardiocentesis to be done to relieve tamponade followed by coronary angiography and subsequent resection of necrotic and ruptured myocardium with primary reconstruction and CABG if required.
3. *Rupture of papillary muscle (acute MR):* Medical treatment (inotropic agent and IABP support) followed by surgical repair/ mitral valve replacement usually accompanied by coronary revascularisation.

B. Management of cardiogenic shock due to other causes

1. *Pericardial tamponade:* Only effective therapy is removal of pericardial fluid either by needle/catheter drainage or by surgery.
2. *Pulmonary embolism:* Read pulmonary embolism as an emergency). Massive pulmonary embolism with shock is treated with thrombolytic therapy, i.e. streptokinase 2.5 lac I.V. over 30 min as a loading dose followed by 1 lac unit/hr for 24–48 hours. Other options are suction embolectomy, mechanical fragmentation of the thrombus or surgical embolectomy with cardiopulmonary bypass.

Shock or Acute Circulatory Failure

33

SHOCK OR ACUTE CIRCULATORY FAILURE

Definition

It is a clinical syndrome of low cardiac output characterized by hypotension (systolic BP <90 mmHg and mean arterial pressure <60 mmHg, peripheral vasoconstriction, oliguria and impairment of consciousness. The basic underlying mechanism is low cardiac output followed by vasoconstriction and hypoperfusion of vital organs such as brain, lungs and kidneys. It is low cardiac out, low CVP and low pulmonary capillary wedge pressure shock.

Aetiopathogenesis and Classification

Adequate organ perfusion, depends on arterial pressure which is determined by cardiac output and peripheral vascular resistance. Normally when cardiac output falls, systemic peripheral resistance rises to maintain a systemic pressure to perfuse vital organs. Cardiac output is a product of stroke volume and heart rate. The stroke volume is dependent on *preload, afterload and myocardial contractility.* Hence, organ perfusion may be compromised by a decrease in cardiac output or its maldistribution. However, when mean arterial pressure falls to <60 mmHg organ dysfunction occurs.

Vascular resistance is proportional to length of vessel and viscosity of blood and inversely proportional to fourth power of the radius of the vessel, therefore, cross-sectional area of the vessel is major determinant of vessel resistance. Vascular resistance is regulated by arterial tone which depends on neural (sympathetic system), hormonal (adrenal) mechanisms and intrinsic or local factors (a variety of vasoconstrictor, e.g. endothelin-II, angiotensin-II) and O_2 free radicals and vasodilators, e.g. endothelial derived relaxation factor eicosanoids, etc. The balance between vasoconstrictive and vasodilatory factors determines local perfusion.

Microcirculatory failure is critical in pathogenesis of shock. Normal blood supply to an organ does not guarantee the fulfillment of adequate metabolic demands of all segments of that organ. Adhesion of leucocytes and platelets to the damaged or activated endothelium causes occlusion of microvasculature, activation of coagulation cascade and fibrin deposition (microthrombi) also contribute to vessel occlusion. Shunting of blood and decreased deformability of RBCs through vessel are also contributory factors for microcirculatory failure.

Microvascular flow depends on the balance between colloid osmotic pressure and capillary hydrostatic pressure, which, in turn, determines the balance between intra-vascular and extravascular fluid. Sympathetic stimulation decreases the capillary hydro-static pressure by constricting the precapil-lary resistance vessels, results in movement of fluid from the extravascular compartment to intravascular compartment. As severe tissue hypoxia and acidosis supervene, then this sympathetically mediated responses are overcome by metabolic vasodilatation and this response along with vasoconstriction can cause extravasation of fluid into interstitial space resulting in reduction of effective circu-latory volume. In addition, circulating toxins, adhesions of activated leucocytes can increase capillary permeability and further increase the tissue oedema. This process is increased by further loss of plasma proteins into the interstitium resulting in reduction of colloidal osmotic pressure, intravascular volume and tissue perfusion.

An aetiological classification of shock is given in Box 1.

The causes of acute circulatory failure are divided into two groups:

i. Those associated with low central venous pressure (CVP) such as hypovolaemic shock, anaphylaxis and septic shock.

ii. Those associated with raised central venous pressure such as cardiogenic shock, pulmonary embolism and cardiac tamponade.

Central venous pressure measurement (Fig. 33.2) before and during management of shock is mandatory.

Clinical Manifestations

Some symptoms and signs are similar for all types of shock, characterised by low cardiac output, hypotension (SBP <90 mmHg and MRP <60 mmHg) and low tissue perfusion (Fig. 33.1). They are enumerated in Box 2.

Other manifestations are specific to the type of shock. They are given in Table 33.1.

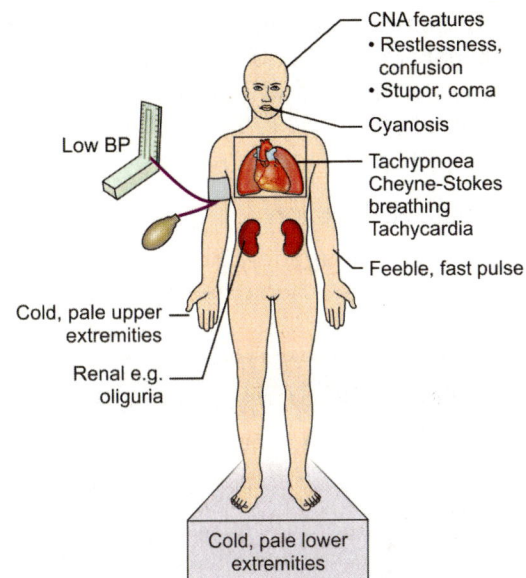

Fig. 33.1: Clinical features of shock syndrome

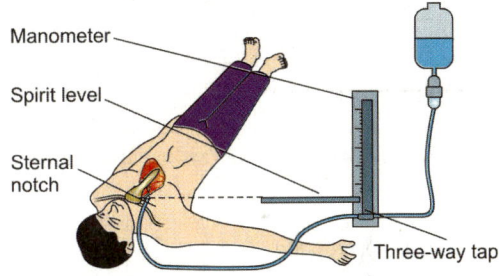

Fig. 33.2: Central venous pressure measurement using a manometer system. The reading must be referred to the level of the right atrium (indicated by the axillary fold or, provided the patient is supine, the sternal notch) using of spirit level.

Hypovolaemic Shock

It results from loss of fluids or blood resulting in hypovolaemia. The causes are given in Table 33.1. The cilinical features are given in Box 2 discussed below.

Mild hypovolaemia (≤ 20% of blood volume) produces only mild tachycardia with few external signs, i.e. cold extremities, diapho-resis, anxiety.

Moderate hypovolaemia (20–40% loss of blood volume)

• Patient becomes anxious, tachypnoic and tachycardiac in addition to above features.

- Normal BD maintained in supine position, but there may be signified postural hypotension, tochycardia and oliguria.

  Severe hypovolaemia, (>40% reduction in blood volume).

Diagnostic Evaluation

Shock is an emergency, needs full clinical assessment to understand the shock and target

Table 33.1   Symptoms and signs of specific forms of shock

1. **Cardiogenic shock** (symptoms or signs of heart disease will be present)

• Raised JVP	• Pulsus alternans, muffled heart sounds
• Gallop rhythm	
• Pulmonary oedema (tachypnoea, Cheyne-Stokes breathing)	• Basal crackles

2. **Hypovolaemic shock** (Box 1) (history of blood loss or fluid loss)

• Dehydration	• Haemoconcentration
• Extreme pallor	• Collapsed jugular veins

3. **Mechanical (compressive cardiogenic) shock**

- Elevated JVP, hypotension
- Pulsus paradoxus and muffled heart sound in cardiac tamponade
- Kussmaul's sign (JVP rises in inspiration) in cardiac tamponade
- Signs of pulmonary embolism (if present)

4. **Anaphylactic shock**

   i. Signs of profound vasodilatation
     • Warm extremities   • Low BP
  ii. Erythema, urticaria, angioedema, pallor, cyanosis
 iii. Bronchospasm
 iv. Oedema of face, pharynx, larynx
  v. Pulmonary oedema
 vi. Hypovolaemia due to capillary leak
vii. Nausea, vomiting, abdominal cramps, diarrhoea

5. **Septic shock**

- Pyrexia, rigors or hypothermia, tachypnoea
- Nausea, vomiting
- Warm extremities (vasodilatation)
- Bounding pulse, hypotension
- Other signs, e.g. jaundice, coagulopathy or coma

Box 1   Aetiologic classification of shock

1. **Hypovolaemic shock** (Low CVP; low PCWP, low cardiac output)

   - *Haemorrhage* (external or internal), loss of plasma (burns)
   - *Fluid loss* e.g. gastrointestinal (diarrhoea, vomiting); renal (diabetes mellitus, insipidus, and diuretics), and cutaneous (burn, perspiration)
   - *Internal sequestration* e.g. pancreatitis, acute intestinal obstruction, haemothorax, ascites, hemoperitoneum

2. **Cardiogenic shock:** (Read as a separate emergency) (raised CVP, raised PCWP low cardiac output)

3. **Obstructive shock** (extracardiac obstruction) (raised CVP, raised PCWP, low cardiac output)

   - Pulmonary embolism
   - Cardiac temponade
   - Cardiac tumor
   - Stenotic valvular heart disease (MS)
   - Tension pneumothorax
   - Dissecting aneurysm of aorta

4. **Distributive shock** (Low CVP, low PCWP, high cardiac output)

   - Septic shock
   - Anaphylaxis (type I hypersensitivity reaction)
   - Neurogenic shock
   - Endocrinal shock (e.g. Addisonian crisis, thyrotoxic crisis, myxoedema)
   - Anaesthesia
   - Ganglion-blocking drugs

Box 2   Clinical manifestations of hypovolaemic shock

1. **Cardiovascular**

   - Fast and feeble pulse   • Feeble heart sounds
   - Systolic BP <90 mmHg or a drop of >50 mmHg from the baseline in hypertensive patients and mean arterial pressure (MAP < 60 mmHg)

2. **Respiratory**

   - Tachypnoea   • Cyanosis
   - Cheyne-stokes breathing

3. **CNS**

   - Listlessness, restlessness   • Stupor and coma
   - Confusion, disorientation

4. **Renal**

   - Oliguria (urine output < 20 ml/hr)

5. **Skin**

   - Cold, pale extremities   • Perspiration

therapy to the cause. A practical approach is to make a clinical diagnosis based on the clinical features and a rapid diagnostic evaluation by specific diagnostic procedures directed towards determining the cause as well as severity of shock. Hypovolaemic shock can be readily diagnosed when there are signs of haemodynamic instability and the source of volume loss (fluid or blood) is obvious i.e. from nose, GI tract, kidneys.

Investigations

1. A complete haemogram and blood culture.
2. X-ray chest
3. ECG
4. Measurement of arterial blood gas.
5. Serum electrolytes (Na^+, K^+, Ca^{++}, Mg^{++})
6. Haemodynamic parameters such as central venous pressure (CVP—Fig. 31.2). A CVP <5 mmHg suggests hypovolaemia, pulmonary capillary wedge pressure (PCWP) and cardiac out (CO) are also low.

They are given in Box 3 in relation to specific shock.

Management of Hypovlaemic Shock

Goals of Treatment

1. To maintain adequate arterial BP above 90 mmHg to ensure adequate tissue perfusion.
2. Reduction of elevated serum lactate levels.
3. Specific therapy directed against the cause.

1. Initial Resuscitation

Delay in making the diagnosis and initiating treatment as well as inadequate resuscitation may lead to multiorgan failure, hence, must be avoided. The initial resuscitation includes:

- Procure intravenous line and start fluid administration unless the patient is in pulmonary oedema.
- Maintain patent airway, e.g. endotracheal tube may be inserted as it will prevent aspiration of the gastric contents.
- A Foley's catheter may be put to measure urine output.

Box 3	Haemodynamic changes in different types of shock			
Diagnosis	CVP	PCWP	CO	Systemic vascular resistance
Cardiogenic shock	↑↑	↑↑	↓↓	↑
Cardiac temponade (pericardial effusion)	↑	↑	↓ or ↓↓	↑
Pulmonary embolism	N or ↑	N or ↑	↓↓	↑
Hypovolaemic shock	↓↓	↓↓	↓↓	↑
Septic shock	↓ or N	↓ or N	↑ or N rarely ↓	↓
Anaphylactic shock	↓ or N	↓ or N	↑ or N	↓

↑↑ or ↓↓ designates moderate to severe increase or decrease

↑ or ↓ designates mild to moderate increase or decrease

- CVP is central venous pressure N means normal
- PCWP is pulmonary capillary wedge pressure
- CO is cardiac output

Blood volume is a critical factor in hypovolaemic shock hence 'fluid first' strategy to be adopted for all patients irrespective of aetiology.

2. Monitoring

Once initial resuscitation has been started, efforts should be made to find out the underlying cause and to recognise the pattern of shock by haemodynamic studies (already discussed). Based on the CVP, cardiac output and pulmonary capillary wedge pressure measurements, hypovolaemic shock can be defined. Monitor the following:

I. *Clinical parameters,* i.e. vitals, level of consciousness, urine output.

II. *Biochemical parameters,* i.e. blood urea, creatinine, blood lactate, haemoglobin, O_2 saturation, coagulation profile (platelets, PTI, PTTK)

III. *Haemodynamic monitoring* (CVP, cardiac output, PCWP).

3. Fluid Therapy

Fluid therapy is to restore adequate ventricular filling pressure to optimal levels promptly and adequately without inducing pulmonary oedema and compromising oxygenation. Volume replacement is mandatory in hypovolaemic shock.

In hypovolaemic shock (low CVP, low PCWP and low CO) the most important step is to replace fluids lost from the circulation quickly (in minutes or hours) to reduce tissue damage and to prevent acute renal failure. Fluid is administered through a wide-bore intravenous cannula to allow large amount to be given quickly and the effect is continuously monitored.

> *Care must be taken to prevent fluid overload with a risk of pulmonary oedema.*

Choice of fluid

Crystalloids either normal saline or Ringer's lactate are used for initial resuscitation for most forms of hypovolaemic shock. Patient may need several litres of crystalloid to replace fluid deficit. Colloids such as albumin or starch solution has been advocated after initial treatment with crystalloids to maintain colloid osmotic pressure. However, they are expensive and numerous studies have not revealed convincing results.

> *The goal of fluid therapy is to restore systolic BP above 80 mmHg in a previously normotensive person and CVP to be kept around 8–12 mmHg but should not exceed 18 mmHg, hematocrit of 30% and venous O_2 saturation on >70%.*

Initially, it matters a little whether isotonic, saline, blood or plasma are given, but when large amount of fluid is to be used then the nature of fluid lost should determine the nature of its replacement.

> *When large transfusions are needed rapidly, it is important to warm the fluid to body temperature before use.*

In haemorrhagic shock, if Hb is <10 g% the blood or packed RBCs are transfused to maintain haemoglobin concentration of 10 g/dl.

4. Vasopressor Agents

Following severe and/or prolonged hypovolaemia, vasoactive drugs dobutamine, dopamine, noradrenaline are employed in treatment of shock but only after restoration of blood volume. *Dopamine* or *dobutamine* are the inotropes of choice in most critically ill patients. Most patients respond to an infusion of dopamine 2.5–10 µg/kg/min. The combination of dopamine and noradrenaline is currently popular for the management of patients who are in shock with a low systemic resistance. Dobutamine is substituted to achieve an optimal cardiac output, once arterial pressure is restored while noradrenaline is used to restore an adequate BP by reducing vasodilatation. However, this combination can only be used safely when guided by full haemodynamic monitoring. *Large doses of steroids (hydrocortisone 400 mg 4–6 hourly)* have been used to restore the response to endogenous catecholamines and to retain salt along with water due to their salt-retaining properties.

5. Treatment of Precipitating Factors and Underlying Illness

Following immediate improvement of perfusion in patients with shock, efforts should be made to findout the cause and to treat it such as gastrointestinal haemorrhage, gastroenteritis, diabetic ketoacidosis or septicaemia. *Metabolic acidosis* is corrected by administration of sodabicarb to restore normal pH and serum electrolytes. Gram-negative septicaemia to be treated with appropriate antibiotic after culture and sensitivity. Tissue hypoxia is to be corrected by administration of 100% O_2 through nasal catheters.

6. Care of Other Systems

- To prevent acute tubular necrosis and acute renal failure, renal perfusion pressure must be maintained by adequate hydration. Acidosis and electrolyte disturbance must be corrected.
- To prevent the development of progressive hypoxia and subsequent development of *ARDS*, oxygen therapy should be given to maintain oxygen saturation more than 90%.

Mechanical ventilation may be required as respiratory support.
- Resuscitated patients are often coagulopathic due to deficient clotting factors in crystalloids and packed RBCs. Early administration of component therapy during massive transfusion improves survival. In extreme emergencies, type-specific or O-negative packed red cells may be transfused.

Heart Failure (HF)

34

Definition

Heart failure is designated term to describe a state when heart is not able to maintain its cardiac output (pump action) to meet the demands of the body despite normal venous return, or can do so only at the expense of raised filling pressures. It may be mild or severe. In mildest form, cardiac output is adequate at rest but becomes insufficient during stress or exercise. The **American Heart Association guidelines** define it as a complex clinical syndrome which results from structural or functional impairtment of ventricular filling or ejection of blood, which in turn leads to symptoms of dyspnoea, fatigue and signs of heart failure (HF) namely oedema and rales.

Pathophysiology

Cardiac output depends on (i) *preload,* (ii) *afterload* and (iii) *myocardial contractility.* The heart failure results due to interactions of these three basic mechanisms depending on the *Starling law of forces* which states that 'overstretching of the heart leads to deterioration of its functions'.

Heart failure is frequently, but not always caused by a defect in the myocardial contractions following an index event leading to a fall in cardiac output. The index event may be of abrupt onset such as AMI or insidious onset as a result of haemodynamic pressure or volume overloading or may be hereditary such as cardiomyopathies. The event activates counter- regulatory neurohormonal mechanisms such as:

i. *Activation of renin-angiotensin-aldosterone system.*

ii. *Sympathetic nervous system.*

At first, both these systems try to compensate normal cardiac function by altering the preload, afterload, and augmenting myocardial contractility. Later on, these mechanisms become counterproductive and often reduce cardiac output by increasing peripheral vascular resistance which further stimulates renin-angiotensin-aldosterone system other vasodilatory molecules and adrenergic system. Thus a vicious circle is set up in heart failure.

Retention of salt and water due to secondary hyperaldosteronism leads to development of peripheral oedema. In addition activation of certain vasodilatory molecules such as *atrial natriuretic peptide* (*ANP*) and *brain natriuretic peptide* (*BNP*), *prostoglandins* (*PGE$_2$ and PGI$_2$*) and *nitric oxide (NO)* try to overcome the excessive peripheral vascular resistance.

The failure of all compensatory mechanisms results in depressed ejection fraction resulting in systolic heart failure. Ejection fraction in diastolic heart failure remains preserved for longtime due to LV remodelling.

Heart failure may be *right sided* or *left sided* or *both*. *Left heart failure* due to elevated pulmonary pressure (pulmonary hypertension) can lead to *right heart failure*.

Causes

For management of congestive heart failure, it is important to identify the underlying cause of the heart disease and also the precipitating factors of heart failure. The causes are given in Table 34.1.

Table 34.1　Causes of a heart failure
1. Ventricular pressure overload
i. Left ventricular pressure overload • Systemic hypertension • Aortic stenosis
ii. Right ventricular pressure overload • Pulmonary hypertension (cor pulmonale) • Pulmonary stenosis
2. Disturbance in ventricular filling
• Mitral stenosis (left ventricular inflow obstruction) • Tricuspid stenosis (right ventricular inflow obstruction) • Endomyocardial fibrosis (stiff ventricles) • Constrictive pericarditis and pericardial effusion.
3. Ventricular volume overload
• Mitral regurgitation, mitral valve prolapse • Aortic regurgitation • ASD and VSD (Eisenmenger's syndrome and complex)
4. Depressed myocardial contractility
• Myocarditis • Cardiomyopathy • Myocardial ischaemia/infarction
5. High output states
• Thyrotoxicosis, beriberi, systemic arteriovenous shunting, chronic anaemia, pregnancy, Paget's disease

Precipitating Factors

A patient with compensated heart failure (impaired cardiac function without an overt heart failure) becomes decompensated with development of frank signs and symptoms of heart failure under the effect of acute illness such as an infection or development of an arrhythmia which jeopardies the ventricular function. Patients with chronic heart failure follow a remitting and relapsing course, with period of stability and episodes of decompensation leading to worsening of symptoms and repeated hospitalisation. The precipitating factors are summarised in Box 1.

BOX 1　Precipitating factors that aggravate CHF in patients with pre-existing heart disease
• Infection • Myocardial ischaemia or infarction • Thyrotoxicosis • Rheumatic and other forms of carditis • Pulmonary embolism • Inappropriate reduction or discontinuation of therapy for CHF • Anaemia • Arrhythmias (e.g. atrial fibrillation) • Pregnancy • Infective endocarditis • Drugs e.g. beta blockers, calcium channel blockers, NSAIDs, etc. • High sodium intake, blood transfusion, fluid overload, emotional stress, etc. • Uncontrolled HT.

Clinical Features

Most symptoms and signs are due to low cardiac output and congestion of viscera.

Symptoms

1. **Dyspnoea and orthopnoea:** Dyspnoea is the earliest symptom of CHF, occurs as a result of increased effort in breathing, first observed during strenuous exercise, then with progression of heart failure, it appears first with less exertion and then at rest. This is due to reduced compliance of the lung and increased cost of breathing. *Orthopnoea* (dyspnoea in recumbent position) occurs later than exertional dyspnoea. Patients with orthopnoea may elevate their heads on several pillows at night to get relief. Frequently, they feel short of breath and cough at night when their head slips off their pillow and disturb their sleep. The breathlessness is usually relieved by sitting upright since this position reduces venous

return and pulmonary venous congestion. In advanced heart failure, patient with orthopnoea cannot lie down at all and may spend the whole night in sitting position. On the other hand, long standing left heart failure may lead to right heart failure which relieves the pulmonary congestion and breathlessness (dyspnoea).

2. **Paroxysmal nocturnal dyspnoea (PND):** Attacks of breathlessness and coughing occur at night, usually awaken the patient from sleep and is not relieved by sitting position. The term *cardiac asthma* relates to PND is characterised by wheezes secondary to bronchospasm, hence, resembles bronchial asthma from which it has to be differentiated.

3. **Cough with or without expectoration and wheezing:** This is due to pulmonary congestion and oedema. The cough and wheezing accompany the dyspnoea, hence the term *cardiac asthma* is used.

4. **Cheyne-Stoke respiration:** It is periodic (cyclic) breathing in which periods of apnoea alternate with periods of hyperventilation. It is a sign of CHF, can also be seen in raised intracranial tension, respiratory failure and uraemia.

5. **Fatigue, weakness, poor effort tolerance:** These are nonspecific but common symptoms of heart failure, are related to low cardiac output with hypoperfusion of skeletal muscles.

6. **Oliguria and nocturia:** Oliguria is a sign of HF, occurs due to hypoperfusion of kidneys leading to acute renal failure. Nocturia is due to increased renal perfusion in recumbent position, results in excretion of fluid retained during the day. It is an early symptom.

7. **Cerebral symptoms:** Disturbed consciousness, confusion, impairment of memory, headache, insomnia, difficulty in concentration are due to low cerebral perfusion.

8. **Gastrointestinal symptoms,** e.g. nausea, vomiting, early satiety, abdominal pain and fullness. This is due to congestion of liver and intestines.

9. **Cardiac cachexia:** Severe chronic HF produces weight loss and cachexia.

Physical Signs (Fig. 34.1)

The **general physical examination** reveals, pallor, anxious look, cyanosis, anaemia and pitting oedema over legs, sacrum, abdominal wall. Jaundice may be present.

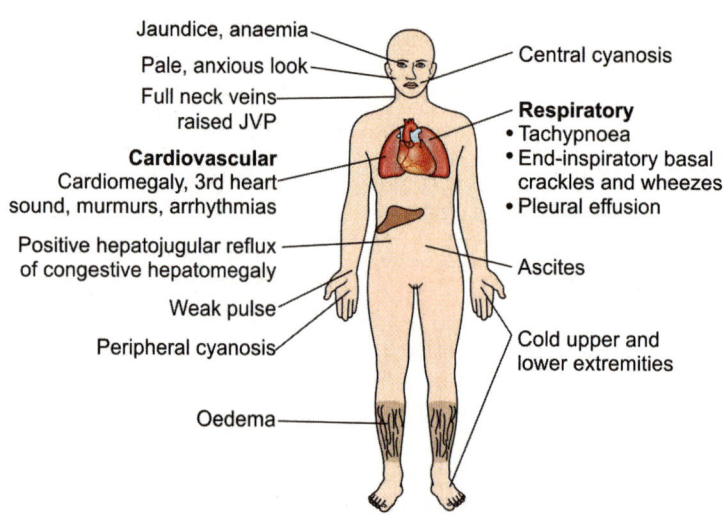

Jaundice, anaemia
Pale, anxious look
Full neck veins raised JVP
Cardiovascular
Cardiomegaly, 3rd heart sound, murmurs, arrhythmias
Positive hepatojugular reflux of congestive hepatomegaly
Weak pulse
Peripheral cyanosis
Oedema

Central cyanosis
Respiratory
• Tachypnoea
• End-inspiratory basal crackles and wheezes
• Pleural effusion
Ascites
Cold upper and lower extremities

Fig. 34.1: Physical signs of congestive heart failure

Neck veins are full and JVP is raised (Fig. 34.2). *Cardiovascular system examination* shows cardiomegaly, parasternal lift, sustained L.V. impulse, 3rd heart sound, murmurs, arrhythmia. **Respiratory system examination** reveals tachypnoea, end-inspiratory basal crackles and wheeze. Pleural effusion is seen in severe cases. *Abdominal examination* may reveal congestive hepatomegaly (tender liver) oedema and ascites.

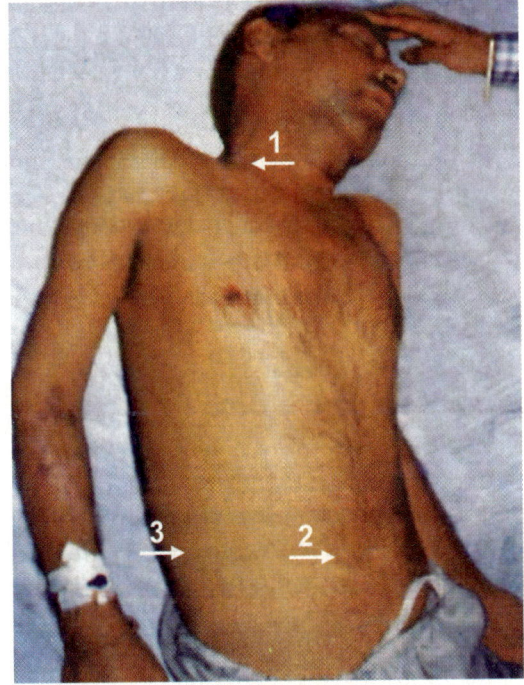

Fig. 34.2: Congestive cardiac failure in a 40-year-old male. (1) An arrow at the level of neck shows distended veins and raised JVP, (2) an arrow at abdomen indicates ascites, (3) an arrow at right hypochondrium indicates tender hepatomegaly, (4) pitting oedema at ankle and leg is not visible.

The **NYHA class of HF based on functional status** is categorised into:
- **Class I** (asymptomatic). Patient with cardiac disease but no symptom.
- **Class II** (symptomatic with moderate activity). Patients with cardiac disease are comfortable at rest and after mild activity, but moderate activity results in dyspnoea, palpitation and fatigue.

- **Class III** (symptomatic with mild activity). Patients with cardiac disease have marked limitation of physical activity. Less than normal activity results in fatigue, dyspnoea and palpitation.
- **Class IV** (symptomatic at rest). Patients are dyspnoic at rest, activity further increases the discomfort.

Diagnosis

The diagnosis of CHF may be established by observing some combinations of the clinical manifestations of heart failure together with findings characteristic of underlying heart disease and precipitating illness/factor. The *Framingham criteria* for diagnosis of CHF are given in Box 2. The functional class categorization by NYHA has already been discussed.

Box 2	Framingham criteria for diagnosis of CHF
Major	**Minor**
• Paroxysmal nocturnal dyspnoea	• Peripheral oedema
• Distended neck veins	• Nocturnal cough
• Rales	• Exertional dyspnoea
• Cardiomegaly	• Congestive hepatomegaly
• Acute pulmonary oedema	• Pleural effusion
• S3 gallop	• Reduced vital capacity by one-third
• Increased venous pressure (>16 cm H$_2$O)	• Tachycardia (HR >120 min)
• Positive hepatojugular reflux	• Weight loss

Δ *For diagnosis:* At least one major and two minor criteria are required.

Differential Diagnosis

HF has to differentiated from:
1. Acute renal failure with volume overload.
2. ARDS
3. Bronchial asthma (acute attack)
4. Angioneurotic oedema.

Investigations

These are done to establish the nature and severity of the disease and to detect complications.

1. **Electrocardiogram:** It will reveal ventricular hypertrophy, arrhythmias and myocardial ischaemia/infarction.
2. **Chest X-ray** will show enlargement of heart, peripheral lung congestion, presence of *Kerley's lines*, pulmonary oedema, hydrothorax, pulmonary hypertension, double atrial shadow in mitral valve disease and calcification of valves.
3. **Two-dimensional doppler echocardiography** is useful to detect unsuspected valvular lesion, assessing the chamber dimensions and ejection fraction (EF), left atrial myxoma and a thrombus or aneurysm or pericardial effusion. **Cardiac MRI** is now the gold standard for assessing LV mass and volumes as well as for determining the cause of HF (amyloidosis, cardiomyopathies, harmachesomatosis).
4. **Blood urea, creatinine and electrolytes** for renal failure and electrolyte disturbance.
5. **Biomarkers:** The circulating levels of brain natriuretic peptide (BNP) are elevated in CHF and it guides therapy in heart failure. A normal level of natriuretic peptide in untreated patients excludes the diagnosis of CHF hence, it differentiates dyspnoea due to heart failure from non-cardic causes. Other biomarkers, e.g. troponins (T and I), C-reactive protein, uric acid are also elevated. The newer biomarkers are soluble ST_2 and galactin-3.
6. **Cardiac catheterisation:** Left heart catheterization may be useful to define the presence or extent of CAD. Coronary angiography can also be performed.

Right ventricular catheterisation is done to monitor the therapy in refractory heart failure.

Management

Aims of Treatment

- Identification and removal of precipitating factor(s).
- Correction of underlying cause.
- Control of congestive state.

To control congestive heart failure, following measures are taken:

1. General measures.
2. Reduction of afterload on the heart.
3. Improvement of myocardial contractility.
4. Control of salt and water retention.

1. **General measures:** Patient is advised to stop smoking and limit the consumption of alcohol (two standard drinks/day). Extremes of temperature and heavy exercise are to be avoided. Avoid use of NSAIDs as far as possible. Hospitalisation of all severe cases is essential to control the heart failure as early as possible.
2. **Reduction of cardiac workload:** The heart size can be decreased by reducing physical activity or by enforcing rest at home or in the hospital for 1–2 weeks in patients with overt heart failure. Anxiety is to be relieved by anxiolytics and reassurance. Meals should be small. In many cases, bed rest and sedatives often result in effective diuresis.
3. **To improve myocardial contractility:**
   A. *Digitalis:* It is a cardiac glycoside, acts by increasing the force of contraction (positive inotropic action), delays conduction through AV node, slows the heart rate (negative chronotropic effect) and increases the excitability of heart, hence, is a proarrhythmic agent also.

   It is useful in CHF (grade III and IV) to improve ventricular emptying, i.e. it improves cardiac output, ejection fraction, reduces end-diastolic pressure, thus improves symptoms resulting from pulmonary vascular congestion. It is most beneficial in patients in whom myocardial contractility is impaired secondary to chronic ischaemic heart disease, hypertensive heart disease or when valvular or congenital heart disease imposes an excessive volume overload. It is not useful in CHF due to high output states (thyrotoxicosis, beriberi, cor pulmonale) or CHF due to stenotic valvular lesions or myocarditis. However, digoxin is used to slow ventricular rate in atrial fibrillation or to convert atrial fibrillation to atrial flutter due to any cause. Digital investigation group (DIG) trial though have found no benefit or harm with digitalis, hence, recommends its use in CHF in patients who remain symptomatic in spite of adequate volume control.

Dose and route: The digoxin is used orally in lower doses, i.e. 0.5 mg followed by oral maintenance dose 0.125 mg to 0.25 mg daily. In chronic heart failure, maintenance dose may be given thrice or 5 times a week.

Toxic effects: These occur due to large dose administration. Hypokalaemia, hypothyroidism, renal and hepatic failure potentiate digitalis effects as well as toxic effects. They are given in Box 3.

> *The clinical digoxin toxicity occurs when its serum level is >2.0 ng/ml.*

Treatment of digitalis toxicity if develops, includes its discontinuation along with diuretic and administration of potassium to treat hypokalaemia; and phenytoin or lidocaine for digitalis-induced arrhythmias. A specific antidote for digitalis toxicity is digoxin-specific antibody (*Fab fragments*). Electrical cardioversion for arrhythmias should be avoided in digitalised patients.

B. *Amrinone:* It is a noncatecholamine, non-cardiac glucoside that exerts positive inotropic effect similar to digitalis and is a vasodilator. It reverses major hemodynamic abnormalities associated with heart failure by stimulating the cardiac contractility and dilating the vascular bed. It is indicated in selected patients not responding to digoxin, because it may worsen myocardial ischaemia or ventricular ectopy.

4. **Control of fluid and salt retention:**

A. *Salt restriction:* Considerable improvement in symptoms and signs occurs by restricting the dietary intake of salt by 50% of normal intake, i.e. simply by excluding salt-rich foods and *no use of salt at the table in any form.* In moderate to severe heart failure, dietary intake of salt should be less than 2.0 g. Fluid restriction is unnecessary unless the patient develops hyponatraemia (Na^+ <130 mEq/L). Caloric supplementation is recommended in patients with cardiac cachexia.

B. *Diuretics:* They are usually the first line of treatment for grade II and IV HF. Diuretics increase urine volume and sodium excretion leading to reduction of preload and improvement in symptoms and signs of pulmonary and systemic venous congestion. Of the commonly used agents, furosemide, torasemide and bumetanide act as loop diuretics, hence, are potent to be used during an emergency. Whereas thiazide, metolazone and potassium-sparing agents act in the distal tubule.

Dose: For mild to moderate heart failure, oral hydrochlorthiazide

---

BOX 3 Digitalis (digoxin) toxic effects

A. Cardiac
- Arrhythmias, e.g. ventricular nodal or atrial ectopics, ventricular bigeminy, non-paroxysmal atrial tachycardia with block, ventricular tachycardia or fibrillation
- Bradycardia
- AV blocks (e.g. first degree) second degree and complete AV block

B. Extracardiac
- Gastrointestinal, e.g. nausea, vomiting, anorexia
- Gynaecomastia
- Yellow vision, blurring vision
- Cachexia
- Neuralgia
- Fatigue, headache, confusion, hallucinations

25–100 mg or chlorthalidone 25–50 mg are sufficient. For patients with moderate to severe heart failure, oral furosemide 20–80 mg or torsemide 10–20 mg daily in single or divided doses is sufficient. For severe or advanced congestive heart failure furosemide 40–100 mg or torsemide 10 mg I.V. may be given initially and then to be repeated 8 hourly depending on the response. Large single daily doses are to be avoided because of risk of acute reduction in blood volume. The ethacrynic acid is given as 50–100 mg I.V. 2 or 3 times a day. Potassium is to be monitored during furosemide therapy. For long-term management, a combination of a loop diuretic and potassium-sparing diuretic is useful. Aldosterone antagonist spironolactone and eplerenone is specially recommended in addition to diuretics, (β-blockers, and ACE inhibitors in moderate to severe HF. Ultrafiltration and dialysis are used in cases with refractory HF not responding to diuretics.

5. **Reduction of afterload by vasodilators:** The vasodilators reduce afterload, left ventricular end-diastolic pressure and volume, and raise cardiac output, hence are useful in all grades of HF (NYHA class). Vasodilators are contraindicated in CHF with hypotension.

   i. *Angiotensin-converting enzyme (ACE) inhibitors* are potent vasodilators (dilatation of both venous and arterial bed), act by antagonising the action of stimulated renin-angiotensin system in CHF, therefore, all patients with heart failure due to LV systolic dysfunction (EF < 40%) should receive an ACE inhibitor.

      Dose: Treatment with ACE should be initiated at very low doses because of risk of first dose hypotension followed by gradual increments in dose. The starting dose, i.e. captopril 6.25 mg, enalapril 2.5 mg, lisinopril 2.5 mg should be given twice or thrice a day for 3–5 days and then dose may be increased if needed. Renal function and potassium should be assessed during the therapy.

      The side-effects of ACE inhibitors include hypotension, worsening renal function and hyperkalaemia, intractable cough and angioedema. Less common side-effects are rash, mouth ulcers, taste disturbance and blood dyscrasias.

      Contraindication: Intrinsic renal disease, bilateral renal artery stenosis and systemic hypotension are their contraindications. In case of cough and angioedema due to ACE, another class of drug, angiotensin receptor blockers (losartan, irbesartan, candesartan) may be used whose effects are similar to ACE.

   ii. *Nitrates:* Intravenous nitroglycerine or sodium nitroprusside are primarily used for acute or severely decompensated chronic heart failure especially associated with hypertension or myocardial ischaemia. The starting dose of nitroglycerine is 10 µg/min titrated upwards to 10–20 µg/min infusion to achieve desired effect. The dose of nitroprusside is 0.3 to 0.5 µg/kg/min with upwards titration to maximum of 10 µg/kg/min.

      Oral nitrate or nitrate transdermal patches are effective in long-term management.

   iii. *Nesiritide:* This agent, a recombinant form of human BNP is a potent vasodilator, improves cardiac out. Its haemodynamic effects resemble those of I.V. nitroglycerine. The ASCEND trial has found it useful in improving symptom of CHF. In clinical studies, nesiritide (administered as 2 µg/kg I.V. bolus injection followed by an infusion of

0.01 µg/kg/min which may be titrated upwards) produced rapid improvement in dyspnoea and hemodynamic parameters.

The role of nesiritide may be primarily in patients who continue to be symptomatic after treatment with diuretics and nitrates.

iv. Recombinant human relaxin 2 or serelaxin is being tried in acute discompensated heart failure. It reduces dyspnoea and symptoms and signs of congestion.

6. **Other drugs:**

A. *Anticoagulation:* Congestive heart failure is a potent risk factor for thromboembolism especially in the presence of atrial fibrillation and in patients with recent AMI, hence these groups of patients may be anticoagulated with warfarin for 3 months, otherwise anticoagulants should not be used in patients with normal sinus rhythm without history of thromboembolism.

B. *Beta-adrenergic receptors blocker:* So far beta-blockers were considered to be contraindicated because of blunting of sympathetic and catecholamine response in CHF, but recent clinical trials have shown this blunting response to have beneficial effects. Out of several beta-blockers, only carvedilol, bisoprolol and nebivolol have been approved by FDA for management of class II or III chronic heart failure. Treatment with beta-blockers should be initiated in very low doses followed by gradual increments in dose if lower doses have been well-tolerated. For example, therapy should be started at a dose of 3.125 mg of carvedilol twice daily, 12.5 to 25 mg sustained release metoprolol, 1.25 to 2.5 mg bisoprolol daily followed by doubling the dose after 2 to 4 weeks. Patients should be monitored closely for evidence of hypotension, bradycardia, fluid retention (weight) or worsening heart failure.

There is strong recommendation that stable patients with any grade of heart failure (mild moderate, severe) should be treated with beta-blockers unless there is any contraindication.

C. *Antiarrhythmic and assist device therapy:* Because patients with heart failure have frequent and complex ventricular arrhythmias, and being at high risk of sudden death, may require antiarrhythmics therapy (amiodarone, dafetilide) for their suppression, but recent recommendation is to use them only in life-threatening ventricular arrhythmia refractory to treatment in haemodynamically stable patients. The results of use of a device-implantable cardioverter defibrillator (ICD) in treating recurrent VT/VF in patients with HF are promising in clinical trials, in cardiac arrest survivors and high risk postinfarction patients, but at present there is little evidence that ICD placement prevents sudden death or prolongs life in patients with chronic heart failure who have asymptomatic arrhythmias.

D. *Biventricular pacing:* Although pharmacotherapy is the primary therapy for patients with heart failure, the use of biventricular pacemakers (cardiac resynchronisation) to improve cardiac haemodynamics is well documented. Despite promising initial results, controlled studies have not verified the benefits of dual-chamber pacing in a non-selected population of severely symptomatic congestive heart failure.

7. **Cardiac transplantation for advanced HF:** Because of poor prognosis of patients with advanced heart failure, cardiac transplantation has become widely used, and 5 years survival have been claimed over 70% patients. It is costly and done at few specialised centre.

Left Ventricular Failure (Acute Cardiogenic Pulmonary Oedema)

35

LEFT VENTRICULAR FAILURE (ACUTE CARDIOGENIC PULMONARY OEDEMA)

Definitions

Left ventricular failure (LVF) is defined as failure to maintain an effective left ventricular output for a given pulmonary venous or left atrial pressure or can do so at the cost of an elevated left atrial filling pressure. Acute pulmonary oedema is a haemodynamic consequence of LVF.

Acute Pulmonary Oedema

It refers to collection of fluid into alveoli, its wall and alveolar sacs due to transudation as a result of elevated pulmonary capillary venous pressure (> 25 mmHg) consequent to elevated left atrial pressure. This is called backward failure. Acute pulmonary oedema can be cardiogenic or noncardiogenic. Cardiogenic pulmonary oedema will be discussed here. The elevated hydrostatic pressure within capillaries more than oncotic pressure leads to transudation from capillaries into lungs (Fig. 35.1).

Pathophysiology

Left ventricular output depends on *preload, afterload* and *myocardial contractility*. Left ventricular failure occurs due to interactions of these complex mechanisms. Low cardiac output due to LVF leads to complex neuroendocrine changes in which there is stimulation of renin-angiotensin-aldosterone system as well as stimulation of sympathetic system. At first, these try to optimise the left ventricular function called *compensatory mechanism'*, but when these mechanisms also fail, then LVF sets in. The activation of renin-angiotensin-aldosterone system increases *afterload* due to vasoconstriction and salt and water retention. Stimulation of sympathetic system increases both preload and afterload (peripheral vasoconstriction). This also increases myocardial contractility. By these complex mechanism LVF is produced.

By backward failure mechanism, due to rise in left ventricular end-diastolic pressure/volume due to increased afterload, there is rise in left atrial pressure and subsequently rise in pulmonary venous and capillary pressure (>25 mmHg). This raised pulmonary venous pressure is more than plasma oncotic pressure in the capillaries leading to transudation and development of acute pulmonary oedema (Fig. 35.1). In long standing cases or in chronic heart failure, hypoxia produced by edematous lungs is potent vasoconstrictor of pulmonary vessels leading to pulmonary arterial hypertension and ultimately oedema is relieved slowly. Development of pulmonary arterial hypertension is protective mechanism for acute pulmonary oedema.

Causes and Precipitating Factors

They are given in Table 35.1. The precipitating factors patients with pre-existing heart disease are infection, anaemia, acute coronary ischaemia, pregnancy, tachyarrhythmias rapid I.V. infusion, hypervolaemia and undue physical exertion.

Clinical Features

The clinical features result from low cardiac output, pulmonary venous congestion and rise in left ventricular end-diastolic volume/pressure. They are given in Table 35.2.

Investigations

1. **Full blood count,** blood urea, creatinine, electrolytes, etc.
2. **Arterial blood gas analysis** may show low PaO_2 with normal or low $PaCO_2$ and low blood pH (metabolic acidosis).
3. **The ECG** may show LVH, arrhythmias, evidence of ischaemia or myocardial

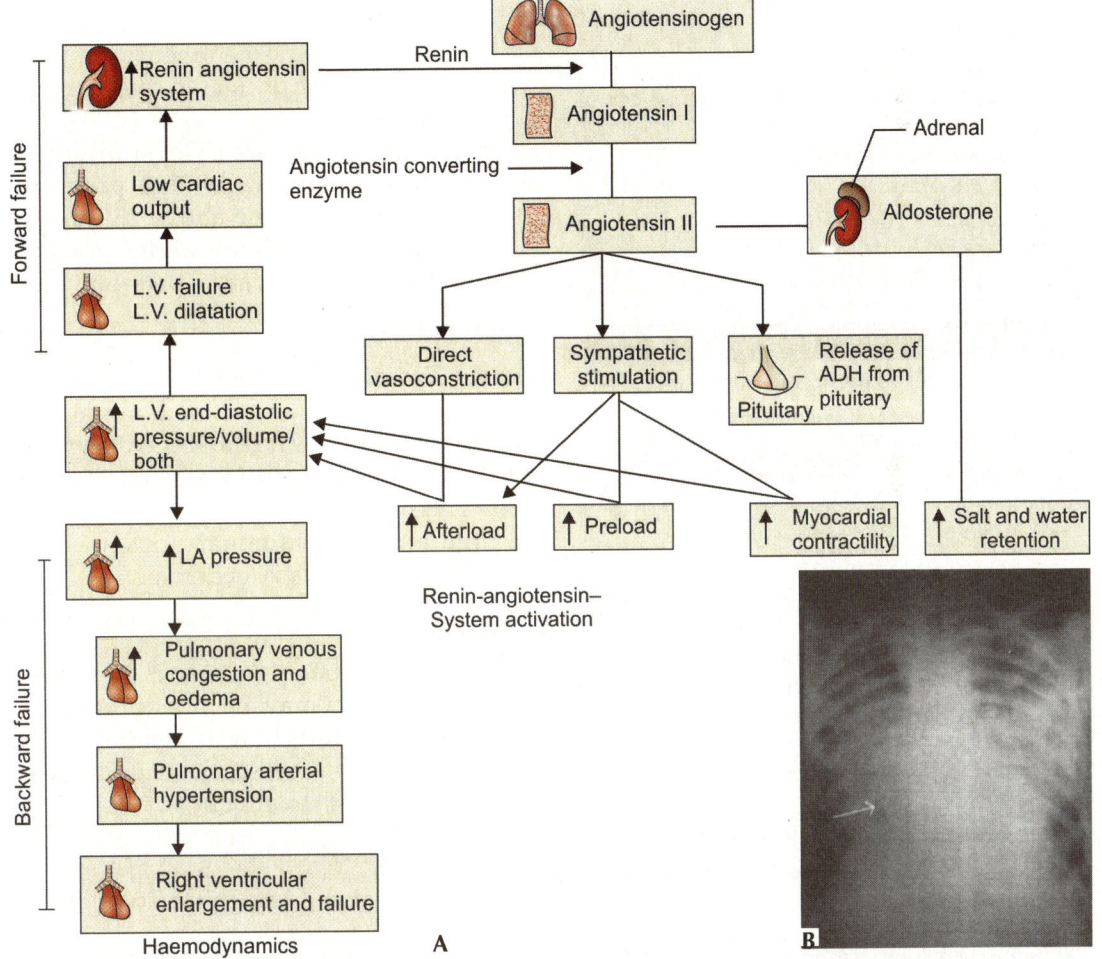

Fig. 35.1: (A) Pathogenic mechanism and haemodynamics of left ventricular failure. LA: left atrium, LV: left ventricle ↑: increase or stimulation. (B) Acute cardiogenic pulmonary oedema. Chest X-ray (PA view) shows enlarged heart shadow. There is bilateral diffuse haze extending from hila to periphery. An arrow indicates outline of right border of the heart

Table 35.1 Causes of left ventricular failure

1. **Left ventricular outflow obstruction (pressure overload)**
   - Systemic hypertension.
   - Aortic valvular stenosis (congenital or acquired).
   - Hypertrophic cardiomyopathy.

2. **Left ventricular inflow obstruction**
   - Mitral stenosis.
   - Left atrial myxoma.
   - Endomyocardial fibrosis (left ventricle).

3. **Left ventricular volume overload**
   - Mitral regurgitation or mitral valve prolpase.
   - Aortic regurgitation (rheumatic and non-rheumatic).
   - Ventricular septal defect.
   - Patent ductus arteriosus.
   - High output states (anaemia, thyrotoxicosis, beriberi, AV fistula, Paget's disease).
   - Papillary muscle dysfunction.

4. **Reduced left ventricular contractility**
   - Dilated cardiomyopathy (LV predominant).
   - Anterior wall MI
   - Myocarditis and left ventricle endocarditis.

Table 35.2 Symptoms and signs of LVF

1. **Symptoms and signs due to rise in left ventricular end-diastolic volume or pressure and subsequent rise in left atrial pressure**
   - Tachycardia
   - Murmurs depending on the cause
   - Low BP
   - Gallop rhythm
   - Low volume pulse or pulsus alternans
   - Heaving apex beat

2. **Symptoms and signs due to pulmonary venous hypertension, pulmonary congestion/oedema**
   - Dyspnoea, orthopnoea, PND, tachypnoea
   - Cough, haemoptysis (pinkish, frothy sputum)
   - Basal pulmonary crackles and rales
   - Central cyanosis
   - Hydrothorax/pleural effusion
   - Cheyne-Stokes respiration

3. **Symptoms and signs due to low cardiac output leading to hypoperfusion and hypoxia of various organs**
   - Oliguria and nocturia
   - Cerebral symptoms, e.g. confusion, difficulty in concentration, anxiety, insomnia, etc.
   - Fatigue and weakness
   - Peripheral cyanosis
   - Pale, cold extremities

infarction, LBBB or ventricular strain pattern depending on the cause of LVF.

4. **Chest X-ray:** It will show pulmonary oedema [haziness extending from the hilum to periphery (Fig. 35.3)] and cardiomegaly. Kerley's B lines may be seen due to alveolar oedema. Hydrothorax or left-sided pleural effusion may be evident.

5. **Echocardiogram:** It is most useful investigation and is mandatory in all patients with acute cardiogenic pulmonary oedema. It gives valuable information regarding:
   i. Unsuspected yet correctable valvular lesion(s).
   ii. Unsuspected cardiac aneurysm.
   iii. Hypertrophic or dilated cardiomyopathy.
   iv. Systolic or diastolic LV dysfunction.

6. **Pulmonary capillary wedge pressure:** It is elevated, may be above 25 mmHg. The pulmonary capillary wedge pressure indirectly reflects left atrial pressure.

Differential Diagnosis

It has to be differentiated from bronchial asthma. Acute pulmonary oedema is also called *cardiac asthma*. The differences between bronchial asthma and cardiac asthma are given in Box 1. It has be differentiated from ARDS and high altitude pulmonary oedema and other types of pulmonary oedema.

Management

Cardiogenic pulmonary oedema is life-threatening emergency, may be precipitated by arrhythmias and infection in a patient with pre-existing heart disease, need immediate attention and urgent treatment.

Aims of Treatment

1. To reduce venous return (preload) to the heart.
2. To lower pulmonary capillary pressure and decrease transudation.
3. To improve myocardial contractility by digitalis if systolic LV dysfunction is the cause.

Box 1	Differentiation between cardiac and bronchial asthma	
Cardiac dyspnoea (asthma)	**Bronchial asthma (dyspnoea)**
1. History	
• Clinical evidence of heart disease	• Clinical evidence of respiratory disease
2. Symptoms	
• Acute onset	• Gradual onset or there can be an acute exacerbation of chronic asthma
• Non-seasonal, no evidence of atopy	• Atopic or nonatopic and seasonal
• Associated symptoms e.g. chest pain, orthopnoea, palpitation, sweating	• Associated symptoms include e.g. cough, wheeze, haemoptysis, stridor
• Attacks of PND are common, relieved by sitting or recumbent position	• Attacks of PND are less common, relieved by cough and expectoration
• Wheeze is less frequent	• Wheezing is marked and even audible
• Dyspnoea is out of proportion than cough	• Cough is out of proportion than dyspnoea
Signs	
• Tachypnoea, tachycardia, cyanosis (central, peripheral)	• They are less marked
• Trachea central, normal in length	• Trachea is central but palpable part is decreased
• No retraction of supraclavicular fossae or intercostal spaces	• Retraction of supraclavicular fossae and/or intercostal spaces is marked
• Percussion note is dull at the bases	• Hyper-resonant note may be present
• Crackles at the bases	• Both crackles and rales throughout the lungs
• Apex beat is normal or displaced	• Apex beat may not be visible or normal
• Breath sounds are normal	• Normal breath sounds with prolonged expiration
• 3rd heart sound (gallop rhythm) may be present	• No 3rd heart sound
Investigations	
• Chest X-ray shows cardiomegaly with acute pulmonary oedema	• Heart size normal, or may be tubular. There is increased translucency of lungs with low flat diaphragm
• ECG may show LVH, LBBB, MI, arrhythmias or conduction defect	• Sinus arrhythmia
• Echocardiogram shows depressed ejection fraction, enlarged LV	• Normal ejection fraction
• Arterial blood gases; low PaO_2 and $PaCO_2$	• PaO_2 low but $PaCO_2$ is normal

4. To reduce afterload by vasodilators.
5. To find out the precipitating cause such as arrhythmia, ischaemia / infarction or infection and treat them appropriately.

Steps of Management

1. Measure to reduce preload

- *Upright or prop up posture of the patient on the bed* with legs dangling along the side of the bed, if possible. This reduces venous return.
- *Morphine* is used to relieve anxiety and dyspnoea. It is given I.V. in dosage of 5–10 mg with an antiemetic (metoclopramide 10 mg I.V.) and repeated frequently as desired. This drug leads to arteriolar and venous dilatation (capacitance vessels) thereby reduces venous return (**preload**). Naloxone (an antidote to morphine) should be available in case respiratory depression occurs.

2. Measures to lower pulmonary capillary wedge pressure

- *Oxygenation:* There is arterial hypoxaemia due to lowered oxygen diffusion as a result of alveolar oedema, hence, 100% O_2 should be given through the mask preferably under positive pressure (it will stop transudation of fluid into alveoli by reducing venous return and thereby lowering pulmonary capillary pressure). Positive pressure ventilation has been found beneficial in refractory cases of pulmonary oedema.

- *Bronchodilatation:* Sometimes amino-phylline (theophylline ethylenedi-amine), 240 to 480 mg given I.V. is effective in relieving bronchospasm, and in addition may lower pulmonary venous pressure. It has also a mild diuretic and positive inotropic effect (augments myocardial contractility).

- *Inotropic and inodilators:* The inotropic agents (dopamine, dobutamine) and inodilator (milrinone) are indicated in cardiogenic pulmonary oedema with severe L.V. dysfunction.

- *Diuretics:* The high potency loop diuretics such as fursemide (40–100 mg I.V.) or bumetanide (1 mg) or torsemide 10 mg I.V. may be given to reduce the circulating blood volume and clear fluid overload by profuse diuresis. Fursemide, when given I.V. also exerts vasodilator action, thereby reduces venous return (preload).

3. **To reduce afterload**
- *Vasodilators:* Intravenous sodium nitro-prusside 20–30 µg/min may be given to reduce afterload in patients whose systolic BP is above 100 mmHg.

- *Nitrates:* Nowadays, sublingual nitrate (0.4 mg every 5 min up to 3 tablets) is considered as first line therapy for acute cardiogenic pulmonary oedema, I.V. nitroglycerine (starting at 10 µg/min) can be given if patient is not in hypoten-sion.

- *ACE inhibitors:* They reduce both preload and afterload, hence, are recommended in hypertensive patients with acute LVF.

- *Natriuretic peptides:* They also reduce **afterload** (*vasodilator*). Intravenous recombinant brain natriuretic peptide

(*nesiritide*) is useful in cardiogenic pulmonary oedema. It is potent vasodi-lator with diuretic properties.

4. **To improve ventricular contractility**
- *Digitalis:* It is given to improve left ventricular myocardial contractility, hence, is useful in patients of LVF due to systolic dysfunction. If the patient has not taken digoxin within the last 5–6 days then 0.5 mg I.V. may be given stat followed by 0.25 mg (half the initial dose) after 6 to 8 hours, if necessary, to a maximum of 1 mg/24 hours. This therapy is also beneficial if pulmonary oedema has been precipitated by one of supraventricular tachyarrhythmia such as supraventricular tachycardia or atrial fibrillation with rapid ventricular rate.

5. **If above measures fail, rotating tourni-quets** may be applied, but its efficacy is doubtful.
- *Intra-aortic balloon counterpulsation:* Intra-aortic balloon counterpulsation (IABP) is useful to relieve cardiogenic pulmonary oedema during cardiac surgical repair, e.g. acute mitral regur-gitation, VSD.

6. **To find out the underlying cause and to treat it:** After instituting the above measures, attempt should be made *to find out the precipitating factor* such as an arrhythmia or infection which should be treated by appropriate anti-arrhythmic and antibiotic therapy respectively.

7. **For future management:** The diagnosis of underlying disease must be established and if possible to be removed such as mitral valvotomy for MS, or surgical treatment for atrial myxoma, aneurysms or papillary muscle dysfunction.
- After discharge from the hospital, patient should be advised salt restric-tion, avoid exertion; and the dose of a diuretic, digitalis and an ACE inhibitor should be properly adjusted to prevent further episode.

Management of Tachyarrhythmias

Definitions

Tachycardias result from disorders of impulse propagation and disorders of impulse formation. Tachycardias due to disorders of impulse propagation (re-entry) are generally considered to be most common (Fig. 36.1). Disorders of impulse formation can be subdivided into tachycardias caused by enhanced automaticity and those caused by triggered activity. Sinus tachycardia, escape rhythms, accelerated AV nodal rhythms and ectopic tachycardias are its examples.

TACHYARRHYTHMIAS

Definition

Any arrhythmia with heart rate more than 150/min is defined as an *tachyarrhythmia*. They occur more often in diseased rather than normal hearts. Those tachycardias that are initiated by an APC or a VPC are considered

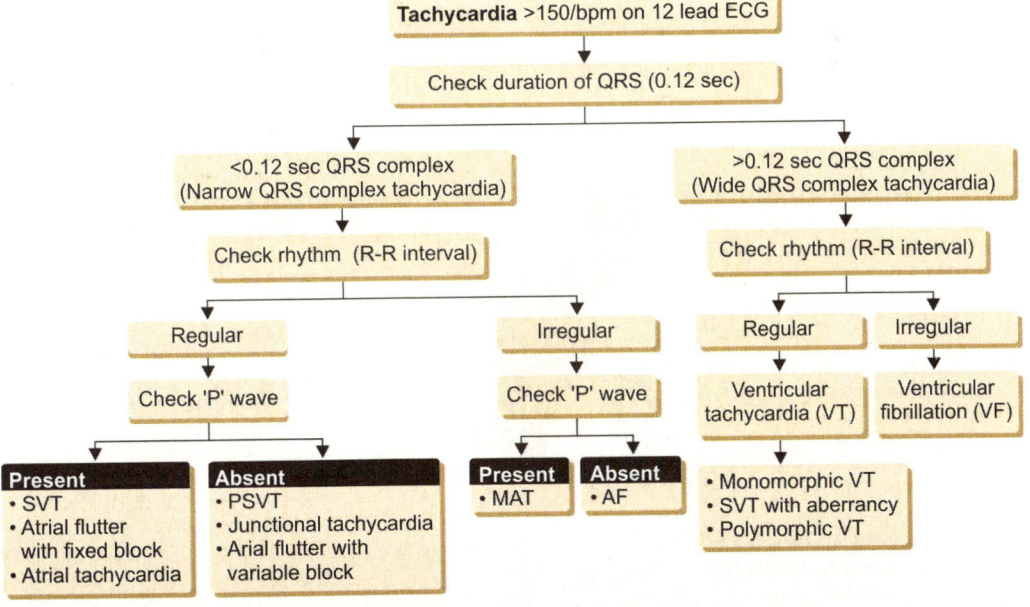

Fig. 36.1: How to identify tachyarrhythmias

to be due to an re-entry mechanism except digitalis induced arrhythmias which are due to triggered activity.

In a haemodynamically stable patient, an attempt should be made to find out the mechanism and origin of tachycardia by examining the patient clinically and by recording a 12 lead surface ECG (Fig. 36.1). This is important for appropriate therapeutic decision.

The ECG will give informations regarding:

1. The presence or absence of P-wave, frequency, morphology and regularity of P-waves as well as QRS complexes.
2. Relationship of P-waves to QRS complexes.
3. A comparison of QRS morphology can be made during sinus rhythm and during an episode of tachycardia. It is useful to summon the ECG before tachycardia, i.e. recorded during sinus rhythm.
4. If necessary, an oesophageal lead may be used to define supraventricular tachycardia by the recording the atrial activity (P waves).

5. The response to carotid sinus massage or other vagomimetic maneuvers such as Valsalva maneuver, immersion of face in cold water and administration of 5–10 mg edrophonium.

Clinical Observations

1. Examination of jugular venous pulse is important because 'a' wave will be absent in atrial fibrillation.
2. Arterial pulse will reveal regularly irregular pulse in ventricular ectopy and irregularly irregular pulse in atrial fibrillation. The pulse deficit is <10 beats/min in frequent VPCs but is > 10/min in atrial fibrillation.
3. Cannon 'a' wave suggests AV dissociation, complete AV block and nodal rhythm.
4. Variable intensity of first heart sound during an arrythmia suggests AV dissociation, or heart block or atrial fibrillation.

The classification of antiarrhythmics is given in Table 36.1. The sites of action of antiarrhythmics are depicted in Fig. 36.2.

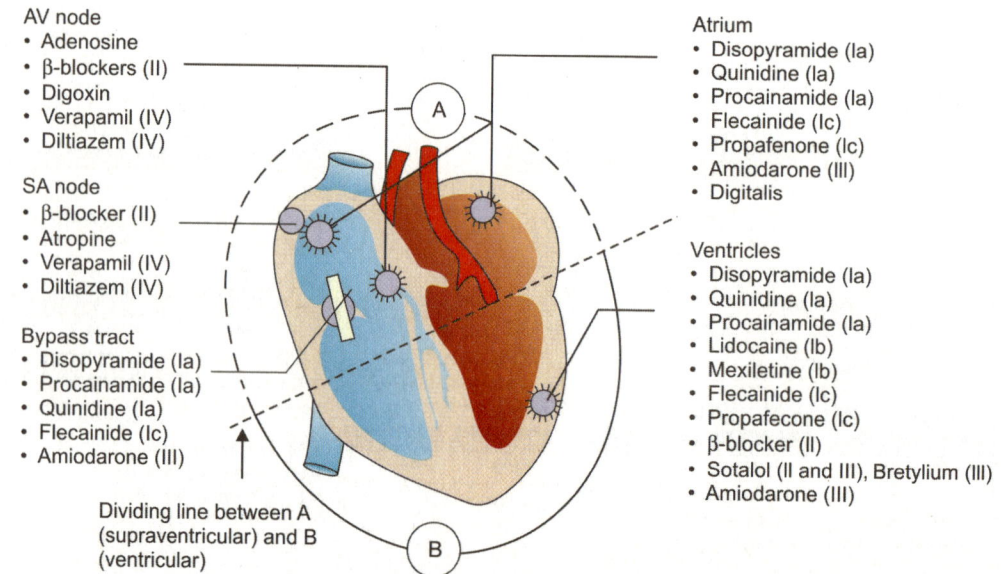

AV node
- Adenosine
- β-blockers (II)
- Digoxin
- Verapamil (IV)
- Diltiazem (IV)

SA node
- β-blocker (II)
- Atropine
- Verapamil (IV)
- Diltiazem (IV)

Bypass tract
- Disopyramide (Ia)
- Procainamide (Ia)
- Quinidine (Ia)
- Flecainide (Ic)
- Amiodarone (III)

Atrium
- Disopyramide (Ia)
- Quinidine (Ia)
- Procainamide (Ia)
- Flecainide (Ic)
- Propafenone (Ic)
- Amiodarone (III)
- Digitalis

Ventricles
- Disopyramide (Ia)
- Quinidine (Ia)
- Procainamide (Ia)
- Lidocaine (Ib)
- Mexiletine (Ib)
- Flecainide (Ic)
- Propafecone (Ic)
- β-blocker (II)
- Sotalol (II and III), Bretylium (III)
- Amiodarone (III)

Dividing line between A (supraventricular) and B (ventricular)

Fig. 36.2: Tachyarrhythmias. Division into A (supraventricular) and B (ventricular) indicates their origin. The drugs acting at different sites are depicted with their classification (given in the bracket)

Table 36.1 Vaughan William's classification of antiarrhythmics

Class I: They block fast Na+ channels

A. Prolong action potential duration
  • Quinidine, procainamide, disopyramide
B. Shorten duration of action potential
  • Lidocaine, phenytoin, tocainide mexiletine,
C. No effect on action potential, slow the conduction
  • Flecainide, encainide, propafenone

Class II: Beta-blockers

Propranolol, metoprolol, atenolol, timolol, sotalol

Class III: They block K+ channel

• Amiodarone, sotalol, bretylium

Class IV: Ca++ channel blockers

• Verapamil, diltiazem

PAROXYSMAL SUPRAVENTRICULAR TACHYCARDIA (PSVT)

Supraventricular tachycardias (*atrial* or *nodal in origin*, Box 1) occurring in paroxysms (paroxysmal) are due to re-entry (*circus movement*); while **non-paroxysmal supraventricular** tachycardia is digitalis induced.

It is the most common tachycardia characterised by regular narrow QRS complexes at a rate of 120 to 250/min. It occurs commonly in females. Age is no bar. It is invariably initiated by an APC with prolonged P-R interval (marked AV nodal conduction delay-prolonged AH interval) which may be visible on ECG followed by narrow QRS complexes with embedded P-waves or distortions of QRS at the terminal parts by P-waves. It is an re-entrant tachyarrhythmia at AV node called **AVNRT (AV nodal re-entrant tachycardia).**

The **pathogenesis** is explained by dual pathway hypothesis, AV node has two pathways—(i) *a beta (fast) pathway* and (ii) *slow alpha pathway*. During sinus rhythm, only conduction over the fast pathway manifests resulting in a normal P-R interval. An atrial premature complex (APC) with critical coupling interval is blocked in beta pathway but is conducted slowly through alpha pathway. This beat while passing through alpha pathway may find beta pathway recovered, gets conducted through it

Box 1 Supraventricular tachycardias

1. *AV nodal re-entry* (atrioventricular nodal re-entrant tachycarida, AVNRT). This is the commonest form of PSVT.
2. *Atrioventricular re-entry:* (atrioventricular re-entrant tachycardia-AVRT). This is less common. It may be:
   • *Orthodromic AVRT:* In this type, impulses are conducted to the ventricles via AV node, and the retrogradely back to atria through an accessory pathway. This is a narrow QRS complex tachycardia.
   • *Antidromic AVRT:* In this type, impulses are conducted abnormally through an accessory pathway, and then retrogradely via AV node. This produces wide QRS tachycardia simulating VT.
3. SA nodal or atrial re-entrant tachycardias.
4. Non-paroxysmal supraventricular tachycardia. It is commonly due to digitalis.

retrogradely into atria resulting in setting up of a vicious circle resulting in sustained paroxysonal supraventricular tachycardia.

Clinical Features

It may produce palpitation, syncope and heart failure depending on the rate and duration of an arrhythmia. The signs and symptoms of underlying heart disease are present. Hypotension may occur due to loss of atrial boost to ventricular filling due to rapid rate. There may be visible cannon 'a' wave due to simultaneous atrial and ventricular contractions.

Treatment (Fig. 36.3)

1. **Vagal maneuvers** (e.g. carotid sinus massage, lowering the head between knees Valsalva maneuver, immersion of face in cold water induce coughing) can be performed to block the conduction in the AV node. They may terminate tachycardia. Carotid sinus massage is done by the physician avoiding it in old persons with atherosclerosis. Firm pressure applied for 10–20 seconds on one side if unsuccessful, then apply on other side. Continuous. ECG or auscultatory monitoring for heart rate is done.

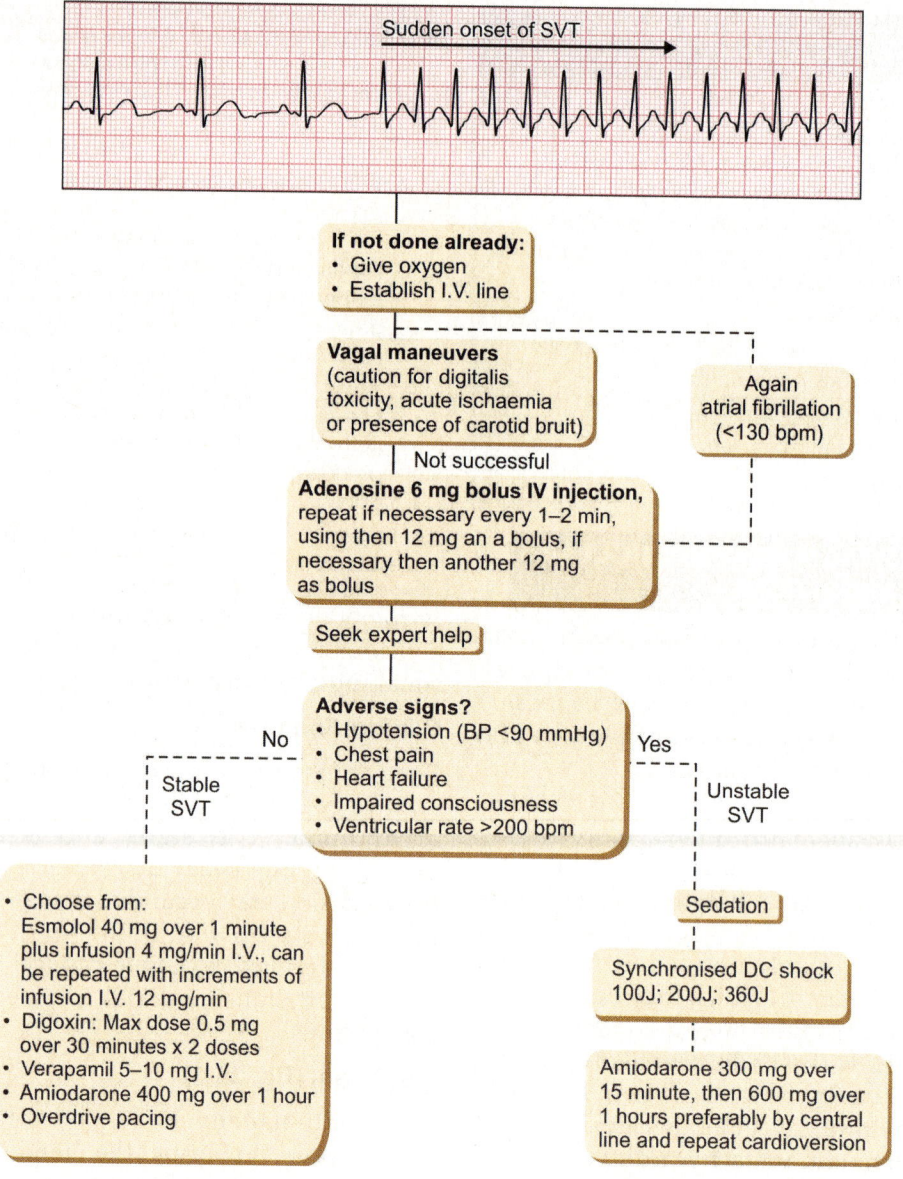

Fig. 36.3: Algorithm for treatment of narrow QRS complex tachycardia (Adapted from *European Resuscitation Council* endorsed by *British Resuscitation Council*)

2. If vagal maneuvers are unsuccessful, the intravenous injection of a drug that prolongs the refractory period of AV node (adenosine, verapamil, diltiazem) and digitalis may be administered. Out of these, *adenosine* which interrupts the AV circuit is preferred because of its extremely short half-life and less side-effects, other drugs constitute second line agents. The dose of I.V. adenosine is given in Fig. 35.3. The flushing, bronchospasm and chest discomfort are its side effect. Calcium channel blocker, e.g. *verapamil* can be given as an alternative in the dose of 2.5 mg bolus

followed by another 2.5 mg every 1–3 min. till tachycardia is reverted or maximum dose of 20 mg is achieved. I.V. *diltiazem* 0.25 mg/kg over 2 minutes followed by second bolus of 0.35 mg/kg if necessary then I.V. infusion (5–15 mg/hr) *Esmolol* I.V. (500 mg/kg) as bolus then 25–200 µg/min as infusion is also effective (Fig. 35.3).

3. When these drugs fail to terminate the tachycardia or when tachycardia is recurrent but patient is still hemodynamically stable, atrial or ventricular pacing via a temporary pacemaker may be used to terminate tachycardia called *overdrive suppression.*

4. If the patient is symptomatic and has compromised state due to unstable tachycardia (e.g. hypotensive or in acute distress), synchronised cardioversion (100–200 J) may be performed immediately.

5. For chronic recurrent PSVT, **radio-frequency ablation** of micro re-entry circuit may be indicated.

The chronic drug therapy includes use of beta-blocker or calcium channel blocker in absence of heart disease and class 1A, class 1C and class III (amiodarone) antiarrhythmic drugs for patients with underlying heart disease.

NON-REENTRANT ATRIAL TACHYCARDIA

Nonparoxysmal atrial tachycardia is commonly digitalis-induced or may be associated with severe pulmonary or cardiac disease, with hypokalaemia or with administration of theophylline or adrenergic drugs. Multifocal atrial tachycardia (MAT) is not digitalis induced, occurs commonly following theophylline administration.

It is **diagnosed** by narrow QRS complex tachycardia with irregular heart rate. The P-waves have three or more different morphology in more than two contiguous heads.

Treatment is withdraw digoxin, theophyline if found to be the cause, otherwise:

- Treat underlying cause, i.e. pulmonary disease
- One can use metoprolol or verapamil I.V. or oral as desired.

ATRIAL TACHYCARDIA

The *atrial tachycardia* is characterised by atrial rate of 150–200/min and the P-wave contour is different from that of sinus P-wave. As atrial rate increases, the degree of AV block increases and Wenckebach second degree AV block may ensue, i.e. atrial tachycardia with block (a manifestation of digitalis toxicity).

The **ECG** shows isoelectric line between the P-waves which are abnormal in shape and differ from sinus P-waves. The ventricular complexes are narrow and there is normal intraventricular conduction.

Treatment

1. Digoxin withdrawl is sufficient to terminate it if it is the cause of the arrhythmia.

2. Automatic atrial tachycardia not caused by digitalis is difficult to terminate. Radio-frequency ablation should be attempted since control of this form of tachycardia with drugs such as digitalis, beta-blockers, calcium channel blockers is usually unsuccessful.

JUNCTIONAL TACHYCARDIA/NODAL TACHYCARDIA

It is a narrow QRS complex tachycardia with enhanced automaticity of AV node either due to digitalis toxicity or excessive use of exogeneous catecholamine.

It is **diagnosed** by tachycardia with narrow QRS complexes where P waves are either obscured or may propagate antegrade or retrograde with origin at the juction, hence, P-wave may proceeds or follow QRS,

Management

- Cardioversion is harmful if it is digitalis induced. Otherwise also cardioversion is unsuccessful.

- I.V. beta-blockers are effective in symptomatic JT.
- I.V. dilitiazem, Verapamil or Procainamide are resonably good in acute cases.

ATRIAL FIBRILLATION (AF)

It is characterised by rapid atrial rate >350 beats/min, uncoordinated atrial contractions and irregular rapid ventricular response. It is a common supraventricular arrhythmia which may occur in paroxysms (paroxysmal atrial fibrillation) and persistent forms (chronic atrial fibrillation). Atrial re-entry is the common underlying mechanism.

In atrial fibrillation, the AV node is bombarded by numerous excitatory stimuli from the atria (atria re-entry) but all supraventricular (atrial) impulses do not reach the ventricles due to refractoriness of AV node which produces physiological block to these impulses and protects the ventricles from going to chaos. On the other hand, if AV node is bypassed such as in accessory pathway conduction (WPW syndrome), then the atrial fibrillation will be dangerous because there will be 1:1 conduction without any AV nodal interference.

Causes

They are given in Box 2.

Box 2 Causes of atrial fibrillation	
• Rheumatic heart disease (MS, MR etc.)	• Thyrotoxicosis
• Mitral valve prolapse	• Congenital heart disease (ASD, Ebstein's anomaly)
• Hypertensive heart disease	• Constrictive pericarditis
	• Cor pulmonale
• Cardiomyopathy, alcohol induced (holiday heart syndrome)	• Left atrial myxoma
	• Idiopathic (lone atrial fibrillation)

Clinical Features

Atrial fibrillation (AF) may produce palpitation, syncope fatigue due to rapid ventricular rate. AF may lead to hypotension, precipitate angina pectoris in susceptible individuals.

It may manifest as systemic embolisation in patients with underlying rheumatic or ischaemic heart disease producing stroke (hemiplegia, monoplegia) peripheral gangrene and infarction of various organs.

Patients with AF exhibit loss of 'a' wave in the jugular venous pulse and variable pulse deficit (>10 bpm). The *arterial pulse* is *irregularly irregular*. The *first heart sound varies in intensity*. In addition, there may be signs of underlying heart disease.

Diagnosis

It is made on *ECG* which shows fibrillatory (f) waves instead of normal P waves, undulating baseline, atrial rate >400 bpm and ventricular rate >100/min. The R-R intervals are variable due to irregular ventricular response. The morphology of QRS is narrow unless there is phasic aberrant ventricular conduction called *Ashman's phenomenon*. On *echocardiography*, the left atrium is frequently enlarged and may even contain a thrombus.

Treatment

1. Find out the precipitating factor or cause and treat it accordingly.
2. If the patient's clinical status is haemodynamically unstable, cardioversion is the treatment of choice for patients with shock or hypotension, an initial shock of 100–200 J is given, if it fails an additional shock of 360 J is indicated.
3. In the absence of cardiovascular compromise, drug therapy to slow the ventricular rate and anticoagulation to prevent thromboembolism is indicated. Beta-blockers (propanolol, metoprolol), amiodarone and calcium channel blockers (verapamil, diltiazem) may be used for this purpose. Digoxin may be added to rate-controlling drugs in acute AF.
4. If medical therapy (rate control measures) fails to convert AF within 24 hours, electrical cardioversion is useful.
5. In situations where AF has been present for 48–72 hours or more in patients who have

known risk factor(s) for stroke or when there is evidence of systemic embolisation, anti-coagulants (warfarin) may be used indefinely with INR 2–3. Recently *dabigatran* (a thrombin inhibitor was used orally (150 mg twice a day) found safe and effective than warfarin.

6. In patients of AF with enlarged (giant) left atrium, it is difficult or even impossible to convert AF into normal sinus rhythm, in such patients, drug therapy may be used to control the rapid ventricular response.

7. In occasional patient, it may not be possible to slow the ventricular rate by drugs what to talk of conversion of AF to sinus rhythm. Such a case may require creation of complete heart block by radiofrequency ablation of the AV node followed by implantation of permanent pacemaker. Catheter ablative therapy also holds promise in patients with severe or persistent AF.

8. Once sinus rhythm is restored by any means described above, dafetilide (500 µg bid or flecainide (50–150 mg twice daily orally) or propafenone (1C) (150–300 mg, 80–160 mg 8 hourly) or sotalol (class III) may be used to prevent recurrence.

ATRIAL FLUTTER (AF)

It is a supraventricular arrhythmia characterised by rapid atrial rate (250–350/min) due to intra-atrial re-entry (*circus movement*), involves commonly the right atrium. The arrhythmia occurs commonly in patients with organic heart disease. Flutter may be paroxysmal induced by pericarditis, acute respiratory failure, or it may be persistent. Atrial flutter if lasts for more than a week, it will usually convert into atrial fibrillation.

Causes

The causes of atrial flutter are more or less same as that of atrial fibrillation with the exception that pericardial disease, severe pulmonary disease commonly lead to atrial flutter than atrial fibrillation.

Diagnosis

It is diagnosed on ECG which shows narrow QRS complex tachycardia (atrial rate of >300 bpm) with ventricular rate either half or one-third (2:1, 3:1 block) which is regular. The P-waves produce *saw-tooth appearance* of the baseline between R-R intervals.

Treatment

When the diagnosis of atrial flutter is made, then there are three therapeutic modalities to treat it:
- Drug therapy for ventricular rate control.
- DC cardioversion.
- Catheter ablative therapy.

Conversion of atrial flutter to sinus rhythm: First of all ventricular rate is controlled with those drugs which are used in atrial fibrillation. Conversion of atrial flutter to sinus rhythm with class 1A (quinidine, disopyramide, procainamide) or 1C flecainide is difficult to achieve. The class III agent ibutilide has been more successful in converting atrial flutter. About 50–70% revert back within 1 year of treatment.

Out of other options, DC cardioversion or pacing is the preferred treatment because class I and III drugs are less effective than these techniques. The initial effective treatment in acute setting is low-energy DC shock (25–50 J) under mild sedation. Higher energy 100J shock is virtually always successful and never harmful, hence, may be considered as initial shock. Precardioversion anticoagulation is not necessary in atrial flutter.

VENTRICULAR TACHYCARDIA (VT)

Definition

It is a wide QRS (>0.12 sec) tachycardia consisting of 3 or more consecutive ventricular premature beats at a rate of >100 bpm. The sudden onset of a wide QRS tachycardia usually rings an alarm bell if the patient is symptomatic. If left untreated, VT may degenerate into fatal ventricular flutter. VT may be sustained (persists for >30 seconds) or nonsustained (does not persist beyond 30 seconds). The sustained VT requires termination because of haemodynamic consequences. Repeated episodes (>2 in 24 hours) of VT require external cardioversion/defibrillation or DC shock therapy.

Causes

VT generally accompanies some form of structural heart disease. The causes are:

1. Acute myocardial infarction or ischaemia.
2. Cardiomyopathy (ischaemic or idiopathic).
3. Electrolyte disturbance (e.g. hypokalaemia, hypomagnesemia).
4. Drugs (e.g. digitalis and other proarrhythmics)
5. Myocarditis, mitral valve prolapse.
6. Reperfusion.
7. Ventricular aneurysm.
8. Pacemaker mediated (e.g. DDD pacemaker).
9. Mechanically induced by a pacing catheter or flow directed pulmonary artery catheter.
10. Idiopathic.
11. Miscellaneous such as right ventricular dysplasia, Bergada syndrome, sarcoidosis.

Clinical Features

Sustained VT occurs in association with a cardiac disease; while *nonsustained VT* can occur in the absence of heart disease. Sustained VT is almost always symptomatic; while nonsustained VT (3 VPCs in a row or VT lasting for <30 seconds) does not produce symptoms. Sustained monomorphic VT is commonly encountered in patients with chronic or old myocardial infarction. A fixed anatomical lesion producing ischaemia is responsible for recurrent sustained monomorphic VT.

The symptomatic patients of sustained VT present with *palpitations, dizziness, syncope* or even a *cardiac arrest*. The presence of cannon waves, changing intensity of first heart sound with rapid ventricular rate suggest AV dissociation and favour the diagnosis of VT. A history of previous infarction and first episode of tachycardia after infarction is highly suggestive of VT; while long history of tachycardia with frequent attacks, absence of organic heart disease and presence of pre-excitation suggest PSVT with aberrant conduction.

Diagnosis

The ECG helps in the diagnosis. Wide QRS complexes (>0.14 seconds), at a regular rate of >100 bpm with presence of AV dissociation (independent P-wave not related to wide QRS complexes), concordant pattern, superior QRS axis, capture beats and fusion complexes favour the diagnosis of VT. It may be *monomorphic* (all QRS complexes alike originating from a single focus) or *polymorphic* (QRS complexes are not alike suggestes organ from multiple foci). *Torsades de pointee* is a form of polymorphic VT. It must be stressed here that in spite of all these criteria, the ECG diagnosis of VT is not only difficult but may be impossible to differentiate it from PSVT with aberrant conduction (another common cause of wide QRS tachycardia) because there is no single electrocardiographic sign which confirms the diagnosis of VT.

The causes of wide QRS tachycardia are given in Box 3.

Box 3   Common causes of wide QRS tachycardia

- Ventricular tachycardia
- Supraventricular tachycardia with aberrant intra-ventricular conduction (common)
- Supraventricular tachycardia with pre-existing bundle branch block (less common)
- Atrioventricular tachycardia (antidromic WPW conduction)

Management

See the algorithm for wide QRS tachycardia (Fig. 36.4).

Treatment of VT depends on the clinical setting and the ability of the patient to tolerate it. Proceed as follows:

1. First of all establish intravenous line and give oxygen.

2. **Check the pulse:** If there is no pulse in presence of VT on ECG (pulseless VT), treat it as for ventricular fibrillation (see the algorithm of cardiac arrest—Chapter 41).
3. If there is pulse, evaluate vital signs and clinical symptoms. Look for adverse signs:

- If patient is not tolerating the tachycardia and adverse signs (BP <90 mm, ischaemic chest pain, heart failure, unconsciousness, ventricular rate >150 bpm) are present, attempt to convert rhythm with a single precordial thump (*thump-version*) if onset of VT is witnessed on monitor and then proceed

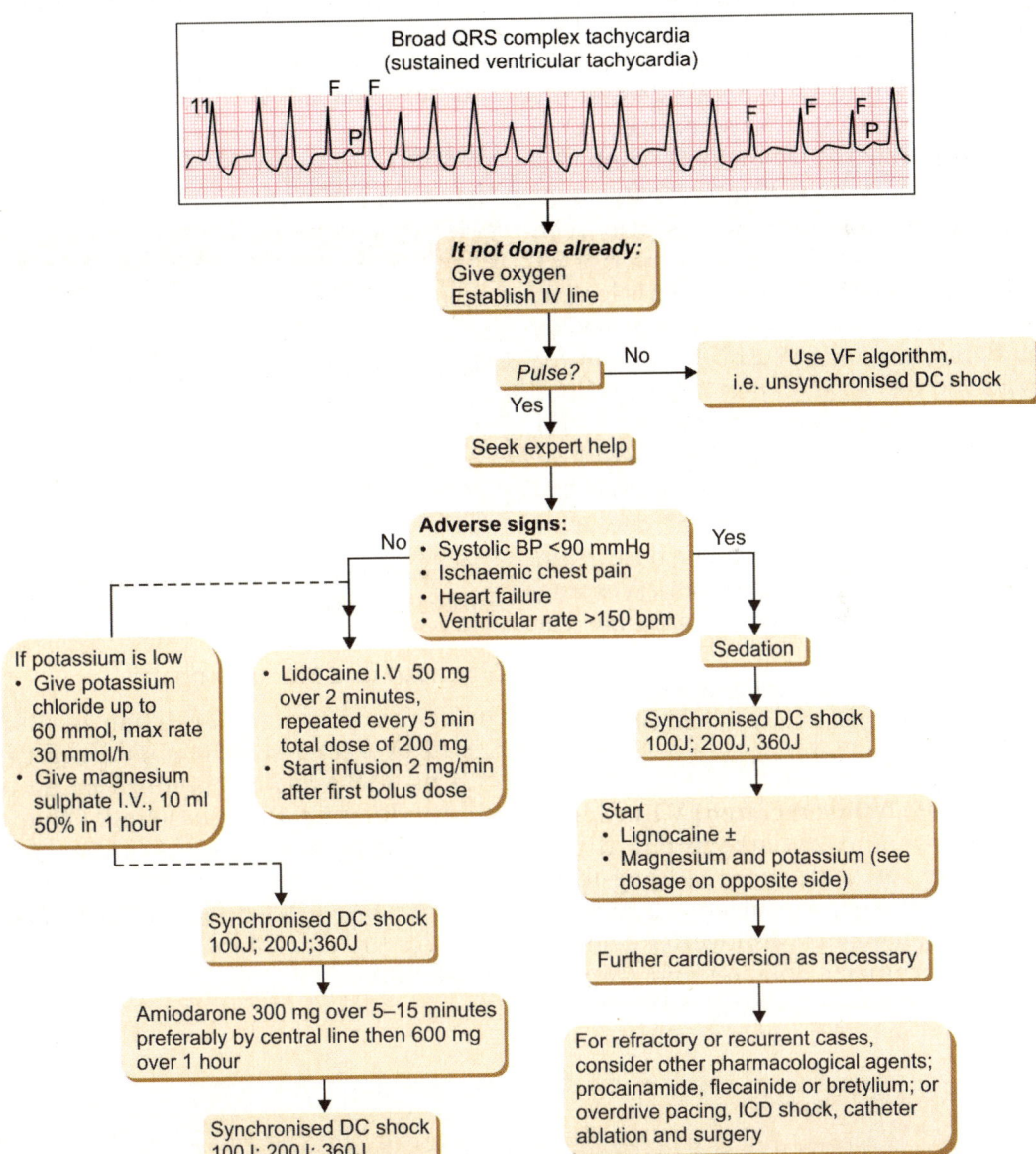

Fig. 36.4: Algorithm for treatment of broad QRS complex tachycardia

immediately with synchronised DC cardioversion. After that begin therapy with xylocaine or bretylium.

- If patient is tolerating the tachycardia and no adverse signs present, then proceed with drug therapy.

The efficacy of procainamide, and amiodarone is higher than lidocaine. Procainamide can be given as I.V. bolus in the dose of 10–15 mg/kg at a rate of 50 mg/min, following which a maintenance infusion dose of 2–6 mg/min is necessary. During procainamide therapy monitoring of BP (for hypotension), QRS duration (prolongs QRS) and QTc interval (prolongs the QTc interval) is necessary.

Intravenous amiodarone has also been found most successful for management of VT but the time taken for the response is longer. The usual intravenous dose is 150 mg as bolus over 10 minutes followed by 1 mg/min for 6 hours and then 0.5 mg/min for next 1 hour for next few days. Empiric treatment with magnesium sulphate (1–2 g IV) may help.

Alternatively intravenous lidocaine (50–100 mg) is given as bolus over 2 minutes with second injection of one half of the dose given after half an hour (total dose not exceeding 200 mg). The infusion has to be maintained at 1–4 mg/min.

If unresponsive to drug therapy, sedate the patient and perform cardioversion (100 J: 200 J: 360 J).

Treatment of chronic recurrent VT includes therapy with oral antiarrhythmic drugs beta-blocker or amiodarone. Long-term treatment options for recurrent VT include the use of implantable cardioverter defibrillator (ICD), catheter ablation and surgery after specialised electrophysical studies and endocardial mapping.

VENTRICULAR FIBRILLATION (VF)

It is a catastrophic arrhythmia characterised by a rapid, irregular, disorganised ventricular rhythm resulting in lack of cardiac output, absent pulses and unrecordable BP. In the absence of ECG monitoring, VF cannot be distinguished from ventricular asystole because both rhythm disturbances result in clinical cardiac arrest.

Causes

They are given in Box 4.

Box 4 Causes of ventricular fibrillation	
• Myocardial ischaemia/ infarction	• Cardiomyopathy
• Electrolyte disturbance (e.g. hypokalaemia, hypomagnesaemia)	• Drugs (digitalis, proarrhythmics)
• Electric shock	• Failure to proper synchronisation of cardioversion
• Atrial fibrillation with rapid ventricular rate may degenerate to VF	
• Congenital prolonged QT syndrome	• As a terminal cardiac event in dying heart
• Severe hypothermia	

Diagnosis and Management

On ECG ventricular fibrillation is characterised by very fast (>300/bpm) heart rate with no identifiable waveform or pattern with undulating wavy baseline. Clinically it is indistinguishable from cardiac arrest, hence, management is like cardiac arrest with unsynchronised DC shock called *defibrillation stock* (*see* the algorithm of cardiac arrest—Chapter 40).

Management of Bradyarrhythmias and Stokes-Adams Attacks

MANAGEMENT OF BRADYARRHYTHMIAS

Definitions

Arrhythmias with slow ventricular rate (<60/min) are defined as *bradyarrhythmias*. These occur due to disorders of SA node and AV node.

1. **Sinus node dysfunction (sick sinus syndrome)**
   - First degree sinoatrial block.
   - Second degree sinoatrial block.
   - Third degree sinoatrial block.
   - Bradycardia-tachycardia syndrome.

2. **AV conduction disturbances**
   - First degree AV block.
   - Second degree AV block.
   - Third degree AV block.
   - AV dissociation.

SINUS NODE DYSFUNCTION

1. **Sinus node dysfunction:** The sinus node is a natural dominant pacemaker. Its intrinsic rate of discharge is highest (60–100 bpm) than other potential cardiac pacemakers (e.g. atrium, AV node, ventricle), hence, it suppresses the activity of all other pace-makers, hence called *king of his own empire*. It is influenced by autonomic nervous system; alterations in autonomic nervous system is responsible for the normal acceleration of heart during exercise and the slowing during rest and sleep. Sympathetic stimulation increases its discharge rate; while parasympathetic stimulation slows the discharge rate. In case the SA node

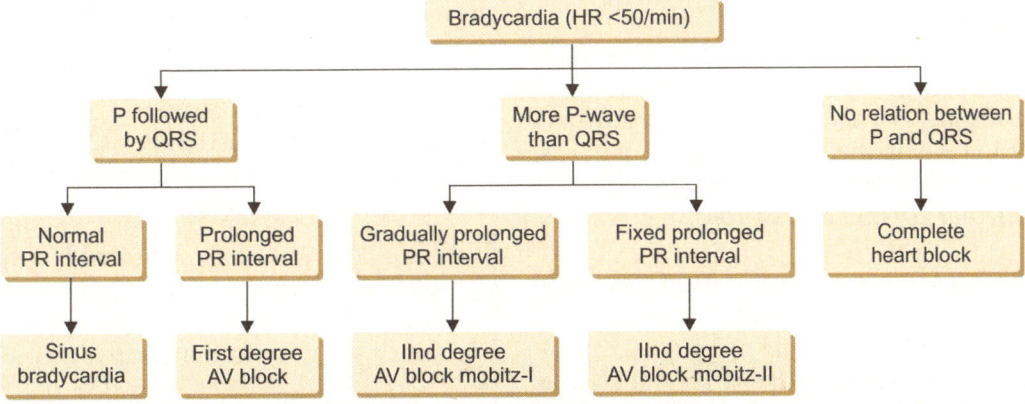

Fig. 37.1: Analysis of bradycardia and determination of various types of heart blocks

Sick sinus syndrome: ECG lead shows' intermittent sinus pause with nodal escape beat (N)

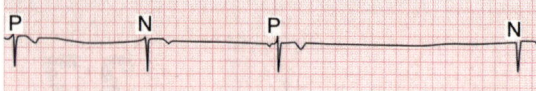

Fig. 37.2: Sick sinus syndrome that cause syncopal attacks

defaults, the lower subsidiary pacemaker, i.e. AV node or ventricle may take up the control of cardiac rhythm. The SA node lies in the right atrium and has dual blood supply. The causes of structural sinus nodal disease are given in Box 1.

Box 1 Causes of structural nodal disease
• Acute MI (inferior wall infarction) • Cardiomyopathies • Metastatic disease involving the heart (right atrium) • Primary muscular dystrophies • Amyloid heart disease • Tuberculosis involving the heart • Degenerative fibrotic disease of atria

Clinical Manifestations

The clinical manifestations of sinus node dysfunction are sinus pauses due to inter-mittent sinus arrest or sinoatrial exit block. In either case, the ECG manifestation is prolonged pause (>3 sec) of atrial asystole. The symptoms include *weakness, fatigue, paroxysmal dizziness* or *syncope, confusion* and *congestive heart failure*.

In some patients, there may be abnormality both in SA node and AV node conduction (*dual nodal disease*) hence, there is failure of the AV node to take up the control of rhythm in case the sinus node defaults resulting in periods of ventricular asystole and *syncope*.

Sick sinus syndrome is a hallmark of sinus node dysfunction, refers to include a combination of symptoms (dizziness, confusion, fatigue, syncope and CHF) and manifested by marked sinus bauses (Fig. 37.2) bradycardia, SA blocks, or sinus arrest, or bradycardia–tachycardia syndrome on ECG or Holter's monitoring.

Diagnosis

The diagnosis of sick sinus syndrome is suspected on clinical grounds and correlated with ECG manifestations of sinus node dysfunction. SA node dysfunctions manifest SA blocks seen intermittently or constantly on the ECG as a pause created by cessation of atrial activity (the whole P-QRS-T complex is dropped Fig. 37.2). The *tachycardia-brady-cardia syndrome* is also a manifestation of sick sinus syndrome characterised by alternating periods of tachyarrhythmias and bradyar-rhythmias.

The most important step in diagnosis of sick sinus syndrome is to correlate symptoms with ECG manifestations of sinus node dysfunction. While ambulatory ECG (Holter) monitoring remains a mainstay in evaluation of sinus node dysfunction, most of the episodes of syncope are paroxysmal and unpredictable. Single and multiple 24-hour monitoring may fail to record a symptomatic period, therefore, provocative tests (carotid sinus pressure, exercise test and pharmacological tests) are frequently helpful. *Carotid sinus pressure* for 5 seconds producing a sinus pause >3 seconds on ECG indicates sinus node dysfunction. Similarly injection of *atropine* 1–2 mg I.V. will not accelerate the heart beyond 90/min in case of sinus node dysfunc-tion but will do so in vagotonaemia (normal response). Similarly isoprenaline 1–2 mg I.V. may be employed to test structural nodal disease.

Electrophysiological studies (sinus node recovery time and sinoatrial conduction time) help in establishing the diagnosis. The normal values are given below. These parameters are recorded following pacing.

1. *Sinus node recovery time* (corrected for spon-taneous heart rate) normally is <550 ms; prolongation indicates sinus node dys-function in a symptomatic patient.
2. *Sinoatrial conduction time:* It is one half of the difference between the pause following termination of brief period of pacing and the sinus cycle length.

Management

- Treat the underlying cause.
- Administer atropine (if necessary).
- Insertion of permanent pacemaker is the mainstay of treatment for symptomatic patients. Patients with intermittent paroxysms of bradycardia or sinus arrest are usually adequately treated by demand ventricular pacemaker. Patients with symptomatic chronic sinus bradycardia or frequent prolonged episodes of sinus node dysfunction do better with dual chamber pacemakers that preserve the normal AV activation sequence (AV synchrony).

AV CONDUCTION DISTURBANCES AND ITS EVALUATION

The impulses from the SA node travel through atria to AV node where there is slight physiological delay before they are conducted to the ventricles. Abnormalities of conduction of sinus impulses to the ventricles occur due to block at the level of AV node (heart blocks) which can ultimately lead to syncope or cardiac arrest.

The physician must assess, i.e. proximal or distal to bundle of His.

i. The site of conduction disturbance, i.e. proximal or distal to bundle of His.

ii. The risk or possibility of progression to complete heart block.

iii. The probability that an emergence of escape rhythm arising distal to site of block will be haemodynamically stable. This is the most important since the rate and stability of the subsidiary pacemaker will determine what symptoms result from heart block. This is because a pacemaker arising from bundle of His or above will discharge at a rate of 45–60 bpm and will be stable and asymptomatic. On the other hand, pacemaker distal to bundle of His will generate impulses at a slower rate (15–45 bpm), produces wide QRS complexes, and symptoms of syncope, dizziness, and will

be unstable. There will be chances of developing ventricular asystole.

The morphology of QRS determines the site of block in AV node.

Causes of Heart Blocks

1. Vagotonaemia
2. Acute rheumatic carditis
3. Myocarditis (diphtheric, Chagas' disease)
4. Coronary artery disease (e.g. inferior wall infarction, right ventricular infarction).
5. Drugs (e.g. digitalis, beta-blockers, calcium channel blockers anti-arrhythmics).
6. Aortic valve disease (e.g. syphilitic aortitis).
7. Infiltrative heart disease (e.g. amyloidosis, myxoedema).
8. Idiopathic fibrosis of conduction system (*Lenegre's disease*).
9. Idiopathic calcification and sclerosis of fibrous ring of aortic and mitral valve called *Lev's disease.*
10. Electrolyte disturbance, e.g. hyperkalaemia.

Classification of Heart Block

1. **First degree AV block** is characterised by prolongation of P-R interval beyond 0.20 seconds at normal heart rate and 0.22 at heart rate of 60/min (Fig. 37.3). It does not cause any symptoms and is detected on the ECG. It does not require specific treatment except the underlying cause or when bundle of His ECG shows block in the infranodal region.

2. **Second degree AV block (intermittent AV block):** In this block, some of the atrial impulses (P-waves) are conducted while others are blocked. It is of two types, i.e.

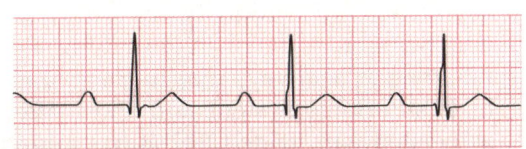

Fig. 37.3: First degree AV block. PR interval is 0.28 seconds.

mobitz type I (Wenckebach) and *mobitz type II* (fixed). In *mobitz type I* (Fig. 37.4), there is progressive lengthening of P-R intervals with each successive beat till one atrial impulse (P-wave) is blocked. In this type, first P-R interval is always shorter than the last P-R interval prior to blocked P-wave. The pause that follows the blocked P-wave is less than twice of the normal sinus intervals. This type of block is always localised to AV node and is followed by normal QRS complex. It occurs transiently in inferior wall infarction or with drugs toxicity, particularly digitalis, beta-blockers, etc. This type of block can occur normally in athletes or normal individuals with high vagal tone. It usually does not progress to complete heart block, except in setting of acute inferior wall infarction. Even when it does, it is well tolerated because the escape pacemaker lies in the proximal part of bundle of His and provides a narrow QRS stable rhythm. As a result, Mobitz type I block rarely requires aggressive therapy (i.e. drug or pacing). Therapeutic decision depends on the ventricular rate and symptoms of the patient. If ventricular rate is adequate and the patient is asymptomatic, observation is sufficient.

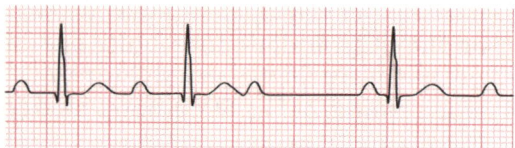

Fig. 37.4: Mobitz type I AV block. There is a progressive lengthening of P–R interval till one P-wave is blocked (not followed by QRS)

In *Mobitz type II second degree AV block*, conduction fails suddenly and unexpectedly without a delay in preceding P-R intervals. It is always due to the disease of His-Purkinje system and most often associated with wide QRS. It has a high incidence of progression to complete heart block, leading to unstable wide QRS (idioventricular) rhythm. Therefore, pacemaker implantation is necessary in this condition.

In *high grade AV block* (Fig. 37.5), there are periods of three or more consecutively blocked P-waves (e.g. >3:1 AV block) but intermittent conduction can be demonstrated. Block is usually in the His-Purkinje system, but simultaneous block in AV node is also present. The escape rhythm arises from the focus below the His-Purkinje system which produces wide QRS (idioventricular) slow rhythm. It is unstable and usually the patient is symptomatic and a cardiac pacemaker implantation is mandatory.

3. **Third degree (complete) AV block** is said to be present when no atrial impulse (e.g. P-wave) is propagated to the ventricles, therefore, there are two independent pacemakers in complete heart block, i.e. one in the atria and other in the ventricle. The duration of QRS decides the site of pacemaker in the ventricle. If QRS duration is normal, and heart rate is 40–55 beats/mm, the pacemaker is situated in the AV node above the bundle of His for example, congenital complete AV block (Fig. 37.6A). If pacemaker lies below the His bundle (block is within His bundle), the escape rhythm is wide (one of the bundle branch block patterns) and is usually less responsive, occurs at a slow rate (15–45 beats/min (Fig. 37.6B) and requires immediate pacemaker implantation.

MANAGEMENT

The analysis of bradycardia and recognition of various heart blocks is presented in Fig. 37.1 on the front page.

The bradycardia (HR < 60/min) or conduction blocks with impending asystole or with an appreciable risk of asystole is important to be recognized from treatment point of view. The following are the situations where the risk of developing asystole is high and there is need to

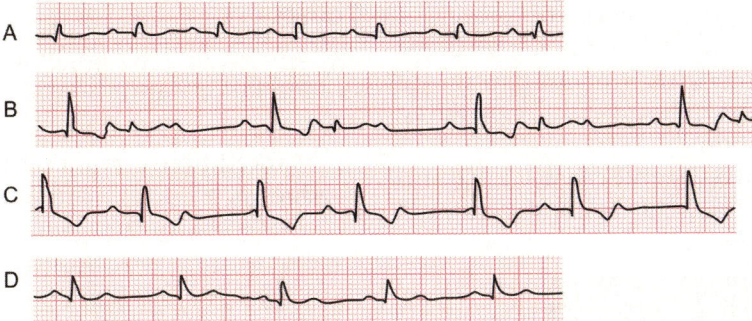

Fig. 37.5: Transient high grade AV block degenerating into complete AV block followed by restoration of normal sinus rhythm with treatment. (A) First degree AV block (P-R interval = 0.24 sec), (B) second degree 3:1 AV block (high grade), (C) complete AV block, and (D) restoration of normal sinus rhythm

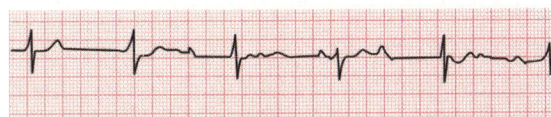

A. Congenital complete heart block. The QRS complex is narrow (0.08s) and the QRS rate is relatively rapid (58 bpm)

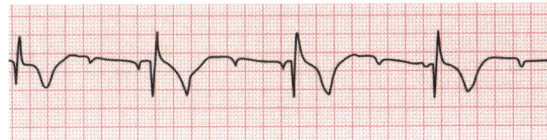

B. Acquired complete heart block. The QRS complex is broad (0.13s) and the heart rate is relatively show 38 bpm The ST is elevated and T is inverted, indicating myocardial ischaemia/infarct as the cause.

Fig. 37.6A and B: Complete heart blocks

recognize them before starting the treatment:
1. History of previous episode of asystole.
2. A pause equal or greater than 3 seconds regard less of the cause.
3. Presence of AV block with idioventricular or nodal rhythm.
4. Dual nodal disease with an idioventricular escape rhythm.
5. Trifascicular and bifascicular block in AMI.

First of all, assess the patient for developing risk of asystole.

1. **When there is risk for asystole:** If there is definite risk of developing asystole, I.V. line should be established and atropine administered as indicated in the algorithm

(Fig. 37.7). In the meantime, arrangements should be made for transvenous pacing. In many cases, expert help will be required for this purpose. If situation demands an early pacing and if necessary equipment is available, then external pacing (Fig. 37.8) should be done. Isoprenaline (initial dose 1 µg/min is used by dissolving 2.5 mg in 500 ml of carrier solution and 0.2 ml/min delivered by an infusion pump) is an alternative mode of treatment. Isoprenaline also increases the O_2 demand and may even cause serious hypokalaemia, therefore, its use must balance the benefits versus risks.

2. **When there is no risk of asystole:** If there is no risk of asystole, proceed on the other side of algorithm and look for the presence or absence of adverse signs.
   a. *When adverse signs are absent,* the patient should be just monitored and observed.
   b. *When one or more adverse signs present,* then atropine should be given I.V. as initial dose of 0.5 mg, increased at an interval of few minutes if required, but not exceeding a total dose of 3 mg. If a satisfactory response to atropine is achieved, then observe the patient; if no response, then proceed for transvenous pacing, if there is likelihood of an appreciable delay in instituting pacing, then interim measures as discussed in the algorithm may be adopted.

When the successful effect of atropine is short-lived or higher doses are required, transvenous pacing will usually be indicated for long-lasting stabilization.

3. **Correction of reversible cause,** e.g. electrolyte disturbance, ischaemia and withdrawl of an offending drug.

STOKES-ADAMS SYNDROME

It is defined as transient loss of consciousness due to hypoxia of the brain as a result of sudden fall in cardiac output.

Causes

The underlying pathogenic mechanism is sudden fall in cardiac output which may be due to:

1. **Marked bradycardia (HR < 30 minutes) due to:**
   - Sinoatrial dysfunction e.g. sinus pauses (Fig. 37.2), sinoatrial block, high grade or complete AV block (Fig. 37.6).

2. **Depressed ventricular contractions,** e.g. ventricular tachycardia, ventricular fibrillation or asystole.

The causes are summarized in Box 2.

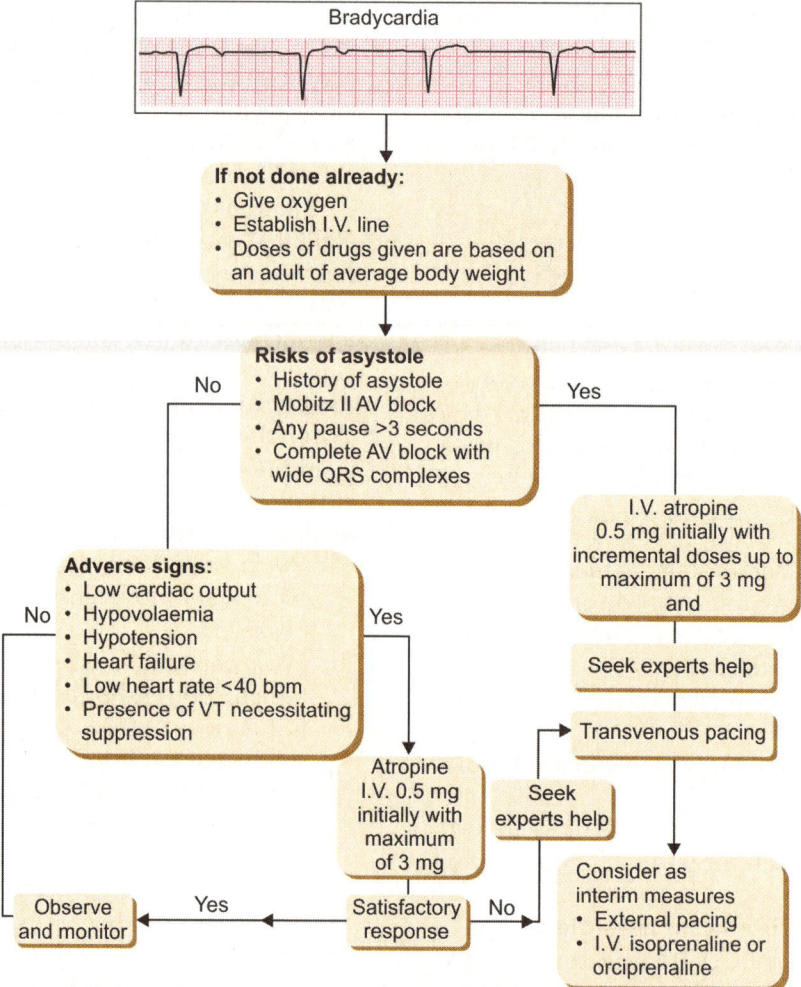

Fig. 37.7: Algorithm for management of bradycardia and conduction blocks

Clinical Features

The typical attacks of Stokes-Adams syndrome are characterised by frequent faintings without any warning symptoms; and in majority of the cases, high grade or complete AV block is detected. In patients with these attacks, the block may be persistent or temporary with a subsidiary pacemaker below the block which either fails to function or functions at slow rate producing bradycardia. If the attacks occur during standing, the patient may fall and hurt himself/herself. Should the attack persists more than 8 to 10 seconds, the patient turns pale, falls unconscious and may exhibit few clonic jerks. If an attack persists with longer period (2–3 minutes) asystole results leading to irregular breathing, cyanosis, fixed pupils, incontinence of urine and bilateral plantar extensor response. The giant T waves in leads V_2–V_4 is virtually diagnostic of recent syncopal attack (Box 3). The recovery from such attacks is also prompt and complete without permanent impairment of mental functions. After recovery, patient does not recall presyncopal symptoms.

Box 3 Pathognomonic sign of Stokes-Adams attacks on ECG

Large, broad, bizarre and inverted T-waves-called giant 'T' in leads V_2–V_4 is visually pathognomic sign of recent syncopal attack; if present. This is associated with prolonged QTc interval.

Diagnosis

In between *Stokes-Adams attacks*, the patient appears normal or may be slightly confused, does not remember what happened before the attack. A careful history, clinical and electrocardiographic evidence of basic heart disease with conduction defect or an arrhythmia help in the diagnosis. If routine ECG fails to reveal an arrhythmia or conduction defect, a 24-hour Holter monitoring may be useful to find out the underlying cause.

Management

1. **Treatment of an attack:** This is just similar to treatment of cardiac arrest, e.g. precordial thump, followed by external cardiac massage and mouth to mouth breathing (see algorithm of cardiac asystole). Most of the attacks are so brief; may not be witnessed by the physician because it may disappear before a physician arrives. In such a situation, the future plan to prevent such an attack is warranted, therefore, find out the underlying cause and treat it.

2. **Treatment in-between attacks:** Most of the patients have either a complete heart block or an arrthythmia as underlying cause for such attacks. Therefore, complete heart block may require pacing; temporary (Fig. 37.8) or permanent depending on the underlying cause. An arrhythmia should be identified and managed accordingly.

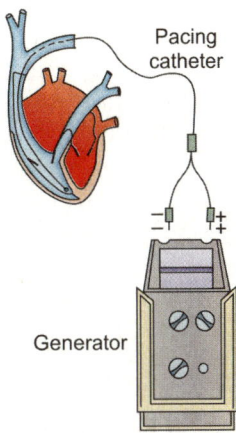

Fig. 37.8: Temporary pacing (diagram). A pacing catheter is connected to a temporary generator. A bridging cable or pacemark extension cord (not shown) can be used between the generator and the catheter

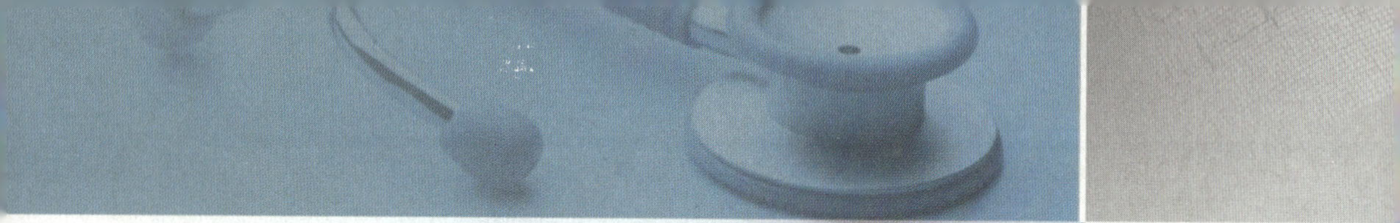

Acute Coronary Syndrome (ACS)

ACUTE CORONARY SYNDROME (ACS)

Definition

Patients of ischaemic heart disease fall into two main categories, i.e. (i) patients with chronic coronary artery disease (CAD) presenting as chronic stable angina and (ii) patients with acute coronary syndrome (ACS) which include patients with ST-elevation myocardial infarction (STEMI) and non-ST-elevation MI (NSTE-ACS) based on ECG on presentation (Fig. 38.1). The later includes patients with unstable angina who by definition do not have myocyte necrosis and patients with non-STEMI having evidence of myocyte necrosis. This distinction guides us to determine which patients need

Presenting symptom	→	Ischaemic chest pain			
Provisional diagnosis	→	Acute coronary syndrome (ACS)			
ECG	→ →	Persistent ST-elevation	Non persistent ST-elevation		Normal
Cardiac markers (CPK + MB, troponin)	→	Positive	Positive	Nega-tive	Nega-tive
Final diagnosis	→	ST-elevation MI (STEMI)	Non-ST-elevation MI (NSTEMI)	Unsta-ble angina	Not ACS

Fig. 38.1: Spectrum of acute coronary events

acute reperfusion therapy. The evolution of cardiac biomarkers allows determination whether myocardial infarction has occurred or not.

Etiopathogenesis

Almost all cases of acute coronary syndrome occur as a result of plaque rupture or haemorrhage, leading to thrombus formation and incomplete occlusion of a major vessel (Figs 37.2A and B). The thrombus often forms over a tear or fissuring on the surface of a cholesterol plaque. A severe narrowing of a coronary artery, i.e. stenosis >70% of the diameter is generally required to produce ACS.

Other causes of ACSs are:
1. Coronary spasm, for example in Prinzemetal's variantangina
2. Progressive atherosclerosis causing mechanical obstruction.
3. Increased myocardial oxygen demand produced by conditions such as fever, tachycardia, thyrotoxicosis in the presence of fixed epicardial obstruction.

Clinical Manifestations/Diagnosis

The diagnosis of NSTE-ACS (unstable angina) is based on clinical presentation. It is diagnosed when chest discomfort is severe and has at least one of the three following features:

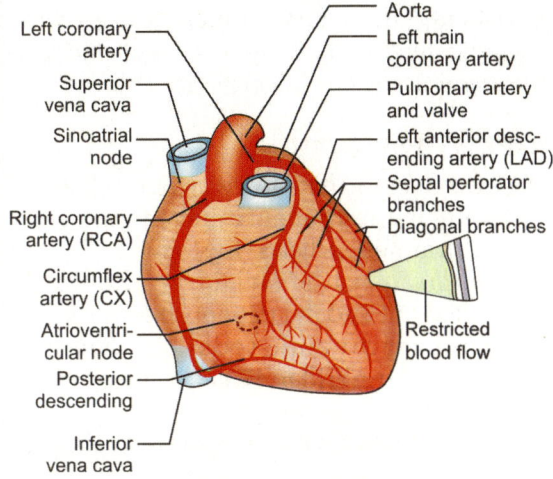

A. Acute coronary syndrome (ACS)

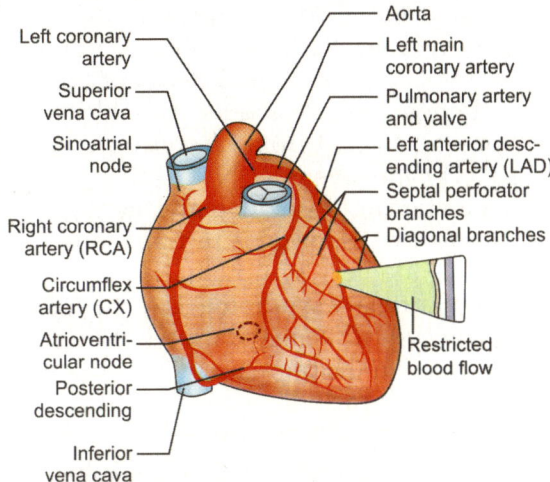

B. Acute myocardial interaction

Fig. 38.2A and B: Pathogenesis of acute coronary artery disease
NB: Stable angina pectoris is not shown.

1. Pain/discomfort occurs at rest or with minimal exertion lasting >10 minutes.
2. It is of recent onset (<2 weeks)
3. It has crescendo pattern, i.e. it is more severe, prolonged and more frequent than previous episodes.

The diagnosis is confirmed by elevated levels of biomarkers of myocardial necrosis (CPK-MB and troponins).

There is usually no physical sign but patients with rest pain frequently develop third or fourth heart sound during the episodes, and in some instances exhibit transient left ventricular failure (murmur of mitral incompetence) due to development of heart failure.

Patients with ACS should be explored for the **precipitating cause** such as **uncontrolled hypertension, anaemia, occult thyrotoxicosis**, and presence of atherosclerosis (carotid, aortic or peripheral artery disease).

Investigations

1. **The electrocardiogram (ECG):** The ECG taken during an episode of pain is highly valuable. Its diagnostic accuracy further improves if a prior ECG is available for comparison.

    ST-segment depression occurs in 20–25% patients. It may be transient and reversible without any evidence of myocardial necrosis or may be persistent for several days in NSTEMI. The T-wave inversion may be either non-specific or specific as deep symmetric inversion.

2. **Biochemical serum cardiac markers:**
    - Troponins (T and I).
    - CPK-MB.
    - Serum myoglobin.
    i. *Troponins:* Immunoassays are used to detect cardiac specific troponins T and I. Both troponins (T and I) have equal sensitivity and specificity in detection of muscle damage. Normally troponins are not present in the blood of healthy persons, elevated troponin indicates muscle damage due to ACS. Small elevations of troponins may occur nonspecifically in conditions like CHF, pulmonary embolism, sepsis, and myocarditis. This is an disadvantages of this test.

    An additional disadvantage of troponins is nonspecific elevation in conditions other than MI such as pulmonary embolism, sepsis, CHF, etc.

ii. *Serum CPK-MB:* It is less sensitive and less specific than troponins for detection of minor myocardial damage (micro-infarct). It is elevated in non-ST segment elevation myocardial infarct in which 25% cases develop acute Q-wave MI (Fig. 38.2). If CPK-MB is elevated, it suggests a significant myocardial damage.

iii. *Serum myoglobin:* Serum myoglobin may be helpful in this situation. Even though it is nonspecific, a negative myoglobin test indicates that raised troponins is not due to acute event.

3. **Stress testing:** It may reveal myocardial ischaemia in patients who have normal resting ECG.

4. **Coronary computed topographic angiography (CCTA)** obstructive lesion in the cornary arterier such a plaque.

> **Note:** The elevated cardiac biomarkers distinguish patients with NSTEMI from those with unstable angina.

Management

The patients with rest pain or who are at medium or high risk should be admitted for observation, further diagnosis and treatment. Concomitant conditions that may accelerate ischaemia such as uncontrolled tachycardia, hypertension, diabetes, thyrotoxicosis, heart failure, cardiomegaly, arrhythmia and any acute febrile illness should be looked for and treated.

Patients with definite or possible acute coronary syndrome are observed with cardiac and haemodynamic monitoring. An ECG, CPK-MB and troponin tests are repeated after 8–12 hours of the onset of symptoms. If the follow up ECG and biochemical markers are also normal, the patient may be discharged.

Acute MI should be ruled out by serial ECGs and measurements of serum cardiac enzymes. A stress ECG may be performed before and after discharge to assess the prognosis. If stress test is negative, then patient is managed as outpatient; if the patient is unable to exercise or has persistent ST-T changes, should undergo dobutamine stress echocardiography.

Steps of Management

1. *Bed rest* should be enforced while ischaemia is ongoing, but patient can sit in a chair and use commode when symptom free.

2. *Continuous ECG monitoring* should be carried out and the patient should receive reassurance and sedation. Sudden ventricular fibrillation is the major cause of death in early period.

3. *Oxygen therapy:* Oxygen therapy is given to improve arterial oxygen saturation.

4. *Intravenous nitroglycerin:* First of all 3 doses of sublingual or buccal nitroglycerine at an interval of 5 minutes are tried to relieve pain. Patients whose symptoms are not relieved with 3 doses of 0.4 mg sublingual nitrate and I.V. beta-blockers, may get benefit from I.V. nitroglycerine (NGT). Intravenous NTG (10 µg/min as a starting dose; increase the dose to titrate the response) is recommended in each and every symptomatic patient of acute coronary syndrome (UA/NSTEMI) to relieve ischaemia and pain. It cannot be given in the presence of hypotension. *Side-effects* include headache, fall in BP and tolerance. To avoid tolerance, intermittent infusion may be used once the patient is free of pain or oral nitrate may be started.

5. *Morphine:* Intravenous morphine sulphate, (2.5 to 10 mg) is recommended for patients whose pain is not relieved by sublingual NTG and anti-ischaemia therapy. It is repeated after 3–5 minutes if needed.

6. *Intravenous beta-blockers:* Beta-blockers reduce myocardial contractility and decrease the oxygen demand of myocardium, hence, are useful in high risk patients and in patients with rest pain. If there is no contraindication (e.g. heart block, asthma, CHF), then I.V. metoprolol (three 5 mg doses 5 minutes apart) may

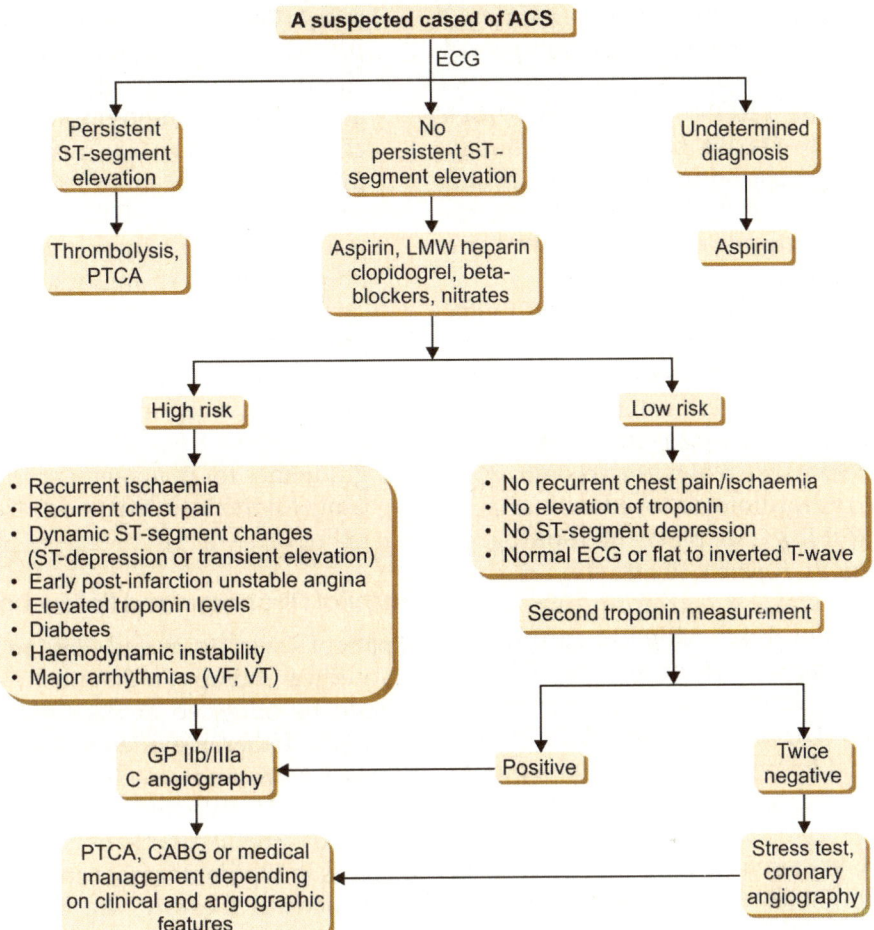

Fig. 38.3: Risk stratification and management protocol for acute coronary syndrome. PTCA: percutaneous transcoronary angioplasty, CABG: coronary artery by pass graft

be used and the patient must be observed carefully to avoid bradycardia, heart failure and hypotension. After initial I.V. dose, it is possible to change to an oral beta-blocker. The target resting heart rate during beta- blockers therapy is between 50–60 bpm.

7. *Calcium channel blocker:* Calcium antagonists are reserved as a third choice after the initiation of nitrates and beta blockers. Definite evidence to their benefit is symptom relief, hence, are used in combination with nitrates or beta-blockers to relieve pain. These drugs may control hypertension in patients with acute coronary syndrome. I.V. verapamil or diltiazem is preferred if calcium antagonist is to be used. Side effects include fall in BP, precipitation of heart failure and heart blocks. Additional medical therapy includes angiotensin converting enzyme, blockers or angiotensin receptor blockers.

8. *Potassium channel openers (e.g. nicorandil):* In one study, nicorandil has been claimed to significantly reduce the number of episodes of transient myocardial ischaemia and arrhythmias.

The majority of the patients (about 80%) improve with such treatment over a period of 48 hours.

9. *Statins:* The PROVE-IT trial provides evidence to start a statin immediately following an episode of ACS. Atorvastatin 80 mg/day regardless of LDL-C levels has improved outcome as compared to 40 mg of pravastatin.

10. *Antithrombotic therapy:* Initial treatment with aspirin 300 mg daily in combination with clopidogrel (300 mg stat, 75 mg daily) should be given. The combination is considered better than aspirin alone. The newer P_2Y_{12} blockers such as *prasugrel* or *ticargeal* are used by cardiologist to reduce mortality and morbidity in place of lopidogrel. *Intravenous heparin* (unfractionated or low molecular, e.g. enoxaprin 1mg/kg SC every 12 hourly) is added to antiplatelet therapy described above to achieve anticoagulation which is mainstay of therapy. The factor Xa inhibitor *fondaparinux* (2.5 mg SC daily) is equally effective. Similarly preliminary data indicate that direct thrombin inhibitor *bivalirudin* is equivalent in efficacy to heparin. *Intravenous GP Ilb/IIIa inhibitors* (*tirofiban or eptifibatide*) and monoclonal antibody inhibitor *abciximab* have been shown to be beneficial in high risk patients in whom intensive management is intended. *Fibrinolytic therapy* should be avoided in NON-STEMI ACS.

11. *Urgent revascularisation:* If angina and/or ECG evidence of ischaemia do not diminish within 24–48 hours of the comprehensive therapy discussed above, then the patient should undergo cardiac catheterisation and coronary angiography if there is no contraindication for revascularisation procedures. If anatomy of coronary artery is suitable, PTCA (percutaneous transluminal coronary angioplasty) can be performed. If angioplasty cannot be done, coronary artery bypass surgery should be considered to relieve symptoms and myocardial ischaemia, and as a means of preventing myocardial damage. European Society of Cardiology guidelines for management of ACS according to risk stratification are depicted in Fig. 38.3.

Hospital Discharge and Follow-up

If patient's symptoms and signs are controlled on medical therapy, a diagnostic stress ECG should be obtained at the time of hospital discharge. If there is evidence of severe myocardial ischaemia and/or a high risk of coronary events, cardiac catheterization should be done followed by revascularisation if needed. Many patients in whom unstable state is controlled with medical therapy, are left with severe chronic stable angina and ultimately require mechanical revascularisation (angioplasty with stenting). Patients with successful revascularisation are advised **life-style modifications**, i.e. *cessation of alcohol, smoking, diet, reduction of weight, daily exercise, BP control* and *lipid management*. They are advised to contine medical therapy as advised.

Cardiac Tamponade

CARDIAC TAMPONADE (Fig. 39.1A to C)

It is defined as clinical syndrome occurring due to rapid accumulation of fluid in the pericardial sac in a quantity sufficient to cause obstruction to the inflow of blood to the ventricles. It is a life-threatening emergency where cure can be achieved by pericardiocentesis (removal of pericardial fluid).

Causes

Three common causes are neoplastic disease, idiopathic pericarditis and renal failure. It can be due to bleeding into pericardial sac with trauma or thoracic injury or due to iatrogenic causes such as anticoagualant therapy, following cardiac surgery, cardiac catheterisation, pacing, etc.

Most cases are subacute or chronic. Tuberculosis is the most common cause followed by viral pericardial effusion. The causes of cardiac tamponade are given in Box 1.

Clinical Features (Fig. 39.2)

The clinical manifestations result due to acute elevation of intracardiac pressure, restricted ventricular filling and reduction of cardiac output. The amount of fluid required

---

Box 1 Causes of cardiac tamponade

Acute cardiac tamponade	*Subacute or chronic cardiac tamponade*
1. **Trauma** • Penetrating or blunt thoracic injury • Iatrogenic, e.g. pacing, catheterisation, pericardial tapping, post-resuscitation, anticoagulant therapy 2. **Cardiac rupture** • Acute MI-free wall rupture • Aortic aneurysm rupturing into pericardium	1. **Infections** • Tuberculosis • Bacterial (pneumococal, streptococcal, staphylococcal) • Viral, fungal, parasitic • AIDS-associated 2. **Malignancy**—secondaries 3. **Uraemic** pericarditis 4. **Systemic** disorders, e.g. SLE, myxoedema, Dressler's syndrome (post-MI or postcardiotomy), amyloidosis 5. **Radiation** 6. **Idiopathic** 7. **Drugs**, e.g. anticoagulants, procainamide, isoniazide hydralazine, daunorubicin, etc.

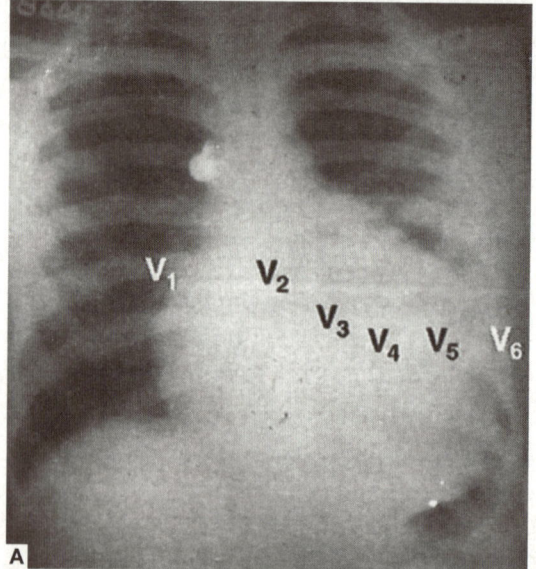

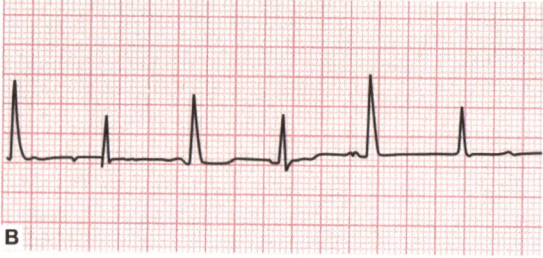

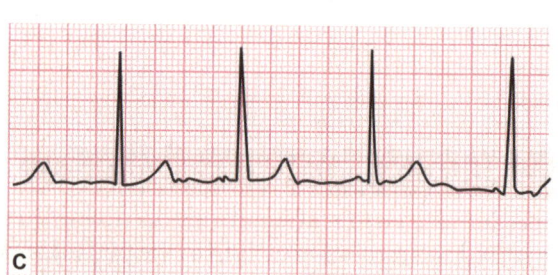

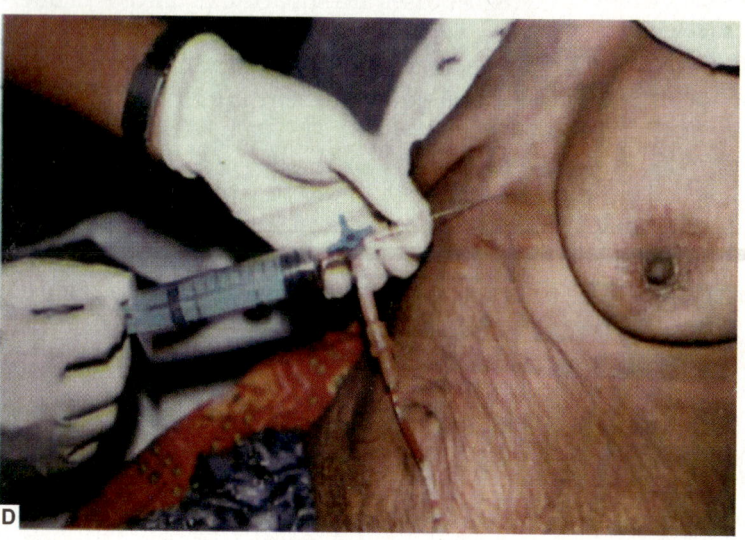

Figs 39.1A to D: Cardiac tampo-nade due to acute massive peri-cardial effusion. (A) The X-ray chest showing pericardial effusion with labelling of ECG leads, (B) the ECG lead taken from a patient with pericardial effusion shows low voltage of QRS complexes and electrical alternans (one short QRS alternates with a large QRS), (C) the same lead repeated after removal of fluid shows normal complexes with reversal of electrical alternans, (D) emergency pericardiocentesis (read the text)

to produce cardiac tamponade may be as small as 200 ml if it collects rapidly or may be 2000 ml if it collects slowly to allow the pericar-dium to stretch and adapt to the increasing volume of fluid.

The **manifestations** of tamponade range from asymptomatic or mild disease to symptomatic disease characterised by *hypoten-sion, soft or absent heart sounds* and *raised JVP with prominent 'x' discent and absent 'y' descent.* Tamponade may also develop more slowly, and the clinical manifestations resemble those of heart failure (e.g. dyspnoea, orthop-noea, congestive hepatomegaly, raised JVP). Tamponade, sometimes, may be so sudden that symptoms may not be experienced or reflect only vague symptoms, The tamponade should even be considered in any patient with hypotension, low volume pulse and raised JVP, a widened area of dullness on percussion on anterior aspect of chest wall, a paradoxical pulse, clear lung fields, dimin-ished cardiac pulsations over precordium, nonvisible apex beat, with no apparant cause of

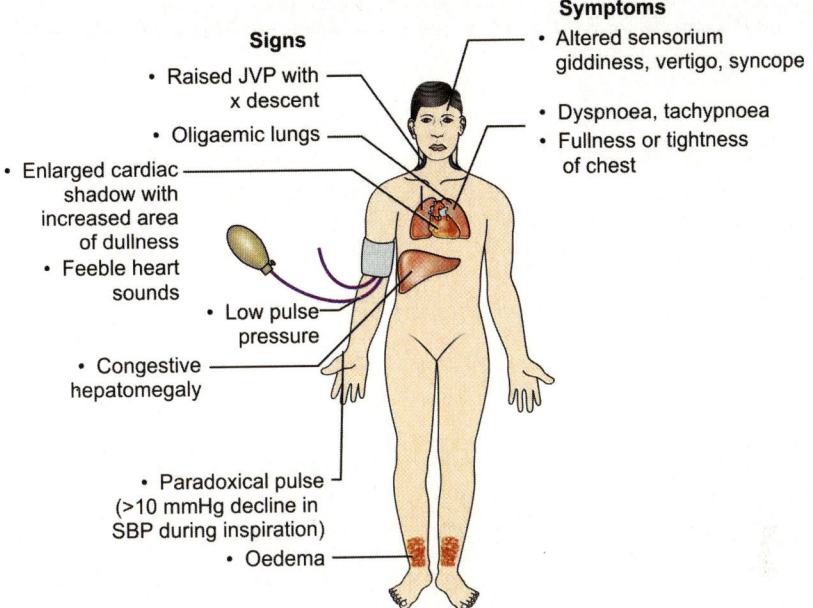

Signs

- Raised JVP with x descent
- Oligaemic lungs
- Enlarged cardiac shadow with increased area of dullness
- Feeble heart sounds
- Low pulse pressure
- Congestive hepatomegaly
- Paradoxical pulse (>10 mmHg decline in SBP during inspiration)
- Oedema

Symptoms

- Altered sensorium giddiness, vertigo, syncope
- Dyspnoea, tachypnoea
- Fullness or tightness of chest

Fig. 39.2: Clinical manifestations of cardiac tamponade (diagrammatic illustration)

pericardial disease. Patient should be subjected to investigations for confirmation of the diagnosis. The clinical features are summarized in Box 2.

Box 2	Clinical features of cardiac tamponade

1. Symptoms

- Progressive dyspnoea, tachypnoea
- Fullness, tightness of chest
- Cerebral symptoms, e.g. altered sensorium, confusion, dizziness, vertigo, syncope
- Pain chest if pericarditis present

2. Signs

- Tachycardia, low blood pressure with low pulse pressure
- Elevated JVP with prominent x descent and absent 'y' descent
- Kussmaul' sign (paradoxical rise in JVP during inspiration) is less common
- Pulsus paradoxus
- Increased area of dullness over anterior chest on percussion
- Feeble heart sounds
- Congestive hepatomegaly
- Dry lung fields on auscultation
- Pericardial knock can sometimes be present

Diagnosis and Investigations

Cardiac tamponade should be suspected in a patient who appears to be in shock but has high jugular venous pressure and distended neck veins. This is especially true in setting of trauma. The physical signs of low cardiac output with silent heart, enlarged area of dullness further strengthen the diagnosis which is confirmed by demonstrating the fluid in the pericardial sac on echocardiography. The **investigations** that help in the diagnosis are:

1. **Chest X-ray** may show enlarged globular heart (money-bag appearance) with oligaemic lungs (Fig. 39.1A).
2. **Fluoroscopy** may show diminished cardiac pulsations with enlarged cardiac shadow.
3. **The electrocardiogram** (Fig. 39.1B) may show low voltage graph, sinus tachycardia and electrical alternans (QRS alternans) (Fig. 39.1C).
4. **The echocardiogram shows:**
   i. Significant anterior and posterior echo-free space.
   ii. Right ventricular and right atrial cavities are reduced in diameter

Table 39.1 Features that distinguish cardiac tamponade from other similar clinical disorders

Feature	Tamponade	Constrictive	Restrictive	CHF
A. Clinical				
• Pulsus paradoxus	Common	Absent	Rare	Absent
• Prominent x descent on JVP	Present	Usually present	Present	Absent
• Prominent y descent on JVP	Absent	Usually present	Rare	Present
• V and Y collapse on JVP	Absent	Absent	Absent	Present
Kussmaul's sign	Absent	Present	Absent	Present
Third heart sound	Absent	Absent	Rare	Present
Pericardial knock	Absent	Present often	Absent	Absent
B. ECG				
• Low voltage graph	May be present	May be present	May be present	May be present
• Electrical alternans	May be present	Absent	Absent	Absent
C. Echocardiography				
• Thickened pericardium	Absent	Present	Absent	Absent
• Pericardial calcification	Absent	Often present	Absent	Absent
• Pericardial effusion	Present	Absent	Absent	May be present in small amount
• RV size	Usually small	Usually normal	Usually normal	Enlarged
• Myocardial thickness	Normal	Normal	Usually increased	Normal or decreased
• Right atrial collapse and RVDC	Present	Absent	Absent	Absent
• Increased mitral flow velocity	Absent	Present	Absent	May be present
• Exaggerated respiratory variations in inflow velocity	Present	Present	Absent	Absent
D. CT/MRI				
• Thickened or calcific pericardium	Absent	Present	Absent	Absent
E. Chest X-ray				
Cardiac shadow	Enlarged	Normal or enlarged	Normal	Enlarged
Cardiac pulsations on fluoroscopy	Absent	Diminished	Diminished	Normal or diminished
F. Cardiac catheterisation				
Square root's sign in ventricular pressure pulses	Absent	Present	May be present	Absent

and there is diastolic inward motion (collapse of RV and RA free wall due to high pericardial pressure).

iii. Enlarged inferior vena cava with absence of respiratory variations.

iv. *Doppler study:* The characteristic and diagnostic feature on Doppler study is the exaggerated respiratory variations in tricuspid and pulmonary valve inflow velocity. Venous flow is prominently systolic with exaggerated respiratory variations in inferior vena cava (IVC) and hepatic vein flow (diminished forward flow during expiration).

5. **CT or MRI:** Cardiac CT or MRI may be necessary to diagnose loculated effusion responsible for cardiac tamponade.

6. **CVP monitoring** helps in the diagnosis, differential diagnosis and serves as a guide to fluid therapy. CVP is raised in pericardial effusion with shock, hence, differentiates

it from hypovolaemic shock where CVP is low.

7. **Other investigations** are done to find out the cause such as biochemical, microbiological (culture for DNA of *M. tuberculosis* by PCR) and cytological examination (RBC, WBCs) of pericardial fluid. Fluid may be transudate, exudate or bloody depending on the cause.

Differential Diagnosis

The conditions (constrictive pericarditis, restrictive cardiomyopathy and CHF) that simulate the cardiac tamponade have to be differentiated from therapeutic point of view. The differential diagnosis of cardiac tamponade is tabulated in Table 39.1.

Management

It includes:

1. **Treatment of shock:** If patient is in shock state, treat it like cardiogenic shock (read cardiogenic shock). After assessment, maintain basic life support measures, i.e. airway, breathing and circulation. Fluid therapy is given to maintain preload under CVP monitoring. Inotropic agent may be used if fluid therapy alone is insufficient to restore the shock. Metabolic acidosis may be corrected.

2. **Pericardiocentesis (removal of pericardial fluid):** It is the mainstay of management because it provides rapid relief and restores the circulation and diastolic filling of the ventricles. Unless situation is immediately life-threatening, tapping should be done by an experienced personnel under echo or fluoroscopic guidance with ECG monitoring.

Procedure: Left subxiphoid approach with patient propped up to 45° is preferred (Fig. 39.1D on front page). Rarely apical or parasternal approach may be required in loculated effusions. The procedure is as follows:

a. The patient is made to lie in propped up position with back rest.

b. The patient is premedicated with atropine and diazepam.

c. The skin over the precordium and upper part of the abdomen is shaved.

d. Under aseptic precautions and local anaesthesia, a large bore long needle or I.V. cannula connected to a syringe is inserted and then connected to a 3-way stopcock for rapid aspiration. The fluid is continuously aspirated. Fluid is removed as much as possible till patient feels relief in dyspnoea and BP is restored above 90 mmHg.

e. If at any stage during procedure, frank blood is seen entering the syringe, the tip of the needle should be repositioned.

f. Always look at the ECG monitor for any VPC as this may indicate the presence of the needle in the myocardium.

g. If the fluid drawn is purulent, then it should be drained by an indwelling catheter connected to an underwater seal.

h. After removal of the fluid, patient is made to lie comfortably on the bed and observed for pulse, BP for few hours. The I.V. line is maintained during this period.

3. **Surgical pericardiotomy or pericardiectomy:** It is indicated for recurrent, frequent, disabling pericardial effusion.

Acute Chest Pain

Definitions

Acute chest pain (*central* or *peripheral*) is a common emergency encountered in clinical practice. Chest pain is a common presentation of cardiac disease, anxiety, or disease of respiratory system, musculoskeletal system or gastrointestinal system. Correct assessment and management is essential because failure to recognise a life-threatening situation such as myocardial infarction may result in unnecessary delay in instituting the treatment resulting in adverse outcome. On the other hand, erroneous diagnosis may result in psychological tension and economic consequences.

Chest pain results due to a variety of causes, has a little correlation with seriousness of the disease, hence, to be taken seriously unless proved otherwise.

Causes

A variety of causes that can lead to chest pain is divided mainly into two major categories, i.e. *central* and *peripheral* (Box 1).

Differential Diagnosis of Acute Chest Pain

A detailed history (regarding quality, location, pattern, provoking and alleviating factors) and physical examination (i.e. vital signs examination of CVS, lungs, abdomen and musculoskeletal system) would help in distinguishing

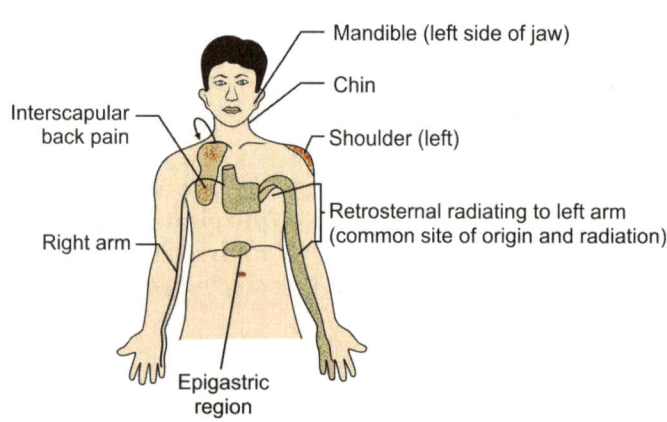

Fig. 40.1: Cardiac chest pain with radiation to other sites

Box 1 Common causes of chest pain

Central	Peripheral
a. Psychological, e.g. anxiety or cardiac neurosis	a. Lungs/pleura
b. Cardiac (42%)	• Pneumonia (consolidation)
• Myocardial ischaemia (angina) (Fig. 38.2A)	• Pneumothorax
• Myocardial infarction (Fig. 38.2B)	• Malignancy
• Myocarditis	• Pleurisy
• Pericarditis	b. Musculoskeletal
• Mitral valve prolapse syndrome	• Osteoarthritis
• Aortic dissection	• Costochondritis (Tietz's syndrome)
• Aortic aneurysm	• Injury (muscle/rib)
c. Gastroesophageal (31%)	• Epidemic myalgia (Bornholm disease)
• Oesophagitis	c. Neurological
• Diffuse oesophageal spasms	• Prolapse intervertebral disc
• Peptic ulcer disease	• Neuralgia, e.g. herpes zoster
• Hiatus hernia	• Thoracic outlet syndrome
• Mallory-Weiss syndrome	
d. Massive pulmonary embolism (2%)	
e. Mediastinal	
• Tracheitis	
• Malignancy	

Note: The musculoskeletal disorder have such a wide clinical presentation that they may produce central and/or peripheral or both types of chest pain.

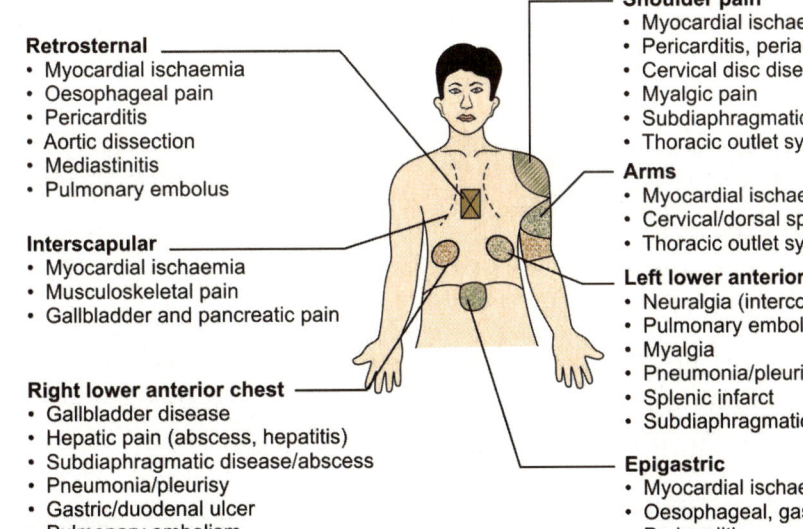

Fig. 40.2: Differential diagnosis of chest pain

cardiac pain from that of non-cardiac chest pain (Figs 40.1 and 40.2). Recording the ECG is essential in each and every case of acute chest pain or discomfort. It is important to differentiate between central and peripheral chest pain as it will help in assessing the cause of origin of pain as already listed in Box 1.

The characteristics of cardiac and noncardiac chest pain are given in Table 40.1.

Once it has become established that it is cardiac chest pain then its cause has to be established as follows:

1. **Anginal pain (stable vs unstable):** Stable angina is defined as chest pain brought

Table 40.1 Differential diagnosis of acute chest pain

Conditions/disorders	Characteristics/Location/pattern	Associated symptoms/signs
1. Ischaemic chest pain	Centrally located, retrosternal or across the chest, radiating to left arm, shoulder, neck, jaw or even right arm. Patient describes such a pain either as discomfort or tightness, pressure, squeezing or like a band (rather than actual constriction pain). Clenching of fist in front of chest (Levine's sign) is highly suggestive of cardiac pain	Diaphoresis, dyspnoea, nausea, fatigue, faintness • Auscultate for murmur • Record vital signs
2. Inflammatory/musculoskeletal		
• Myalgia • Costocondritis (Teitz's syndrome)	There is tenderness of chest on applying pressure. Pain increases on movements and is constant. Tenderness and swelling of costochondral junctions present in Teitz's syndrome	May or may not be associated fever.
3. Neurological		
• Herpetic neuralgia	There are either vesicles or scabs present along the distribution of intercostal nerves. Pain increases with chest movements	Itching, redness
4. Gastrointestinal		
• Hiatus hernia • Reflux esophagitis • Diffuse oesophageal spasms	Pain is retrosternal, occurs during lying down, relieved on sitting or by antacids and H2 blockers. Pain is in the form of heart burn, occurs after heavy meals on lying down. It causes retrosternal pain, intermittent in character, relieved by prokinetic drugs. Sometimes, it is difficult to distinguish it from angina at rest	Nausea, vomiting, sour erectation, dyspepsia, localised tenderness, mass on abdominal examination
5. Cardiovascular		
• Acute aortic dissection	Acute severe 'tearing' pain across the chest, asymmetric pulses, bradycardia are its features. • Look for hypertension. Record BP in both arms. Hear for aortic diastolic murmur	Syncope or presyncope, dizziness
• Pericarditis	Pain varies in intensity, does not increase with respiration. Audible pericardial rub may be present	
6. Respiratory		
• Pleurisy (pleurodynia)	Pain increases with breathing and a pleural rub is present	Haemoptysis, respiratory distress
• Pneumothorax	Sudden onset of pain with breathlessness. Hyper-resonant percussion note (with diminished or absent breath sounds). Chest X-ray is diagnostic	
7. Psychological		
• Cardiac neurosis	Tachycardia, pain not related to exertion but related to anxious moments. They can pinpoint the site of pain. There is sighing respiration	Nervousness, depression, frequent sobbing.

on exertion and relieved by rest and/or sublingual nitrate. The provoking factors include anaemia, thyrotoxicosis, exposure to cold, heavy meals, stress and sexual activity.

Unstable angina is *crescendo angina* or rapidly worsening angina with changing pattern of pain during the past 6 weeks (occurs on minimal exertion or at rest and pain is prolonged) without an evidence of myocardial infarction on ECG or cardiac enzyme elevation (CPK-MB).

2. **Prinzmetal's angina or variant angina**, occurs at rest without any provoking factor and is due to coronary vasospasm. The characteristic features of this type of angina is marked ST segment elevation >4 mm with increase in the height the R-wave in same leads during attack of pain and return of ST-segment to normal with relief of pain.

3. **Acute coronary syndrome:** Prolonged chest pain lasting for 10–20 minutes may be present due to acute coronary syndrome and these patients even have no abnormalities on ECG and cardiac enzymes may be normal in some cases. Others may have ST-T changes with elevation of cardiac markers like Troponin-T or Troponin I.

Exceptions: Atypical anginal symptoms such as fatigue, exhaustion, fainting sensation or dyspnoea may occur. These are called anginal equivalents. Older patients and patients with distress may not have chest pain but may have anginal equivalents as described above.

4. **Myocardial infarction:** It is characterised by central retrosternal pain which is prolonged and severe and is associated with nausea, vomiting, sweating and dyspnoea. Initial ECG and levels of cardiac enzymes may be normal but subsequent ECGs show serial changes of infarction (i.e. ST-segment elevation, q-wave and T-wave inversion in more than 2 leads) and elevation of cardiac markers, i.e. troponin T and I and raised cardiac enzymes (CPK-MB).

5. **Pain due to dissecting aneurysm of aorta:** A centrally located excruciating tearing pain lasting for hours and radiating to the back into thoracic region is a characteristic feature. Examination may show acute aortic regurgitation (early diastolic murmur in the aortic area) and evidence of hypertension (the condition is common in hypertensive). X-ray chest may show mediastinal enlargement. ECG may be normal.

6. **Pain of pericarditis:** Acute pericardial pain is not related to effort, is constant and continuous, not aggravated by deep breathing. The pain is 'sharp' located in the precordial region and may radiate to the left or right shoulder. To relieve pain, patient may sit leaning forward (Muslims' prayer sign). The pericardial rub is often present but its absence does not rule out pericarditis.

7. **Pain of pulmonary embolism:** Only large embolism produce pain similar to myocardial infarction. The triad; pain, hemoptysis and pleuritic pain in a patient with deep veinf thrombosis suggests acute pulmonary embolisms. The pain is mostly peripheral but may be central, gets aggravated by respiration and coughing.

8. **Pneumothorax:** Primary pneumothorax is rare. Secondary pneumothorax due to COPD, asthma, cystic fibrosis produce symptoms of underlying disease. The diagnosis is suspected by localised hyper-reasonant note and confirmation is done on X-ray chest.

9. **Pleural chest** due to pleurisy, pneumonia, malignancy is typical knife-like pain worsened by inspiration and coughing. Pleural rub is diagnostic.

10. **Other noncardiac conditions**, i.e. gastrointestinal, musculoskeletal disorders are described in Table 40.1 and Fig. 40.1.

Investigations

ECG: It is a pivotal for identifying the myocardial ischaemia/infarction with the primary aim of recognising ST-elevation (STEMI). These are candidates for PTCA.

It also helps to detect abnormalities indicative of pulmonary embolism, ventricular hypertrophy, pericarditis, myocarditis, electrolyte imbalance and metabolic disorders.

Chest X-ray: It is performed routinely. The chest X-ray is useful for identifying pulmonary diseases causing chest pain, i.e. pneumonia, pneumothorax. It is also helpful in diagnosis of pulmonary oedema and aortic dissection.

Cardiac biomarkers: Creatinine kinase MB, cardiac troponin is the preferred biomarker for diagnosis of MI.

D-dimer: It helps to exclude pulmonary embolism.

Other non-invasive studies:
- *Echocardiography:* It is not a routine test. It is done for ischaemic dysfunction (i.e. regional wall abnormality) for mechanical complications of MI or for pericardial tamponade. Transthoracic echocardiography is useful for detection of aortic dissection.

CT angiography/MRI: CT angiography of chest, coronary angiography may be done in selected cases. Cardiac MRI is a versatile technique for structural and functional evaluation of the heart and vasculature of chest.

Management

The patients of acute chest pain should be managed appropriately depending on the cause.

Cardiac Arrest and Sudden Cardiac Death

CARDIAC ARREST

It is defined as sudden and complete loss of cardiac pump function leading to no pulse, no respiration and sudden loss of consciousness. Death is virtually inevitable if prompt intervention is not done.

SUDDEN CARDIAC DEATH (SCD)

It is defined as the unexpected natural death due to cardiac causes within a short period of time (usually within 1 hour) from the start of symptoms in an individual who may have pre-existing heart disease but in whom the *time* and *mode* of death are unexpected. *Death means irreversible loss of all biological functions.*

Cardiovascular collapse means loss of sufficient cerebral blood flow to maintain consciousness due to acute dysfunction of the heart and/or peripheral *vasculature*.

Sudden and unexpected cardiac death is usually due to development of a catastrophic arrhythmia (ventricular fibrillation, Fig. 41.1 or pulseless VT) and accounts for 25–30% of cardiovascular deaths.

Risk Factors

1. **Advanced age:** The incidence of sudden cardiac death increases with age in both the sexes and in all races; though it is more common in males.

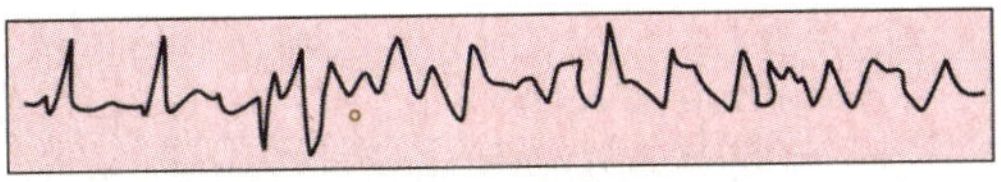

Fig. 41.1: Ventricular fibrillation

2. **Altered coronary anatomy** such as atheroma, plaque rupture or both.
3. **Depressed left ventricular function:** There is an increased risk of sudden cardiac death in patients with cardiac disease having ejection fraction <30%.
4. **Reversible risk factors:** Certain factors such as transient myocardial ischaemia and reperfusion, electrolyte disturbances (hypokalaemia, hypomagnesemia), drugs (diuretics, digitalis), alteration in pH or blood gas may provoke SCD if not taken care of immediately.
5. **Other risk factors are:**
   • Hypertension
   • LVH
   • Conduction defects
   • Hyperlipidaemia
   • Smoking
   • Glucose intolerance
   • Decreased vital capacity.

In *Framingham study,* the incidence of SCD in smokers was two and half times more than in non-smokers.

Causes

Structural coronary artery disease is the single most common cause of SCD (90%). The

Table 41.1 Common causes of sudden cardiac death

1. Coronary artery diseases (80%)
- Myocardial ischaemia
- Acute MI or healed MI
- Previous MI with myocardial scarring
- Anomalous coronary artery anatomy

2. Myocardial diseases
- Ventricular hypertrophy, e.g. LVH, RVH, CHF
- Hypertrophic cardiomyopathy, e.g. obstructive and nonobstructive
- Dilated cardiomyopathy
- Inflammatory or infiltrative diseases, e.g. myocarditis, arrhythmogenic right ventricular dysplasia

3. Valvular heart diseases
- Aortic stenosis/regurgitation
- Mitral valve prolapse
- Endocarditis

4. Congenital heart diseases
- Stenotic lesions (aortic or pulmonary)
- Eisenmenger's syndrome
- Postoperative repair of Fallot's tetralogy

5. Nonstructural heart disease (e.g. electrophysiological abnormalities):
- Prolonged QT syndrome (congenital or acquired)
- Brugada syndrome. It is characterised by a defect in sodium channels function and an abnormal ECG (RBBB and ST elevation in V_1 and V_2 without prolongation of QT interval)
- Wolff-Parkinson-White syndrome (Kent bundle conduction)
- Adverse drug reactions leading to torsade de pointes
- Electrolyte disturbances (severe hypokalaemia)
- Acid-base disturbance, e.g. severe acidosis

6. Miscellaneous
- Massive pulmonary embolism, air embolism
- Aortic dissection
- Cafe coronary

Box 1 Potentially reversible causes of cardiac arrest

4Hs	*4Ts*
• Hypovolaemia	• Thromboembolism
• Hypoxia	• Tension pneumothorax
• Hypo- or hyperkalaemia	• Tamponade
• Hypothermia	• Toxic disturbance or therapeutic disturbances

myocardial causes (cardiomyopathies) account for another 10–15% cases; the remaining are due to other causes given in Table 41.1.

Aetiology of Cardiac Arrest

Cardiac arrest may be due to:
- Ventricular fibrillation
- Pulseless ventricular tachycardia
- Asystole
- Bradyarrhythmia
- Electromechanical dissociation

Ventricular fibrillation (VF) and pulseless ventricular tachycardia: This is most common and most easily treatable cause of sudden death. It is characterised by uncoordinated rapid, bizarre ventricular contractions which are ineffective to produce a pulse. The ECG shows rapid irregular ventricular rhythm with no identifiable complexes (Fig. 41.2). Ventricular tachycardia may also cause loss of cardiac output (pulseless VT) and may further degenerate into VF.

Ventricular asystole: It is characterised by no electrical activity of the ventricles producing more or less straight line on ECG. It is usually due to failure of the conducting tissue or massive ventricular damage complicating MI. A sudden blow to the chest (precordial thump) or cardiac massage can sometimes restore the cardiac activity. An artificial pacemaker may be needed to prevent further attacks (see the algorithm).

Electromechanical dissociation: There is dissociation between electrical activity (it is normal or near normal) and mechanical events (no effective cardiac output). It is mostly due to extraneous causes such as hypovolaemia, tension pneumothorax, cardiac rupture or massive pulmonary embolism. It carries poor prognosis.

Clinical Characteristics of Cardiac Arrest

1. **Prodromal symptoms and signs:** These complaints are nonspecific, presaged by days, weeks or months and are indicative of any major cardiac event. These include

increasing angina, dyspnoea, palpitation, easy fatiguability, etc.

2. **Onset of terminal events:** Any change in cardiovascular status one hour before cardiac arrest constitutes onset of terminal events. The more rapid is the onset of terminal events, the more is the probability of cardiac arrest. Continuous ECG recordings fortuitously obtained at the onset of a cardiac arrest commonly demonstrate changes in cardiac electrical activity (ECG changes of dying heart) within the minutes or hours before the event. Most cardiac arrest occurring by the mechanisms of VF begin with a run of sustained or nonsustained VT degenerating rapidly into VF and asystole.

3. **Disturbed consciousness:** Arrhythmic cardiac arrest (VF) is characterised by likelihood of the patients being awake and active prior to arrest; while on the other hand cardiac arrest due to circulatory failure is characterised by disturbed consciousness, any long duration of terminal illness.

Complete loss of consciousness with no pulse and BP are sine qua non of cardiac arrest.

4. **Forewarning symptoms and signs** may occur in setting of acute MI; such as prolonged angina or pain of AMI, acute onset of dyspnoea, orthopnoea, sudden onset of palpitation, sustained tachycardia or light headedness. In MI, cardiac arrest may be *primary* (no haemodynamic instability) or *secondary* (presence of haemodynamic instability) and has clinical significance because majority or all patients survive with primary cardiac arrest while majority (70%) die in secondary cardiac arrest immediately or during the hospitalization.

5. **Progression to biological death** is a function of the mechanism of cardiac arrest and depends on length of the delay before interventions. VF or asystole without CPR within first 4–6 minutes leads to biological death.

Management

The treatment of a patient with cardiac arrest is divided into 5 stages:

1. Initial evaluation and basic life support; if cardiac arrest is confirmed.
2. Defibrillation (when available)
3. Advanced life support.
4. Post-resuscitation management/care.
5. Long-term management.

Initial Evaluation

The first step is to establish cardiac arrest. Ask the patient, *Hello! Are you OK* and observe the response. Observe for stale of consciousness, respiratory movement, pulse and skin colour, sweating, etc. The absence of pulse and respiration is primary diagnostic criteria and can be confirmed accurately by a trained or lay person. As soon as cardiac arrest is confirmed, call an emergency rescue system/van.

Thumpversion or precordial blow (a sudden discharge of a blow to the precordium) and clearing the airway by head tilt/chin lift, removal of denture and/or foreign body (*Heimlich maneuver* if suspected) are the steps of initial management before CPR can be carried out. A precordial thumb occasionally may revert VT or VF. If respiratory arrest precipitating the cardiac arrest is suspected, a second precordial blow/thump is delivered after the airway is clear. Precordial thump/blow is delivered with a clenched fist to the junction of middle and lower thirds of the sternum.

Basic Life Support (Fig. 41.2)

Basic life support, popularly known as *cardiopulmonary resuscitation (CPR)* is meant to maintain organ perfusion until definite interventions can be instituted. The initial and primary element of CPR is to maintain *circulation (C), airway (A)* and *breathing (B).*

Circulation is maintained by closed chest compressions by placing one palm of one hand over the lower sternum while other palm resting on the dorsum of lower hand. The sternum is depressed with the arms remaining straight at a rate of 100/min. Sufficient force to depress the sternum (4–5 cm) is used and then released abruptly. Airway is kept patent by tilting the head back and lifting the chin and clearing the respiratory passage. *Breathing* (B) is maintained either by mouth-to-mouth or by oropharyngeal airways, or masked ambu bag.

Advanced Life Support Measures (Fig. 41.2)

Advance life support aims at:

1. To restore normal cardiac rhythm by defibrillation when the cause of cardiac arrest is tachyarrhythmias.
2. To restore cardiac output by correcting other reversible causes of cardiac arrest (*4 Hs and 4 Ts*) are given in Box 1
3. To provide additional support to basic life saving measures by administering intravenous drugs
4. Intubation with an endotracheal tube to administer positive pressure ventilation.
5. Insertion of intravenous line.

Measures/Actions

If cardiac arrest is witnessed, a *thumpversion (precordial thump)* may sometime convert VF/VT to normal sinus rhythm. It is of no use if the cardiac arrest has lasted longer than few seconds. Start CAB also called ABC of basic life support.

The priority of advanced life support (ALS) is to assess basic cardiac rhythm by attaching a defibrillator/monitor. *Defibrillation* is indicated if VF or pulseless VT is observed on monitor. Defibrillation is started first with 200 Joules, if normal sinus rhythm is not restored within few seconds, then CPR is done at a rate of 100/min for 2 minutes followed by shock of 200 Joules; if unsuccessful, chest compressions continued followed by a third shock of 360 Joules. If all the three shocks remain unsuccessful, then 1 mg of adrenaline intravenously *plus* CPR is continued for full one minute to prepare the patient for next cycle of three shocks each at 360 Joules (Fig. 41.2). If the patient is less than fully conscious on reversion

or if two to three attempts fail, prompt intubation, ventilation and arterial blood gas analysis should be carried out. Ventilation with O_2 may promptly reverse hypoxemia and acidosis. For acidosis, $NaHCO_3$ may be used. If electromechanical dissociation is the cause of cardiac arrest, then it is treated without defibrillation by only maintaining the CPR and treating or correcting the reversible causes of cardiac arrest (4 Hs and 4Ts) which have already been discussed (Box 1).

Antiarrhythmia Therapy

After initial unsuccessful defibrillation attempt or with persistent/recurrent electrical instability, intravenous amiodarone (150 mg over 10 minutes followed by 1 mg/min up to 6 for and 0.5 mg/min thereafter) is the initial treatment of choice, for cardiac arrest due to VF, a bolus of 1 mg/kg of lidocaine may be given I.V. as an alternative and dose may be repeated after 2 minutes. I.V. procainamide or Intravenous magnesium can be used.

Cardiac Arrest due to Bradyarrhythmias

Cardiac arrest due to bradyarrhythmias or asystole is managed differently. The steps of management are:

- Intubation, I.V. access and suctioning of obstructing secretion. Heimlich manoeuvre for removal of foreign body. Confirm asystole
- CPR is continued.
- Control hypoxemia with O_2 therapy and acidosis by $NaHCO_3$ (1mEq/1 kg I.V.).
- Adrenaline 1 mg or atropine (1 mg) is given I.V. or intracardiac depending on the cause.
- External pacing to establish a regular cardiac rhythm.

Postcardiac Arrest Care

After successful resuscitation of cardiac arrest, the patient is observed in intensive care unit for continuous monitoring for a minimum period of 48–72 hours. Treat the underlying cause if found out.

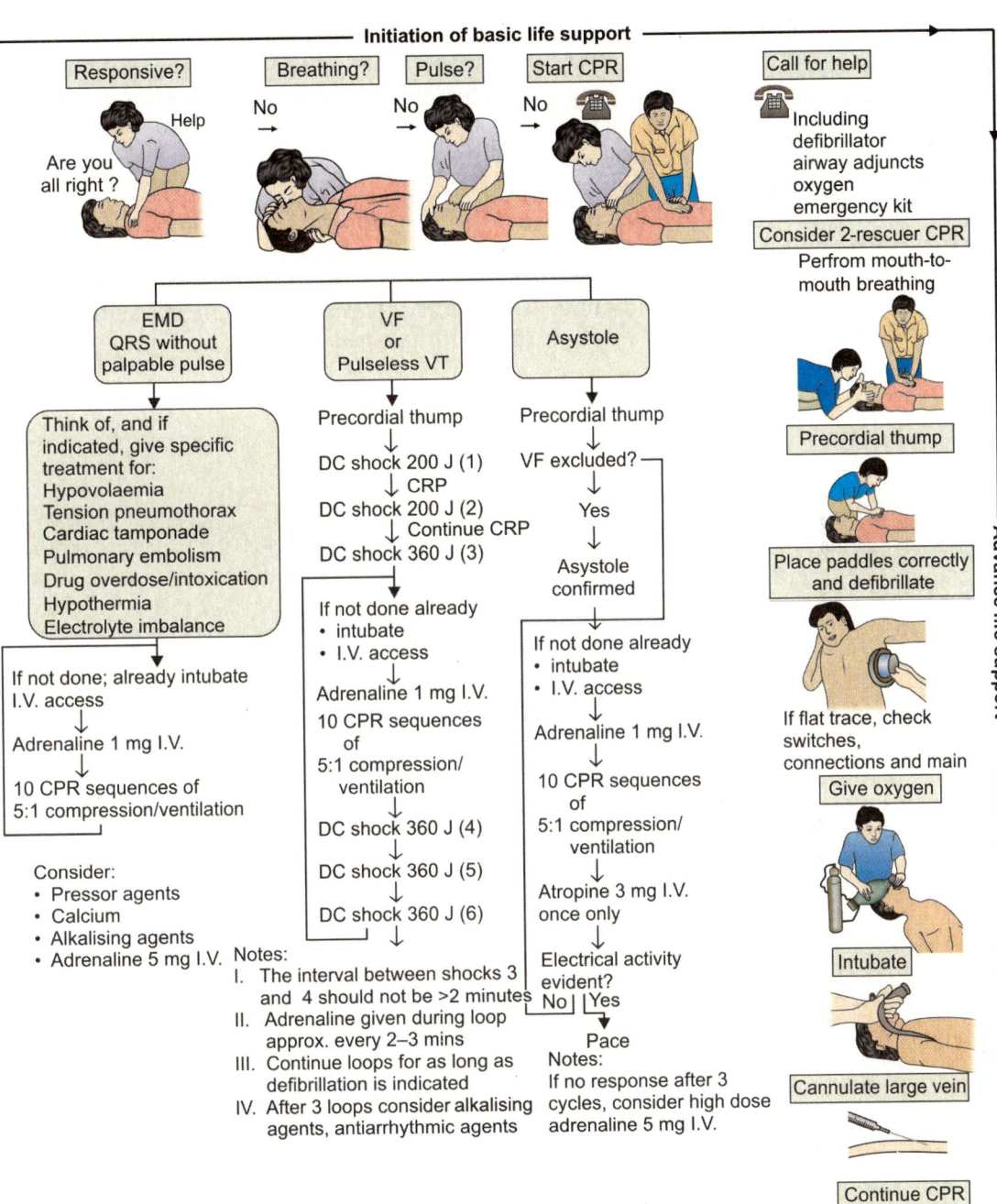

Initiation of basic life support

Responsive? — Are you all right? Help

Breathing? — No

Pulse? — No

Start CPR — No

Call for help — Including defibrillator airway adjuncts oxygen emergency kit

Consider 2-rescuer CPR — Perfrom mouth-to-mouth breathing

Precordial thump

Place paddles correctly and defibrillate

If flat trace, check switches, connections and main

Give oxygen

Intubate

Cannulate large vein

Continue CPR

Advance life support

EMD QRS without palpable pulse

Think of, and if indicated, give specific treatment for:
Hypovolaemia
Tension pneumothorax
Cardiac tamponade
Pulmonary embolism
Drug overdose/intoxication
Hypothermia
Electrolyte imbalance

If not done; already intubate I.V. access
↓
Adrenaline 1 mg I.V.
↓
10 CPR sequences of 5:1 compression/ventilation

Consider:
• Pressor agents
• Calcium
• Alkalising agents
• Adrenaline 5 mg I.V.

VF or Pulseless VT

Precordial thump
↓
DC shock 200 J (1)
↓ CRP
DC shock 200 J (2)
↓ Continue CRP
DC shock 360 J (3)
↓
If not done already
• intubate
• I.V. access
↓
Adrenaline 1 mg I.V.
↓
10 CPR sequences of 5:1 compression/ventilation
↓
DC shock 360 J (4)
↓
DC shock 360 J (5)
↓
DC shock 360 J (6)
↓

Notes:
I. The interval between shocks 3 and 4 should not be >2 minutes
II. Adrenaline given during loop approx. every 2–3 mins
III. Continue loops for as long as defibrillation is indicated
IV. After 3 loops consider alkalising agents, antiarrhythmic agents

Asystole

Precordial thump
↓
VF excluded?
↓
Yes
↓
Asystole confirmed
↓
If not done already
• intubate
• I.V. access
↓
Adrenaline 1 mg I.V.
↓
10 CPR sequences of 5:1 compression/ventilation
↓
Atropine 3 mg I.V. once only
↓
Electrical activity evident?
No | Yes
↓
Pace

Notes:
If no response after 3 cycles, consider high dose adrenaline 5 mg I.V.

If an I.V. line cannot be establised, consider giving double or triple doses of adrenaline via an endotracheal tube
Prolonged resuscitation
Consider alkalising agents, e.g. 50 mmol sodium bicarbonate (50 ml of 8.4%) or according to blood gas results

Post-resuscitation care
Check:
• Arterial blood gases, Electrolyte, Chest X-ray
• Monitor ECG and treat patient in an ICU

Fig. 41.2: Advanced cardiac life support (recommended by the European Resuscitation Council and Resuscitation Council of UK)

Long-term Management

Patients who survive a cardiac arrest caused by AMI need no specific treatment other than routinely given to those recovering from an infarct. Those with reversible causes such as exercise induced ischaemia or aortic stenosis should be treated if possible. Survivors in whom no reversible cause can be found out and are at higher risk of developing another episode, such patients are treated either by antiarrhythmic therapy or implantation of implantable cardioverter defibrillator (ICD). Superiority of ICD over antiarrhythmic drug therapy (predominantly amiodarone) has been shown in AVID trial and in other studies (CIDS and CASH).

> ICD is the initial treatment of choice for long-term management in patients revived from VF in whom no reversible cause could be found out, e.g. right ventricular dysplasia, long QT syndrome and Brugada syndrome.

Hypertensive Emergencies or Urgencies

HYPERTENSIVE CRISES

Terms used Related to Hypertension

Hypertension: The 7th JNC (Joint National Committee) report on prevention, detection, evaluation and treatment of hypertension has defined normal and abnormal values of BP (Box 1) superseding the recommendation of VI JNC report.

The VIIth JNC report describes <120/ 80 mmHg as normal BP in patients aged 18 years or above; beyond 120/80 mmHg is considered either prehypertension or hypertension.

Clinically, hypertension may be defined as that level of BP at which the patient requires treatment to lower it. The JNC VIII has defined this as upper limit of normal, i.e. 140/90 mmHg. Above this limit, patient has to be treated. Otherwise all the guidelines suggest 120/80 mmHg as normal BP in stricker sense.

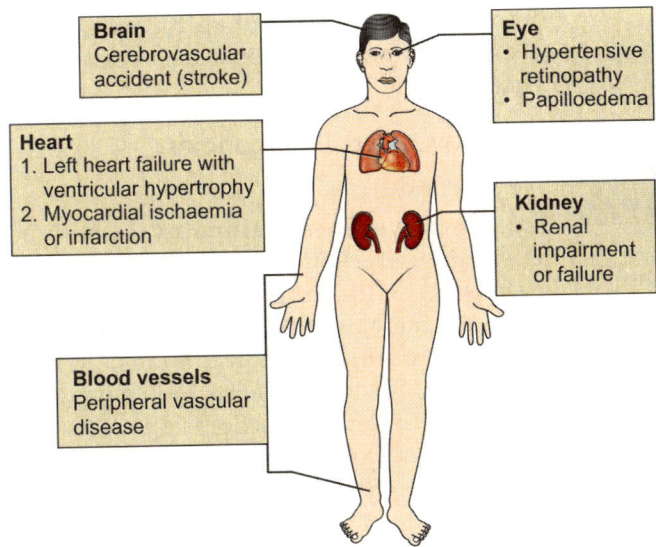

Fig. 42.1: Possible organ damage in hypertensive emergency

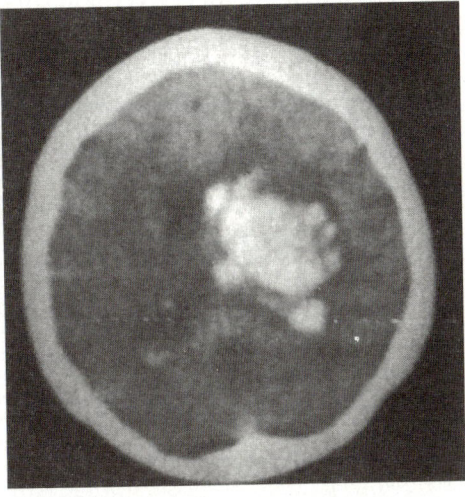

Fig. 42.2: CT scan showing intracranial bleed

Box 1   JNC VII classification of hypertension

Category	Systolic (mmHg)	Diastolic (mmHg)
Normal	<120	<80
Prehypertension (previous term high normal replaced)	120–139	80–89
Hypertension		
Stage 1st	140–159	90–99
Stage 2nd	>160	>100
JNC VIII defining hypertension		
Hypertension	≥140	≥90
Normal	120	80

HYPERTENSIVE EMERGENCIES/ URGENCIES

Hypertensive emergency: According to JNC VI report, a hypertensive emergency was defined as a severely elevated BP diastolic >130 mmHg with signs or symptoms of acute target organ damage (Fig. 42.1), requiring parenteral drug treatment, close observation in ICU and immediate reduction of blood pressure (within one hour) to avoid risk of morbidity or death.

These are patients with severe asymptomatic hypertension with BP >220/120 mmHg with ocular fundal changes (Table 42.1).

Hypertensive urgency: It is a state of severely elevated blood pressure which is not associated with severe symptoms or progressive

Table 42.1   Hypertensive emergencies and urgencies

Emergencies	Urgencies
• Hypertensive encephalopathy or malignant hypertension	• Hypertension associated with coronary artery disease
• Hypertensive nephropathy	• Accelerated hypertension
• Acute aortic dissection	
• Pheochromocytoma crisis	• Severe hypertension in patients with kidney transplantation
• Hypertension with LVF	
• Pre-eclampsia	• Postoperative hypertension
• MAO inhibitors with tyramine interaction	• Uncontrolled hypertension in patients requiring surgery
• Intracranial haemorrhage	

organ dysfunction wherein BP can be reduced within a few hours, often with oral drug therapy given in an outpatient setting with ocular fundal changes (Table 42.1).

JNC VI stressed acute target organ damage irrespective of blood pressure reading as hypertensive emergency rather than urgency.

With this report, previously used term, (i) accelerated hypertension (diastolic BP >130 mmHg and malignant hypertension with diastolic BP >130 mm have been replaced and are covered as hypertensive urgency and hypertensive emergency respectively. The fundoscopic differentiation, between accelerated and malignant hypertension has no relevance with respect to clinical picture and prognosis, hence, may be taken hypertensive emergency or urgency.

Most authors treat hypertensive emergency as hypertensive crisis.

COMMON HYPERTENSIVE EMERGENCIES (TABLE 42.1)

It is the presence of critical multiple end organ injury that determines the seriousness of emergency and the approach to treatment. These include:

Cerebrovascular Emergencies

These include:

Hypertensive encephalopathy is defined as sudden, marked rise in blood pressure associated with encephalopathic features, i.e. headache, vomiting, visual disturbances, transient paralysis, convulsions, stupor and coma. These manifestations have been attributed to spasm of cerebral vessels and to cerebral oedema (read the management at the end). The other examples of hypertensive emergency and urgency are given in Table 42.1.

The *pathophysiological basis* of hypertensive crisis is loss of autoregulation on the vascular beds (*cerebral, cardiac, renal*) with the result they are not able to constrict appropriately to maintain perfusion. This leads to ischaemia and tissue damage. This forms the basis that BP should be lowered as early as possible (within minutes or hours) with parenteral drugs during hypertensive emergency (Box 2) so as to restore autoregulation. The blood pressure should not be drastically reduced to normal because it can give rise to serious consequences, hence, should be kept near normal rather than normal.

Clinical Evaluation

It includes:

1. Careful history with respect to duration, severity of pre-existing hypertension and symptoms of any target organ damage should be asked.
2. Record the type of drug therapy received and compliance of treatment.
3. Examination of BP in both lying and standing positions, in both the arms. Significant difference between two arms suggests aortic dissection.
4. Examine cardiovascular, renal and nervous system for any organ damage.
5. Fundus examination for retinopathy.
6. Blood biochemistry, i.e. urea, creatinine, sodium, K^+.
7. Chest X-ray for cardiomegaly.
8. ECG for LVH, prior MI.
9. Urine examination for proteinuria.
10. CT scan/MRI for neurological damage.

Intracranial bleed (Fig. 42.2) or **subarachnoid haemorrhage** is diagnosed by *altered mental state, signs of meningeal irritation, symptoms and signs of raised intracranial tension*; and confirmed on lumbar puncture, CT scan and MRI. The aim of treatment is to minimise bleeding and blood pressure goals depend on the patient's BP. In normotensive patients the target systolic BP to be achieved is 110–120 mmHg; in hypertensive patients BP should be kept near normal or slightly above normal (≥ 140/90 mm kg). The drug of choice is nicardipine or labetalol.

Acute ischaemic stroke is often associated with marked elevation of BP which will usually resolve spontaneously. In such case antihypertensive should be started if BP exceeds >220/120 mmHg and BP should be reduced cautiously by 10–15%. If thrombolytics are to be given the BP should be maintained <180/110 mmHg during treatment and 24 hours following treatment.

Treatment

The risks and benefits of acute lowering of BP during an acute stroke or cerebrovascular disease are still unclear, but control of BP at intermediate level (<160/100 mmHg) is appropriate for thrombolysis if planned or until the condition has stabilized or improved (JNC report VIII). Sudden drastic lowering of BP in hypertensive emergency is counterproductive, may increase ischaemia of watershed areas of brain. The drug therapy used is discussed at the end for all emergencies. However, a short-acting intravenous drug (Table 42.2) is preferred which can be stopped at ease. Preffered drugs for various hypertensive emergencies are presented in Box 2.

Renal Emergencies (Hypertensive Nephropathy)

Most patients who present as hypertensive emergencies have already dearranged renal functions, i.e. reduction in GFR, rise in serum creatinine, microalbuminuria or overt albuminuria.

The **therapeutic goals** are to slow deterioration of renal functions and prevent cerebrovascular disease (CVD). Hypertension appears in majority of patients and should receive aggressive BP management often with combination of drugs (3 or more) to achieve target BP value of < 130/80 mmHg.

Cardiovascular Emergencies

It includes:

1. **Acute myocardial ischaemia/infarction** in hypertensive patient is diagnosed on ECG and echocardiography. Drug of choice is nicardipine plus on beta-blocker.

Table 42.2 Parenteral drugs used in hypertensive emergencies

Drug	Dosage and route	Onset of action	Duration of action	Side effects
Nitroprusside (Veno-arteriolar dilator)	I.V. infusion 0.25–10 µg/kg/min	Immediate	3–5 minutes	Nausea, vomiting, sweating muscle twitchings, thiocyanate toxicity with high doses for prolonged period
Diazoxide (arteriolar dilator)	50–150 mg I.V. as bolus every 5–10 minutes or 15–30 mg/min I.V. infusions (max 600 mg)	2–4 min	6–12 min	Nausea, hypotension, flushing, tachycardia, chest pain and hyperglycaemia and Na⁺ and water retention
Hydralazine	10–20 mg/I.V. or IM at 30 minutes intervals or 0.5–1 mg/min I.V. infusion	10–20 min	3–8 hours	Tachycardia, flushing, headache, vomiting, aggravation of angina
Nitroglycerin (predominant venous than arteriolar dilator)	Initial 5–10 µg/min I.V. infusion, titrate to higher doses to get the response (max 100 µg/min)	2–5 min	3–5 min	Headache, hypotension methemoglobinaemia, nausea nitrate tolerance requiring an increase in dose
Enalaprilat (ACE inhibitor)	0.625–1.25 mg every 6 hourly	10–15 min	Within 6 hours	Hypotension, angioedema, renal failure (if bilateral renal artery stenosis)
Nicardipine (Ca⁺⁺ channel blockers)	2–8 mg/hour I.V. (max 15 mg/hr)	5–10 min	30–60 min	Tachycardia, headache, hypotension, flushing, rhinitis
Esmolol (beta-blocker)	200–500 µg/kg/min for 4 minutes then 50–300 µg/kg/min	1–2 min	10–20 min	Hypotension, bronchospasm, nausea, bradycardia, AV blocks
Labetalol (alpha and beta-adrenergic blocker)	20–40 mg/I.V. bolus every 10 min up to 300 mg; 2 mg/min I.V. infusion total	5–10 min	3–6 hours	Nausea, vomiting, burning in throat, dizziness, broncho-spasm postural hypotension
Trimethaphan (ganglion blocker)	0.5–5 mg/min I.V. bolus	1–5 min	10 min	Postural hypotension, bowel paresis, blurring of vision and tachycardia

2. **Left heart failure or pulmonary oedema** due to HT is diagnosed on clinical examination, chest X-ray and echocardiogram.

3. **Aortic dissection** is suspected clinically and echocardiogram is helpful in diagnosis.

The *goal of therapy* is to reduce BP <140/90 mmHg. The drugs of choice are vasodilators, i.e. ACE inhibitors and/or angiotensin receptor blockers (ARBs), beta-blockers and diuretics.

In aortic dissection, a BP of <120 mmHg should be achieved quickly within minutes using beta-blockers and a vasodilator to decrease aortic stress. Surgical management thereafter is mandatory.

PREGNANCY AND HYPERTENSION

Pregnancy Related States

1. **Gestational hypertension** is defined as transient hypertension occurring after 20 weeks of gestation in the absence of pre-existing chromic hypertension or proteinuria. Such women need close observation.

2. **Pregnancy-induced hypertension (PIH)** means a previously normotensive woman develops hypertension (≥140/90 mmHg) after 20 weeks of pregnancy. Pregnancy induced hypertension is the earliest sign of pre-eclampsia syndrome. Increasing blood pressure as above prepregnant BP during first half

of pregnancy is more important than any exact figure. In pregnant women, BP should be measured in sitting position and at least 2 readings 6 hours apart must be taken before labelling the patient as hypertensive. BP after delivery returns to normal.

3. **Pre-eclampsia/Eclampsia:** Pre-eclampsia is diagnosed clinically by the development of *hypertension, proteinuria, oedema* which may be associated with *convulsions* (*eclampsia*) or *haemolysis, hepatic dysfunction,* i.e. *elevated liver enzymes* and *thrombocytopaenia* (HELLP syndrome) even in the absence of significant hypertension.

As the risk of eclampsia is real, BP control has to be much stricter in pregnant patients. Patient with mild eclampsia should be managed conservatively with limited physical activity. For women with severe eclampsia (BP>160/110 mmHg) should be treated with I.V. labetalol or hydralazine or nicardipine. Oral nifedipine and methyldopa can be used in patients with chromic hypertension in pregnancy (patients who are hypertensive become pregnant). Therefore, women with hypertension should be followed carefully because of increased risk to mother and foetus. The ACEs and ARBs should be avoided. The target blood pressure to be achieved is <140/90 mmHg by drug therapy.

Drug Therapy for Hypertensive Emergencies

Drugs used for hypertensive emergencies are generally given parenterally in an ICU where the progress can be easily monitored. The

Box 2	Preferred parenteral drugs during hypertensive emergencies	
Emergency	*Recommended drug (drugs of choice)*	*To avoid*
Hypertensive encephalopathy	• Labetolol • Nicardipine, nimodipine • Nitroprusside	• Diazoxide • Methyldopa
Stroke	• Labetolol • Nicardipine • Nitroprusside	• Methyldopa • Diazoxide • Hydralazine
Heart failure	• Enalaprilat plus • Nitro glycerin plus • Loop diuretics (fursemide)	• Labetolol • Beta-blockers (e.g. esmolol)
Coronary artery disease	• Nitroglycerin plus esmolal • Labetolol • Nicardipine plus esmolol	• Hydralazine • Diazoxide
Phaeochromocytoma	• Phenotolamine • Labetolol	All others
Postoperative	• Labetolol • Nitroglycerine • Nicardipine	Trimethophan
Eclampsia/pre-eclampsia	• Hydralazine • Labetolol • Nicardipine	• Nitroprusside • Trimethophan • Diuretics
Aortic dissection	• Nitroprusside plus esmolol • Labetalol • Esmolol plus nicardipine	• Hydralazine • Diazoxide

Note: Sodium nitroprusside is no longer the treatment of choice for acute hypertensive emergencies, in most circumstances, appropriate BP control can be achieved using combinations of nicardipine or elevidipine plus labetalol or esmolol.

drugs (Table 42.2) used are those which have rapid onset and offset of action and their effects can easily be reversed.

Choice of an Antihypertensive Drug during an Emergency

Each drug has its own advantages and disadvantages, hence, choice of an antihypertensive drug during an hypertensive emergency depends not only on its action but its suitability during that situation. The various drugs suited to various hypertensive emergencies are given in Box 2.

Treatment Targets

In the hypertension optimal treatment (HOT) trial, the optimal BP for reduction of major cardiovascular events was found to be 130/80 mmHg, or even lower in patients with diabetes. Nowadays a consensus opinion is to achieve the target BP of <130/80 mm in all patients of hypertension with diabetes, with chronic kidney disease and coronary artery disease.

Drugs Therapy in Hypertensive Urgencies (Box 3)

As already discussed, the hypertensive urgencies require oral administration of drugs to control hypertension as there is no target organ damage. The drugs are:

1. **Oral or sublingual nifedipine:** This was the most common and most popular drug for immediate control of hypertension and is available in gelatinous capsule. It fell into controversy for some period due to its adverse effects (e.g. sudden fall in BP following sublingual use leading to hypoperfusion of organs and reflex tachycardia. Because myocardial infarction and stroke have been reported with its use, hence, its use is not advised.

2. **Oral clonidine:** It is given as oral loading dose of 0.2 mg followed by 0.1 mg every hour thereafter till BP falls to a target level. It can be given on outpatient basis. Sedation and rebound hypertension may occur if the drug is stopped.

3. **Oral captopril:** It can be used in hypertensive urgencies in the dose of 12.5 to 25 mg.

MALIGNANT HYPERTENSION

It is characterised by marked rise in BP (≥220/130 mmHg) in a patient with underlying hypertension or sudden onset of hypertension in a previously normotensive person, with grade IV fundal changes (haemorrhage, exudate and papilledema of optic fundi) and

Box 3	Oral drugs for hypertensive urgencies		
Drug	Dose and route	Duration of action	Side-effects
Amlodipine	5–10 mg	Action starts within 45–60 min. remains for 24 hours	• Hypotension • Tachycardia
Clonidine	0.1–0.2 mg every hour	Action starts within 45–60 min., remains for 6–8 hours	• Dry mouth • Sedation
Captopril or enalapril	6.25–20 mg 10–30 mg	Action starts within 15–30 min, lasts for 4–6 hours	• Acute renal failure, dry cough • Angioneurotic oedema, Hyperkalaemia
Labetolol	100–300 mg	Action within 30–60 min. lasts for 6–12 hours	• Bronchospasm, nausea, vomiting, tingling of scalp
Carvedilol	(2.5–50 mg)	-do-	• burning in throat, dizziness, postural hypotension
Prazosin	1–2 mg	Onset of action 15–60 min; remains for 6 hours	• Flushing • Hypotension
Losartan	25–100 mg	Action starts within half and hour, lasts for 6–8 hours	• ARF, dry cough • Angioneurotic, oedema, Hyperkalaemia

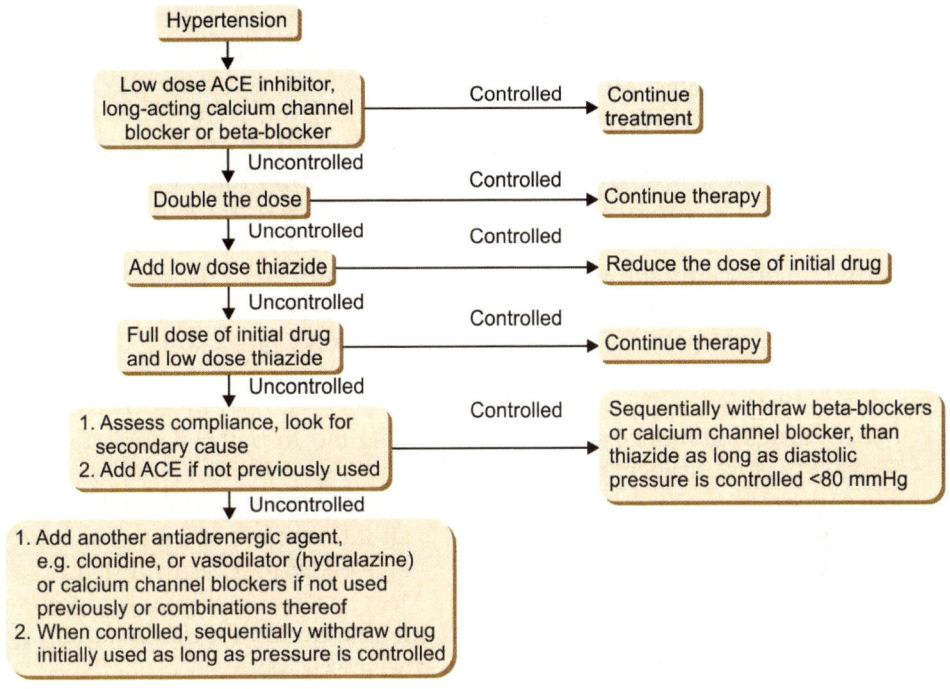

Fig. 42.3: Schematic approach to hypertension (fresh case who does not have volume expansion)

features of hypertensive encephalopathy and / or nephropathy. The characteristic lesions of malignant hypertension are necrotising vasculitis, arterial thrombi and fibrinoid necrosis of walls of small arteries and arterioles.

The clinical manifestations have been attributed to spasms of cerebral vessels and to cerebral oedema (*hypertensive encephalopathy*), deteriorating renal function and *retinopathy* (arteriorar spasm, exudate, hemorrhage and papilloedemo).

Perhaps less than 1% of hypertensive patients develop malignant phase, which can occur in the course of both essential and secondary hypertension. Rarely, it is the first recognised manifestation of hypertension. With the advent of effective antihypertensive therapy, now 50% patients survive more than 5 years after development of malignant hypertension.

Treatment

Therapeutic approach is identical to that used in other hypertensive emergencies (Box 2)

Aims

1. *To reduce the diastolic BP around 160/100 mmHg:* It is unwise to reduce the BP too rapidly because there may occur further deterioration of cardiac, cerebral and renal functions.

2. *Treatment of associated organ dysfunction,* i.e. LHF, encephalopathy or renal impairment.

Steps

- Hospitalise the patient and put the patient on railing bed if there are convulsions.
- Maintain I.V. line; give O₂.
- Drug therapy.

1. *Antihypertensive drug therapy:* The drugs to be used are chosen on the basis of onset of action and availability as I.V. preparation. The first line drug of choice is a rapid acting vasodilator, i.e. *nicardipine* I.V. infusion (5 mg/hr, may increase 1–2.5 mg hour every 15 minutes to 15 mg/hr) but requires constant supervision preferably in an intensive care unit. *Nitroglycerine*

I.V. infusion (5–100 μg/min) is used in treatment of hypertension following coronary bypass surgery, myocardial infarction, left ventricular failure, or unable angina pectoris. *Diazoxide* is an alternative immediate acting drug, can be used as 50–150 mg I.V. rapidly as bolus, can be repeated after every 5–10 min (max dose 600 mg). This drug should not be used in patients in whom aortic dissection or myocardial infarction is being suspected.

Other drugs that have slight delayed action than the drugs mentioned above, can be used in patients without encepholopathy or another catestrophic event such as I.V. enalaprilat (ACE inhibitor), I.M. labetolol (2 mg/min to maximum of 200 mg) or hydralazine (5–10 mg aliquot repeated at half an hour interval; dose titrated according to response). Sublingual nifedipine is nowhere used.

2. *Intravenous furesemide (40–120 mg) or torsemide:* To induce sodium diuresis and thus reduce the BP and to speed up recovery from encephalopathy.
3. *Digoxin:* It is used to treat LHF, if present.
4. *Sedation:* Intravenous diazepam (5–10 mg) is given for effective sedation.
5. In the mean time, investigate the patient and find out the cause such as pheochromocytoma, if suspected. This can be treated by appropriate measures if proved.
6. In patients who fail to respond to above mentioned measures, there is still hope to improve with peritoneal or hemodialysis as removal of extracellular fluid has resulted in better blood pressure control and impairment of renal functions.
7. Once patient comes out of emergency situation, oral conventional antihypertensive drugs may be instituted.

Most cases of malignant hypertension are those that are either inadequately treated or compliance is poor.

A schematic approach to hypertension (fresh case which does not have volume overload) is represented in Fig. 42.3.

Emergency in Neurology

Acute Confusional State (Delirium)

Definition

Acute confusional state or delirium is a state of reduced mental clarity, coherence, comprehension and thinking compounded by inattention and disorientation (Figs 43.1A and B). As this state worsens, there is deterioration in memory, perception, comprehension, decision making, language, praxia and visuospatial functions.

Two subtypes based on psychomotor features have been described.

I. **Hyperactive type:** It is characterised by *agitation, hallucination, hyperarousal* and *automatic instability*. Alcohol withdrawl syndrome (*Delirium tremens*) is a classical example.

II. **Hypoactive type** in which patients are *withdrawn* and *quiet*. There is *apathy* and *psychomotor slowing*. Benzodiazepine intoxication is an example of this type.

In spite of two distinct types, most patients fall in between these two types and fluctuates from one type to other.

Pathophysiology

Acute confusional state of metabolic origin occurs due to interruption of energy substrate delivery. The substrate for neuronal functions is oxygen and glucose. The cerebral blood flow carries these substrate to neurons. Therefore, reduced substrate supply such as O_2 (hypoxia), glucose (hypoglycaemia) or reduced blood supply (ischaemia) or alteration of neurophysiological responses of neurons by drugs or alcohol intoxication, toxic endogenous metabolites, anaesthetics or epilepsy produce acute confusional state and coma by widespread neuronal dysfunction in the cortex (cerebral hemispheres and RAS) and reduces all aspects of mentation.

The reversibility of delirium in *metabolic encephlalopathies* (hepatic failure, renal

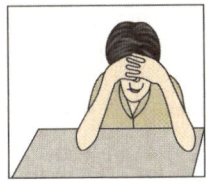
Thought reduced

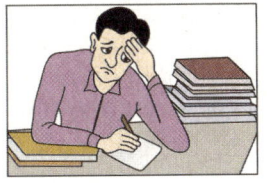
Concentration impaired

Fig. 43.1A: Acute confusional state

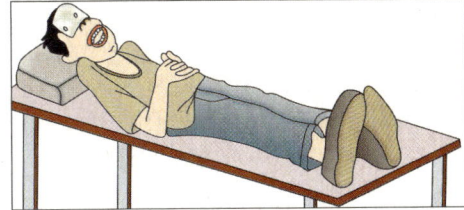

Fig. 43.1B: Delirium due to substance abuse

failure, hypercapnia, diabetic and hyperosmolar nonketotic coma, hypothyroidism, Vitamin B$_{12}$ deficiency, hypothermia), *drugs intoxication* (CNS depressants and anaesthetic) and *postictal phenomenon of epilepsy* is not fully understood, probably is related to interference in cerebral energy metabolism and abnormalities in neurotransmitters, hence recovery occurs when neural metabolic balance is restored.

Causes

They are given in Box 1.

Clinical Features

Acute confusional state is a transient global disorders of attention and consciousness. Dis-orientation with hypoactive presentation is called *confusion*; while hyperactive disoriented patients are called *delirious*. Delirium has an acute onset and fluctuating course. Its characteristic features are:

1. **Impaired consciousness or clouding of consciousness:** Usually, there is decreased awareness of surrounding, decreased ability to respond to external stimuli, disturbance in sleep-wake cycle (insomnia at night with daytime drowsiness).

2. **Disturbance in memory:** There is impairment of registration, and retention of short term memories and recall. Disorientation of time, place and person is the earliest or presenting manifestation, may be associated with inattention and distractibility.

3. **Disturbance in perception:** Normal perceptions are distorted, i.e. objects may appear larger (macropsia) or smaller (micropsia) than normal. Illusions and visual hallucinations are common.

4. **Thought disorder:** Difficulty in thinking and slowness of thought is present. Fleeting delusions are common.

5. **Psychomotor disturbance:** Psychomotor activity is reduced. Speech is slow, slurred and incoherent. Motor and verbal preservation, agraphia and impaired

Box 1	Causes of acute confusional state (delirium)

1. CNS disorders
  A. *Vascular*
   • Cerebral, subarachnoid, subdural, haemorrhage
   • Hypertensive encephalopathy
  B. *Infections*
   • Meningitis, encephalitis
   • Typhoid, malarial encephalopathy
  C. *Nutritional/Vitamin deficiency*
   • Thiamine (Wernicke-Korsakoff syndrome)
   • Vit. B12
  D. *Head injury/trauma*
  E. *Epilepsy (postictal)*
  F. *Degenerative*
   • Multiple sclerosis, Alzheimer's disease
   • Neoplastic disorders e.g. metastases

2. Metabolic
  • Hepatic failure, renal failure
  • Postoperative state
  • Porphyria
  • Fluid and electrolyte disturbance

3. Endocrinal
  • Hypoglycaemia, hyperglycaemia
  • Hypo or hyperthyroidism, hypopituitarism
  • Adrenal crisis (Addison's disease)

4. Cardiopulmonary
  • Myocardial infarction
  • Cardiac arrhythmias
  • Congestive heart failure
  • Respiratory failure (hypoxia, hypercapnia)
  • Shock

5. Systemic illness
  • Substance intoxication or withdrawal (Fig. 43.1B)
  • Systemic infection, e.g. sepsis
  • Heat injury (hypo or hyperthermia)

6. Drugs and toxins
  • Drugs of use having anticholinergic properties, narcotics and benzodiazepines.
  • Drug of abuse, e.g. alcohol intoxication and alcohol withdrawl, opiates, ecstasy, LSD, cacaine, marijuana, etc.
  • Poisons, e.g. inhalants, carbon monoxide, ethylene glycol, pesticides

comprehension are seen. Motor symptoms include tremors and myoclonus.

6. **Emotional changes:** There may be anxiety, irritability and depression. In severe cases, emotional responses become apathetic.

7. **Autonomic disturbance:** Pallor, sweating, tachycardia, dilated pupils, raised temperature, piloerection and G.I. disturbance may occur.

The average duration is about one week with full recovery in most of the cases.

Systemic Findings

• Neuropsychiartric examination
• Assessment of mental status (mini-mental state examination for orientation, language), screening for attentional deficit etc.
• Examine for new focal neurological deficit, (stroke, mass lesion, CVA)
• Look for signs of neurodegenerative conditions, e.g. Parkinsonism (asterixis) and cognitive functions (Alzheimer's disease, dementia)

Diagnosis and Differential Diagnosis

The diagnosis of acute confusional state involves:

1. To find out the cause of confusion / delirium by detailed history and physical examination (Table 43.1).
2. Exclusion of other psychiatric disorders associated with delirium such as acute functional psychosis and dementia (Table 43.2).

Diagnostic Criteria

Feature 1.   Acute onset and fluctuating course (behaviour fluctuation)

Feature 2.   In-attention (difficulty in focussing attention). Patient is distractible.

Feature 3.   Disorganised thinking (thinking is disorganised, irrelevant or incoherent)

Feature 4.   Altered level of consciousness

Note: The diagnosis of delirium requires features 1 and 2 and either of 3 or 4.

Table 43.1 Physical examination	
General sign/findings	*Possible causes of delirium*
Look for the following signs which are dues to the diagnosis:	
Smell of breath	Diabetic ketoacidosis, uraemia, alcohol, aluminium phosphide poisoning
Fever	Septicaemia, thyroid crisis, vasculitis
Autonomic hyperactivity	Anxiety, thyrotoxic crisis, hypoglycaemia
Bradycardia	Hypothyroidism, Stokes-Adam attacks, OP poisoning
Tachycardia	Hyperthyroidism, shock, CHF, infections
Hypotension	Shock, Addison's disease, AMI, drug intoxication, internal haemorrhage, etc.
Hypertension	Encepholopathy, intracranial mass, cerebral haemorrhage, etc.
Tachypnoea	Diabetes, metabolic acidosis, pneumonia, infections
Shallow breathing	Alcohol, acidosis
Dilated pupils	Anxiety, autonomic hyperreactivity
Papilloedema	Hypertensive encephalopathy brain tumour, subarachnoid haemorrhage
Neck rigidity	Meningitis, subarachnoid haemorrhage, meningism
Tongue/Cheek bite	Seizures, postictal delirium
Cardiomegaly/heart murmurs	CHF, hypertensive heart disease
Arrhythmia	Myocardial infarction, CHF
Cyanosis, pulmonary rales and crackles	Pulmonary oedema, CHF, pneumonia
Hepatomegaly or Jaundice	Hepatic failure
Asymmetric deep tendon reflexes	CVA, subdural haematoma, mass lesion
Plantar extensors	Raised intracranial pressure, hypoglycaemia
Primitive reflexes present	Dementia, frontal lobe lesions
Needle pricks	I.V. drug abusers

Table 43.2 Differential diagnosis of acute confusional states

Feature	Acute confusion state	Delirium	Dementia	Acute functional psychosis
Onset	Acute	Acute	Insidious	Sudden
Course	Fluctuating	Fluctuating	Stable	Stable
Consciousness	Clouded	Clouded	Clear	Clear
Attention	Globally impaired	Globally impaired	Globally impaired	Variably affected
Cognition	Globally affected	Globally affected	Globally affected	Selectively affected
Hallucinations	Usually visual and tactile	Usually visual and tactile	Often absent	Mainly auditory
Delusions	Feeding, poor systematized	Fleeting	Often absent	Sustained and systematized
Orientation to time, space and person	Usually impaired	Mostly impaired	Often impaired	May be impaired
Psychomotor activity	Reduced or impaired	Increased	Often normal	Varies from retardation to hyperactivity
Speech	Slow, slurred incoherent	Incoherent, confabulations	Difficulty in finding the words	Normal, slow or rapid
Involuntary movements	Often asterixis flapping tremors	Tremors, delirium tremens	Absent	Absent
Physical illness	Often present	May be present	Absent	Absent
Drug toxicity	May be present	May be present	Often absent	Absent

Investigations

1. **Laboratory investigations:** They are done in all cases with delirium:
   - Complete blood counts.
   - Routine blood biochemistry e.g. sugar, acetone, electrolytes.
   - Lives and kidney functions tests.
   - ECG and X-ray chest.
   - Arterial blood gases analysis.
2. **Additional tests indicated on suspicion of specific conditions:**
   - Urine and blood culture and sensitivity.
   - Blood levels of drugs and their estimations in urine.
   - Serum folate, Vit. B_{12} levels, ammonia.
   - HIV testing.
   - Urinary porphyrins.
   - Tests for endocrinological disorders (T_3, T_4, TSH, LH, FSH, cortisol)
   - *EEG:* Diffuse slowing of EEG has a good correlation with diagnosis of delirium but absence of EEG abnormalities does not rule out the diagnosis. Fast activity is seen in benzodiazepine and alcohol withdrawal delirium.

- Imaging, e.g. CT scan, MRI, etc. for neurological disorders
- *CSF analysis.* Lumbar puncture should be attempted only after exclusion of mass lesion on CT and if infected aetiology of delirium is suspected.

Management

1. **Supportive treatment**
   i. Identification of the cause and its immediate correction, e.g. 25–50% glucose I.V. for hypoglycaemia, O_2 therapy for hypoxia, 100 mg of vitamin B_1 for thiamine deficiency, physostigmine 1 to 2 mg parenterally for anticholinergic overdosage. The fever must be reduced with fans, ice-packs and antipyretics. Appropriate antibiotics should be given for systemic/CNS infection.
   ii. Discontinue medications that may be contributing to the problem.
   iii. I.V. fluids and electrolytes to correct dehydration and electrolyte disturbance. Dehydration is the common cause of delirium is elderly patients.

iv. The patient should be placed near the nurse's station for close observation and monitoring. The patient's safety must be ensured by use of side-rails. The patients who use glasses and hearing aids, the same must be provided to reduce visual and auditory misperceptions. The level of noise in the patient environment should be minimum. A close family member should be advised to stay with the delirious patient. This strategy, if followed, can have calming effect on the patient and help in her/his reorientation.

The patient should not be allowed to sleep in the day by engaging him/her in daytime activities. At night quiet darkroom is necessary for proper sleep.

2. **Specific treatment:** All the current therapy should be reviewed and wherever possible stopped and replaced with drugs which have least psychoactive action.

Antipsychotics

Antipsychotics are the drug of choice for treatment of delirium. Neuroleptics are superior to benzodiazepines in patients with both hyperactive and hypoactive clinical profiles. Haloperidol or droperidol is commonly employed drug because of its short half-life and lower anticholinergic side-effects. It has the advantage of being available as oral, intramuscular and intravenous preparations.

Abrupt discontinuation may result in rebound delirium. The usual starting dose of haloperidol is 2 to 10 mg depending on the level of agitation. Dose may be repeated every 2–4 hours as needed. For elderly patients, dose is 0.5 to 1 mg.

Benzodiazepines: Usually benzodiazepines are useful for the treatment of deliriums caused by withdrawal from alcohol (delirium tremons) or benzodiazepine. They can be used as beneficial adjunctive treatment in patients who cannot tolerate anti-psychotics.

Lorazepam has a rapid onset of action, intermediate half-life and is suitable for patients with impaired liver functions. The standard dose of lorazepam for delirium tremons is 2 mg every 2 hours. For severe agitation, lorazepam 2 mg I.M. may be given every hour until a calming effect is produced. Diazepam may also be used instead of lorazepam. After control of symptoms, the drug should be withdrawn slowly.

Electroconvulsive Therapy (ECT)

It is a standard treatment for delirium in Scandinavia. One to four *ECT* treatments are rapidly effective in the control of delirium regardless of the cause.

The Unconsciousness or Coma

THE UNCONSCIOUSNESS OR COMA (Figs 43.1A and B)

Definition

Coma is defined as persistent loss of consciousness in which the subject lies with eyes closed and shows no understandable response to external stimulus or inner need. The coma may vary in degree; and in deep coma, i.e. corneal, pupillary, pharyngeal reflexes are lost. The tendon and plantar reflexes become also absent. With lesser degree of coma (precoma), pupillary reflexes, reflex ocular movements

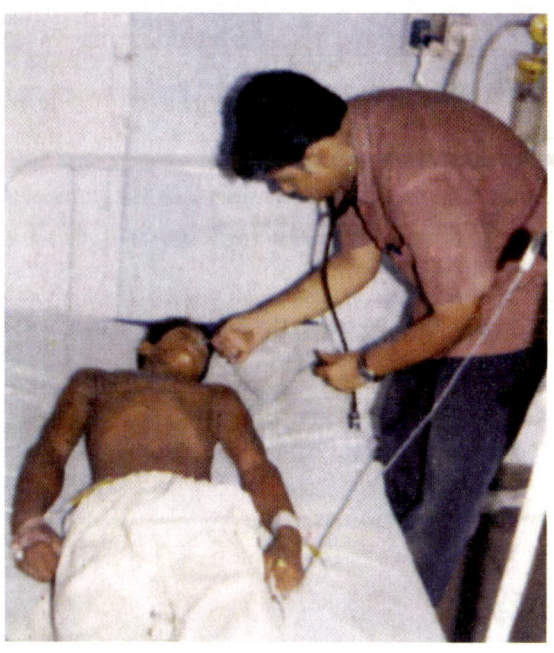

A. Unconscious patient The suction is being done by the resident doctor.

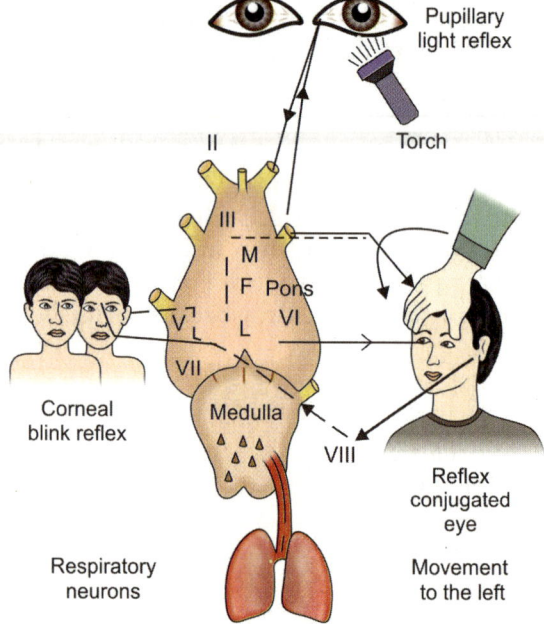

B. Reflexes in coma

Fig. 44.1: (A) Unconscious patient and (B) brainstem reflexes and eye movements in coma examination (read the text)

and other brainstem reflexes are preserved and there may or may not be rigidity of the limbs and extensor plantar response.

The term **coma** refers to a deep sleeplike state from which the patient cannot be aroused. The **stupor** refers to a sleeplike state from which patient can be aroused with vigorous stimuli and patient tries to avoid the stimuli. **Drowsiness** means light sleep-like state from which patient can easily be aroused and there is a brief period of alertness.

Coma-like Syndromes

1. **Vegetative state:** This is state of unresponsiveness in which the eyelids are open giving the appearance of wakefulness. There is an absolute absence of response to commands and an inability to communicate. This is also called 'awake coma'. There may be yawning, grunting and random movements of limbs and head. There are accompanying signs of extensive bilateral cortical damage, i.e. Babinski signs, decerebrate or decorticate limb posturing and absent response to visual stimuli. Respiratory and autonomic functions are preserved. The vegetative state results from global damage to the cerebral cortex most often following cardiac arrest or head injury.

2. **Akinetic mutism:** It refers to the state of partial or full awakefulness in which patient lies immobile (akinetic) with eyes open and is unable to talk (mute). It results from hydrocephalus, mass in the region of third ventricle, bilateral frontal lobe lesions.

3. **Locked-in-state:** It is a state of pseudo-coma in which patient appears to be unconscious, immobile and unresponsive but can open and move the eyes on command. Often these patients communicate with movements of eyes, a form of 'sign language'. These individuals are thus locked in, or imprisoned within their own bodies. It results from infarction or

haemorrhage of ventral pons due to basilar artery occlusion.

4. **Coma vigil:** It indicates a state of impaired consciousness with muttering. It is observed in infectious fevers such as typhoid, dengue or pneumonia.

5. **Catatonia:** It is hypomobile, mute syndrome associated with major psychosis. In its typical form, the patients appear awake with eyes open but make no voluntary or responsive movements. The characteristic feature is that the limbs maintain their posture when lifted or moved in any position by the examiner but may also show waxy flexibility.

6. **Hysterical pseudocoma:** It indicates voluntary attempt to appear comatosed. Patient resists to examination. Eyelid elevation is actively resisted. Blinking occurs to visual threat when the lids are held open. The eyes move concomitantly with head rotation. All these signs belie brain damage.

Pathophysiology of Coma

A normal level of consciousness depends on the activation of the cerebral hemispheres by neurons located in brainstem reticular activating system (RAS). Both these components and the connections between them must be preserved for maintenance of normal consciousness. The principal causes of coma are therefore:

i. Widespread damage to both hemispheres (i.e. disease, ischaemia, trauma),

ii. Depression of cerebral functions by drugs, toxins, hypoxia or metabolic derangements,

iii. Brainstem lesions involving RAS.

Causes

They are given in Box 1.

Clinical Evaluation of a Patient with Coma

Proper management of a case of coma depends on the recognition of the cause of coma, an

> **Box 1**   Common causes of coma
>
> **A. Brainstem and cerebellar lesions**
> - Infarction, haemorrhage of brainstem and cerebellum
> - Tumour, trauma
>
> **B. Lesions of cerebral hemisphere with oedema and brainstem compression**
> - Infarction, haemorrhage
> - Encephalitis, meningitis, brain abscess
> - Tumour, trauma (subdural, extradural)
> - Hydrocephalus
> - Hypertensive encephalopathy
> - Status epilepticus
> - Cerebral malaria
>
> **C. Metabolic abnormalities**
> - Diabetic and hypoglycaemic coma
> - Hepatic failure, renal failure, cardiac failure, respiratory failure
> - Hyponatraemia (severe), hypokalaemia
> - Hyper and hypocalcaemia
> - Hypoxia
> - Myxoedema coma, hypopituitarism
> - Adrenal crisis
> - Vitamin deficiencies (e.g. B1, nicotinic acid, B_{12})
>
> **D. Drugs and physical agents**
> - Anaesthetic agents
> - Drug overdose or poisoning and alcohol ingestion
> - Hyper and hypothermia
>
> **E. Psychogenic/hysteria**

interpretation of certain clinical signs such as brainstem reflexes, proper use of diagnostic tests. It is a common practice that acute respiratory and cardiovascular problems should be attended to on priority basis than neurological examination. Therefore, vital signs must be maintained such as clear airway, pulse, BP before subjecting the patient to further evaluation; otherwise appropriate resuscitative measures should be adopted immediately. The clinical evaluation consists of:

1. **History:** In many cases, the cause of coma is immediately evident (e.g. trauma, cardiac arrest or known drug ingestion); while in others informations have to be gathered from friends, relatives and witnesses accompanying the patient regarding the:

    i. *Mode of onset of coma,* abrupt onset of coma suggests subarachnoid haemorrhage, intracranial bleed, brainstem infarction, etc.

   ii. Details of preceding neurological symptoms (confusion, weakness, headache, seizures, dizziness, diplopia, etc.).

  iii. Use of medications, illicit drugs or alcohol.

  iv. History of liver, kidney, lung, heart disease or other medical illness such as diabetes, hypothyroidism, Addison's disease.

2. **Physical examination:** The temperature, pulse, respiratory rate and pattern, and BP should be noted. The **smell** from the breath may be noted (*hepatic* or *renal failure, diabetic coma*). The clinical clues to the cause of coma are same as already discussed in the earlier chapter on acute confusional state (Table 42.2). **High body temperature 42°C or above** associated with dry skin indicate CNS infection, meningitis heat stroke or anticholinergic drug intoxication or malignant hyperthermia due on anesthetics. **Hypothermia** is observed in alcoholic, barbiturate, sedative or phenothiazine intoxication hypoglycaemia, hypothyroidism, peripheral circulatory failure. Hypothermia causes coma when temperature is <31°C.

Marked hypertension suggests subarachnoid hemorrhage, hypertensive encephalopathy. **Hypotension** is a feature of coma due to alcohol or barbiturates intoxication, MI, sepsis, hemorrhage or Addisonian crisis.

Skin examination:

  a. *Cutaneous petechiae* suggest thrombotic thrombocytopenic purpura (TTP), meningococcaemia, or a bleeding diathesis associated with intracerebral hemorrhage.

  b. *Cyanosis* indiciates respiratory failure.

  c. *Reddish skin* indicates CO poisoning.

d. *Pallor or anaemia* indicates haemorrhage (external or internal).

3. **Neurological examination:** Systemic assessment of the unconsciousness patient is an important part of neurological examination. An application of Glasgow coma scale not only provides a grading of coma by numerical scale but allows serial comparisons to be made for prognostic information particularly in traumatic coma (Box 2). This scale should be applied in each and every patient under observation and should be charted out from time to time for comparison. Under neurological examination:

- Assess the level of consciousness (*Glasgow Coma Scale*).
- Look for signs of head injury, e.g. bruising, wound, fracture, bleeding from nose, ear or other site.
- Check the pupils (size, reaction).
- Look for pattern of respiration, abnormal posturing and ocular movements.
- Elicit the reflexes.
- Examine ocular fundi.

4. **Abnormal posturing:** The patient posture should be observed first without examiner intervention.

- *Decorticate rigidity or posturing* is characterised by flexion of elbows and wrists and arm supination against the rigid body; suggests bilateral cerebral damage above the midbrain.
- *Decerebrate rigidity or posturing* describes extension and adduction of elbows and wrists with pronation; suggest corticospinal damage in the midbrain or caudal to diencephalon.
- *Arms extension with flaccid legs* have been associated with low pontine lesions.
- *Total flaccidity of all the four limbs* and *hypotonia* indicate the involvement of pontomedullary junction.
- *Multifocal myoclonus* is almost always an indication of a metabolic disorder (uraemia, anoxia, drug intoxication).

Box 2   Glasgow Coma Scale

Scale	Score
Eye opening (E)	
• Spontaneous	4
• To loud voice	3
• To pain	2
• Nil	1
Best motor response (M)	
• Obeys	6
• Localises	5
• Withdraws (flexion)	4
• Abnormal flexion	3
• Extensor response	2
• Nil	1
Verbal response (V)	
• Oriented	5
• Confused, disoriented	4
• Inappropriate words	3
• Incomprehensible sounds	2
• Nil	1
Coma score (E+M+V)	
Minimum	3
Maximum	15

Note: Patients with head trauma scoring 3 or 4 have an 85% chance of death or vegetative state; while scores above 11 indicate only 5–10% chance of death or vegetative state and 85% chance of moderate disability or good recovery. Intermediate scores have intermediate prognosis.

- *Rigidity and opisthotonos position* indicate either tetanus or strychnine poisoning.
- *Lack of restless movements on one side* or an out-turned leg suggests hemiplegia.
- *Bilateral asterixis* in a confused or drowsy patients indicate metabolic encephalopathy (hepatic or uremic) or drug intoxication.
- *Neck rigidity* indicates either meningitis or subarachnoid haemorrhage.

5. **Pattern of respiration:** Respiration patterns are of little help in localisation of the lesion:
- *Slow, shallow, regular breathing* suggest metabolic or drug effect.
- *Rapid, deep (kussmaul) breathing* suggests metabolic acidosis, but can occur in pontomesencephalic lesions.
- *Cheyne-Stokes breathing* in classic cyclic form ending with a brief apnoea

suggests bihemispherical damage or metabolic coma.

- *Agonal gasps* (gasping respiration) is a terminal respiratory pattern, suggests bilateral lower brainstem damage.

6. **Brainstem reflexes (Fig. 44.1B):** Assessment includes:

   A. *Pupillary size and reaction:* The size, equality and inequality of pupils and their reaction to light provide valuable information regarding the site of lesion in an unconscious patient.

      - Symmetrically reactive round pupils usually exclude the midbrain lesion.
      - With cortical lesion (encephalopathies, hydrocephalus), the pupils are small but react to light.
      - With early midbrain lesion, the pupils become mid-dilated and non-reactive to light. As the damage increases, the pupils become dilated and fixed. The ciliospinal reflex is also lost at this stage. The use of mydriatic eye drops by a previous examiner, self administration by patient or direct ocular trauma may cause misleading pupillary enlargement.
      - Very small (pinpoint) pupils with reaction to light characterize narcotic or barbiturate poisoning but also occurs in bilateral pontine lesions (haemorrhage). The response to naloxone and the presence of reflex eye movements distinguishes the two.
      - Unilateral 3rd nerve palsy causes unilateral pupillary dilatation with loss of direct and consensual light reflex could be due to ipsilateral lesion (mass lesion of midbrain) or due to contralateral compression of 3rd nerve in midbrain against the opposite tentorial margin (contracoup effect).
      - Unilateral small pupil of a Horner's syndrome is seen in cerebral

haemorrhage that affects the thalamus. (sympathetic system).

   B. *Eye movements:* These are cornerstones of physical diagnosis in coma (Fig. 42.1B).

      - The eyes are first observed by elevating the lids and noting the resting position and spontaneous movements of the globes. (i) Horizontal divergence of the eyes at rest is normally observed in coma. (ii) Conjugate deviation of the eyes to the side suggests either an ipsilateral spherical lesion or a contralateral pontine lesion. (iii) An adducted eye at rest indicates lateral rectus palsy due to 6th nerve in the pons; and when bilateral, it is often a sign of raised intracranial tension. (iv) An abducted eye with pupillary dilatation indicates 3rd nerve palsy in the midbrain.
      - *Skew deviation,* i.e. vertical separation of the eyes (ocular axes) results from pontine or cerebellar lesions. A mesencephalic lesion leads to downward conjugate deviation
      - *Oculocephalic reflex (Doll's eye movement):* Normally sudden passive turning of the head to one side produces conjugate deviation of the eyes to the opposite side. Absence of this reflex in a comatosed patient implies dysfunction of pons where the 6th nerve nucleus or lateral gaze centre is located. However, this reflex does not pinpoint the cause of coma, can occur both in structural and toxic metabolic causes of coma.
      - *Oculovestibular reflex (caloric test):* It tests the integrity of pathway from the labyrinth in the ear to the midbrain via medial longitudinal fasciculus (this connects the 6th nerve and 8th nerve to contralateral 3rd nerve). This reflex is tested by cold water irrigation into a ear. Normally there

is deviation of eyes towards irrigated side and nystagmus to opposite, while opposite happens with warm water irrigation. The acronym used to remind students is 'COWS' which denotes the direction of nystagmus to opposite side with cold water and to same side with warm water. The absence of this reflex carries same significance as oculocephalic reflex, i.e. brainstem lesion.

- *Corneal blink reflex* (Fig. 43.1B): Touching the cornea with wisp of cotton produces blinking is called corneal blink reflex. It indicates intactness of 5th and 7th nerve in the pons. Absence of this reflex indicates pontine lesion.
- *Ocular bobbing* describes a brisk downward and slow upward movements of the eyes, indicates bilateral pontine damage.
- *Ocular dipping* describes a slower downward and faster upward movements of the eyes, denotes anoxic damage to the cerebral cortex.

8. **Motor responses:** Presence of local signs or unilateral paralysis indicates focal structural damage to the brain. The only evidence of paralysis may be abnormal flaccidity on the side affected (hemiplegia). Alteration of deep tendon jerks and plantar extensor response on the paralysed size indicate contralateral corticospinal involvement; but in deep coma, plantar reflexes become extensor on both the sides.

Investigations

1. **Laboratory investigations** done are same as discussed in acute confusional state. Chemical and toxological analysis of blood and urine is must.

2. **Specialised investigations:**
   i. *CT scan and MRI:* The CT scan and MRI give valuable informations regarding radiologically detectable lesions, e.g. haemorrhage, tumours, hydrocephalus, etc. hence, should be done right in the accidental and emergency department. These investigations are not useful in toxic or metabolic causes of coma, but are done to exclude the radiological evident lesion.
   ii. *The EEG:* It gives valuable informations:
   - Diffuse slowing of EEG indicates diffuse encephalopathy.
   - Predominent high-voltage slowing (delta waves) in the frontal regions is typical of metabolic coma (hepatic coma).
   - Alpha waves (8 to 12 Hz activity) called Alpha coma indicates high pontine or diffuse cortical damage,
   iii. *CSF examination* is done in those cases where CT scan has ruled out mass lesion(s) or raised intracranial tension. It is valuable in the diagnosis of meningitis, encephalitis, subarachnoid haemorrhage (xanthochromic CSF), etc.

Differential Diagnoses of Coma

All the causes of coma usually fall into three main categories (Table 44.1).

Management

I. **Immediate treatment:** Hospitalise each and every case of coma. Immediate treatment is to maintain patent airway, I.V. access and to stabilise vital signs, i.e. pulse, BP before proceeding to clinical evaluation. An emergency sample of blood for biochemistry, sugar, electrolytes may be taken. Tracheostomy or endotracheal intubation and frequent suction be done to keep the airway patent (Fig. 44.1A). A Foley's catheter or condom drainage is put in for urine output.

II. **General supportive measures**
   A. *Care of the patient*
      i. *Position the unconscious patient* to one side rather than in supine position to minimise the risk of aspiration.

Table 44.1 Differential diagnosis of coma

Absence of focal or lateralising neurological signs (e.g. CT scan and cellular content of the CSF is normal)	Presence of focal brainstem or cerebral lateralising signs (e.g. CT or MRI is abnormal with or without changes in CSF)	Presence of neck rigidity (meningeal irritation) with or without fever and with an excess of cells (WBCs or RBCs) in CSF; CT scan/MRI excludes mass lesion
• Poisoning, e.g. drugs, alcohol, opiates • Metabolic coma due to hypoxic encephalopathy, uraemia, hepatic coma, diabetic acidosis, hyperosmolar hyperglycaemic coma, hypoglycaemia, Addisonian or thyroid crisis, hypo or hypernatraemia, respiratory failure • Severe infection, e.g. septicaemia, typhoid encephalopathy, pneumonia, malaria, Water-house-Friderichsen syndrome • Peripheral circulatory failure/ shock due to any cause • Status epilepticus • Hypertensive encephalopathy, eclampsia • Hyperthermia or hypothermia • Cerebral concussion • Hydrocephalus or raised ICP	• Hemiplegia with secondary brainstem compression (cerebral haemorrhage) • Brainstem infarct • Brain abscess, subdural abscess • Subdural or epidural haemorrhage • Brain tumour or space occupying lesion • Cerebellar/pontine infarct or haemorrhage • Metabolic coma with pre-existing focal damage • Miscellaneous, e.g. 　– Cortical vein thrombosis 　– Herpes simplex encephalitis 　– Acute disseminated encephalopathy 　– Multiple cerebral emboli 　– Thrombotic thrombocytopaenic purpura	• Subarachnoid haemorrhage (e.g. ruptured aneurysm/ arteriovenous malformation or trauma) • Acute bacterial meningitis • Viral encephalitis • Malarial encephalopathy • Miscellaneous: Fat embolism, carcinomatous and lymphomatous meningitis

ii. *To prevent bed sores:* The position of the patient on bed must be changed frequently (every 1–2 hours) so as to minimise pressure at pressure points to prevent bed sores. A water or air mattress should be used if the course of illness is prolonged.

ii. *Gental movements on the bed:* Cervical injuries must be excluded before attempting neck movements during intubation and oculocephalic reflexes elicitation. The clothes of the patient should be loosened and rings to be removed. The limbs should be kept in optimal position and moved passively through full range frequently so as to avoid contractures and deep vein thrombosis.

iv. *Oral hygiene:* Proper oral hygiene to be maintained by mouth washes and suction.

v. The patient having convulsions should be kept in *railing bed* so as to prevent falling.

vi. *Eye care,* e.g. tapping of lids, prevention of corneal damage.

vii. *Chest physiotherapy* should be carried out as soon as patient improves.

B. **Feeding or nutrition:** Nasogastric feeding (liquid diet of 3000 kcal) should be given if there is no contraindication. The fluid balance should be maintained. I.V. fluids are given if patient does not accept much fluid orally or through Ryle's tube. Serum electrolytes to be monitored and corrected wherever necessary. To avoid aspiration:

• Aspirate the gastric contents before each feed so as to ensure that the tube is in the stomach.

• The patient should be nursed in the sitting or propped up position.

- Each feed should be small (200 ml) to avoid distension of the stomach.

C. *Maintenance of vital signs/parameters*

i. *Respiration:* Adequate respiration must be ensured by patent airway. Denture should be removed and oral airway (mouth gag) inserted to prevent the falling of tongue backwards. Frequent suctions are to be done to remove the secretions. If patient does not have cough reflex and is likely to stay in a coma for a long period, the endotracheal intubation or even tracheostomy may be done for proper removal of secretions. Intermittent O_2 therapy by nasal catheter may be given. In case of severe hypoxia, mechanical ventilation may be required.

ii. *Circulation:* The circulation should be maintained by proper fluid balance and intake and output chart. A positive balance of 600–1000 ml should be kept as insensible loss over and above the daily output.

Drastic changes or fluctuations in the BP are to be avoided. If hypertension is present, it should be treated appropriately. Hypotension should be resuscitated by fluids and inotropic agents.

iii. *Care of bowel and bladder:* Urinary incontinence should be managed by condom drainage in men and indwelling catheter in women. Fecal impaction should be avoided and bowels to be kept open by frequent isotonic enemas or laxatives. Digital removal of fecal impaction may be needed sometimes.

III. **Specific measures** including administration of an antidot.

Specific therapy should be directed against the cause of coma such as dextrose is given for hypoglycaemia, naloxone is administered for narcotic overdose. Thiamine is administered for Wernicke's encephalopathy in malnourished patient and physostigmine is used to treat anticholinergic overdose / poisoning. The cause of coma should be appropriately dealt with. It is not possible to discuss the management of individual condition. If CSF picture suggests meningitis, a third generation cephalosporine ceftriaxone is given before culture and sensitivity.

In cases with progressive cerebral compression due to raised intracranial pressure, decompressive therapy should be instituted. Seizures may be controlled with phenytoin. If these measures fail, surgical decompression may be required.

Acute Headache

Definition

Headache means ache or pain over the head. It can be *acute* or *chronic* and usually a benign symptom. Acute, severe or new onset headache relates to intracranial lesion. Chronic headache may be *primary* (migraine, cluster headache, tension type headache) or *secondary* to some pathology. Even in emergency setting, only 5% patients presenting with acute headache have been found to have serious underlying neurological disorder. Nonetheless, it is imperative that in a patient presenting with headache these serious conditions be recognised and treated appropriately.

Causes (Fig. 45.1)

A useful classification based on the aetiology of headache, adapted from recommendations of the International Headache Society (IHS) is given in Table 45.1.

Groups 1 to 4 cover the primary headaches and from groups 5 to 13 cover the secondary headaches. The IHS classification is much detailed and appears to be difficult to use in clinical practice. Therefore, a simple practical approach to headache is reproduced in Table 45.2.

Pathogenesis

The following are the pain sensitive structures inside or outside the head, the stretching of which leads to pain or headache.
1. Skin, subcutaneous tissue, muscles, arteries and periosteum of the bone.
2. Intracranial dural venous sinuses or veins.
3. Tissues of eye, ears and nasal sinuses.
4. Duramater at the base of brain and the arteries within dura and pia-arachnoid mater.

Headache commonly occurs due to:
i. Distortions, inflammation, distension and dilatation of intracranial or extracranial vessels.
ii. Traction or displacement of large intracranial veins and/or dural sinuses.
iii. Compression, traction and inflammation of cranial and spinal nerves.
iv. Muscle spasms (voluntary or involuntary) or trauma to cranial or cervical muscles.
v. Meningeal irritation and raised intracranial tension. Headache due to mass lesions occurs only if they distort, displace or put traction on the blood vessels, dural structures or cranial nerves, hence, it may occur early before the raised intracranial tension develops, and produce typical bitemporal or bifrontal headache.
v. Cluster headache triggers trigeminal photonomic vascular system.

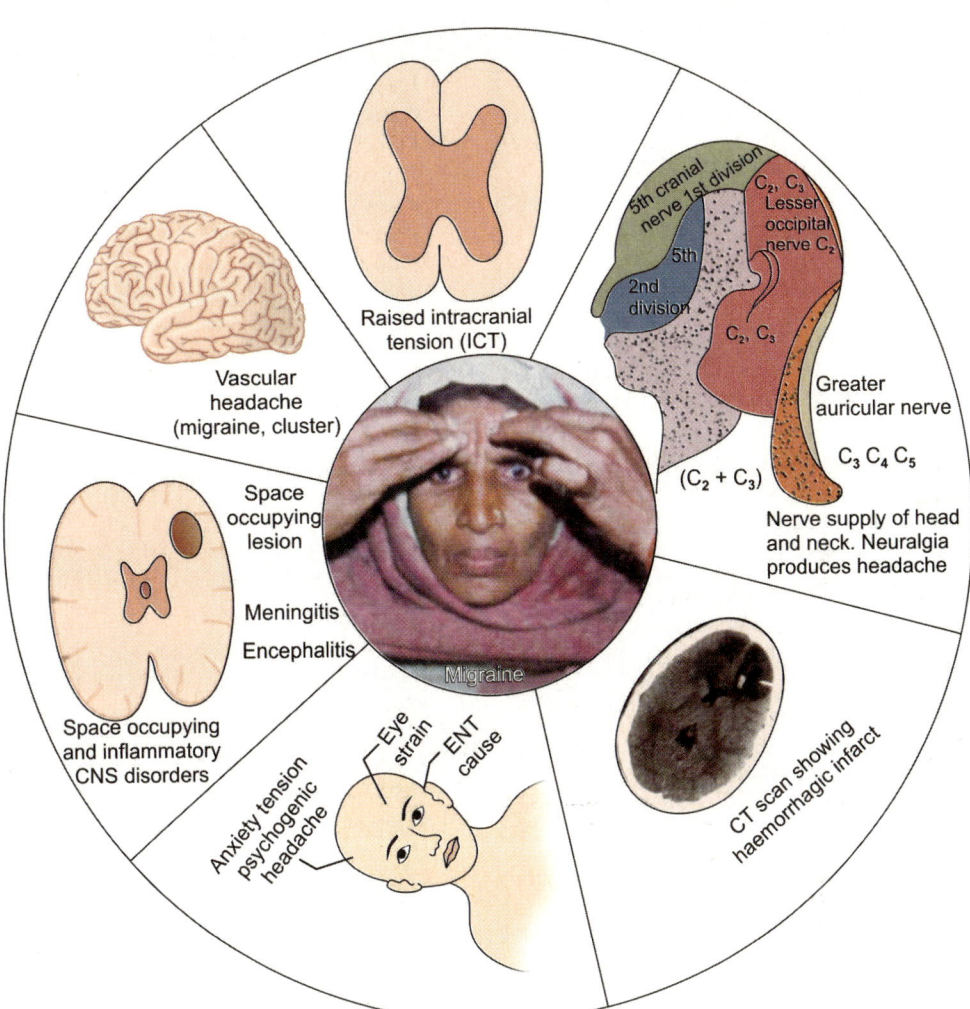

Fig. 45.1: Causes of common headaches. Central figure denotes migrainous headache

Clinical Evaluation of Headache

Headache is a prominent symptom associated with a large variety of disorders, hence, to find out its cause is not only difficult but impossible some time. To establish the diagnosis, one has to go through a long list of causes of headache (Tables 45.1 and 45.2) on history. The main issues to be addressed in a patient with headache are:

1. The diagnosis.
2. To look for the dangerous signals that suggest a serious underlying disorder.
3. Investigational plan.

4. Line of management and the follow up recommendations to prevent recurrence.

History

A careful detailed history is the most important tool in the headache diagnosis. Moreover, headache is complaint, where symptoms outweigh the signs and investigations are obligatory not the rule. Ascertain the followings on the history:

1. **Onset, duration and progress**
   i. Acute severe headache commonly suggests subarachnoid haemorrhage and meningitis.

Table 45.1 Classification of headache (modified vesion of IHS, 1988)

PRIMARY HEADACHES	7. Headache associated with nonvascular intra-cranial disorder

PRIMARY HEADACHES

1. Migraine
- Migraine without aura
- Migraine with aura
- Ophthalmoplegic migraine
- Basilar migraine
- Retinal migraine
- Childhood migraine syndromes
- Complications of migraine, e.g. status migrainosus, migraine associated with stroke

2. Tension-type headache
- Episodic tension-type headache
- Chronic tension-type headache

3. Cluster headache and chronic paroxysmal hemicrania
- Cluster headache (episodic, chronic)
- Chronic paroxysmal hemicrania

4. Miscellaneous headache not associated with structural lesion
- Idiopathic stabbing headache
- External compression headache
- Cold stimulus headache
- Benign cough headache
- Benign exertional headache
- Headache associated with sexual activity (coital cephalgia)

SECONDARY HEADACHES

5. Post-traumatic headaches

6. Headache associated with vascular disorders
- Acute ischaemic cerebrovascular disorders
- Intracranial haematoma
- Subarachnoid haemorrhage
- Unruptured vascular malformations
- Arteritis, e.g. giant cell arteritis
- Venous thrombosis
- Arterial hypertension

7. Headache associated with nonvascular intra-cranial disorder
- High CSF pressure syndromes, e.g. benign intra-cranial hypertension, hydrocephalus
- Low CSF pressure syndrome, e.g. postspinal headache, CSF fistula
- Intracranial infections, e.g. meningitis, brain abscess
- Sarcoidosis and other non-inflammatory diseases
- Intracranial neoplasm

8. Headache associated with substances or their withdrawl
- Acute use or exposure
  – Nitrate, nitrite-induced
  – Monosodium glutamate induced
  – CO-induced
  – Alcohol induced
- Chronic use or exposure
  – Ergotamine-induced
  – Analgesic abuse headache

9. Headaches associated with noncephalic infection
- Viral infection
- Bacterial infection
- Other infection

10. Headache associated with metabolic disorders
- Hypercapnia
- Mixed hypoxia and hypercapnia
- Hypoglycaemia
- Dialysis

11. Headache or facial pain associated with facial or cranial structures
- Disorders of cranial bone, eye, ear, nose, sinuses, teeth, mouth, etc.

12. Cranial neuralgias
- Persistent pain of cranial nerve origin
- Trigeminal neuralgia
- Glossopharyngeal neuralgia
- Occipital neuralgia
- Central causes of headache and facial pain

13. Headache not classifiable

ii. Progressively worsening headache suggests raised intracranial pressure or uncontrolled systemic disease. Focal or lateralizing signs make the diagnosis easier.

iii. A chronic recurrent headache or chronic non-progressive daily headache represents a primary headache such as migraine, cluster headache or tension-type headache.

iv. Headache that develops over weeks or months (slowly evolving recurrent headache) may have a benign cause such as migraine or tension type headache or it could even be due to a serious underlying cause (unruptured aneurysm).

Table 45.2 A practical classification of headache

1. Acute primary headaches
- Migraine
- Benign exertional headache
- Cluster headache
- Tension-type
- Benign orgasmic headache

2. Secondary headaches

A. Intracranial causes
- Vascular disorders, e.g. embolic thrombotic stroke; arterial or venous haemorrhagic stroke.
- Infections, e.g. meningitis, encephalitis, sinusitis, brain abscess
- Inflammation, e.g. vasculitis, arteritis
- Brain tumours, e.g. primary, metastatic
- Non-vascular disorders, e.g. benign intracranial hypertension, postspinal headache, post-traumatic headache

B. Extracranial causes
- Eye, ear, sinuses, teeth, neck, temporomandibular joint involvement

C. Systemic illnesses and acute intoxications

3. Neuralgias, e.g. trigeminal, glossopharyngeal and occipital

v. Some headaches may show nocturnal frequency and awaken the patient at night or may occur at the same time of the day (cluster headache) or at specific occasion such as during menstruation or may increase towards the evening such as tension-type (psychogenic) headache.

vi. Acute positional headache (occipito frontal) following lumbar puncture or epidural injection is due to low CSF volume or pressure headache as a result of CSF leak. It occurs on sitting relieved by recumbency.

The age of the patient is also a prime importance as migraine generally begins at a younger age, cluster or tension headache is more common in middle age and headache originating in older persons are usually due to organic causes.

2. **The frequency and duration of headache.** It also help to differentiate the *episodic headaches* from *chronic progressive headaches*. Many attacks of unilateral periorbital pain

or headache of short duration in the day with ipsilateral nasal congestion, rhinorrhea, lacrimation, red eyes and Horner's syndrome would favour the diagnosis of cluster headache or chronic paroxysmal hemicrania (a variant of cluster headache).

3. **Site and quality of pain**
   i. Unilateral pulsating/throbbing headaches are usually vascular such as migraine and cluster headache (occur at the same location unilaterally).
   ii. Bilateral diffuse dull headache is usually of tension-type headaches.
   iii. With secondary headaches of organic cause, the nature, location and severity of headache vary according to cause and mechanism of production.

4. **Associated symptoms**
   i. Associated features such as nausea, vomiting, hypersensitivity to light and noise along with headache suggest migraine.
   ii. Fever, arthralgia and malaise suggest a systemic illness or meningitis.
   iii. Transient visual symptoms (auras) is characteristic of migraine but can occur in transient ischaemic attacks, vascular anomalies or focal epilepsy secondary to space occupying lesions.
   iv. Behaviour following an acute attack of headache distinguishes migraine (patient tries to sleep undisturbed in a dark room) from cluster headache in which a patient is up and moving about.
   v. Headache may be related to menstruation, more common in morning (hypertensive) and worst on bending (sinusitis related), may occur towards the evening (eye strain headache) or follow a period of inactivity (cervical pain), or mood change/depression (psychological headache).

5. **Provoking and relieving factors:** Primary headaches such as migraine or cluster headache can be triggered by various stimuli including food items (Box 1).

Headache due to intracranial pathology or raised intracranial tension worsens during coughing, straining or adopting the head in low posture.

Box 1	Provoking factors for migraine (cluster headache)
1. *Food item*	Cheese, dairy products, fruits, chocolates, ice-cream etc.
2. *Food additives*	Caffeine (coffee), nitrates
3. *Alcohol*	Beer, red wine
4. *Hormonal changes*	Menstruation, pregnancy, ovulation, oral contraceptive
5. *Visual triggers*	Bright lights, glare
6. *Auditory triggers*	Noise and music
7. *Olfactory triggers*	Perfumes, odours
8. *Sleep, hunger, exertion, head and neck trauma, stress and anxiety, cough*	

Note: The clinical interview of an acute headache patient should be quick and systematic including onset, location of pain, the character, severity, duration of pain, precipitating and relieving factors. Past history of similar episodes, history of trauma, exertional aspect of headache, physical tests done earlier, any treatment taken earlier and relief obtained therefrom should be noted.

Physical Examination

A thorough physical and neurological examination includes:

1. **The physical examination** should evaluate vital signs (pulse, BP), the cardiac status, the extracranial structures (to palpate over the head and neck for detection of tender spots , to auscultate over the skull, carotid vessels for bruit, to palpate the temporal artery for pulsation) and cervical spine for pain and limitation of movements. Examine the nose and sinuses, the teeth and temporomandibular joint, the ear and throat.
2. **The neurological examination:**
   - Mental status and level of consciousness.
   - Cranial nerve examination including optic fundi.
   - Motor system examination, e.g. power, tone, reflexes, etc.
   - Look for neck stiffness and other signs of meningitis.

Investigations

Certain features in the history or examination should raise the suspicion of ominous disease warranting investigations. These danger signals are listed in Box 2.

Box 2	Danger signals warranting testing
1. First severe headache ever
2. Subacute worsening or progressive over days and weeks
3. Disturbs sleep or presents immediately after awaking
4. Abnormal neurological examination
5. Fever, nausea, vomiting or other systemic signs
6. Headache precipitated by Valsalva maneuver (cough, sneeze, bending, straining, position change, exercise and sexual activity)
7. New-onset headache in adult life (>40 years) or a significant change in a long-standing headache problem.

The investigations to be done are:
1. Complete blood count, ESR and blood biochemistry.
2. **CSF examination:** CSF examination is indicated in acute onset of headache with fever or when there are associated cranial nerve involvement. The lumbar puncture should be done after a CT scan has ruled out the possibility of raised intracranial tension.
3. **Neuroimaging:** The choice of MRI or CT scan will depend on the clinical suspicion. MRI or CT scan is indicated in patients of recent onset headache or headache with abnormal neurological examination (e.g. neck stiffness, focal deficits, diminished consciousness, signs of raised intracranial pressure) or progressive worsening headache, acute first severe headache, etc. An MR scan has advantage over CT scan in a patient with headache of organic cause. It helps in identification of the lesions in

the brainstem and pituitary region better than CT scan. It also helps in ruling out or confirming the nature of the lesions, i.e. demyelinating, ischaemic or inflammatory disease.

4. **EEG:** It is not of great value in the investigation of headache.

5. Temporomandibular joint and dental evaluation for malocclusion of teeth. **X-rays or MRI of TM** joint is useful for displacement.

Management

1. **Symptomatic relief of pain:** Treatment is dictated by the specific diagnosis for patients with serious secondary causes of headache. Acute migraine, tension-type headache and cluster headache need to be treated with both standard analgesics and specific drugs.

   Patients need symptomatic relief when the headache is severe or incapacitating or there is an acute exacerbation of an underlying primary headache or an acute infective neurological disorder or some more sinister underlying disorder.

   - *Analgesics and simple analgesic combinations* are more useful for mild to moderate headache such as migraine, tension-type or cluster headache. Aspirin, acetoaminophen and opiates are some of the drugs used. Aspirin should be avoided in children (potential to produce Reye's syndrome).

   - *Non-steroidal anti-inflammatory drugs (NSAIDs)* such as naproxen, indomethacin, diclofenac meclofenamate, ketorolac are useful drugs to treat mild to moderate headache. Some of them are available in parenteral preparation, e.g. diclofenac, ketorolac can be used in acute situation.

   - *Use of corticosteroids:* Corticosteroids (4–6 mg dexamethasone I.M. or I.V.) are recommended in acute headache due to raised intracranial pressure. Prednisolon (60 mg daily for 5 days followed by gradual withdrawl over 7 days) is effective for cluster head prophylaxis.

   - *Anticonvulsants,* e.g. carbamazepine, phenytoin, topiramate or gabapentine may be needed to control trigeminal neuralgia and migraine in addition to analgesics.

   - *Ergot derivatives and triptans:* The ergot derivatives (ergotamine and parenteral dihydroergotamine) or cafergot (combination of ergotamine and caffeine) are useful in symptomatic relief of moderate to severe **migraine, cluster headache** and **intractable chronic daily headache**, dihydroergotamine (DHE) can be given I.M. or I.V. (0.5 to 1 mg) alone or in combination with promethazine and dexamethasone (1 mg DHE plus 50 mg promethazine and 4 mg dexamethasone I.M.) to abort most migraine headaches. All ergotamine preparations produce nausea, vomiting, muscle cramps, paraesthesias and precipitate angina. Anticonvulsants such as topiramate, valproate are also useful in migraine. Triptans (sumatriptan, zolmitriptan, naratriptan, rizatriptan) are useful in the treatment of migraine and cluster headache. Sumatriptan (25–50 mg orally or 6 mg subcutaneously) or zolmitryptain 5 mg orally or nasal spray gives fastest relief in acute attack of migraine.
   Tryptans are contraindicated in pregnancy, hemiplegic or basilar migraine, in patients with risk factors for stroke and coronary and peripheral vascular disease.

   - *Neuroleptics* (e.g. metoclopramide and domeperidone) are useful to control the associated nausea and vomiting associated with migraine and cluster headache.

2. **Specific management**
   - Subarachnoid haemorrhage needs angiographic confirmation and surgical intervention.

- Meningitis needs confirmation by CSF and aggressive antibiotic therapy.
- Raised intracranial tension needs diagnostic evaluation by CT scan or MRI. For control, I.V. mannitol or steroids may be helpful. Benign intracranial hypertension is treated by acetazolamide, topiramate or CSF removal.
- For suspected temporal arteritis, corticosteroids are beneficial.
- Use of oxygen by a mask at 8 to 10 L for 10–15 min for acute cluster headache.
- Low CSF volume or pressure headache can be relieved by bed rest, I.V. caffeine (500 mg in 500 ml of saline infused over 2 hours), abdominal binder etc. Oral theophylline is alternative in intractable cases.
- Management of medically intractable headache is difficult. Currently neuromodulatory approaches such as *occipital nerve stimulation* has been found useful in chronic cluster headache. *Single pulse transcranial magnetic stimulation* is in use in Europe and is approved for migrane with aura in USA.
- In medication overuse headache, analgesic use should be slowly reduced and eleminated.

3. **Long-term management and follow-up:** One must plan to prescribe non-habituating therapy.

Acute Syncope/Faint

Definition

It is defined as sudden self-limited transient loss of consciousness usually leading to fall (Fig. 46.1). It is due to acute reduction in cerebral blood flow, followed by spontaneous recovery. There is no or minimal injury, no incontinence and no abnormal movements. Exceptionally, there can be few clonic jerks.

Presyncope or near syncope is defined as premonitory symptoms such as feeling of weakness, nausea, visual blurring, light headedness, tinnitis, sweating, pallor and heaviness of lower limbs that occur before syncope. These symptoms increase in severity until consciousness is lost or ischaemia to the brain is corrected often by assuming the recumbent posture.

Pathogenesis and Pathophysiology

Syncope results from transient ischaemia of the brain usually in upright position, brought about by reduction in cardiac output or hypotension

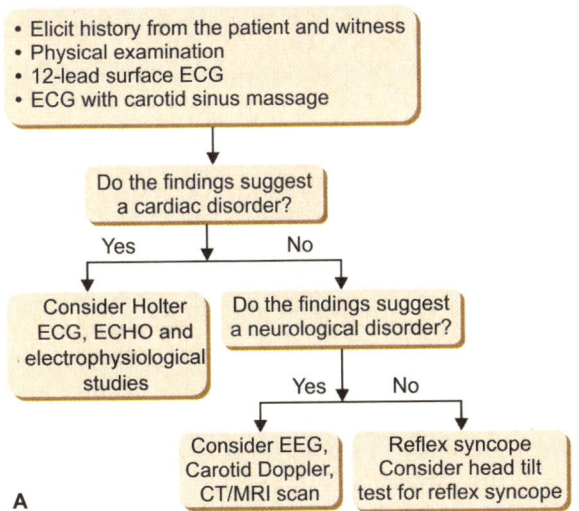

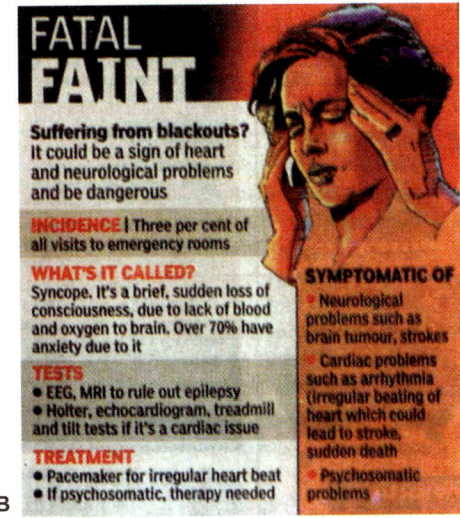

Fig. 46.1: (A) A valuable guide to investigations, diagnosis and differential diagnosis of syncope (B) Fatal faints/blackouts called syncope: The summary of incidence, investigations, main causes and proposed investigation

due to any cause. Depending on the pathophysiologic mechanisms, syncope may be naturally mediated syncope (vasovagal, neurocardiogenic), postural (orthostatic) and cardiac. The causes of syncope are given in Table 46.1. The underlying mechanisms in syncope are:

i. Inadequate vasoconstrictive response. Examples are vasodepressor, postural syncope.
ii. Reduced venous return, i.e. cough, micturition, defecation syncope.
iii. Reduce cardiac output, i.e. myocardial and pericardial diseases, obstructive valvular lesions and arrhythmia.
iv. Altered state of blood, e.g. anaemia, hypoxia, etc.

Clinical Features

It includes:

1. Symptoms and signs of syncope *per se.*
2. Symptoms and signs of the underlying disease/cause.
1. **Symptoms and signs of syncope:** A syncopal attack begins when the patient is usually in an upright position (sitting or standing) except in Stokes-Adam attack (this can occur in any position). The patient is warned of impending faint by premonitory symptoms:

- There may be a sense of giddiness or vertigo (swaying of the floor or surrounding objects) patient may even-fall during syncope (Fig. 46.2)
- Confusion, yawning and blurring of vision.
- Perspiration or ashen-gray colour of the skin.
- Nausea, headache, light headedness may occur.

In some patients, syncope occurs without warning symptoms. The onset varies from 10–30 seconds, rarely longer.

The depth and duration of unconsciousness varies, i.e. partly awareness to profound coma. The patient remains in the state for few seconds to minutes. Usually during the attack, patient lies motionless

Table 46.1 Causes of syncope

A. **Naturally mediated (reflex or vasovagal)**
 1. **Vasovagal**, e.g. due to fear, pain, anxiety, intense emotion, unusual scene, unpleasant odour, stress etc.
 2. **Reflex syncope**
  - *Pulmonary,* e.g. cough, sneeze
  - *Urogenital,* e.g. micturition, urinary tract instrumentation, prostatic massage
  - *Gastrointestinal,* e.g. swallow syncope, defecation syncope, G.I. tract instrumentation etc.
  - *Cardiac* e.g. cardiac outflow obstruction
  - Carotid sinuse, e.g. carotid sinus massage
  - Ocular, e.g. ocular pressure, ocular surgery

B. **Orthostatic hypotension**
  - *Primary autonomic failure,* e.g. Parkinsonism, Shy-Droger syndrome
  - *Secondary autonomic failure,* e.g. diabetes, amyloidosis, hereditary sensory, autonomic neuropathy, Sjogren's synrome, paraneoplastic autonomic neuropathy, postprandial hypotension, iatrogenic (drug-induced) or volume depletion, prolonged bed rest.

C. **Cardiac syncope**
 1. **Arrhythmias**
  - Sinus node dysfunction
  - AV node dysfunction
  - Supraventricular tachycardias
  - Ventricular tachycardias
 2. **Cardiac diseases**
  - Valvular heart disease, AMI, atrial myxoma, cardiomyopathies, pericardial effusion and taemponade.

D. **Cerebral syncope**
  - Cerebrovascular accidents, i.e. TIA
  - Vertebrobasilar insufficiency
  - Hypertensive encephalopathy
  - Altered state of bend to the brain, e.g. anaemia, hypoxia, hyperventilation

but sometimes a few clonic jerks may be noticed in the beginning of unconsciousness. There is no incontinence. The eyes typically remain open and deviated upwards. Pupils are dilated. Roving eye movements can occur. Pulse is feeble and BP is low to undetectable and breathing is stertorous. Following recovery in recumbent position, the volume of pulse improves, improves, colour of skin begins to return,

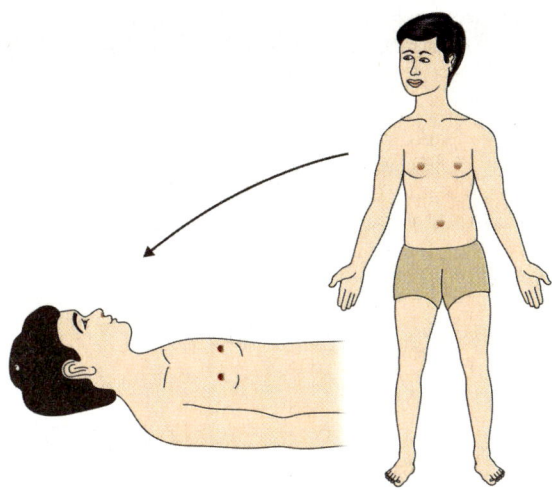

Fig. 46.2: A fall during syncope

breathing becomes quicker and deeper and consciousness is regained. There is recovery with no residual symptoms.

2. **Symptoms and signs of underlying disease/condition** such as cardiac disorders with low cardiac output, arrhythmias or infarction with pump failure. There may be an evidence of hypovolaemia or dehydration. Certain syncopes are related to specific circumstances, e.g. cough, alcohol, intake, menstruation, posture, pain, sight of blood, venepuncture instrumentation etc. There may be history of cerebrovascular disease, i.e. TIAs.

Diagnosis

Diagnosis may be difficult but analysis of patient symptoms by careful analysis of history is useful. For example, a history of vertigo is suggestive of labyrinthine or central vestibular disorder.

History

Whenever possible, an accurate description of the attack (already discussed) should be obtained from the patient, relative or attendant and a witness. Particular attention should be paid to the predisposing factors or triggers such as *medication, sight of blood, slight pain, venepuncture, intense emotion, exercise,*

alcohol etc., the period of unconsciousness and the recovery phase.

In vasodepressor (vasovagal) syncope called orthostatic hypotension or common faint, there may be history of prolonged standing, fatigue, venepuncture, minor surgery and painful stress, etc. while certain situations, e.g. cough, micturition, menstruation are related to an attack of syncope. There is fall of 20 mm in systolic BP within 3 minutes of standing or head up tilt on a tilt table. It indicates sympathetic vasoconstrider (autonomic) failure. In *cardiac syncope*, there may be history of structural heart disease or the presence of an arrhythmia at the time of an attack.

The period of recovery is important. Patients with cardiac syncope recover fast without residual symptoms; the patients with vasovagal syncope often feel nauseated and unwell for several minutes and patients with neurogenic syncope usually take more than 5 minutes to recover.

The typical features of four common types of syncope are summarised in Table 46.2.

The syncope has to be differentiated from an epileptic attack (Table 46.3).

Physical Examination

1. **Observations** of pulse rate, BP, and symptoms in the recumbent and after 3 mintues of standing position for postural or orthostatic hypotension (a fall of 20 mm in systolic BP and 10 mm in diastolic BP on standing suggests postural hypotension).
2. **Valsalva manoeuvre** to induce cough syncope, if suspected.
3. **Carotid sinus** massage for vasodepressor syncope. It is done under BP and ECG control commonly in supine position. Generally massage is done for 5 seconds on one side, bilateral massage must never be done. Reproduction of the symptoms indicate carotid sinus hypersensitivity. If there is 50 mmHg or more fall in systolic BP associated with bradycardia, vasodepressor response is diagnosed.

Table 46.2 Salient features of common syncope

Feature	Cardiac syncope	Vasovagal syncope	Neurogenic syncope	Orthostatic hypotension
1. Premonitory symptoms	• Light headedness • Palpitation • Chest discomfort • Breathlessness • Convulsions may occur	• Nausea • Perspiration • Pallor • Light headedness	• Headache • Confusion • Hyperexcitability • Visual or olfactory hallucinations • Aura	• Headedness • Dizziness • Fainting on sudden posture change • Weakness, fatigue • Headache, visual blurring, neck pain
2. Predisposing/provocative factors	Arrhythmias, conduction defects, heart failure medications, basic heart disease	Motionless upright posture, dehydration, alcohol ingestion, anaemia, pain, sight of blood venepuncture, intense emotion, anxiety, hyperventilation, fear, stress.	• Head injury, trauma, TIA, pain, emotional disturbance, vertebro-basilar insufficiency	• Diabetes, autonomic disturbance (familial, acquired), drugs, arrhythmias, cardiac disease (outflow tract obstruction), old MI
3. Period of unconsciousness	Extreme, death like pallor with transient unconsciousness	• Pallor, Ashen-grey skin with short duration dizziness	• Prolonged (>1 minute) unconsciousness • Motor-seizure activity • Urinary incontinence • Tongue-biting	Slight dizziness
4. Recovery	Rapid recovery	• Slow recovery with nausea and light headedness	• Prolonged confusion • Headache • Focal neurologic signs	Rapid recovery after assuming recumbent position

Table 46.3 The distinguishing feature between syncope and epilepsy

Feature	Syncope	Epilepsy
• Precipitating factors	• Emotional, painful or stressful event	• Unusual
• Position	• Upright (usual)	• Any position
• Diurnal pattern	• Daytime	• Day and night
• Onset	• Subacute or gradual	• Abrupt
• Aura	• Absent	• Present
• Motor symptom and signs	• Motionless, flaccid, may have short clonic spasms or jerks	• Often tonic or tonic-clonic, clonic movement
• Colour of skin	• Pale or ashen-gray	• Pale or flushed
• Cyanosis	• Absent	• May be present
• Breathing	• Slow, shallow foaming	• Stertorous
• Incontinence of urine and stool	• Rare	• Common
• Biting of tongue	• Rare	• Common
• Injury from falling	• Rare	• Common
• Post-ictal	• Rare, physical weakness and clear sensorium are characteristics	• Confusion, headache, drowsiness, sleep
• Period of unconsciousness	• Brief (few seconds)	• Short (few minutes) but longer than syncope
• Return of consciousness	• Prompt	• Slow

4. **Head-up tilt table testing** (autonomic testing) is useful provocative technique for diagnosis of autonomic testing. Upright lift to a maximum of 60 to 70° in conjunction with isoproterenol infusion (sympathetic testing) or sublingual nitroglycerin (parasympathetic testing) usually precipitates symptomatic hypotension or syncope within 30 to 60 seconds in patients with autonomic failure. Autonomic testing is helpful to uncover objective evidence of autonomic failure and also to demonstrate a predisposition to vasovagal (naturally mediated) syncope. Valsalva monoeuvre can be performed for dysautonomia in patients with diabetes and familial dysautonomia.

> *Bradycardia, hypotension or both indicate a positive result on upward head tilt*

Investigations

1. **Blood levels:** Measurements of electrolytes, haematocrit, glucose is indicated. Toxological screens for alcohol and drugs if suspected. Hormonal levels if endocrinal disorder is the cause.
2. **Resting ECG and stress testing:** Resting ECG may be helpful in diagnosis of arrhythmias or coronary artery disease. However, a normal ECG does not rule out these as a cause of syncope. ECG done during carotid sinus massage indicates positive response (vasodepressor syncope) if a sinus pause of 3 seconds or more is produced. Echocardiography should be performed in patients with history of heart disease or evidence on physical examination.

   Exercise testing can be done when symptoms are associated with exertion or stress.
3. **Holter monitoring:** Ambulatory ECG (Holter ECG) is mainly useful to correlate the symptoms with arrhythmias recorded on Holter ECG which could not be recorded on resting or serial ECGs. Continuous loop event recorders can be used for long-term monitoring for weeks to months; these are activated by the patient at the time of symptoms, freezing in its memory for analysis. In particularly difficult cases, tiny implantable ECG recorders may be used.

4. **Signal-averaged ECG:** It is helpful in detecting the late potentials for predicting inducible sustained VT.
5. **Electrophysiological studies:** In cases with recurrent syncope of unknown aetiology where Holter monitoring is noncontributory and there is underlying heart disease particularly ischaemia or prior MI, the detailed electrophysiological studies like sinus node recovery time (for sick sinus syndrome). His bundle electrocardiography for conduction delays and inducible VT by prolonged stimulation may be helpful.
   Electrophysiological clues to syncope
   • SNRT (sinus node recovery time) >3 seconds or more
   • Pacing induced infranodal block
   • HV interval >100 msec on His-bundle ECG
   • Paroxysmal SVT with symptoms
6. **EEG and CT scan** not helpful except in differentiating syncope from epilepsy.
7. **Psychiatric evaluation for anxiety disorders** may reveal hyperventilation and syncope.

A simple guide to investigations, diagnosis and differential diagnosis of syncope is given in Fig. 46.2A.

Treatment

It depends on the aetiology. Wherever possible, the precipitating or triggering factors should be avoided.

1. **General supportive emergency measures:** During an attack of syncope, the patient should be placed in a position which allows maximal blood flow to the brain, i.e. with head lowered between the knees, if sitting; or, preferably in the supine position. Clothings of the patient should be

loosened. Head is turned to one side so that tongue does not fall back into the throat. Peripheral irritation such as sprinkling of cold water over face or application of cold moist towel may be helpful. If temperature is subnormal, the body should be covered with warm blanket. Aspiration of vomitus may be prevented by turning the patient to one side and nothing is allowed orally until the patient regains consciousness. Patients should not be allowed to rise immediately after regaining consciousness but should be observed for few minutes in supine position so that physical weakness has passed off.

2. **Treatment of the specific cause:**

   A. *Cardiogenic syncope:* In elderly patients, a sudden faint without obvious cause, should arouse the suspicion of complete heart block or a tachyarrhythmia, even though all findings are negative when the patient is examined. The treatment of cardiogenic syncope includes treatment of underlying structural mechanical disorder and appropriate management of arrhythmias (brady or tachyarrhythmias) and conduction defects (permanent pacing for documented conduction defects).

   B. *Carotid sinus syncope:* It is better prevented than treated. Patient is advised to avoid measures that cause pressure on the carotid sinus such as tight cervical collar. Patient is advised to turn the whole body rather turn the head alone when looking to one side. Atropine or the ephedrine group of drugs should be used if there is profound bradycardia or hypotension during attacks. Dual-chamber pacing relieves the symptoms due to bradycardia unresponsive to other measures.

   C. *Vasovagal (reflex) syncope:* This is mediated by the Bezold-Jerisch reflex and is usually triggered by a reduced venous return due to prolonged standing, excessive heat or a large meal. Some variants of vasovagal syncope occur in the presence of identifiable and remediable triggers (e.g. cough syncope, micturition syncope, etc.) are collectively called *situational syncope.*

   Treatment is unnecessary in mild cases where leg crossing, hand grip, arm tensing may be useful as these manoeuvre raise the BP. Tilt training (standing and leaning against a wall for progressively long periods each day) tone up the reflexes, hence useful. In severe cases, beta-blockers or disopyramide (a vagolytic agent) may be helpful. Cardiac pacing alone is rarely indicated. A dual-chamber pacing may be used in case profound bradycardia is the cause of intractable symptoms. Finally, patients with salt depletion syndrome (urinary excretion of less than 170 mmol/24 hours) may respond to salt loading or hydrofludrocortisone (a salt retaining hormone) proamatine (2.5–10 mg b.i.d) is effective and used as first line therapy for such cases either alone or in combination. Paroxetine (a selective serotonine reuptake inhibitor) has been found effective in refractory vasovagal syncope.

   D. *Postural/orthostatic syncope:* Whenever possible, the underlying cause should be found out and treated such as control of diabetes. Dehydration should be avoided. Simple measures such as keeping the head-end of the bed elevated (30°); gradual arising from the recumbent position, avoidance of prolonged standing flexing the calf muscles during standing to improve venous return, wearing a snug elastic abdominal binder and elastic compression stockings and volume expansion by liberal salt intake or 9α-fluorohydrocortisone (oral dose 0.1–0.2 mg/day) may be helpful.

Acute Vertigo

ACUTE VERTIGO

Definition

Vertigo is sense of self or environmental movement, most commonly due to a disturbance in the vestibular system (Fig. 47.1).

It is important to differentiate *true vertigo* from more common symptom of *'dizziness'* which is most often not due to vestibular causes.

Dizziness is common and often vexing symptom that patients use to describe a variety of sensations such as light-headedness, faintness, spinning, giddiness, imbalance

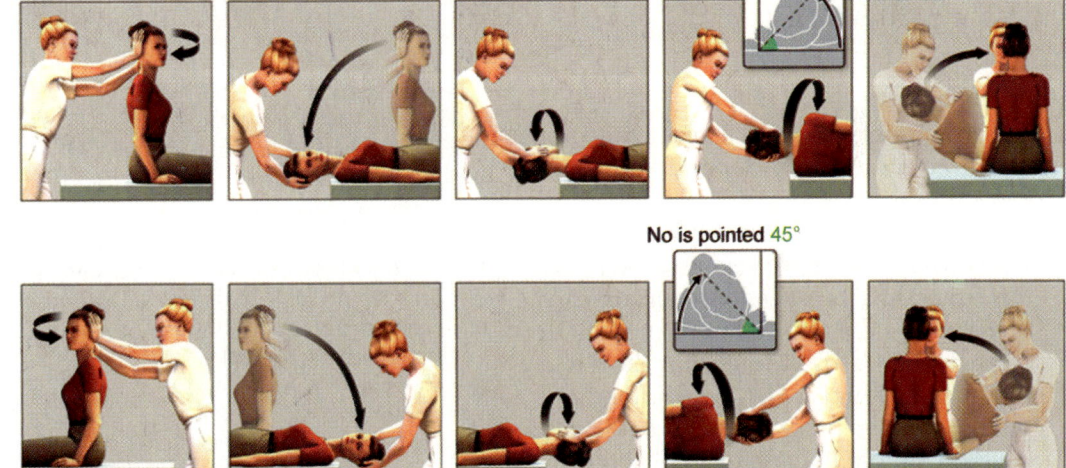

Fig. 47.1: Steps of modified Epley manoeuvre for treatment of benign paroxysmal positional vertigo of the right (top panels) and left (bottom panels) posterior semicircular canals. **Step 1.** Make the patient sit, turn the head 45° toward the affected ear. **Step 2.** With the head turned, lower the patient to the head-hanging position and keep it for at least 30 seconds and until nystagmus disappears. **Step 3.** Without lifting the head, turn it 90° toward the other side. Hold for another 30 seconds. **Step 4.** Rotate the patient onto her side while turning the head another 90°, so that the nose is pointed down 45°. Hold it again for 30 seconds. **Step 5.** Make the patient sit up on the side of the table. After brief rest, the manoeuver should be repeated to confirm successful treatment.

etc. Operationally, dizziness is classified into four categories: (i) faintness, (ii) vertigo, (iii) miscellaneous head sensations, and (iv) gait disturbances.

Causes

Vertigo can occur in normal persons (physiological) when brain is subjected to undue rotation/motion, abnormal head/neck positions or following a spin. It can be pathological; could be due to involvement of vestibular system, visual involvement (new or in correct spectacles or weakness of extraocular muscles) and somatosensory system (peripheral neuropathy and myelopathy).

Vertigo is a symptom complex of any type of vestibular lesion whether situated in the vestibular receptors (semicircular canals, the utricle and saccule) or in the pathways (vestibular nerves) called peripheral vertigo or projections to the cerebral cortex via thalamus-called 'central vertigo'.

The causes of both central and peripheral vertigo are given in Table 47.1.

Pathophysiology

The spatial orientation and maintenance of posture and equilibrium depends on three sensory systems:

1. **Vestibular system:** There are two basic vestibular system reflexes subserving this function: (i) vestibulo-ocular reflexes that stabilise the position of the eyes with respect to space so that images on the retina remain stationary, (ii) vestibulospinal reflexes that stabilise the head and body position for maintaining upright posture.
2. **Visual system** (retina to occipital cortex) that conveys the informations from the eyes to the cortex.
3. **The somatosensory system** that conveys peripheral informations from the skin, joint muscle receptors.

The three stabilising systems overlap sufficiently to compensate for each other deficiencies.

Vertigo may represent either physiological stimulation or pathological dysfunction in any of the three systems.

Table 47.1 Common causes of vertigo
I. Peripheral
1. Labyrinthine and vestibular causes
A. Hereditary
B. Acquired
i. Physiological
• Motion sickness
• Height vertigo
• Space sickness
ii. Pathological
• Infections, e.g. labyrinthitis, vestibular neuronitis, meningitis
• Benign paroxysmal positional vertigo
• Meniere's disease/syndrome
• Post-traumatic
• Drugs induced e.g. ototoxic (aminoglycosides), nerve involvement (diuretics)
• Cerebropontine angle tumours e.g. acoustic neuroma, meningioma, cysts (epidermal or arachnoid)
• Vascular compression of vestibular nerves
• Toxic, e.g. ethyl alcohol
2. Visual causes
• In correct or new spectacles
• Extraocular muscles paresis
3. Somatosensory causes
• Peripheral neuropathy
• Myelopathy
II. Central (brainstem and cerebellum causes)
• Brainstem ischaemia/infarction, embolism, haemorrhage
• Transient ischaemic attacks
• Multiple sclerosis
• Vertebro-basilar insufficiency
• Acute cerebellitis
• Posterior fossa tumour
• Migraine (basilar artery)
• Epilepsy (temporal lobe focus)

Nystagmus is useful indicator of vestibular dysfunction in patients with vertigo. Inhibition of the canals (caloric test) results in nystagmus to the side of the lesion, while excitation of canals results in nystagmus away from the canals (lesion).

Clinical Evaluation of a Patient with Vertigo

When evaluating patients with vertigo, consider the following:

1. Is it dangerous (e.g. arrhythmia, TIA, stroke etc.?)
2. Is it vestibular or nonvestibular (gait disorder, visual disorders)?
3. If vestibular, is it peripheral or central?

A careful history and examination will provide answers to these questions.

a. **Checking for orthostatic hypotension.** Duplication of symptoms during orthostatic hypotension indicate cerebral ischaemia.
b. **Valsalva manoeuvres** exacerbate vertigo in patients with cardiovascular disease.
c. Sudden turns when walking or spinning the patients while standing reproduce true vertigo (vestibular).
d. The simplest provocative test for vestibular dysfunction is *rapid rotation and abrupt cessation of movement in a swivel chair.* This always induces vertigo that the patient can compare with the symptomatic dizziness.
e. **Hyperventilation** is the cause of dizziness in many anxious patients. Forced hyperventilation for 1 minute is indicated for patients with enigmatic dizziness and normal neurological examination.

Once, it has been established that it is vestibular (true) vertigo rather than dizziness, then find out whether vertigo is central in origin or due to peripheral causes. Rapid unilateral injury to either peripheral or central vestibular structures produces the acute vestibular syndrome consisting of severe vertigo, nausea and vomiting, spontaneous nystagmus and postural instability.

The **time course** and **duration of vertigo** also help in the diagnosis:

1. Recurrent episodes of brief positional vertigo (lasting less than a minute) indicate *benign positional vertigo, or post-traumatic vertigo.* It can be *psychogenic.* They are provoked by changes in head and body position.

2. Recurrent spontaneous vertigo lasting for minutes or hours indicates *Meniere's disease, vertebrobasilar insufficiency, migraine* or *autoimmune ear disease.*
3. Spontaneous prolonged attacks of vertigo lasting for a day or longer suggest *labyrinthitis, multiple sclerosis* or *infarction in the vertebrobasilar artery territory.*

The differences between peripheral and central vertigo are given in Box 1.

Central vertigo as the cause can be suspected in elderly patients with positive history of hypertension, smoking, IHD and past history of CVA. Patients with central vertigo cannot stand or walk and direction of fall is variable. Central nystagmus is multidirectional (nystagmus that changes direction with direction of gaze, i.e. gaze evoked) in the brainstem and cerebellar disorders. Vertical nystagmus (upbeat-or downbeat nystagmus) is almost pathognomonic of brainstem or midline cerebellar disorders. Most common central disorders producing vertigo are vascular (brainstem ischaemia/infarction or basilar artery insufficiency or inferior cerebellar infarction).

A peripheral vertigo is suspected when there is a history of ear discharge or pain, unilateral deafness or tinnitis. Peripheral nystagmus due to labyrinthine disorders results in unidirectional nystagmus with slow phase (component) moving towards the affected ear and fast phase (component) opposite to the lesion. Vertigo is severe with direction of spin towards fast phase, while tendency to fall is toward slow phase. The nystagmus is spontaneous and unidirectional with a torsional component. It continues in the same direction when the direction of gaze changes. It increases in intensity as the eyes are deviated towards the normal ear. Visual fixation inhibits nystagmus and vertigo—a bedside diagnostic test.

Bedside Test used for Evaluation of Vertigo

1. **Visual fixation:** The effect of visual fixation is tested at the bedside with an ophthalmoscope focussed on the optic disc of one eye while the patient covers and uncovers

Box 1 Differentiation between central and peripheral vertigo

Feature	Peripheral vertigo	Central vertigo
• Postural instability (imbalance)	• Mild	• Severe
• Direction of nystagmus	• Unidirectional, fast phase opposite to lesion (ear)	• Bidirectional or unidirectional i.e. nystagus changes with direction of gaze.
• Purely horizontal nystagmus without torsional component	• Uncommon	• Common
• Vertical or torsional nystagmus	• Never present	• May be present
• Visual fixation and vertigo	• Inhibits nystagmus and vertigo	• No change
• Direction of spin	• Towards fast component	• Variable
• Direction of fall	• Towards slow component	• Variable
• Nausea and vomiting	• Severe	• Mild to moderate
• Tinnitis and/or hearing loss	• Often present	• Usually absent
• Duration of symptoms but recurrent	• Finite (minutes, days, weeks), acute	• May be chronic
• Neurological dysfunction	• Rare	• Common
• Common causes	• Read Table 47.1	• Read Table 47.1
• Head impulse test (vestibulo-ocular reflex)	• Positive	• Negative

the other (fixating) eye. The intensity of the nystagmus and velocity of its slow phase are increased by covering the fixating eye in peripheral vestibular lesions.

Dynamic visual acuity is a functional test for assessing vestibular function. Visual acuity is measured with head still and head rotation (back and froth). A drop in visual acuity during head motion of more than one line on a near chart or Snellen chart is abnormal and indicates vestibular dysfunction.

2. **Caloric test:** Caloric stimulation test is applied to each ear separately. The test is performed by making the patient in recumbent position and head flexed at 30°. Cold water stimulation normally induces horizontal nystagmus with slow phase towards the cold water stimulation and fast phase to the opposite side. Warm water stimulation has opposite effect. A reduced response indicates vestibular disorder on the same side. An inability to induce nystagmus with ice water denotes a 'dead labyrinth'.

3. **Head impulse test (vestibulo-ocular reflex):** It is assessed by multiamplitude

rapid head rotations. While patient fixes on a target, the head is rotated to right and left and look for nystagmus after rotation. If head impulse test is negative, the rotation is followed by nystagmus in the opposite direction (leftward nystagmus) after a rightward rotation, if positive then to the same side of rotation.

4. **Dix-Hallpike manoveuvre** for benign positional paroxysmal vertigo (BPPV).

5. **Auditory testing:** It gives informations regarding the hearing loss or tinnitus or other auditory symptoms that accompany vertigo in peripheral nerve lesions. CNS disorders rarely accompany auditory symptoms.

Electronystagmography is done for recording the sponatoneus nystagmus for positional vertigo.

6. **MRI imaging:** If a central aetiology is suspected, MRI should be done.

Specific Common Vertigo

Benign paroxysmal positional vertigo (BPPV): Positional vertigo is precipitated by a recumbent head position either to the left or to the right. BPPV is the most common positional vertigo. Benign positional vertigo is common in middle aged females and the episodes are precipitated by turning over in bed, getting in or out of bed, bending over and straightening up, extension of neck to look upwards, to reach an object placed overhead shelf. The duration of vertigo lasts for less than one minute. It generally abates spontaneously after weeks and months. The common causes of BPPV include idiopathic, post-traumatic and viral neurolabrinthitis.

Diagnostic Clue to BPPV

The most important positive sign in paroxysmal positional nystagmus is elicited by Dix and Hallipike method. A rapid change of position from sitting to a sudden head hanging to left or right positions (30–45° on one side) induces nystagmus within 2 seconds. This nystagmus has fast component away from the undermost ear and disappears within few seconds.

The recognition of positional nystagmus by above described method is important from therapeutic point of view, because specific repositioning manoeuvres can cure it dramatically. The **Epley manoeuvre** is commonly used procedure to treat BPPV (Fig. 47.1).

The vertigo and accompanying nystagmus have a distinct pattern of latency, fatiguability and habituation that differs from the less common central positional vertigo due to lesions in and around the fourth ventricle (Table 47.2).

Vestibular neuronitis: It is an acute, nonpositional (constant) vertigo with nausea, vomiting, oscillopsia (motion of visual scene) and imbalance. It can be central as well as peripheral. In peripheral lesion, the nystagmus is unidirectional with fast phase away from the lesion and head impulse test is positive. Central vestibular neuronitis is characterised by gaze-directional nystagmus and there are associated symptoms of CNS involvement (diplopia, weakness or numbness, dysarthria, etc.)

Table 47.2 Distinguishing features between benign paroxysmal positional vertigo and central positional vertigo

Feature	Benign paroxysmal positional vertigo (BPPV)	Central positional vertigo
Frequency	Common	Less common
Latency*	3–40 sec.	None, immediate vertigo and nystagmus
Fatiguability**	Yes	No
Habituation +	Yes	No
Intensity of vertigo	Severe	Mild
Reproducibility ++	Variable	Good

*   Time between achieving head position and onset of symptoms

** Disappearance of symptoms with maintenance of offending position

\+   Lessening of symptoms with repeated trials

++ Reproduction of symptoms during each examination

Most patients with vestibular neuronitis improve spontaneously, glucocorticoids and vestibular suppressants can improve acute symptoms. Antiviral treatment is indicated in herpes zoster infection (*Ramsay Hunt syndrome*), otherwise it is given on empirical basis. Vestibular rehabilitation therapy is given later onto accelerate improvement.

Management

Aims

1. To abolish vertigo.
2. To enhance vestibular compensation to allow brain to find a new sensory equilibrium despite a vestibular lesion.

Treatment of acute vertigo consists of bedrest and vestibular suppressant drugs such as antihistaminics (meclizine: 12.5 to 50 mg every 4–6 hours; dimenhydrinate: 25–50 mg every 8–12 hours, promethazine 25 mg I.M. 6 hourly or suppository), centralacting anti-cholinergics (scopolamine), homatropine histaminergic drugs (betahistadine—an antivertigo drug causing vasodilation of micro-circulation of internal ear), or a tranquiliser with GABA-nergic effects (diazepam) or calcium channel antagonists (flunarizine, cinnarizine). If the vertigo persists beyond few days, most authorities advise ambulation, despite short-term discomfort to the patient.

Antiviral agent: An antiviral therapy is indicated in herpes zoster oticus (Ramsay Hunt syndrome, i.e. vertigo with vesicles around the ear) otherwise, it is not useful. Most of the physicians use it on empirical basis.

Corticosteroids: They are useful in vestibular neuronitis during acute phase (within 3 days), to improve symptoms.

Vestibular rehabilitation: Vestibular exercises should begin as early as possible as the acute phase ends; and vestibular suppressants should be avoided because dizziness is required for compensation. The exercise programme should be systematized to facilitate compensation. While nystagmus is present, fixation should be exercised in the direction with greatest dizziness. When nystagmus decreases then eye-head coordination exercises should be done.

BPPV is often self-limited, when present may respond dramatically to repositioning exercise programs, one of these exercises, the Epley procedure (Fig. 47.1) is useful.

The treatment of recurrent spontaneous vertigo depending on the cause is summarised in Box 2. Prophylactic measures to prevent vertigo are variably effective. Antihistamines are commonly utilised.

Box 2 Treatment of recurrent spontaneous vertigo	
Disease	*Treatment*
Meniere's disease	Low salt diet
	Diuretics
Migraine	Anti-migraine treatment
Autoimmune inner ear disease	Steroids and immuno-suppressants
Vertebrobasilar insufficiency	Antiplatelets
TIAs	Anticoagulants
Syphilitic labrynthitis	Antibiotics
	Steroids

Acute Ischaemic Stroke | **48**

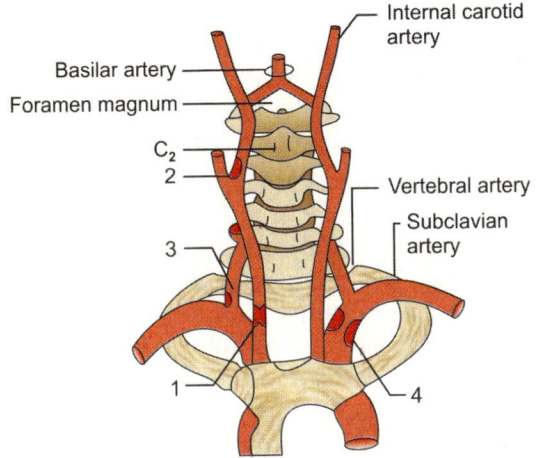

Fig. 48.1: The principal sites of atheroma in extracerebral vessels: (1) common carotid artery; (2) internal carotid artery; (3) vertebral artery and (4) subclavian artery

STROKE OR CEREBROVASCULAR ACCIDENT (CVA)

Definitions

Stroke is defined as sudden onset of focal neurological deficit resulting from focal disease of the cerebral vasculature, lasting for more than 24 hours or brain infarction demonstrated on brain imaging. The standard definition of *transient ischaemic attack (TIA)* implies complete recovery of such as neurological deficit within 24 hours without evidence of brain infarction

on brain imaging (MRI). Most of the TIAs last for <1 hour. CVA is the largest single cause of morbidity and disability in developing countries after cancer and heart diseases.

Pathophysiology

A decrease in cerebral blood flow to zero leads to brain death within 4–10 minutes. **Ischaemic stroke** results due to occlusion of a cerebral artery or less often due to reduction in perfusion due to severely stenosed cerebral artery (atherosclerosis). When the cerebral blood flow is critically reduced below 20 ml/100 g/min, the resulting cerebral ischaemia without infarction unless prolonged for hours or days results in loss of neuronal electrical excitation due to failure of Na^+, K^+ and ATP mechanism lead to cytotoxic oedema. This stage is reversible.

Further fall of cerebral blood flow to below 10 ml/100 g/min causes cerebral infarction with failure of cellular aerobic metabolism and lactic acidosis and ultimately death. This stage is irreversible.

Truely speaking, in any infarction, there is central core where the cerebral blood flow is drastically reduced (<10 ml/100 mg/min) which cannot be salvaged. A large area surrounds this area where cerebral blood flow is sufficiently reduced (between 10–50 ml/100 g/min) and the clinical symptoms are as a result of this reduction. The area is salvageable, if adequate timely intervention is done to improve the perfusion. This area is called *'ischaemic pneumbra'* which can be rescued.

The variable effects of reduction of cerebral blood flow is given in Table 48.1. The area with blood flow of about 20 ml/100 g/min is salvageable, hence, efforts should be directed to improve circulation in this area to provide neuroprotection.

Therapeutic time window (window period): This is a period between reversible stage (ischaemic pneumbra) to irreversible stage of cellular death (homeostatic failure). This period is important from therapeutic point of view because intervention at this stage can protect the brain from damage (neuroprotection is possible). This window period is one to three hours which means that all intervention should be done within 3 hours and the earlier it is done the better are the results. However it is not possible to reach the hospital within this period soon after the stroke, some studies include patients up to 6 hours of stroke. It is estimated that about 50% pneumbra may still survive up to 72 hours.

Brain Ischaemia and Free Radicals Mediated Toxicity

Cellular ischaemia leads to cascade of free radicals mediated changes which are deleterious to the vital functions of tissues. Ischaemic depolarisation results in membrane failure and in an uncontrolled release of excitatory neurotransmitters which are neurotoxic. A lot of substances such as prostaglandins, thromboxanes and leukotrienes are also released which are toxic to cell membrane causing lysis and generation of free radicals. The free radicals lead to neurotoxicity.

An inflammatory response to ischaemic neuronal damage leads to elaboration of interleukins, leucocyte adhesion, production of arachidonic acid and toxic free radicals formation.

Reperfusion either achieved by endogenous thrombolysis, thrombus migration

Table 48.1 Progressive reduction in cerebral blood flow and their variable effects

Cerebral blood flow	Effects
1. >55 ml/100 g/min	Normal
2. ≤20 ml 100 g/min *(Ischaemia without infarction)*	Cytotoxic oedema, failure of Na⁺, K⁺, ATPase mechanism. The stage is reversible.
3. 10–20 ml/100 g/min *(infarction within an hour)*	Ischaemic pneumbra (read text). This can be rescued with timely intervention
4. ≤10 ml/100 g/min *(Brain death)*	Cellular failure or cellular dealth. This stage is irrevesible

or therapeutic intervention may aggravate ischaemic damage by production of toxic free radicals from reperfused tissue.

Causes

Three types of major strokes are now recognised. These are:

1. **Ischaemic (thrombotic and embolic) stroke:** It is characterised by new cerebral infarction resulting from atherothrombosis or embolism to cerebral vessel regardless whether symptoms persist or not. The transient ischaemic attack (TIA) implies cerebral ischaemia with subsequent complete recovery within 24 hours. This results from platelet fibrin microemboli (embolic hypothesis) which get dislodged and gap reopens the occuded vessel with recovery.

   Lacunar or small vessel strokes are deep, small, cerebral infarcts located deep in the basal ganglion or cerebral white matter resulting from lipohyalinosis of small penetrating vessels leading to its obliteration.

2. **Haemorrhagic stroke:** It results from bleeding within central nervous system, occurs due to ruptured aneurysm in the young and hypertensive intracerebral bleed in the elderly.

3. **Stroke due to undetermined origin**

The causes of various types of stroke are given in Table 48.2.

Ischaemic Stroke (Fig. 48.1)

Ischaemic stroke results from thrombotic or embolic occlusion of a cerebral vessel or may

result due to prolonged systemic hypotension with underperfusion of cerebral vessels (ischaemic-anoxic encephalopathy). In the latter group, the areas of the brain with marginal blood supply are commonly affected.

Depending on the time course and reversibility of neurological signs, ischaemic stroke is divided into:

1. **Transient episode of ischaemia (transient ischaemic attacks**—TIA). This is reversible within 24 hours.
2. **Reversible ischaemic neurologic deficit:** This is an infrequently employed term, denotes an ischaemic event in which the neurological deficit usually recovers over a period of 24 to 72 hours but may take even one week to resolve.
3. **Completed stroke (thromboembolic stroke):** It evolves with a maximum neurological deficit at the onset (within few hours). Often, the patient awakens with a completed deficit. A completed stroke may be thrombotic or embolic, is sometimes heralded by one or more TIAs in the preceding days, weeks or months. The mechanism of ischaemic stroke revolves around the pathophysiology mechanisms responsible for TIAs.

Thrombotic strokes (completed stroke) are generally due to underlying atherosclerosis (Fig. 46.2); while embolic stroke results as a result of embolism from the proximal atherosclerotic vessel (ruptured plaques, clot) or the heart (cardiovascular cause).

Clinical Features

Symptoms and signs of TIAs: These are brief episodes of focal neurological symptoms or deficit of vascular origin, lasting for less than 24 hours without any residual sign. The episodes may be isolated and infrequent, or may occur many times a day and tend to be consistent in their symptomatology in affected individuals suggesting that recurrent ischaemia consistently involves the same side of the brain. Recovery is the rule in TIA.

Table 48.2 Causes of stroke	
Common causes	*Uncommon causes*

1. **TIAs (transient ischaemic)**
 2. **Thrombosis attacks)**
 • Small vessel (Lacunar stroke)
 • Large vessel (atherosclerotic)
 • Dehydration
 3. **Embolism**
   i. Artery to artery (carotid bifurcation, aortic arch)
   ii. From heart to cerebral artery
     • Mural thrombus
     • Atrial fibrillation
     • AMI
     • Valvular lesions
     • Cardiomyopathies
     • Prosthetic valves
     • Bacterial endocarditis
   iii. Paradoxical embolism
     • Patent foramen ovale
     • Eisenmenger's syndrome
 4. **Haemorrhages**
   • Hypertensive cerebral haemorrhage
   • Subarachnoid haemorrhage
	1. **Hypercoagulable disorder**
	 • Protein C and protein S deficiency
	 • Antithrombin III deficiency
	 • Antiphaspholipid syndrome
	 • Factor V Leiden inhibitor
	 • Sickle cell anaemia
	 • Malignancies
	 • Homocysteinemia
	 • DIC
	 • Thrombotic thrombocytopenic purpura
	 2. **Vasculitis**
	 • PAN, SLE
	 3. **Cardiogenic**
	 • Atrial myxoma
	 • Intracardiac tumour
	 • Libman-Sacks and marantic endocarditis
	 4. **Cerebral**
	 • Vasospasm (eclampsia, migraine)
	 5. **Stroke due to undetermined cause:**
	 • Moyamoya disease
	 • Multi-infarct dementia
	 • Fibromyalgia
	 6. **Infections**
	 • Meningitis, encephalitis, tubercular endarteritis

The embolism of platelet—fibrin clot formed over atheromatous plaques within a great vessel is the most common (90%) cause of TIAs.

Attacks are more common in older persons. The clinical features depend on the vascular system (carotid, vertebrobasilar) involved (Box 1). TIAs cause sudden loss of function in one region of the brain, symptoms reach their peak within seconds and last for minutes or hours but not beyond 24 hours (by definition). Consciousness is usually preserved.

Physical signs: As signs may recover completely within a short period, hence, the clinical examination may be normal. Therefore, the description of the event that led to an attack may be diagnostic. In addition, there may be clinical evidence of a source of embolus such as:

1. Carotid atheroma may lead to arterial bruit.
2. Arrhythmia (atrial fibrillation) may produce irregularly irregular pulse.
3. Evidence of valvular heart disease, myocardial infarction (fresh or old) or endocarditis.
4. Difference of blood pressure between two arms suggesting dissecting aneurysm or subclavian stenosis.

In addition, there may be clinical evidence of associated disease such as:

- Atherosclerosis of carotid artery leading to weak pulsation.
- Hypertension, diabetes, arteritis, polycythaemia.
- Postural hypotension, low cardiac output.

Thrombotic Stroke

Thrombosis with arteriosclerosis accounts for most of the cases of thrombotic stroke. Atherosclerosis affects extracranial and intracranial arteries at a specific locations (at branchings or divisions and curve of large vessels). The thrombus forms in the vessels where plaque narrows the lumen most. The platelet fibrin-endothelial clot is formed due to (i) fragmentation of endothelial lining by underlying atherosclerosis and the divided surface acts a nidus for thrombus formation, or (ii) there is dissection of plaque by blood column forming an ulcer crater that acts a nidus, or (iii) an hemorrhage within a plaque critically narrows a vessel and leads to superadded thrombosis.

Risk factors for thrombosis are same as that of coronary thrombosis, i.e. diabetes, hypertension, hyperlipidemia, arrhythmias, smoking, hypercoagulable states, old age and positive family history.

Thrombosis of a major cerebral vessel typically produces a large stroke; whereas occlusion of a small penetrating artery results in a small infarction called *(lacunar stroke)*. The clinical pictures varies in these two types:

1. **Thrombotic stroke due to a large vessel involvement:** The clinical picture varies depending on the size and site of infarction. In about 60% cases, prodromal warning symptoms may precede in the form of TIA. In some cases, the stroke evolves slowly in a stepwise fashion, i.e. *stroke-in-evolution*, the symptoms may appear in each limb in succession or simultaneously. The *stuttering* or *intermittent*

Box 1 Features of transient ischaemic attacks	
Carotid system	*Vertebrobasilar system*
• Amaurosis fugax (sudden transient loss of vision in one eye due to embolisation of retinal artery)	• Diplopia, vertigo, vomiting, dysarthria
	• Hemianaesthesia and analgesia
	• Hemianopic visual loss
• Aphasia	• Transient global amnesia (loss of memory)
• Hemiparesis	• Quadriparesis
• Hemianaesthesia and analgesia	• Disturbed consciousness (rare)
• Hemianopic visual loss	

manifestation is characteristic of thrombotic infarction. Not infrequently, the stroke may manifest as a sudden *completed stroke* (a catastrophic event). The major neurovascular syndromes resulting from major arterial occlusion are given in Table 48.3.

2. **Lacunar stroke (occlusion of small vessels):** Lacunar stroke results either from thrombotic occlusion of deep penetrating branches of carotid or vertebrobasilar system. Any of the perforating or penetrating branch can get blocked at its origin or by marked lipohyalinosis of intima in patients with hypertension. The infarcts produced in such a way are small ranging from 3–4 mm to 1–2 cm, often

Table 48.3 Clinical features of major vascular syndromes due to thrombotic occlusion of large vessels

1. **Internal carotid artery syndrome**
   - May be asymptomatic
   - Symptomatic cases have *warning symptoms* such as brief episodes of confusion, speech disturbance (aphasia, dysarthria) and paraesthesias (sensory symptoms) with or without contralateral hemiplegia
   - Transient monocular blindness (*amaurosis fugax*) on the same side with contralateral hemiplegia or hemianaesthesia is pathognomonic of carotid occlusion
   - Bilateral lesion produces quadriplegia with coma, a picture indistinguishable from basilar artery syndrome
   - In fact, the clinial symptoms and sign of acute carotid occlusion resemble acute middle cerebral artery syndrome (read middle cerebral syndrome)
   - Feeble carotid, poor pulsations of retinal vessels with or without optic atrophy, dilated pupil on the side of lesion and a cervical bruit are diagnostic clues to carotid artery occlusion

2. **Anterior cerebral syndrome**
   - Sensori-motor weakness of opposite lower limb (monoplegia) with or without weakness of upper limb (incomplete hemiplegia)
   - Mental features
   - Urinary incontinence
   - Gait disturbances
   - Appearance of primitive reflexes (sucking, grasp)
     Occlusion of unimpaired (single) artery
   - Cortical type of paraplegia, cortical sensory
   - Urinary incontinence
   - Akinetic mutism

3. **Middle cerebral syndrome**
   - Contralateral hemiplegia
   - Contralateral hemianaesthesia
   - Homonomous hemianopia may or may not be present on opposite side
   - Paralysis of the conjugate gaze to opposite side

   - *Global aphasia* if dominant hemisphere is involved
   - Aparxia, agnosia and neglect, all found non-dominant hemisphere involved.
   A. *Occlusion of upper division:*
      - Contralateral hemiplegic
      - Contralateral hemianaesthesia
      - Expressive aphasia (*Broca's aphasia*)
   B. *Occlusion of lower division*
      - All above features with Wernicke's aphasia
   C. *Occlusion of perforating(s)*
      - Lacunar (pure sensory or pure motor syndrome)

4. **Posterior cerebral artery syndrome**
   - Contralateral homonomous hemianopia
   - Visual disturbances, e.g. distorted vision, visual agnosia, dyslexia
   - Central vision is spared even in bilateral disease The pupillary reflexes are preserved
   - Contralateral hemiplegia
   - Thalamic syndromes
   - Memory loss (amnesia)

5. **Verbetrobasilar (brainstem infarction syndromes)**
   - Hemiparesis or quadriparesis (pyramidal tracts involved)
   - Sensory loss due to involvement of medial leminscus and spinothalamic tracts
   - Diplopia (3rd nerve involvement)
   - Facial numbness (5th nerve involvement)
   - Nystagmus, vertigo (vestibular connections involvement)
   - Dysphagia, dysarthria (9th and 10th cranial nerves involvement)
   - Ataxia, dysarthria and hiccups (brainstem and cerebellar connections)
   - Horner's syndrome (sympathetic fibres involvement)
   - Altered consciousness or coma (reticular formation involvement)

cavitate leaving small holes traversed by fine fibrous strands—'lacunae' hence, the name lacunar infarcts. Such infarcts are primarily located in basal ganglia or pons.

The symptoms and signs of lacunar infarct varies with size and site. Small infarct $< 1 \text{ cm}^3$ are usually asymptomatic. Larger infarcts produce the following clinical syndromes:

1. *Pure motor hemiplegia* due to lacuna in internal capsule or pons on the side opposite to hemiplegia.
2. *Pure sensory stroke* (hemianaesthesia) results due to lacuna in posterior limb of internal capsule or thalamus of opposite side.
3. *Ataxic-hemiparesis stroke* results due to lacuna in opposite pons or internal capsule.
4. *Sudden dysarthria and clumsy hand syndrome.*
5. *Pseudobulbar palsy* due to brainstem infarct.

Embolic Infarct (Stroke)

On account of sudden impaction of an embolus, compensatory mechanisms do not get sufficient time to come into action to protect the brain from ischaemia, hence, the neurological deficit is instantaneous and maximum at the onset. Frequently, these embolic plugs break away thereby restoring the normal circulation, hence, recovery is almost complete in these patients of strokes.

The clinical feature is similar to thrombotic infarct (stroke) but differs in some aspects (Box 2).

Haemorrhagic Stroke

This is discussed separately as intracerebral bleed.

Investigations

The preliminary investigations done to find out the cause in a patient with stroke are given in Box 3.

Box 3	Preliminary tests in stroke

- Urinalysis and blood glucose for diabetes mellitus
- Haemoglobin, platelets for polycythaemia
- WBC count for any evidence of infection
- ESR and C-reactive protein for inflammation
- Serological tests for neurosyphilis
- Estimation of protein C and protein S, homocysteine levels and factor V Leiden inhibitors
- X-ray chest for neoplasm, tuberculosis, etc.
- ECG for an evidence of myocardial infarct, ventricular aneurysm and arrhythmias
- Antinuclear factor (ANF), double stranded DNA, anticardiolipin antibodies for stroke in young patients
- Blood culture for endocarditis in patients with underlying heart disease

Box 2	Differentiation between thrombotic and embolic strokes	
Feature	*Thrombotic stroke*	*Embolic stroke*
Prodromal symptoms	Often present	Absent
Onset of stroke	Slow onset, stuttering or intermittent progression or may be sudden	Acute catastrophic
Neurological deficit	Slowly evolves • Step-ladder fashion called stroke-in-evolution • Symptoms and signs may appear intermittently	• Deficit is maximum at the onset
Consciousness	Confusion, disorientation may be present. Coma may supervene	Consciousness is usually preserved
Convulsion	Common, occur during the course or at the onset	Uncommon
Cause	Underlying atherosclerosis of a large vessel with or without thrombosis	Cardiac source or artery to artery embolisation
Recovery	Incomplete recovery may occur with residual symptoms and signs	Recovery is complete Residual symptoms and signs are rare

Further investigations done in patients with stroke are:

1. **Cerebrospinal fluid (CSF) examination:** It is done for inflammatory disease of the brain or for haemorrhagic infarct. It is useful in 80% cases of haemorrhagic strokes and in 90% of subarachnoid haemorrhage, where CSF contains blood. A three vials test should be done to rule out traumatic tap. Red cells and leucocyte counts/mm³ of CSF in three vial citrated blood will differentiate traumatic tap. The availability of CT scan and MRI have obviated the need of invasive lumbar puncture except in subarachnoid haemorrhage or inflammatory cerebral lesions.

2. **CT scan:** This is now widely available and is indicated in usually all patients with stroke or TIA. CT scan will demonstrate the site of the lesion and will also differentiate between haemorrhage and an infarction. It will detect an unexpected space occupying lesion, i.e. tumour, abscess, hematoma, parasitic cyst. It can also detect surrounding oedema and less consistently haemorrhagic infarction. It cannot differentiate early (within 6 hours) ischaemic tissue from normal tissue, nor can it detect cases of early infarction (less than 24 hours) hence CT scan obtained within first few hours of infarction may be normal. Detection rate increases over the succeeding few days and 90% of all infarcts are detected at one week.

    CT scan with angiography (contrast CT scan) will differentiate enhancing from nonenhancing lesions.

3. **Carotid Doppler study:** This ultrasound study is of value in screening for carotid artery disease (TIA, reversible ischaemic neurological deficit). In skilled hands, it is highly useful in demonstrating internal carotid artery occlusion.

4. **Cerebral angiography or digital substraction angiography:** It is gold standard for detection of atherosclerotic stenoses of cerebral vessel. It is most useful than Doppler study. It may demonstrate aneurysm(s) or an angiomatous malformation. Angiography should not be done in a ruptured intracerebral aneurysm. It carries risk of arterial hemorrhage embolic stroke hence should be reserved for select cases.

5. **Magnetic resonance imaging (MRI):** It is supplement to CT scan documents the extent and location of infarction in all areas of brain. MRI can often visualize anoxic lesions missed on CT scan. It usually becomes abnormal within few hours of cerebral infarction, hence, useful in early diagnosis because the peri-infarction parenchyma which appears normal on CT scan often shows abnormality (ischaemic demyelination) on MRI. **MR angiography (MRA) in hyperacute** (within 6 hours) **ischaemic strokes** defines the extent and severity of cerebral lesions which are usually missed on CT. Thus, MRI and MRA help a great deal in taking decision about thrombolytic therapy.

6. **Perfusion studies:** Xenon CT and positron emission tomagraph (PET) can quantify the cerebral blood flow, but are reserved tools for research.

Management of Stroke

Goals of Therapy

To prevent the development of cerebral infarction, but if present already, then to retard its progression or recurrence.

General Measures and Intensive Care

In a patient with stroke, maintenance of vitals (pulse, BP, temp, respiration), patency of airway, fluid and electrolyte balance and prevention of complications such as lung aspiration, seizures, thrombophlebitis and bedsores are essential. The treatment in early stage in intensive stroke care unit is beneficial:

i. *Ventilation:* Cerebral hypoxia predisposes to cerebral oedema, raised intracranial pressure and brain herniation. *Patent airway* must be maintained to prevent accidental aspiration and for continued suction of tracheobronchial secretions to prevent hypoxia.

ii. *O₂ administration* (4–6 litres / min) through a nasal catheter or venturi mask is advocated. Ventilatory support in a comatosed patient is necessary if signs of hypoxia secondary to hypoventilation are present, or there is rising $PaCO_2$. Long-term ventilatory support warrants tracheostomy.

iii. *Blood pressure:* In acute stage of cerebral ischaemia / infarct, blood pressure should not be lowered less than the target value (140/90 mmHg) despite the decongestive therapy and diuretics. On the other hand, in hypertensive CVA with encephalopathy, or malignant hypertension or when BP is >180/110 mmHg a parenteral beta blockers (esmolol) and diuretics may be employed to reduce the blood pressure to target value. Hypotensive episode may be treated by vasopressors (dopamine), I.V. fluids and corticosteroids.

iv. *Cardiac arrhythmias:* In acute CVA, the pulse can be irregular. Frequent ventricular pre-mature beats may be treated by diphenylhydantoin sodium (100 mg three times a day). Bradyarrhythmias may point to raised intracranial pressure or cerebral oedema which will disappear with parenteral fursemide or 100 ml bolus dose of mannitol.

v. *Fluid and electrolyte balance:* Ischaemic tissue with break in blood brain barrier retains fluid, predisposes to cerebral oedema. Judicious restriction of fluids intake (oral or parenteral) during first 2–3 days or even a negative balance is beneficial. On the other hand, excessive diuresis should not be attempted which may produce cerebral hyponatraemia.

vi. *Reduction of cerebral oedema and increased intracranial pressure:* In first week of massive cerebral infarction, IV. mannitol is used to reduce the vasogenic cerebral oedema. High doses of corticosteroids can reduce cerebral oedema but their role in treatment of ischaemic strokes is doubtful. A controlled trial of IV glycerol infusion in acute stroke has demonstrated reduced mortality in treated patients probably due to reduction in cerebral oedema.

vii. *Measures to improve cerebral blood flow:* Hyperviscosity reduces cerebral blood, if present, should be treated with low molecular dextran, or 5% albumin infusion to bring down the hematocrit 30–33%. Such treatment if employed, should be monitored in patients with cardiovascular disease and in those at risk of developing cerebral oedema.

viii. *Treatment of risk factor,* e.g. avoidance of smoking cessation of drug(s) responsible for stroke, tight control of blood sugar in diabetes, and Statins in patients with history of previous stroke with or without elevated LDL.

Specific Management

A. **Medical therapy:** It is directed against the cause and to prevent recurrence and complications.

    i. *Antiplatelet agents:* Antiplatelet agents (aspirin, dipyridamole, ticlopidine, clopidogrel) are used to inhibit platelets aggregation and useful in cerebral thrombotic infarction, embolism and transitory ischaemic episodes. Aspirin is widely employed drug for primary and secondary prevention of strokes. The dose is 75–150 mg / day.

      Ticlopidine (a thienopyridine derivative) though more effective than aspirin has been largely replaced because of its adverse effects (neutropenia and thrombotic thrombocytopenic purpura).

      Clopidogrel is marginally more effective than aspirin, causes neutropenia. Nowadays, a combination of clopidogrel plus aspirin is preferred over either alone. The glycoprotein IIa / IIIb receptor inhibitor (abciximab) held promise as an acute treatment in a trial but trial was stopped because of excess intracranial haemorrhage.

ii. *Anticoagulants:* Parenteral heparin or low molecular heparin and long-term oral anticoagulants have extensively been tried in acute ischaemic stroke to prevent extension of thrombosis but its value in completed or established atherothrombotic stroke is doubtful, and its use is often fraught with dangers. Its use has been recommended in recurrent TIAs, thrombosis-in-evolution, in cerebral embolisation due to atrial fibrillation or a cardiogenic cause or carotid artery thrombosis.

> **Danger:** *A diagnosis of ischaemic infarct must be confirmed on the CT scan and CSF examination before start of anticoagulation therapy, otherwise, haemorrhagic complications will pose a danger.*

During heparinisation, PTI is kept 2–3 times than control. Heparin (3000–5000 units) is given after every six to eight hours or an I.V. bolus dose of 100 units/kg body weight followed by continuous infusion of 1000 units/hour for 24 hours is recommended under supervision in acute care unit. Oral anticoagulant warfarin (2–5 mg/day) is generally given keeping the INR 2–3 times. Oral therapy can be continued up to 6 months or longer. A bleeding ulcer, malignant hypertension, hepatic failure and poor compliance constitute its contraindication. The anticoagulation in atherothrombotic stroke has no role.

- *Intravenous thrombolysis:* Intravenous thrombolysis with rtPA (recombinant tissue plasminogen activator) has been found useful in acute ischaemic stroke within 3 hours of onset (window period in patients with no evidence of haemorrhage/oedema on CT scan).

iii. *Use of oral thrombin inhibitor dabigatran* in two doses trials (110 mg/day and 150 mg/day) have been found useful equivalent to anticoagulation, hence is recommended in patients who cannot take oral anti-coagulation. This drug is convenient to take and does not require monitoring to titrate the dose and its effect is independent of intake of vitamin K. Once daily oral direct factors *Xa inhibitor* (*rivaroxaban, endoxaban*) have similar efficacy to warfarine, hence are alternatives to it.

iv. *Treatment of complications:* Infections (chest, urinary, etc.) dehydration, hyponatraemia, hypoxaemia, seizures, hyperglycaemia, deep vein thrombosis may occur and they should be treated appropriately. Avoid pressure sores by frequent turning and good nursing care. Use lexative for constipation.

B. **Surgical treatment:** Endovascular mechanical thrombectomy has been recommended as an alternative or adjunct therapy within few hours or days after acute ischaemic episode in select number of cases who are ineligible or have contraindication to thrombolysis. Best results are obtained when it is combined with best medical care. During the immediate postoperative period, higher doses of aspirin and control of all risk factors are mandatory. Carotid endovascular revascularisation is useful for TIAs caused by carotid stenosis.

Extracranial to intracranial bypass surgery has been proven ineffective than endartrectomy in atherosclerotic occlusion of either internal carotid or middle cerebral artery.

Recently, percutaneous balloon angioplasty (endovascular therapy) with stent placement is being used in carotid artery stenosis with good results. In carotid stenosis, angioplasty may open accessible stenotic lesions and in postoperative stenosis and maintain their patency.

Table 49.1 Causes of subarachnoid haemorrhage (SAH)	
Spontaneous (nontraumatic)	*Traumatic SAH*
• Ruptured cerebral aneurysm (congenital or saccular and mycotic)	• Skull fracture (cerebral contusion and laceration)
• Arteriovenous malforma-tion(s)	• Penetrating foreign body
• Leakage of intracerebral bleed into subarachnoid space	• Bleeding from traumatic AV fistula
• Haemorrhagic cerebral infarction/hypertensive haemorrhage	• Traumatic aneurysms (false aneurysm)
• Rupture of atherosclerotic vessel	
• Bleeding or clotting disorder	
• Vasculitis	

Ehler-Danlos syndrome, Marfan's syndrome and Rendu-Osler-Weber syndrome.

2. **Acquired**

   i. *Traumatic aneurysms:* They form as false aneurysms of meningeal vessels as a complication of major head injury. True aneurysms in the internal carotid or anterior or middle cerebral artery can occur from penetrating brain injury or bony fractures when intima herniates through the musculoelastic layers. These are rare.

   ii. *Mycotic aneurysms:* They are secondary to infective microemboli (bacterial endocarditis) in the *vasa nervosa* of an artery which in turn predisposes to septic degeneration of its muscular and elastic coats.

   iii. *Arteriosclerotic aneurysms:* These aneurysms arise from weakness of arterial wall due to extensive arterio-sclerotic degeneration in the large arterial trunks (basilar, internal carotid and middle cerebral). These aneurysms vary in appearance such as 'fusiform', globular or diffuse. They seldom rupture. They cause neuro-logical deficit by compressing the nearby structures. They predispose to throm-bus formation within its sac.

   iv. *Dissecting aneurysms:* Primary dissec-tions between intima, media, or adven-titia of internal carotid, middle cerebral or vertebro-basilar arterial walls have now been documented in the absence of injury or atherosclerosis. They present like stroke syndrome without S AH. Such dissections can be treated by 'trapping' of its proximal vessel some time by a by pass procedure.

   v. *Giant aneurysms* (>25 mm in diameter) may be congenital or atherosclerotic, represent 5% of all aneurysms. They produce symptoms due to mass effect like space-occupying lesion.

Pathogenesis of Aneurysms

The most common mechanism of aneurysms formation is thus a combination of several causes as discussed, starting with a congenital defect in the media at the bifurcation of cerebral vessels. These weak spots are present at branch-ings of these vessels. Hemodynamic stress in the form of local turbulance of blood at this site causes hyperplasia and splitting of internal elastic lamina. This combination of a congenital defect with acquired loss of elastic membrane under the effect of blood pressure may predis-pose to outpouching of the fragmented elastica leading to saccular aneurysm formation which produces clinical features due to its rupture at the weakest spot. Aneurysms >7 mm in diameter and those located at the top of basilar artery and at the origin of posterior communi-cating artery are at greater risk of rupture.

Sites of Aneurysm (Box 1)

Box 1 Sites of aneurysms
1. Anterior communicating artery (30.1)
2. Midele cerebral artery (20)
3. Internal carotid artery (7.5%)
• Posterior communicating artery (25.1)
• Posterior inferior cerebellar artery (4.12)
• Basilator tip (7%)
• Others 6.1

Clinical Features

Most aneurysms are asymptomatic until rupture. They may cause focal neurological deficit by compression of adjacent structures. Symptoms are divided into:

1. Symptoms and signs during acute phase.
2. Symptoms and signs in later phase (delayed neurological deficit).

1. **Symptoms and signs in acute phase of SAH:** Most aneurysms rupture without a warning and the most frequent presentation is sudden (thunderclap) unexplained headache if rupture is small; while aneurysmal rupture with major subarachnoid haemorrhage (Fig. 49.3A and B) produces rise in intracranial pressure leading to severe headache, vomiting and sudden loss of consciousness (patient may collapse suddenly on the floor). The headache at the time of rupture or immediately after that is so severe that patient describes it as 'the worst headache of my life' and is unforgettable. Fundus examination may show subhyaloid haemorrhage. The symptoms of SAH in order of frequency are given in Box 2.

Box 2 Symptoms of SAH in order of frequency	
Symptoms	*Percentage*
Headache	>50%
Sudden loss of consciousness	20–22% (approx)
Convulsions	5% (approx)
Funny feeling in head	4% (approx)
Pain in back and limbs	2% (approx)
Paralysis or paresis	2% (approx)
Confusion	1% (approx)
No information	4% (approx)

Physical signs depend on the site of an aneurysm, amount of bleed and rapidity with which subarachnoid haemorrhage develops. Sudden death from massive bleed is not uncommon. Majority of the patients develop initial coma, wake up from coma, and continue to remain confused, disoriented and may have transient amnesia for few days. During this period intermittent lethargy and headaches are common. Although sudden headache without focal neurological symptom is the hallmark of rupture of an aneurysm but focal neurological deficit may occur in addition due to formation of hematoma that may produce mass effect. In posterior communicating

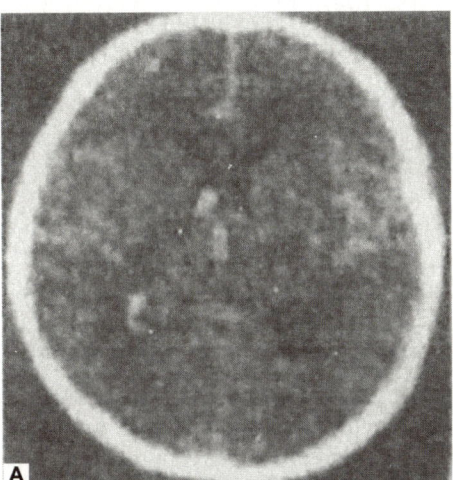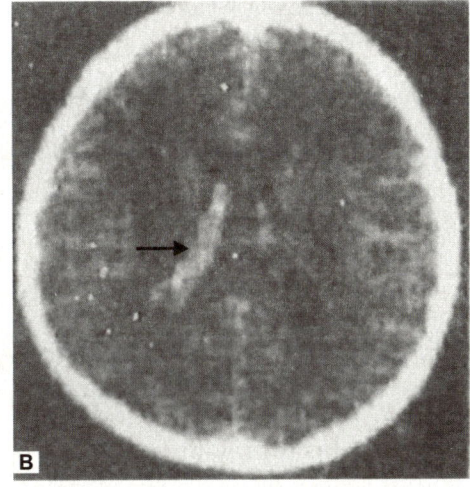

Fig. 49.3A and B: Subarachnoid haemorrhage. CT axial images without contrast show hyperdensity in the subarachnoid spaces due to extravasated blood. (A) More pronounced collection of blood is seen in the anterior part of the frontal interhemispheric cistern indicating the source of haemorrhage which was a ruptured anterior communicating artery aneurysm. (B) Intraventricular blood (→) is seen in the third and lateral ventricles

aneurysmal bleed, 3rd nerve palsy is common and dilatation of pupil on side of lesion is the earliest sign. In SAH of internal carotid or middle cerebral aneurysmal bleed, hemiplegia with or without aphasia and slow mentation (abulia) has been described. Temporary paraplegia, urinary incontinence and akinetic mutism indicate aneurysmal rupture of anterior communicating artery. In aneurysmal bleed of vertibrobasilar system produce lower cranial nerve palsies with pyramidal signs. The clinical findings in SAH are given in Box 3.

Box 3   Common clinical findings in SAH

- Neck stiffness or rigidity (meningismus)
- Pyrexia (fever)
- Transient hypertension
- Bradycardia (HR <60 min)
- Pre-retinal (subhyaloid) haemorrhage
- Confusion, restlessnes, memory loss, coma
- Symptoms and signs of raised intracranial pressure, i.e. headache, vomiting, papilloedema, pupillary change, 6th nerve palsy, bilateral plantar extensor response
- Irregular respiration (Cheyne-Stoke breathing)
- ECG shows nonspecific ST-T changes. There may be deep, symmetric T wave inversion, QTc pro-longation, the cause of which is unknown
- Hyponatraemia (cerebral salt wasting)

---

2. **Symptoms and signs in later phase (delayed neurological deficit):** These are primarily due to:
   i. *Re-rupture:* The risk of re-rupture in untreated aneurysm is maximum within first 2–3 days; but few cases may have re-rupture within 4 weeks. Early surgery eliminates this risk.
   ii. *Hydrocephalus:* Acute hydrocephalus due to intraventricular bleeding may cause stupor and coma. Subacute hydrocephalus (developing over few days) produces progressive drowsiness and lethargy with incontinence. Chronic hydrocephalus (developing over few weeks or months following bleed) presents with gait difficulty,

incontinence, slow mentation and lack of interest in surroundings.
   iii. *Vasospasm:* Vasospasm usually occurs 2 to 14 days following SAH due to focal arterial spasm. It causes symptomatic ischaemia or infarction, presents with symptoms referable to arterial territories involved as follows:
      a. Spasm of middle cerebral artery causes contralateral hemiplegia and aphasia (if dominant hemisphere is involved).
      b. Proximal anterior cerebral artery vaso-spasm causes abulia (slow mentation) and incontinence.
      c. Vasospasm of posterior cerebral artery produces characteristic hemianopia.
      d. Basilar or vertebral artery vasospasm produces variable focal brainstem signs.
      e. Cerebral oedema.
   iv. *Hyponatraemia with hypovolaemia called cerebral salt-wasting syndrome* develops within 2 weeks following SAH. It is attributed to natriuresis and water loss caused by atrial and brain natriuretic hormones.

Investigations

1. **CSF examination:** A uniform blood stained or sanguinous CSF under raised pressure is diagnostic, to be done if CT scan does not show bleed or signs of raised intracranial pressure or this facility is not available. Microscopically, it may show RBCs (crenated) and pleocytosis. On standing, CSF supernatant is xanthochromic.

   SAH can be differentiated from a traumatic lumbar puncture by the lack of clearing of RBC from the first and fourth tube of CSF or by presence of xanthochromia. RBC count $<2000 \times 10^6/L$ is unlikely due to SAH.

2. **Cerebral angiography (carotid or vertebral):** Cerebral angiography or digital substraction angiography is not

only diagnostic but defines the site of bleed and outlines the aneurysm if seen. If angiograms show no abnormality, the examination should be repeated after 2 weeks because vasospasm or thrombus may have prevented detection of an aneurysm or other vascular anomaly during acute phase.

3. **CT scan:** CT scan is diagnostic. Contrast CT (CT angiography) demonstrates the aneurysm. Over 75% cases of SAH are detected on non-contrast CT within 48 hours of rupture.

4. *MRI* is better than CT scan in imaging the aneurysm.

5. **Transcranial doppler:** It is useful for proximal, middle, anterior and vertebrobasilar system flow detection and response to management of vasospasm.

6. **ECG:** The ECG frequently shows tall T waves, or deep symmetric inversion of T waves, widening of QRS and prolongation of QTc.

7. Electrolyte monitoring may reveal hyponantremia.

Complications of SAH

I. **Neurological**
   - Raised ICT or hydrocephalus
   - Intracerebral hematoma
   - Cranial nerve palsies
   - Cerebral oedema

II. **Systemic**
   - Diabetes insipidus
   - Hyponatraemia
   - Infections (secondary)
   - DVT and pulmonary embolism
   - Pulmonary oedema, cardiac failure

Management

Aims of Treatment

1. Stabilisation of patient and protection of airway.
2. Prevention of recurrence of bleeding.
3. To control cerebral vasospasm.

4. Treatment of symptomatic hydrocephalus.
5. Treatment of hyponatraemia.

1. **Stabilisation of patient:** Patient is stabilised by:
   - Complete bed rest in a quiet room for 3–4 weeks if surgical treatment is not done.
   - All sorts of physical strains (coughing, sneezing straining at stool) or manipulations must be avoided.
   - Mild sedation may be prescribed for anxiety and to prevent acute elevation of BP.
   - A laxative or stool softness to avoid constipation.
   - General nursing and medical care as discussed in management 'acute ischaemic stroke'.
   - Blood pressure should be lowred slowly but not below a diastolic level of 100 mgHg
   - *Seizures are not uncommon in SAH and can be catastrophic.* Prophylactic anticonvulsants (phenytoin in a loading dose of 15–20 mg/kg given over one hour period followed by main-tenance of 300 mg/day) are recommended in all cases of SAH.
   - To control severe headache, analgesics may be used.
   - In stuporous or comatosed patients, the general measures for unconscious patients may be applied (oxygen therapy, patent airway, maintain adequate oxygenation, if need assisted ventilation, monitoring for vital signs and pre-vention of bed sores).
   - *Raised intracranial pressure or tension (ICT)* occurs with large hemorrhage can be controlled by mannitol in I.V. boluses (0.5 to 1.0 g/kg). Dexamethasone 4 mg IV every 6 hourly helps to reduce pressure. Induced hyperventilation can be instituted to lower ICP in patients with midline shift.
   - *Monitoring:* Blood pressure, heart rate, temperature, intake and output balance,

arterial blood gases and electrolytes must be monitored.

2. **Prevention of rebleeding:** The main complication of SAH is rebleeding which is often disabling or fatal. Blood pressure should be brought gradually by nicardipine, labetolol or esmolol. *Microsurgical clipping* is the gold standard in the management of intracranial aneurysms. Though surgical clipping of an aneurysm can be attempted during first 48 hours but usually undertaken after about 10–14 days of SAH to prevent symptomatic vasospasm in postoperative period. Recently introduced endovascular treatment (coil embolisation) is an alternative for aneurysms not amenable to surgery.

Surgical treatment in patients with arteriovenous malformations consists of excision of malformations, if inoperable, then embolisation is the treatment. Two other techniques are injection of occlusive polymer and permanent occlusion of the bleeding vessel. Stereotactic radiosurgery with the gamma knife is useful in the management of inoperable arteriovenous malformation.

3. **Control of Vasospasm:** Intravenous nimodipine (a brain calcium channel blocker) infusion is started as 1 mg/hour and if there is no precipitous fall in BP, then it is increased to 2 mg/hour infusion for few days followed by oral dose of 60 mg every 4–6 hourly for 2–3 weeks. Intravenous $MgSO_4$ sufficient to raise serum levels between 5 and 6 mg/dl reduced the risk of vasospasm and vasospasm-induced cerebral infarction. However, symptomatic vasospasm can be treated by increasing cerebral perfusion pressure by inducing hypertension with phenylepinephrine or norepinephrine, hypervolaemia with plasma or volume expanders and haemodilution with fluids. This method is called **triple 'H'** therapy. Triple H therapy is contraindicated in cardiac patients.

4. **Symptomatic hydrocephalus:** It can develop acutely and needs a ventriculostomy (ventricular drainage). Chronic hydrocephalus is best treated by ventricular CSF shunting which is its definite treatment if symptomatic.

5. **Symptomatic hyponatraemia:** It can be treated with oral salt intake or by hypertonic saline infusion. Free water restriction is contraindicated. Daily monitoring of sodium prevents this complication.

6. **Hypopituitarism:** It may occur as a late complication of SAH.

Status Epilepticus

Definition

It is defined as continuous seizural motor activity for more than 30 minutes or recurrent seizures without recovery of consciousness between seizures. During seizures, patient may hurt himself/herself (Fig. 50.1) and there may be soiling of clothes with urine and faeces. Status epilepticus is a medical emergency as it has potential for neural damage and brain death, therefore, prompt and appropriate treatment is essential. Status epilepticus has many sub-

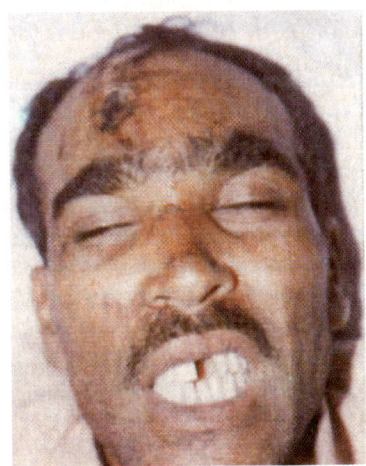

Fig. 50.1: A patient with status epilepticus. Note the injury on the head sustained during convulsions along with a fall of incisor during clenching of teeth

types, i.e. recurrent tonic-clonic seizures (generalised convulsive status epilepticus Fig. 50.2), partial motor status, complex partial status and absence status.

Nonconvulsive status epilepticus: In some cases, status epilepticus presents not with convulsions but with fluctuating abnormal behaviour, confusion, impaired responsiveness and automatism. EEG establishes the diagnosis. The **treatment** is similar to status epilepticus.

Classification

The clinical classification of status epilepticus is given in Box 1.

Box 1 Clinical classification of status epilepticus
1. Convulsive status epilepticus (Fig. 50.2)
A. Primary generalised convulsive status epilepticus • Tonic-clonic status • Myoclonic status B. Simple partial status epilepticus C. Generalised major motor status with partial onset
2. Nonconvulsive status epilepticus
• Complex partial status • Absence status epilepticus (typical or atypical)

Aetiology

It is most common in children, the mentally handicapped individuals and in those with

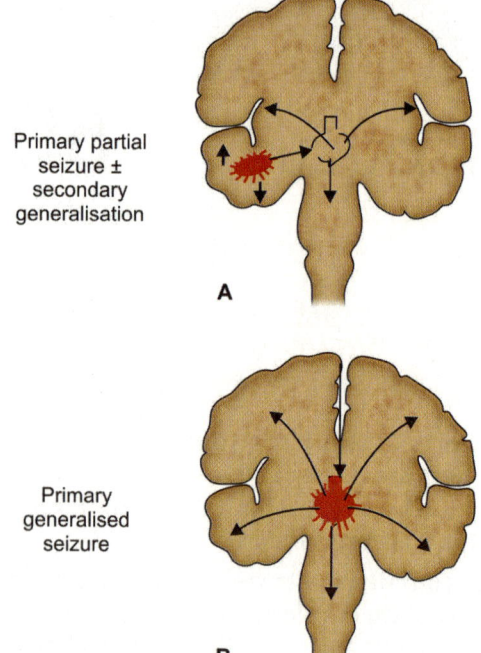

Primary partial
seizure ±
secondary
generalisation

A

Primary
generalised
seizure

B

Fig. 50.2A and B: Types of seizure associated with status epilepticus. (A) A partial seizure originates from a paroxysmal discharge in a focal area of the cerebral cortex and then subsequently spreads to rest of the brain through diencephalon—called secondary generalisation, (B) in primary generalised seizure, the focus of excitation or discharge originates from the midline (diencephalic activating system) and then spreads bilaterally in symmetric fashion simultaneously (indicated by arrows)

organic disease of the brain. In established epilepsy, status can be precipitated by factors given in Box 2.

In children infection with fever is by far the most common cause of status.

Diagnosis

Diagnosis of overt tonic-clonic status epilepticus is not difficult when two or more convulsions occur consecutively without regaining of consciousness between seizures in the absence of intake of benzodiazepines. However, after 30 to 45 minutes of uninterrupted seizures, the signs may become subtle. Patient may have mild clonic jerks of only fingers, or fine,

Box 2 Precipitants for status epilepticus
• Withdrawal of antiepileptic drugs or inadequate drug treatment. It is the most common identifiable precipitating factor for generalised convulsive status epilepticus. • Intercurrent illness/infections • Alcohol use • Acute stroke • Hypoxia/anoxia • Metabolic abnormalities • Progression of underlying disease • Trauma to the brain • Tumours of brain

rapid movements of eyes. There may be paroxysmal episodes of tachycardia, hypertension pupillary dilatation. In such cases, EEG is the only method to establish the diagnosis. Thus, if the patient stops having overt seizures, yet remains comatosed, an EEG should be performed to rule out ongoing status epilepticus.

The diagnosis of *nonconvulsive status epileptics* is often difficult because partial depression of consciousness or abnormal behaviour or confusion may mimic a psychiatric disorder. The diagnosis is confirmed by demonstration of ictal activity on EEG, therefore EEG also helps to differentiate nonconvulsive status epilepticus from hysterical behaviour or a psychiatric disorder.

Investigations

1. **The EEG:** All cases of status epilepticus should ideally be managed using simultaneous recording of EEG. It is also essential for diagnosis of status when convulsive movements have stopped and the patient has not recovered consciousness or when patient having a single convulsion fails to regain consciousness. It is actually indispensable investigation for nonconvulsive status.

2. **Biochemical profile,** e.g. blood urea, blood sugar, serum creatinine, liver function tests, serum electrolytes, Ca^+ and phosphorous to find out any metabolic cause of epilepsy.

3. Complete blood counts (TLC and DLC). C-Reactive protein, chest X-ray for evidence of any infection or aspiration.
4. Toxicological screening of blood and urine samples.
5. Antiepileptic drug levels.
6. **CT and MRI scan:** These imaging techniques help to find out the cause. These are done to find out any structural lesion. Most clinicians routinely order MRI (if not contraindicated) in all patients with new onset of seizure what to talk of status epilepticus. It is done as soon as seizure are under control.

   Indications for imaging are:
   • Epilepsy starts after the age of 20
   • Focal seizures
   • Abnormal EEG with focal seizure source
   • Refractory or resistant seizure
7. **Lumbar puncture:** It is indicated when either an infective cerebral or meningeal disease is being suspected and there is no evidence of raised intracranial pressure or CT/MRI scans are non-contributory towards its cause. The CSF should be sent for biochemistry, cytology and culture.
8. **Serology for syphilis, HIV, collagen vascular disease.**

Management

Aims

1. Termination of status epilepticus.
2. Prevention of recurrence.
3. Treatment of potential precipitating cause(s), such as 25–50 ml of 50% glucose I.V. in case hypoglycaemia is the cause.
4. Treatment of complications and underlying conditions.

Termination of Status Epilepticus

The measures are:
A. **General:** *Immediate or first-aid* measures.
   • Move the patient away from danger (fire, water, machinery, etc.).
   • After convulsions, put the patient in semiprone position. In hospital, put the patient on railing bed.

• Ensure clear patent airway.
• Do not insert anything in mouth (tongue biting occurs at seizure onset and cannot be prevented by observer).
• Secure intravenous line and start dextrose drip 5%.
• Blood samples should be drawn for haematology, serum biochemistry and antiepileptic drug concentration studies.
• Give diazepam 10 mg I.V. (or rectally), repeat once only after 10 min, if necessary or lorazepam 4 mg (0.1 mg/kg I.V. stat repeat after 10 minutes) if necessary or midzolam (10 mg stat I.M., repeat after 10 minutes), if necessary.
• Transfer the patient to intensive care unit (ICU) for monitoring neurological condition, blood pressure, respiration and blood gases.
• Person may be drowsy and confused for 30–60 minutes after an epileptic attack hence, should not be left alone.

B. **Pharmacological treatment**
   i. Regardless of response to lorazepam or diazepam, initiate long term seizure control as follows:
      • Start intravenous infusion (with cardiac monitoring) with one of the following:
         • *Phenytoin* I.V. infusion in saline of 15 mg/kg at a rate of 50 mg/min.
         • *Fosphenytoin* (it is converted to phenytoin) I.V. infusion of 15 mg/kg at a rate of 100 mg/min. in any solution It causes less local reaction.

            During phenytoin infusion, ECG and BP monitoring is essential.
   ii. *If seizure still continue then:*
      • Consider to add sodium valproate 25 mg/kg/I.V. Levetiracetam 20–30 mg/kg I.V. over 15 minutes or *phenobarbitone* a loading dose of 10–20 mg/kg I.V. at a rate of 100 mg/min.

iii. *If seizures still continue after 30–60 minutes (refractory status):*
- Start treatment with intubation and ventilation.
- Give general anaesthesia using I.V. propofol (1–2 mg/kg as bolus followed by an infusion 2–15 mg/kg/hr) or thiopental 15 mg/kg I.V. followed by 0.5–4 mg/kg/hr) or midazolam (0.2 mg/kg loading dose followed by 0.05–0.2 mg/kg/hr infusion).

> **Note:** The treatment is continued for 12–24 hours after last seizure, then withdrawn slowly.

Prevention of Recurrence

Once status is controlled, patient may be put on long-term antiepileptic treatment with one of the following:
- Sodium valporate 100 mg/kg I.V. over 3–5 mins, then 800–1200 mg/day orally.
- Phenytoin is given in a loading dose I.V. if already not given, then 300 mg/day orally.
- Carbamazepine 400 mg by nasogastric tube, then 400–1200 mg/day orally.
- Often, patients with severe brain injury require more than one antiepileptic drug at higher doses.
- Monitoring of drug level and the toxic effects is essential.
- Find out the cause and treat it accordingly.

Discontinuation of Medication

Only when adult patients have been seizure-free for 2–3 years, an attempt should be made to discontinue medication. Dose reduction should be gradual and drugs should be withdrawn one at a time. If recurrence occur, same treatment is reinstituted.

Complications

Status epilepticus, if unattended can lead to profound life-threatening systemic, metabolic and physiological disturbances (Box 3). The mortality rate in status epilepticus has decreased tremendously because of better therapeutic manoeuvres.

Box 3 Complications of status epilepticus
• Sudden death
• Hyperpyrexia
• Peripheral circulatory failure
• Aspiration pneumonia
• Hypoxia, acidosis, hyperkalaemia, renal failure
• Intellectual impairment

Advise after Discharge and Follow Up

Until good control of seizure has been obtained, the epileptics have not to do certain activities (Don't) and has to adhere to certain things (Do's). These are given in Box 4.

Box 4 Advise to epilepticus
Don't
• Not to operate dangerous machinery
• Not to sit near open fires
• Not to swim in pools
• Not to lock the bath room from inside during bathing
• Avoid mountaineering
• Driving and even cycling should be discouraged during first 6 months of treatment and then during period of withdrawl from antiepileptic drugs
Do's
• Take the antiepileptics regularly
• Continue treatment for at least 2–4 years
• Withdraw the drug slowly over a period of next 3–6 months

Epilepsy and Pregnancy

Guidelines of therapy:
- Epilepsy worsens during pregnancy in 30% patients especially in the last trimester as levels of anticonvulsants tend to fall, therefore, monitoring of drug levels is mandatory during pregnancy.
- All antiepileptic drugs are associated with foetal abnormalities except newer ones, e.g. lamotrigine and gabapentine.
- To prevent neural tube defect during antiepileptic therapy, folic acid 5 mg daily should be started 2 months before conception. To

reduce the incidence of haemorrhagic disease of newborn by antiepileptic treatment especially by enzyme-inducer drugs, maternal vitamin K supplement (20 mg orally/day) in the last month of pregnancy and intramuscular injection of vitamin K (1 mg) at birth for infant are advised.

- Breastfeeding as usual should be encouraged.

- Alternative form of contraception instead of oral contraceptive should be advised if patient is taking antiepileptic drugs.
- **Catamenial epilepsy** (increased frequency of seizures at the time of menses) is treated by adding acetazolamide (250–500 mg/dl) for 5–7 days till bleeding stops. Some patient may benefit from increase in dose of antiepileptic drug(s) during this period.

Acute Meningitis

ACUTE MENINGITIS (Fig. 51.1)

Acute meningitis is an inflammatory response to infection of leptomeninges (pia-arachnoid matter) with exudation into the cerebrospinal fluid (CSF) in the subarachnoid space. Acute meningitis may be *bacterial* (septic or pyogenic and tubercular), *viral* or *fungal*, etc.

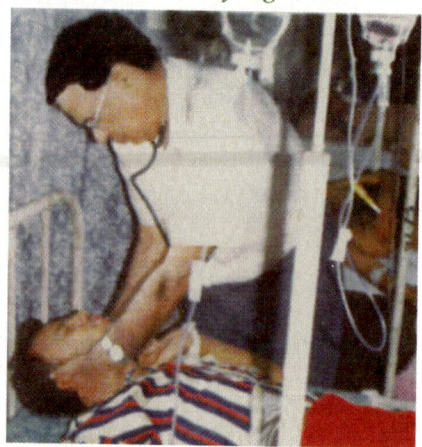

Fig. 51.1: Acute meningitis. Marked neck stiffness is present. Kernig's sign was positive in this patient

BACTERIAL MENINGITIS (NONTUBERCULAR)

It is an acute purulent infection within subarachnoid space. The meninges, subarachnoid space (CSF) and the brain parenchyma are involved in meningo encephalitis.

Pathogenesis

The common pathogens are given in Table 51.1.

Table 51.1 Pathogens for acute pyogenic meningitis

Common (>80% cases)	Less common
• *Haemophilus influenzae*	• Listeria monocytogenes.
	• It causes meningitis in neonates, elderly, alcoholics, immuno-compromised state, etc.
• *Streptococcus pneumoniae*	• Aerobic gram-negative bacilli (*E. coli, Klebsiella, Pseudomonas aeruginosa, B. proteus*). They produce meningitis at extremes of life, debilitating diseases, e.g. diabetes, cirrhosis, UTI and neuro-surgical procedures
• *Neisseria meningitidis*	

S. pneumoniae is the most common pathogens in children and adults in USA and other developed nations. In India, meningococcal meningitidis is the most common cause of bacterial meningitis.

S. Pneumoniae, N. meningitidis and *H. influenzae* are transmitted by air-borne route by droplets or exchange of saliva. These bacteria initially colonise the nasopharynx, attach to the mucosal epithelial cells, secrete IgA protease enzymes that breakdown the protective mucosal layer to enter into the blood stream producing bacteremia. From the blood they reach to CSF by breaching the blood-brain barrier. Once the bacteria reach the CSF, they have an excellent chance of survival and multiplication because humoral defense mechanism depending on the immunoglobulins and complement activity, is absent.

However, bacterial meningitis can occur by hematogenous spread or through congenital neuroectodermal defects, craniotomy sites, middle ear, dental and sinus infection, and skull fractures.

Rarely, intracerebral abscess may rupture into the ventricle or subarachnoid space producing meningitis.

The lysis of bacteria with release of their cell wall components into subarachnoid space incite inflammatory response and the formation of purulent exudate in CSF. The inflammatory response is mediated by cytokines and chemokines. The inflammation of cerebral vessels (vasculitis) produces ischaemia, infarction, thrombosis and thrombophlebitis of cortical veins resulting in cerebral oedema, raised ICT and coma.

Precipitating Factors

These are given in Box 1.

Box 1	Predisposing factors/conditions for bacterial meningitis
• Old age	• Hypogammaglobulinaemia
• Pneumonia	• Alcoholism, diabetes
• Otitis media, sinusitis, mastoiditis	• Immunocompromised state
	• Cirrhosis of liver
• Bacterial endocarditis	• Multiple myeloma
• Splenectomy or asplenic state	• Head trauma with basilar skull fracture and CSF rhinorrhea

Clinical Features

These include:
1. **Symptoms and signs of infection:** Fever, malaise, headache, aches and pains, vomiting, tachycardia, tachypnoea, convulsions in children.
2. **Symptoms and signs of meningeal irritation:** Pain in the neck, neck stiffness

(Fig. 51.1), positive Kernig's and Brudzinski's signs.
3. **Symptoms and signs due to raised intracranial pressure:** Headache, projectile vomiting, photophobia, blurring of vision, false localising signs (bilateral 6th nerve palsy, unilateral or bilateral fixed and dilated pupils, Cheyne-Stokes breathing, bilateral plantar extensor response, etc.) may be present. In addition to this there may be decreased level of consciousness, lethargy and coma, decorticate and decerebrate rigidity. All these are ominous prognostic signs. Papilloedema is rare.
4. **Focal neurological signs:** These are common in pneumococcal meningitis and complicate 15–25% of patients. Focal neurological signs (unilateral cranial nerve palsies, hemiplegia, monoplegia, etc.) are due to cortical vein thrombosis, cerebral artery spasm, subdural empyema or rarely brain abscess. The focal seizures are also common in these patients.
5. **Symptoms and signs due to infecting organisms:**
   • Morbilliform/purpuric/petechial skin rash, ecchymoses and lividity of skin in meningococcal meningitis. DIC is common complication of meningococcal meningitis.
   • Associated lung, ear, sinus infection in pneumococal meningitis.
   • Upper respiratory and ear infection in children associated with meningitis due to *H. influenzae*.
6. **The alteration of symptoms and signs in elderly and immunocompromised states:** The symptoms and signs in these two categories of patients are minimal in the form of fever, confusion and behavioural changes. The tonic-clonic seizure may occur.

Diagnosis

It is suspected when classic triad of meningitis, i.e. *fever, headache* and *neck rigidity* are present. Confirmation is done by CSF.

Investigations

1. **Total and differential leukocytes count** may reveal polymorphonuclear leucocytosis.
2. **Blood culture** may be positive is some cases.
3. **CSF examination:** It is an essential procedure for confirmation of the diagnosis. Fundus examination should be done before to exclude papilloedema. It is not essential to perform CT or MRI before lumbar puncture if patient is not comatosed or does not have focal neurological signs. **The CSF changes** include:
   i. The CSF pressure is raised.
   ii. Fluid may be turbid and contains many neurophils (>1000 cells/mm³). It may be clear if patient is already taking antibiotics.
   iii. The protein content is elevated >45 mg/dl (may be up to 500 mg/dl).
   iv. The sugar content is markedly low, may be less than 30 mg% (sugar is lower than tubercular meningitis). The value of CSF glucose is best determined by the ratio of CSF and serum glucose. The normal CSF to serum glucose ratio is 0.6. In majority of patients with pyogenic meningitis this ratio is < 0.4.
   v. *Gram's staining of CSF sediment (positive in >60%)* is extremely helpful as it allows rapid and accurate identification of microorganisms and forms the basis for empirical antibiotic therapy.
   vi. *CSF culture:* The CSF cuture is positive in >70–80% case of bacterial meningitis. The possibility of negative CSF culture increases if patients has already received antimicrobial therapy.
   vii. *CSF serology:* The CSF latex agglutination test or PCR to detect bacterial antigen are sensitive but not specific, hence positive test is virtually diagnostic but negative test does not exclude infection.
   viii. *Limulus amebocyte lysate assay* to detect gram-negative endotoxin in CSF is diagnostic (>90%) if positive but false positive tests do occur.

4. **X-ray chest:** It may show a patch of consolidation in pneumococcal meningitis.
5. **CT scan/MRI (Fig. 51.2):** It is helpful to diagnose hydrocephalus and brain abscess as a complication of meningitis, i.e. cerebral oedema and ischaemia. Tuberculema(s) may be seen in tubercular meningitis (Fig. 51.2). Neuroimaging of brain should also be considered if the patient is comatosed or there are focal neurological signs or focal seizures and before lumbar puncture if treatment is delayed. MRI shows diffuse pus collection and meningeal enhancement after administration of gadolinium. It is due to increased blood–brain barrier permeability, hence is not diagnostic as it may occur in other CNS diseases.

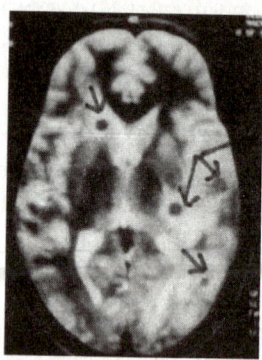

Fig. 51.2: CT scan showing multiple tuberculomas (arrows) in a patient with tubercular meningitis

Management

Acute bacterial meningitis is a grave medical emergency, needs early diagnosis and early institution of antibiotic therapy to prevent significant mortality and morbidity associated with the disease. Any patient with suspected meningitis needs hospitalization.

1. **Antibiotic therapy:** Empirical antibiotic therapy should be started soon after the diagnosis is suspected or confirmed with characteristic CSF findings without waiting for the isolation or identification of the causative pathogen.
   A. *Empirical therapy:* The choice of antibiotic depends on the age, underlying

health status of the patient and its penetration into the CSF. In most patients, vancomycin 10–15 mg/kg I.V. every 12 hourly and third generation cephalosporins (cefotaxime or ceftriaxone 2 gm I.V. every 12 hourly) or fourth generation cephalosporin (cefepime) are recommended. In elderly patients (>50 years), a combination of third generation cephalosporin with broad spectrum penicillin (ampicillin) and vancomycin are recommended. Patients with head trauma and immunocompromised hosts need broader antibiotic coverage such as a combination of cafepime plus vancomycin and ampicillin.

Table 51.2 Empirical antibiotic therapy in acute bacterial meningitis

Age and clinical setting	Likely pathogen	Choice of antibiotic
A. Immuno-competent • Above 50 years	• S. pneumoniae • N. meningitidis • L. monocytogenes • Gram-negative bacilli	Vancomycin plus ampicillin plus cefotaxime/ ceftriaxone
• 18 to 50 years	• S. pneumoniae • N. meningitidis • H. influenzae • L. monocytogenes	Vancomycin plus ceftriaxone
B. Immuno-compromised adults	• L. monocytogenes • Gram-negative bacilli • S. pneumoniae	Ampicillin (2 g I.V. 6 hourly) plus vancomycin plus cefepime or meropenem
C. Penetrating head trauma and ventricular shunt in adults (neurosurgical patients)	• L. monocytogenes • Gram-negative bacilli • S. pneumoniae • Staphylococcus	Vancomycin (2 g every 12 hourly) plus meropenem plus cefepime (2 g every 8 hourly)
D. Otitis media, mastoiditis sinusitis	• Gram-negative anaerobes	Add metronidazole to the empirical regimen

Merepenem may be added to sterilise CSF in neurosurgical conditions. Metronidazole may be added to empirical regime to cover anaerobic infection as cause of meningitis following otitis media and *mastoiditis* (Table 51.2). The antibiotic therapy should be modified as soon as the result of CSF culture and antibiotic-sensitivity report becomes available.

The antibiotic regimen depending on the pathogens isolated is depicted in Table 51.3.

B. *Duration of antibiotic therapy:* The antibiotic therapy for bacterial meningitis is variable depending on the organism isolated and antibiotic sensitivity. The duration of antibiotic therapy for the three common pathogens (*S. penumoniae, N. meningitidis* and *H. influenzae*) is 1–2 weeks; and for *L. monocytogenes* and gram-negative bacilli, it is 2–3 weeks (Table 51.3). It is essential that antibiotic therapy is continued in full dosage throughout this period because the penetration of these antibiotics is better with meninges inflammed, declines with improvement.

C. *Response to treatment:* In responsive patient, the CSF becomes sterile 1 to 3 days after antibiotic therapy. The fever disappears within few days but may persist for several weeks. Dead bacteria may be seen on Gram's staining of CSF for several days. Repeat CSF should not be done if clinical recovery is satisfactory. It is warranted only in meningitis caused by gram-negative bacilli or when therapeutic response is inadequate or when complications arise.

2. **Adjuvant steroids therapy:** Corticosteroids (dexamethasone) have been shown to have some benefit in adults and children of hearing loss in meningitis caused by *H. influenzae*. Adjunctive dexamethasone therapy (10 mg I.V. 15–20 minutes before

Table 51.3 Antibiotic regimen based on isolation of organism in bacterial meningitis

Organism	Antibiotic	CSF penetration	Dose	Duration
S. pneumoniae	• Penicillin G or	3 +	4 million units I.V. every 4 hourly	10–14 days
	• Ceftriaxone or	3 +	2 g I.V. 12 hourly	
	• Ceftriaxone *plus* vancomycin	3 +	2 g I.V. 12 hourly plus 500 mg I.V. 6 hourly	
N. meningitidis	Penicillin g or ampicillin	3 +	4 million units I.V. 4 hourly or 2 g I.V. 6 hourly	7 days
	Vancomycin	3 +	2 g/day in divided does e.g. 500 mg 6 hourly	
	Ceftriaxone	3 +	2 g I.V. 12 hourly	
H. influenzae	–do–	–do–	–do–	
L. monocytogenes	Ampicillin *plus*	3 +	2 g I.V. 4 hourly	14–21 days
	vancomycin *plus*	3 +	500 mg I.V. 6 hourly	
	cefepime	3 +	2 g after every 8 hourly (6 g/day)	14–21 days
Gram-negative bacilli	–do–	–do–	–do–	
P. aeruginosa	–do–	–do–	–do–	

or with antibiotic dose and continued every 6 hourly for 4 days) reduces morbidity and mortality.

3. **Supportive therapy:** It is symptomatic treatment and include:
   - Analgesic for headache and backache.
   - Careful nursing in a dark room if photophobia present.
   - I.V. fluids to maintain hydration. Electrolytes to be monitored and appropriately corrected.
   - In patients with signs of raised intracranial pressure, 20% mannitol or glycerol may be used to reduce the pressure. Elevation of head to 30–45°, intubation and hyperventilation repeated lumbar punctures and placement ventricular catheter are other measures to reduced raised ICP.
   - In some patients, treatment of shock and DIC may be required (*N. meningitidis*).
   - Steps of treatment of unconscious patients are same as for any other unconscious (coma) patient.

Prophylaxis: The measures used for prophylaxis of meningococcal meningitis in close contacts include:

1. *Drug,* e.g.
   A. Rifampicin
      - Adults 600 mg bid × 2 days
   B. Ciprofloaxcin (750 mg daily for 2 days) or Azithromycin 500 mg daily for 2 days.
2. *Vaccination:* Vaccine is not available.

Complications

1. Cerebral arteritis producing hemiplegia.
2. Venous sinus thrombosis.
3. Cerebritis and ventriculitis.
4. Subdural effusions / empyema.
5. Hydrocephalus.
6. Brain abscess (rare).

ACUTE VIRAL MENINGITIS

Infection of the meninges and subarachnoid space by viruses is called *viral meningitis.* Viruses are the most common cause of aseptic meningitis—a generic term used for cases of meningitis in which bacteria cannot be isolated from the CSF. Viral meningitis is an acute, benign, self-limiting illness without any sequela or residual deficit. Less commonly, virus may produce recurrent or chronic meningitis.

Viruses causing aseptic meningitis: Under the modern diagnostic techniques, it can be shown that up to 85% of cases of acute aseptic meningitis are caused by *enteroviruses* (*echo* 3–7, 9, 11, 21, 30 and *Coxsackie* (Ag and B 1–5) and human *enteroviruses* 68–71). The remainder, are caused by other viruses (California encephalitis virus, St. Louis encephalitis virus, Western and Eastern equine encephalitis viruses), varicella-zoster virus, herpes viruses; HIV and mumps viruses (Box 2).

Box 2	Virus causing aseptic meningitis	
Common	*Less common*	*Rare*
• Enteroviruses (Coxsackie viruses, echo viruses and human entero-viruses 68–71)	• HSV1 • Lymphocytic chorio-meningitis virus • Mumps virus	• Adenoviruses • Cytomegalo virus • Epstein-Barr virus • Influenzae A, B • Measles • Parainfluenzae • Rubella, etc.
• Arboviruses • HSV2		

Clinical Features

The cardinal features of viral meningitis include *fever, headache, photophobia* and *neck rigidity*. The constitutional symptoms such as nausea, vomiting, abdominal pain, malaise and myalgia are common. The symptomatology of aseptic (viral) meningitis is less marked than bacterial meningitis. The presence of altered mental status, seizures and focal neurological deficits are less common and indicate parenchymal involvement rather than meningitis alone. The disease is self-limiting and symptoms resolve within a period of 10 days.

Investigations

1. **CSF examination:** The CSF in viral meningitis shows (i) *lymphocytic pleocytosis*, (25–500 cell/μL), (ii) *normal or slightly elevated proteins* level and (iii) *normal glucose content* except in certain situations as discussed below. (a) Polymorphonuclear response in CSF may be seen in first 48 hours of illness especially in enteroviral, echovirus 9 or Eastern Equine virus infection. Repeat CSF after 12 hours may differentiate whether polymorphonuclear leucocytosis is due to viral or bacterial meningitis. A shift to mononuclear cytosis indicates viral; while persistent CSF polymorphonuclear cytosis indicates bacterial meningitis. The total cell count in CSF is less than 1000 cell/ml. (b) The glucose content is normal, may be decreased in meningitis due to mumps, lymphocytic choriomeningitis virus (LCMV); echo virus and other enteroviruses, and herpes simplex virus 2. (c) The conditions producing CSF pleocytosis with low sugar are; fungal listerial tubercular neoplastic some groups of viral meningtis.

2. **CSF culture:** The overall results of CSF are disappointing in viral meningitis. Similarly culture of other specimens such as urine, stool, blood yield negative results.

3. **Polymerase chain reaction (PCR):** Amplification of viral specific DNA or RNA from CSF using PCR amplification is an important method of diagnosing viral meningitis. Studies using CSF-PCR suggest that most cases of benign recurrent lymphocytic meningitis are caused by HSV-2.

4. **Serological test:** The diagnosis is retro-spectively made by viral antibody titre in CSF during acute and convalescent phase. The rise in CSF of viral antibody titre index (IgG index) in paired sera of serum and CSF more than 1.5 indicates CSF infection. The presence of CSF IgM antibody is also useful.

CSF/Serum antibody index >1.5 or presence of IgM antibody is suggestive of viral CSF infection.

5. **Other tests:**
   - Total and differential leucocyte count and ESR.
   - Platelets count.
   - Liver function tests.

- Blood biochemistry (urea, electrolytes, glucose, creatinine, enzymes, etc.).
- Neuroimaging is not necessary, but is performed in patients with altered consciousness, seizure and focal neurological deficits.

Management

- Symptomatic treatment with analgesics, antipyretics and antiemetics.
- Fluid and electrolyte balance.
- Bed rest.
- Acute viral meningitis caused by HSV 1 or 2, EBV and VZV may be treated with intravenous acyclovir (15–30 mg/day in 3 divided dose) followed by an oral acyclovir (800 mg 5 times daily) or oral famciclovir (500 mg tid) or oral valacyclovir (1000 mg tid) for 7–14 days although data supporting their efficacy is anecdotal.
- Acute HIV meningitis may respond to combined anti-retroviral therapy with zidovudine, a reverse transcriptase inhibitor and a protease inhibitor.
- Patient with deficient humoral immunity (X-link agammaglolinemia) should receive a trial of I.V. gammaglobulin. Most cases recover within 7–10 days. Resolution of CSF findings takes several weeks.
- A new drug pleoconaril has shown efficacy against a variety of enteroviral infections.
- Vaccination against viruses (varicella zoster) is the only method to prevent meningitis.

Tubercular Meningitis (TBM)

Tubercular infection of the meninges (TBM) usually has a subacute or chronic onset, but occasionally presents in *acute form* similar to pyogenic meningitis. Most often the diagnosis is delayed until the patient develops impairment of consciousness or develops focal neurological signs/deficit. At this stage, patient's condition warrants an emergency management.

TBM is generally considered a disease of child-hood, however, in recent years an increasing incidence has been observed in adults which account for about 50% of cases, develops commonly in those who are infected with HIV.

Tubercular meningitis results from the hematogenous spread of primary or post primary pulmonary disease, as a part of miliary tuberculosis or from the rupture of subependymal tubercular focus into subarachnoid space. In more than 50% of cases, there may be an evidence of a pulmonary lesion or miliary tuberculosis on X-ray chest.

Pathogenesis

Tubercular bacilli spread from the lungs to the brain via blood stream during the stage of primary complex formation and settle in different areas of the brain to form small subarachnoid or subepen-dymal tubercles, the so-called *Rich's foci.* Most common site of tubercle formation is choroid plexus. One or more of such tubercles may rupture into subarachnoid space discharging *M. tuberculosis leading* to tubercular meningitis. The development of meningitis depends on the virulence and number of the bacilli and the immune response of the host.

Pathology

The disease commonly involves the basal meninges. Secondary involvement of vessels (vasculopathy) and parenchymal lesions of the brain are equally characteristic and are important clinically.

1. Basal meningeal exudate involves the *cranial nerves* (palsy) at the base of brain (II, III, IV, VI, VII, VIII) to a varying degree.
2. **Underlying encephalitis:** In the region of menin-geal exudate, there is underlying encephalitis. TBM is thus pathologically a meningoencephalitis rather than meningitis.
3. **Vasculopathy:** Blood vessels of all types (artery, capillary and veins) are involved in vasculopathy associated with meningitis. The brunt is more on the arteries, and the lesions include periarteritis, fibrinoid

necrosis, panarteritis (panvasculitis with intimal proliferation and luminal narrowing). Focal and diffuse ischemic brain changes develop due to occlusion of both small and medium-sized cerebral arteries.

4. **Tuberculoma formation:** The site of tuberculoma is commonly the cerebellum in children and cerebral hemispheres in adults (Fig. 51.2).

5. **Hydrocephalus:** A communicating hydro-cephalus is common, develops due to blockage of basal cisterns in interpeduncular fossa by dense exudate or granulation tissue. At times, the obstruction may develop at the level of interventricular foramine, aqueduct of sylvius or foramina of *Luschka* and *Magendie*.

6. **Tuberculous encephalopathy** has been described in children where there is diffuse brain involvement due to perivascular demyelination with extensive oedema in the absence of above-mentioned pathological phenomenon to tuber-culoprotein.

Clinical Features

The diseases has an insidious onset, evolves slowly over a period of 1–2 weeks—a course longer than that of bacterial meningitis. The **initial symptoms** are vague till the symptoms of meningeal irritation develop. They include listlessness, apathy, irritability, anorexia, nausea, vomiting and abdominal pain. There may be low grade fever. In about 10–15% in children and 25% adults, there is no history of fever. Acute onset of illness can occur in 50% of children but uncommon in adults. When meningeal irritation sets in, then there will be headache, vomiting becomes severe and signs of *meningitis* (*neck rigidity*, *Kernig's sign*) appear. Even meningeal signs may develop late in the disease or even may not appear.

The disease if untreated passes through three clinical stages:

Stage I (early disease): Patients presenting purely with meningitis with no disturbance in consciousness and without any neurological signs.

Stage II (moderate disease): Patients have signs of meningitis *plus* consciousness is disturbed and focal neurological signs are apparent. The focal neurological signs include; *hemiparesis*, *cranial nerve palsies* (II, III, IV, VI, VII, VIII) and *involuntary movements*. Raised intracranial pressure may occur secondary to hydrocephalus (hypertensive hydrocephalus). In infants, there is bulging of fontanellae and the enlargement of head; while in adults papilloedema develops.

Stage III (advanced disease): The patient is deeply comatosed with signs of brainstem dys-function, i.e. decorticate and decerebrate rigidity, fixed dilated pupils, Cheyne-Stokes respiration with slow pulse rate or bradycardia.

Other modes of presentation of TBM include: acute meningitis, behavioural and intellectual chan-ges, covulsions, visual failure due to (optochias-matic arachnoiditis), isolated cranial nerve palsy, stroke and raised intracranial pressure.

Atypical or modified clinical picture occurs in vaccinated children. Clinical manifestations of TBM in HIV-infected individuals are same as for TBM otherwise, though picture develops more rapidly. Involuntary movements (fine resting tremors, dystonic posturing of limbs and choreiform movements) are common in children and usually subside after 4–6 weeks. Epileptic seizures may be present at any stage, more common in children than adults.

Investigations

1. **CSF examination:** The typical CSF findings in TBM are:
   - Clear or straw coloured fluid (when allowed to stand, forms a cob-web).
   - Raised proteins (100–500 mg/dl). Marked rise in CSF protein >1 g/dl indicates spinal block.
   - Low sugar (<40 mg/dl or 50% of blood sugar at that time). The sugar in CSF starts rising with antitubercular

treatment (ATT), indicates response to treatment.

- Raised cell count (mononuclear leuco-cytosis ≥500 cell/μl, but in acute stage there can be polymorphonuclear leuko-cytosis).

2. **Demonstration of tubercular bacilli** in direct smear or culture of CSF (gold standard) is the only method for establishing the diagnosis of TBM. Detection rate of AFB is poor in these specimens, even after centrifugation of CSF or staining the cob-web. Because of difficulties in isolating the organism, there is need for some simple, specific and rapid diagnostic test for accurate diagnosis. Numerous tests given in Box 3 have been devised but none is acceptable in clinical practice.

3. **Other tests:** Brain imaging may show hydrocephalus, brisk meningeal enhancement on enhanced CT/MRI and/or intracranial tuberculomas.

Management

As soon as the diagnosis is made or strongly suspected, antitubercular drug therapy should be started to prevent death and permanent neurological sequelae. Treatment is usually started with the four first line drugs because they are well absorbed orally giving peak serum concentration at 2 to 4 hours, have bactericidal

Box 3 Test for diagnosis of TBM	
A. Indirect tests	**B. Direct tests (detection of chemical components or antigens of AFB)**
• Adenosine deaminase (ADA) level in CSF	• CSF tuberculostearic acid (gas chromato- graphy or mass spectroscopy)
• Bromide partition test	• *M. tuberculosis* anti-gen in CSF (ELISA)
• Antibody to AFB in CSF	• *M. tuberculosis* DNA (PCR)

and sterilizing activity, low rate of induction of drug resistance and better penetration into CSF. The drugs, their dosage and side-effects are given in Table 51.4. The four drugs to be given for 2 months followed by two drugs (isoniazide plus rifampicin) for one to one and half years.

Drugs should be given as a single daily dose before breakfast. In general, tuberculosis is treated for longer period in patients with concurrent HIV infection (i.e. for 2 years or more).

Response to treatment: It is monitored by repeated CSF examinations. With effective ATT, the following changes occur:

i. The CSF glucose rises,

ii. The elevated proteins fall,

iii. The CSF cell count fluctuates considerably, but over a period of weeks, it declines (unlike acute pyogenic or viral meningitis

Table 51.4 First line antitubercular drugs for TBM					
	Isoniazid	*Rifampicin*	*Pyrazinamide*	*Streptomycin*	*Ethambutol*
Mode of action	Cell wall synthesis inhibitor	DNA transcription inhibitor	Unknown	Protein synthesis inhibitor	Cell wall synthesis inhibitor
Dose	4–6 mg/kg/day (usual 300 mg/ day for an adult)	10–12 mg/kg/day (usual 450–600 mg/ day for an adult)	30 mg/kg/day (usual 1–1.5 g/ day for an adult)	20 mg/kg/day (usual 0.75 g/day for an adult)	15 mg/kg/day (usual 800 mg/ day for an adult)
Major adverse effects	• Peripheral • Neuropathy • Hepatitis • Rash	• Febrile reactions • Hepatitis • Rash • GI disturbance	• Hepatitis • GI disturbance • Hyperuri-caemia	• Deafness • Rash	• Retrobulbar neuritis • Arthralgia
Less common side-effects	• Lupoid reactions • Seizures • Psychosis	• Interstitial nephritis • Thrombocytopenia • Haemolytic anaemia	• Rash • Photosensi-tivity • Gout	• Nephrotoxicity • Agranulocy-tosis	• Rash • Peripheral neuropathy

where it declines rapidly within days or a week).

In some cases, there may be relapse after satisfactory remission following treatment. The relapse is often due to stoppage of drugs, may develop even when adequate therapy is continuing. This may occasionally be due to development of drug resistance. It must be remembered that response to treatment may also cause deterioration of neurological signs due to healing process of tuberculosis (fibrosis) itself. Thus, progressively increasing hydrocephalus or spinal cord compression may be as result of adhesive arachnoiditis. If drug resistance is suspected, the four drug regime should be continued with addition of two new drugs (e.g. cycloserine and ciprofloxacin).

Role of corticosteroids: There is lot of controversy regarding their use routinely in TBM, but, however there is some agreement on their use under specific clinical situations:
 i. Evidence of rising intracranial pressure.
 ii. Progressive hydrocephalus.
 iii. Tuberculous encephalopathy in children.
 iv. Development of focal neurological deficit.
 v. Evidence of archnoiditis on neuro-imaging.

The dose of prednisolone is 1 mg/kg daily for 4 to 6 weeks . Some authorities use steroids in stage II and III disease in all patients.

Surgery

Surgery is indicated for prompt drainage of hydro-cephalus. Deterioration of consciousness level plus suspicion of an enlarging obstructive hydrocephalus are indications for surgical drainage.

Cryptococcal Meningitis

Cryptococcal meningitis follows cryptococcal infection of lungs by inhalation of the aerosolized infection particles. The exact nature of the particles is unknown. Little is known about the pathogenesis of initial infection, but inhalation of cryptococcal cells and/or spores during childhood can be followed by either clearance or development of the latent stage in the lung. The mechanism by which fungus undergoes extrapulmonary dissemination and enters the CNS remains poorly understood. The cryptococcal meningitis is usually chronic meningitis occurs in patients who are immunocomrpomised and have a focus of fungal infection in the lungs. Cryptococcal infection elicit little or no inflammatory response, but its capsule is antigenic which interferes with local immune responses.

Clinical Features

The clinical features are similar to tubercular meningitis, i.e. fever, headache, lethargy, sensory deficits, memory deficits, visual defects, cranial nerve palsies and neck rigidity (rare).The cryptococcal meningitis differs from bacterial meningitis with long duration of symptoms and lack of meningismus.

Diagnosis

Visualisation of the capsule of the fungal cells in CSF mixed with India ink is useful rapid diagnostic test. *Culture of CSF* and *blood for cryptococcal cells* are diagnostic of cryptococosis. The *CSF findings* include increased protein levels with normal to low sugar. There is mononuclear pleocytosis. *Serological tests* (PCR) assay can detect polysaccharide antigen in CSF and blood.

Treatment

In immunocompetent persons, initial treatment recommended is amphotericin B (0.5 to 1 mg/kg I.V.) *plus* flucytosine (100 mg/day orally) for 6–10 weeks. Alternatively patient can be treated with amophoterician B and flucytosine for 2 weeks then with fluconzole 400 mg daily for 10 weeks.

In patients with HIV infection aggressive therapy, i.e. amphotericin B (0.5–1 mg/kg I.V. and fluncytosine (100 mg/day/oral) for 2 weeks followed by flucona zole (400 mg/day) for 10 weeks, followed by life long maintenance therapy with fluconozole 200 mg/day.

Acute Viral Encephalitis

ACUTE VIRAL ENCEPHALITIS

Definition

Viral invasion and inflammation of the brain parenchyma is called *viral encephalitis.* It is an acute febrile illness with some evidence of meningeal involvement and symptoms and signs of diffuse and/or focal brain substance involvement. Some patients have involvement of meninges and brain parenchyma called *meningoencephalitis.* If spinal cord is involved along with, then it is termed *encephalomyelitis.* It is far more serious than viral meningitis.

Causes

The causes are enumerated in Box 1.

Pathogenesis and Pathology

The viral entry and replication of the virus at extra neural locations leads to an interaction between the virus and host cells. Various host factors such as pH, mucosal integrity and local immunoglobulins influence the ability of viruses to invade the host and replicate efficiently. Most of the viruses follow blood route to reach the CNS. Neural route of transmission is applicable to rabies, neonatal HSV encephalitis and poliomyelitis. Upon reaching the CNS, the replication of the virus within nerve cells leads to cellular dysfunction and may lead to cell death. Certain viruses produce mild cellular dysfunction such as mumps virus; while others such as HSV-1 often leads to widespread damage to nerve cells. Immunosuppression is associated with an increased risk of reactivation of latent HSV infection in CNS.

Microscopic examination reveals perivascular and parenchymal infiltration with mononuclear cells and glial proliferation with

Box 1 Causes of viral encephalitis		
A. Immunocompetent individuals		
Common	*Less common*	*Rare*
• Arboviruses (Japanese, St. Louis, Western Equine, Califormia and WNV) • Herpes simplex virus HSV-1 and HSV-II	• Cytomegalovirus (CMV) • Ebstein-Barr virus (EBV) • Human immunodeficiency virus (HIV) • Measles virus	• Adenovirus • Influenza and parainfluenza • Lymphocytic choriomeningitis virus (LCMV)
• Mumps		• Rabies, rubella
B. Immunocompromised individuals, e.g. HSV, VZV, CMV, EBV, human herpes virus-6		

nodules formation. Inclusion bodies may be seen in the cytoplasm or nucleus of brain cells. *Negri bodies* are inclusion bodies specifically seen in rabies.

Clinical Features

It includes:

1. **A prodromal phase of systemic symptoms and signs which may or may not precede the encephalitic phase:** This phase lasts for few days; includes nonspecific symptoms such as mild fever, bodyache, headache and malaise. In addition, there may be specific symptoms and signs indicating the specific virus infection such as skin rashes of coxsackie and echoviruses, upper respiratory symptoms (cough, coryza) are common with respiratory viruses (influenza, parainfluenza). Mumps may present with acute abdominal colic (pancreatitis) or parotid swelling (parotitis). The characteristic skin lesions of chickenpox, rubella and measles are evident before the encephalitis develops due to these viruses.

2. **After prodromal phase:** There is a short period of a febrile illness followed by encephalitic phase. This biphasic pattern is characteristically seen in arboviral encephalitis.

3. **The encephalitic phase:** The onset of encephalitis starts with fever, headache, photophobia, nausea, vomiting, signs of meningeal irritation. There is altered state of consciousness ranging from confusion, disorientation, stupor and coma. Convulsions which are common shown in Fig. 52.1. *Focal neurological deficits* include; *aphasia, ataxia, upper or lower motor neuron pattern of weakness, involuntary movements, sensory deficits, visual field defects* and *cranial nerve palsies.*

Hypothalamic involvement can lead to diabetes insipidus and autonomic instability. *SIADH* (syndrome of inappropriate secretion of ADH) is a common manifestation. In severe cases, there can be cerebral oedema, signs of raised intracranial pressure and brainstem dysfunction.

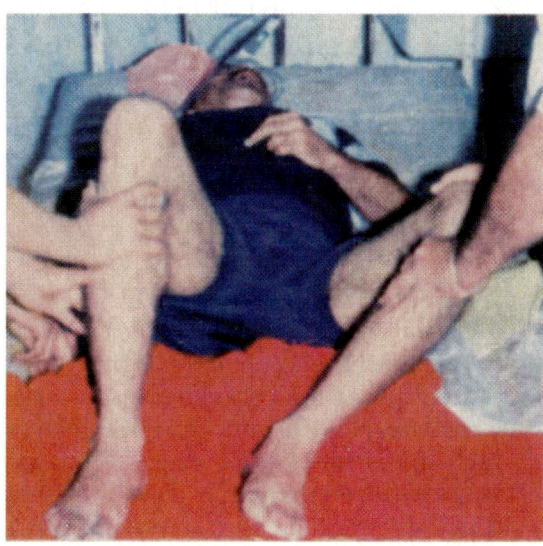

Fig. 52.1: Acute viral encephalitis being treated in the hospital. Patient is violent and has convulsions

Investigations

1. **Blood count** may show atypical lymphocytosis in EBV infection. Increased number of plasmocytoid or mollaret-like large mononuclear cells have been reported in WNV encephalitis.

2. **CSF examination:** CSF is done in all cases. The characteristic findings are similar to viral meningitis. These are include:
   • CSF lymphocytic pleocytosis.
   • Moderate rise in protein content.
   • Normal to mildly reduced sugar.

3. **Serological tests:** Demonstration of WNV IgM antibodies is diagnostic of WNV-encephalatis as IgM antibodies do not cross the blood brain barrier. Optimal detection of both HSV antibodies and antigen in CSF typically occurs after first week of illness, hence, has limited utility in acute diagnosis. Similarly in VZV infection, CSF antibody test may be positive when PCR fails to detect viral DNA antigen, hence, both tests should be performed as they are complementary to each other.

4. **Virus culture** from CSF and serum is disappointing and negative in >95% cases.

5. **CSF-PCR:** Detection of herpes simplex virus (HSV), CMV and EBV by a method of nucleic acid amplification using the polymerase chain reaction is sensitive (98%) and specific (100%) for diagnosis of herpes simplex encephalitis. The role of this test for viruses other than HSV is not defined. The CSF HSV PCR may be negative in first 72 hours of encephalitis.

6. **Imaging studies:** CT scan may show temporal and frontal lobe focal changes in herpes simplex encephalitis (HSE) but MRI is preferred over CT scan for this purpose. Characteristic MRI findings in HSE include high-signal intensity T2 weighted images in the medial and inferior temporal lobes (Fig. 52.2), focal areas of low absorption, mass effect and contrast enhancement on CT. In Japanese encephalitis, MRI shows altered signal intensities in thalami, pons and basal ganglia region. In *VZV encephalitis*, multiple areas of hemorrhage and infarctions are seen rather than enceplalitic changes.

7. **EEG:** It may show bilateral slowing of background rhythm or diffuse/focal epileptiform discharge. In HSE, the EEG in addition to above changes, shows periodic lateralised (focal) epileptiform discharges localized to the temporal lobes.

8. **Brain biopsy:** Though it is the most definitive procedure for diagnosis but is reserved for those patients in whom CSF-PCR study fail to lead to specific diagnosis or who have focal abnormalities on MRI and who continue to show progressive disease despite acyclovir treatment.

Management

Viral encephalitis is a medical emergency. Early diagnosis and early management is essential.

1. **General supportive management:** These include:
   - Treatment of fever with antipyretics.
   - Airway should be cleared and an I.V. line

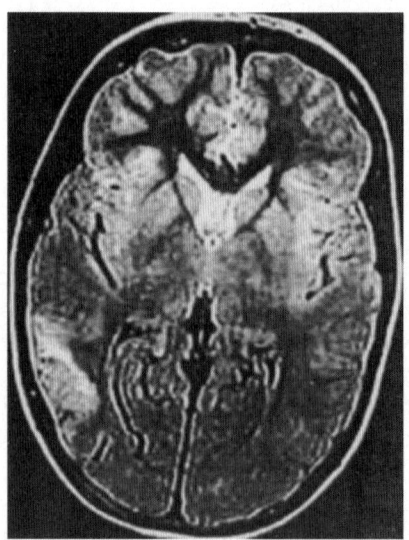

Fig. 52.2: Viral encephalitis. On MRI, the single, T2-weighted image of the brain shows abnormal asymmetric increased signals at the right temporo-parietal grey matter. There was little enhancement of the abnormal area after intravenous gadolinium contrast administration (not shown). This appearance of edema involving the temporal lobe was suggestive of viral encephalitis. The patient promptly received a course of antiviral therapy and recovered strength in her left upper extremity. Herpes simplex virus (HSV) was later confirmed as the causative agent by a rise in the cerebrospinal fluid antibody titre

established. A self-retaining catheter may be put

- The general management of an unconscious patient should be applied here if patient is in coma. Monitor vital signs (pulse, BP, respiration, temp.)
- Maintain fluid restriction and avoidance of hypotonic intravenous solutions
- *Seizures* should be controlled with phenytoin or carbamazepine, even prophylactic therapy with anticonvulsant, may be considered.
- *Cerebral oedema* may be decreased by using mannitol in a dose of 0.5 g/kg of 20% solution I.V. over 20 minutes every 4–6 hours. Steroids may also be used to reduce cerebral oedema. Glycerol is also effective in reducing cerebral oedema.

Box 2	Drug treatment of other viral encephalitis	
Virus	**Drug and dose**	**Toxic effects**
Varicella zoster	Acyclovir; 10–15 mg/kg I.V. every 8 hourly for 10 days	• Renal toxicity • Thrombocyto-penia • GI toxicity • Neurotoxicity
Cytomegalo virus (CMV)	Ganciclovir; 5 mg/kg over one hour after every 12 hours I.V. for 2–3 weeks then maintenance dose of 5 mg/kg daily	• Bone marrow suppression • CNS toxicity, nausea, vomiting
	Foscarnet (60 mg/kg I.V. 8 hourly) for 2–3 weeks, then maintenance dose of 60 mg/kg daily	• Renal toxicity • Hypokalaemia and hypocalcaemia
	Cidofovir (5 mg/kg I.V. weekly for 2 weeks then biweekly for 2–3 more doses). Patient should be well hydrated during treatment	
Influenza	Amantadine (200 mg/day orally for 5–7 days)	• Depression • CHF • Nausea, vomiting • CNS toxicity
California encephalitis virus	I.V. ribavirin (15–25 mg/kg/day in 8 hourly divided dosage)	• Haemolytic anaemia

• *Monitoring* of BP and ICP (intracranial pressure).
• *Care of unconscious patient*, i.e. is change of posture, skin care, care of indwelling catherer etc.

2. **Specific antiviral treatment:** The details of chemotherapy available for some viral encephalitis is given in Box 2. The recommended empirical treatment of suspected herpes simplex encephalitis (HSE) is intravenous acyclovir in a dose of 10 mg/kg infused slowly over one hour, then after every 8 hours for 2–3 weeks. Adequate hydration must be maintained. The complications of the therapy include: (i) rise in blood urea, hence, its dose should be adjusted in renal insufficiency, (ii) thrombocytopenia, GI toxicity (lethargy, confusion, agitation, tremors, hallucinations, seizures). Care should be taken to avoid extravasation of the drug as it can lead to phlebitis. Both ganciclovir and foscarnet are also effective in CMV related CNS infection (Box 2). and cidofovir is an alternative drug. Interferon-α has been found effective in a trial on Japanese B encephalitides but is not a recommended treatment.

Note: The efficacy of oral antiviral drugs in encephalitis has not been proved.

Response to acyclovir in HSE: According to recent reports, a diffusion-weighted MRI (DW-MRI) can be used to follow the effect of acyclovir. The increased signal intensities seen in HSE seem to disappear with effective treatment despite persistent abnormal signals detected on conventional T_2-weighted images.

Sequelae

• Cognitive impairment
• Weakness/paresis/paralysis (hemiparisis)
• Movements disorders e.g. tremors, myoclonus, parkinsonism.
• Seizures
• Ataxic disorders

Acute Transverse Myelitis | **53**

ACUTE TRANSVERSE MYELITIS

Definition

Transverse myelitis is an acute or subacute monophasic inflammation of the spinal cord over a variable number of segments. It presents with acute onset paraplegia or quadriplegia with sensory deficit and sphincter paralysis.

Causes

It results from an autoimmune response triggered by infection and not from direct infection of the spinal cord. It can be due to demyelinating disorders, neuromyelitis optica, postinfectious, sarcoidosis and systemic autoimmune diseases. The causes are given in Box 1.

Clinical Features

Patient may be of any age, presents with acute onset of neck or back pain followed by paraplegia or quadriplegia with a variable combinations of paraesthesias, sensory loss, motor weakness and sphincter disturbances, evolving within hours to several days. The sensory symptoms precede the motor symptoms. Sensory symptoms may be mild only or there may be a devastating functional transection of the cord. Paraesthesias may begin in one lower limb (starting from the foot) followed by other limb and ascend symmetrically or asymmetrically to the trunk where transverse involvement of the cord produces a sharp girdle like pain (a band of constriction around the abdomen or trunk) with a sharply defined spinal cord level indicating the myelopathic nature of the process—this feature differentiates it from acute Guillain-Barré syndrome.

Sensory symptoms are followed by motor system involvement with upper motor neuron signs (exagerated deep reflexes). In severe cases, the deep tendon jerks or reflexes may be absent due to spinal neuronal shock, but persistence of areflexia over few segments of spinal cord indicates acute necrotic myelitis.

Physical Signs (Figs 53.1 and 53.2)

A. *Signs below the level of cord involvement*

1. *Upper motor neuron type of paralysis* (paraplegia or quadriplegia) with hypertonia, hyperreflexia and bilateral extensor plantar response below the level of lesion. This is due to interruption of descending corticospinal tracts. Areflexia with bilateral plantar extensor response indicate **spinal shock**, seen in severe cases. Deep tendon jerks may be variable, i.e. normal to exaggerations.

2. *Sensory loss:* There will be a variable degree of sensory loss below the level of the lesion due to interruption of

Box 1	Causes of acute transverse myelitis

A. Viral infection
- Poliomyelitis
- Postpoliomyelitis syndrome
- Acute encephalomyelitis (viral)
- Herpes zoster, HSV type 2
- Rabies, EBV and CMV
- HTLV-1
- AIDS-related myelitis

B. Bacterial infection
- Acute suppurative myelitis with spinal abscess
- Tubercular myelitis
- Symphilitic myelitis

C. Lyme disease
- Fungal—rare

D. Parasitic, e.g. cysticercosis, schistosomiasis, malaria

E. Postinfectious (measles, mumps influenza, myco-plasma CMV and EBV) and postvaccinal myelitis (tetanus, smallpox, rabies, poliomyelitis)

F. Demylinating disorders
- Multiple sclerosis
- Neuromyelitis optica
- Acute disseminated encephalomyelitis

G. Paraneoplastic (non-metastatic manifestation of malignancy)

H. Toxic
- Contrast media
- Intrathecal injections
- Triorthocresyl phosphate toxicity

I. Immune mediated
- SLE, MCTD and vasculitic syndrome
- Neurosarcoidosis

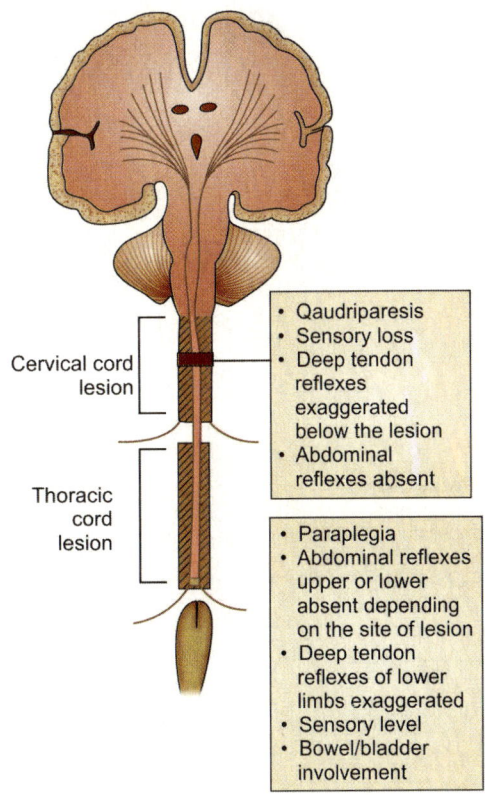

Fig. 53.1: Pattern of motor and sensory loss in transverse myelitis at cervical and thoracic level

ascending spinothalamic and posterior column sensory tracts.

3. *Bladder and bowel disturbances:* Incomplete lesion of the spinal cord affects the inhibitory fibres of the sympathetic system leading to difficulty in holding the urine (*precipitate micturition*), can also interfere with the descending fibres for voluntary control of micturition from cerebral cortex causing retention of urine or *hesitancy* of micturition. Retention of urine can also occur due to spinal shock.

> *Hesitancy or retention of urine is a common bladder disturbance in acute transverse myelitis.*

4. *Impairment of sweating or vasomotor control* below the level of the lesion due to interruption of autonomic fibres.

B. *Signs at the level of cord involvement*
1. *Root pain and root anaesthesia* at the level of the lesion due to nerve root irritation/compression.
2. *Segmental lower motor neuron* signs (a reflex level). There may be fasciculations, wasting or areflexia involving few segments due to interruption of reflex arc or damage to the anterior horn cells.

> **Note:** Acute transverse myelitis is an inflammatory lesion which is not uniformly distributed process, hence partial or incomplete cord lesions are common which tend to produce less severe or partial deficit depending on the tracts involved.

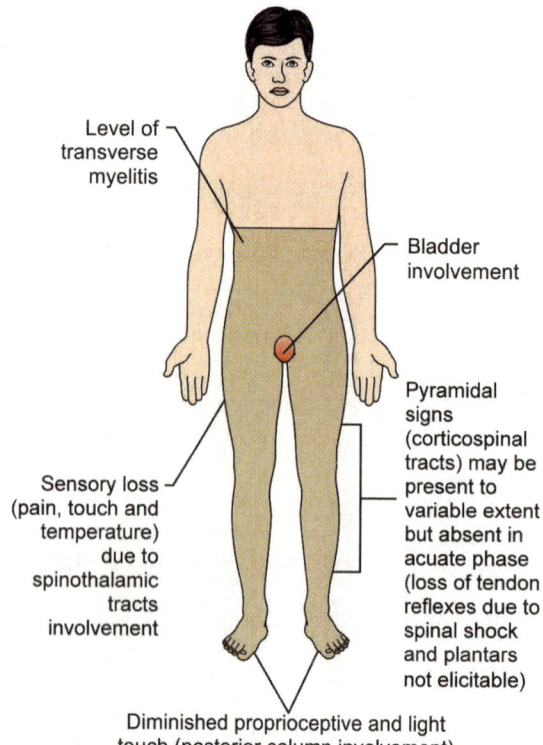

Level of transverse myelitis

Bladder involvement

Pyramidal signs (corticospinal tracts) may be present to variable extent but absent in acuate phase (loss of tendon reflexes due to spinal shock and plantars not elicitable)

Sensory loss (pain, touch and temperature) due to spinothalamic tracts involvement

Diminished proprioceptive and light touch (posterior column involvement)

Fig. 53.2: Clinical manifestations of acute transverse myelitis

Spinal shock: It occurs due to acute neuronal injury leading to loss of reflex activity below the site of the lesion. It has to be differentiated from LMN type of paralysis. Flaccid paralysis below the level of the lesion along with sensory loss and urinary/fecal retention with bilateral plantar extensor response indicate spinal shock due to acute spinal cord injury rather than a LMN type of paralysis. Spinal shock may persist for 1–6 weeks, hence, acute paraplegia due to transverse myelitis may be misdiagnosed as Guillain-Barré syndrome or acute severe peripheral neuropathy but so extensive global sensory loss with bladder dysfunction are rare in a GB syndrome.

Localisation of the lesion in transverse myelitis. It is tabulated in Table 53.1.

Investigations

The purpose of the investigations is to determine the site and the nature of the lesion.
1. **TLC, DLC** may show lymphocytosis. ESR may be raised.
2. **X-ray** chest to rule out tuberculosis or malignancy lung in patients suspected to

Table 53.1 Localisation of spinal cord level in transverse myelitis (Fig. 53.1)	
Cervical cord (Quadriplegia)	*Thoracic cord (Paraplegia)*
• *High cervical cord lesions (C₁–C₄)* are characterised by UMN type of quadriparesis with or without respiratory muscles or diaphragmatic paralysis. Patient may complain of suboccipital pain radiating to neck and shoulder.	• *Lesion above T₆* produces paraplegia with exaggrated deep tendon jerks and loss of abdominal reflexes. The upper most level of the lesion is decided by sensory loss over the chest.
• *Lesions of C₄–C₅* produces UMN type of quadriparesis with preserved respiratory function.	• *Lesions of mid thoracic cord (T₆–T₉)* produces loss of upper abdominal reflexes. The umbilicus is pulled downwards due to contraction of lower abdominal muscles. There is UMN type of paraplegia (deep jerks are variable or brisk)
• *Lesion of C₅–C₆* causes quadriplegia with loss of biceps and supinator jerks while other jerks (triceps and lower limbs) are exaggerated and abdominal reflexes are lost.	
• *Lesion of C₇* produces quadriparesis with loss of triceps jerks, normal biceps and supinators; and exaggerated lower limb jerks and loss of abdominal reflxes	• *Lesions at T₉–T₁₀* produces paraplegia with loss of lower abdominal reflexes with preserved upper abdominal reflexes. There is upward movement of umbilicus due to contraction of upper abdominal muscles. There is UMN paraplegia.
• *Lesions of C₈* causes loss of finger flexion with exaggeration of deep tenden jerks in the lower limbs. Other upper limb tendon reflexes are normal. Abdominal reflexes are lost.	

Note: Motor signs not the sensory level decide the site of the lesion. Lesion may not be exactly localised, may extend over few segments in acute transverse myelitis.

be having tubercular myelitis or paraneo-plastic syndrome.

3. **X-ray spine** (dorsal/lumbosacral) may show an evidence of tubercular osteitis if acute tubercular myelitis is suspected, otherwise X-ray spines are noncontributory.

4. **MRI:** It is an ideal investigation for detecting areas of demyelination, diagnosing myelitis or cord swelling due to inflammatory or toxic myelopathies. MRI distinguishes myelitis from other causes of compressive myelopathy.

5. **CSF examination:** Ideally an MRI scan should precede lumbar puncture to rule out compressive myelopathy (spinal cord compression). The CSF findings in myelitis may be normal or may show rise in CSF proteins with mononuclear cells. Initially there may be polymorphonuclear pleocytosis. The oligoclonal banding is a variable finding; when present, is associated with future evolution of multiple sclerosis.

6. **Visual evoked potential:** There may be accompanying optic neuritis if myelitis is suspected to be a part of demyelinating disease (Devic's disease).

Management

1. **General measures**
   - *Care of the skin:* Proper cleanliness and frequent change of position every 2–3 hourly is necessary to prevent bedsores.
   - *Care of bowel and bladder:* Initially use a condom catheter drainage in man or a permanent indwelling catheter in either sex. Bowel is evacuated either by glycerine suppository or manually.
   - *Care of respiration:* High cervical cord lesions of acute ascending transverse myelitis may cause varied degree of respiratory failure requiring artificial ventilation. Patient should be daily followed for respiratory movements; if there is suspicion of impending respiratory paralysis, the patient may be shifted to respiratory intensive care unit. In the meantime, endotracheal intubation may be done. Continuous suction is necessary.
   - *Care of the joints and limbs:* The paralysed limbs must be passively moved daily to prevent contractures.
   - *Prevention of deep vein thrombosis* by calf compression devices.
   - *Adequate fluid and hydration.*
   - *Psychological support* to keep up the morale of the patient by explaining the reversible nature of the disease.

2. **Specific therapy**
   - *Find out the cause and treat it accordingly.* In a large number of cases, no cause is found out. For herpes zoster, HSV and EBV myelitis, use acyclovir (10 mg/kg tid for 10–14 days) or oral valacyclovir 2 g tid for 10–14 days. For CMV myelitis, ganciclovir (5 mg/kg I.V. bid) plus foscarnet (60 mg/kg I.V. tid) or cidofovir (5 mg/kg/week for 2 weeks) may be used.
   - *High-dose corticosteroids* (1 mg/kg/day) for 2 weeks then taper off the dose. High dose methylprednisolone is effective. The steroids are useful in postinfectious, postvaccinal and demyelinating type of acute transverse myelitis. Preliminary data recommend azathioprine, mycophenolate or anti-CD20 for neuromyelitis optica.

Acute Spinal Cord Compression

Definition

The spinal cord is nothing but tubular extension of medulla oblongata starting at C_1 level (its junction with medulla) and ends at the vertebral body of L_1 (the conus medullaris) and is enclosed in a bony spinal canal. The spinal cord may be compressed by expansion from within (cord disease) or compressed from outside by the diseases of vertebral body and surrounding meninges. The clinical presentation is *paraplegia* or *quadriplegia*.

Acute spinal cord compression is one of the most common neurological emergencies encountered in clinical practice, emergency investigations and surgical intervention is done if needed.

Causes

The clinical expression of cervical cord compression is spastic quadriplegia and that of thoracic cord compression is *spastic paraplegia*. The causes of acute spinal cord compression (acute compressive myelopathy) are given in Table 54.1. A space occupying lesion within the spinal canal may damage the nervous tissue either directly by expanding inside pressure or indirectly by interfering with blood supply (vasculopathy) or oedema from venous obstruction. The early stages of the spinal cord damage before neuronal death is reversible, hence, early diagnosis and treatment is essential.

Table 54.1 Causes of spinal cord compression

1. **Extradural compression** (involvement of vertebral bodies and intervertebral disc). It comprises 80% cases of compression
   A. Vertebral bodies
      - Trauma (fracture dislocation), whiplash injury
      - Metastatic carcinoma (e.g. breast, bronchus, prostate, lymphoma, thyroid)
      - Myeloma
      - Tuberculosis
   B. Disc lesion
      - Intervertebral disc prolapse (degenerative)
      - Trauma
   C. Inflammatory
      - Epidural abscess
      - Cold abscess
      - Granuloma
      - Arachnoiditis
   D. Epidural haemorrhage
2. **Intradural extramedullary compression:** It constitutes 15% cases of compression
   - Tumours, e.g. meningioma, neurofibroma, ependymoma, metastasis, lymphoma, leukaemia
   - Subdural abscess
3. **Intradural intramedullary:** It constitutes 5% of the cases
   - Tumours, e.g. glioma, ependymoma, metastasis
   - Haematomyelia

Clinical Features

Symptoms of Spinal Cord Compression

The onset of symptoms of spinal cord compression are usually slow evolving over days and weeks but can be **acute** as a result of trauma or metastases, especially if there is associated arterial occlusion (ischaemic myelopathy). Symptoms are given in Box 1.

Pain and sensory symptoms appear early; while motor symptoms and sphincter disturbance appear late.

Signs of Cord Compression

The signs vary according to the site of compression and the structures involved. There may be tender-ness over the spine if there is vertebral disease, and this may be associated with local kyphosis.

The signs of spinal cord compression are given in Box 2 and diagrammatically represented in Figs 54.1 and 54.2. Total cord transaction results in immediate flaccid paralysis and loss of sensation below the level of lesion and spinal shock.

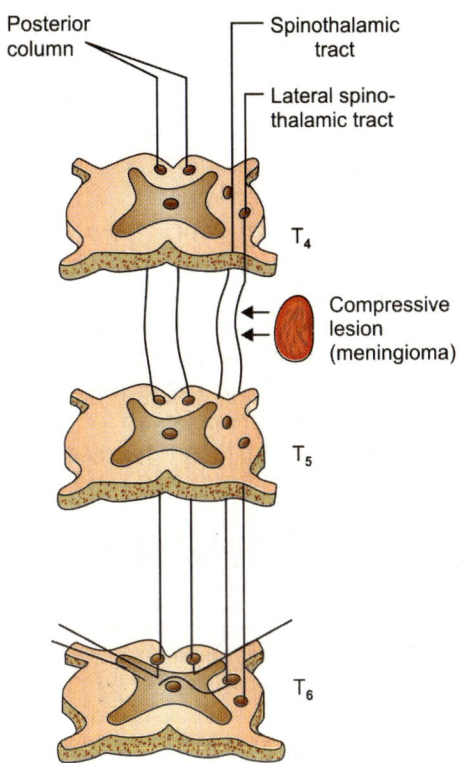

Fig. 54.2: Diagrammatic representation of the tracts compressed by meningioma (indicated by double arrows) in between T_4 and T_5 segments

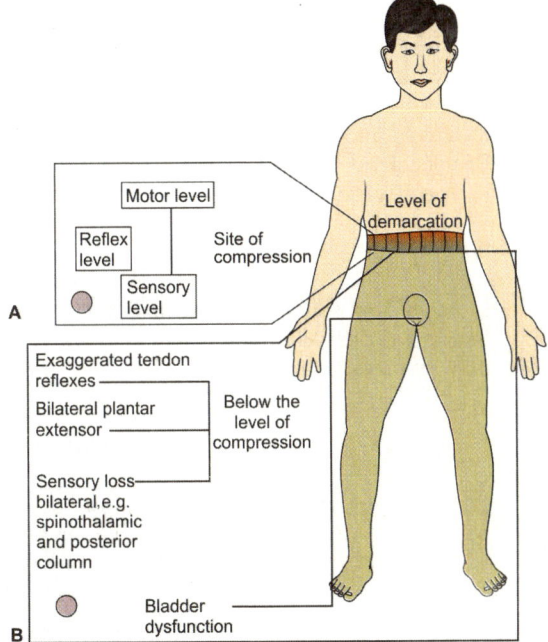

Fig. 54.1: Spinal cord compression showing signs. (A) At the level and (B) below the level of compression. A level or demarcation is must between normal and abnormal signs in spinal cord compression

Box 1   Symptoms of spinal cord compression

1. *Pain:* It may be localised over the spine or may be in the form of radicular pain that increases with sneezing, coughing, bending and straining
2. *Sensory:* Paraesthesias, numbness or cold extremities especially the lower limbs, which spreads proximally symmetrically or asymmetrically towards the site of compression. Over days and week, a sharply demarked spinal cord level of sensory loss indicate myelopathic nature of the lesion
3. *Motor:* Weakness, heaviness or stiffness of limbs most commonly of the legs in paraplegia and all the four limbs in quadriplegia
4. *Sphincters:* Urgency or hesitancy of micturition leading to acute retention of urine in severe compression

Spinal shock: Acute spinal cord injury may produce depression of the reflex activity resulting in areflexia and retention of urine and faeces—a state called *spinal shock*. It may last for days to weeks, hence, may mimic LMN type of paralysis of Guillain-Barré syndrome from which it has to be differentiated. It is however rare for Guillain-Barré syndrome to produce a total and global loss of sensory function below a given level.

As stage of spinal shock passes off, the reflexes return to exaggerated level and plantars become bilateral extensors leading to spastic paraplegia or quadriplegia. The bladder and bowel function also return. As spasticity increases, flexor or extensor spasms (or both) result in paraplegia-in-flexon or paraplegia-in-extension. With lesser degrees of injury spastic paraplagia or quadriplegia with limb weakness, distal sensory disturbance or both with sphincter disturbance (urinary urgency or incontinence occurs).

Comrepressive myelopathy due to intramedullary or extramedullary pathology produces different clinical syndromes (Table 54.2). A central cord lesion may lead to LMN deficit and loss of pain and temperature with preservation of posterior coherent funtions.

Specific Localisation of the Lesion

When there are UMN signs in the lower limbs or in all four limbs with sensory loss, then one has to decide about the site of the lesion (Table 54.3).

Table 54.2 Differences between extramedullary and intramedullary compression

Feature	Extramedullary compression	Intramedullary compression
Type of compression	Compression is from outside, symptoms arise due to pressure effects on roots and spinal cord	Compression is from within due to expansion of the lesion, symptoms arise due to compression of grey matter and white matter directly or by their destruction
Extent of involvement	Involves few segments, produces focal signs	Involve multiple segments and may even involve the whole cord producing widespread signs
Root pain	Root pain is a characteristic feature	Poor localised burning pain instead of root pain
Sacral sensory loss with spastic paralysis	Early	No sacral sensory loss (sacral sparing)
Bowel and bladder involvement	Late	Early
Dissociated sensory loss	Absent	Dissociated sensory loss present, characteristically seen in syringomyelia
Spinal deformity	Visible, palpable or radiographic evidence of vertebral destruction, e.g. cold abscess or 'gibbus'	Bony changes are unusual
Radiological findings • Plain X-ray spine	• Erosion of the pedicles (an early sign of neurofibroma) • Reduction of intervertebral space is characteristic of Pott's disease • Preservation of intervertebral space is diagnostic of secondaries	No change in the bones
• CT myelogram	• A classic 'meniscus sign' in intradural compression (tumours) • A 'brush border sign' is characteristic of extradural compression (tumours)	'Expansion sign' is diagnostic of syringomyelia

Box 2 Signs of spinal cord compression

1. **Signs at the site of compression: Involvement of the roots at the level of compression produces:**
   i. Dermatomal sensory loss due to nerve root compression.
   ii. Segmental lower motor neuron signs i.e. loss of a reflex, fasciculations, and wasting due to interruption of a reflex arc or damage to anterior horn cells.

2. **Signs below the level of compression:**
   A. *UMN type of motor paralysis* (due to involvement of pyramidal tracts)
      • Hypertonia (spastic paraplegia/quadriplegia)
      • Hyper-reflexia (deep tendon jerks are exaggerated)
      • Loss of superficial reflexes (abdominal, cremasteric)
      • Bilateral plantars extensor response
   B. *Sensory signs*
      • Loss of superficial sensations, e.g. pain, touch and temperature due to interruption of spinothalamic tracts
      • Loss of posterior column sensations (e.g. position, vibration and joint sense)
      • Bladder dysfunction, e.g. distension of the urinary bladder

Note: Partial or incomplete cord lesions tend to produce less severe or partial neurological deficit involving posterior columns or spinothalamic tract.

Investigations

The purpose of investigations is to establish the site and the nature of the lesion. These are:

1. **TLC and DLC for infective lesion:** The ESR is raised in infective pathology especially tuberculosis.
2. **X-ray chest:** It is done to rule out tuberculosis or bronchogenic carcinoma in patients suspected with Pott's disease or metastases.
3. **X-ray spine (AP and lateral):** X-rays of spine (cervical, thoracic, lumbosacral) are done to find out the vertebral fracture/collapse in patients with injury, disc prolapse (in old patients), bony erosions (seen in metastases) or evidence of tubercular osteitis.

4. **MRI spine:** It is a special tool to differentiate compressive from noncompressive myelopathy, defines the spinal lesion clearly and helps to plan emergency treatment if needed. It has replaced CT and myelography in the diagnosis of spinal cord masses and can differentiate malignant lesions from other masses.
5. **CT myelography:** It localises the lesion, helps to differentiate extramedullary and intramedullary compression and defines the extent of compression. It has been super seded by MRI.
6. **CSF examination:** The CSF should not be done except at the time of myelography. In cases of complete spinal block, CSF shows a normal cell count with a markedly elevated proteins producing yellow discoloration of the fluid (Froin's syndrome). Acute deterioration may develop after myelography for which it is essential to alert the neuro-surgeon in advance.
7. **Needle biopsy of the tumour** may be required before radiotherapy to establish the histological diagnosis.

Differential Diagnosis

The conditions producing acute paraplegia are briefly discussed individually:

1. **Traumatic myelopathy:** Acute trauma may cause cord compression or angular deformity of the cord by fracture/dislocation of cervical or thoracic spine, is commonly associated with spinal neuronal shock. In less severe injury, signs and symptoms of extradural compression will appear. CT scan confirms the diagnosis of bony lesion; while MRI may be done for detecting damage to the discs, ligaments and pre or paravertebral tissue.
2. **Nontraumatic spinal cord compression:** It may include infection of bone, subdural or epidural space, disc prolapse, neoplastic compression, epidural hematoma etc.
   i. *Infection:* Acute infection of subdural or epidural space' results in an abscess formation, may or may not

be associated with osteomyelitis. Pyogenic osteomyelitis (due to staphylococci, streptococci, *E. coli*, salmonella, etc.) is common in the West while tubercular osteitis is common in Asia and Africa. Risk factors include depressed immunity, I.V. drug abuser and infection of skin and or other tissues. Epidural abscess is characterised by fever, roots pain, spinal tenderness and other signs of infection followed by paraplegia or quadriplegia within

Table 54.3 Specific sites of the lesion with corresponding signs and symptoms

Site	Motor symptom/signs	Sensory symptoms/signs	Horner's syndrome
At or Above C_4 level	• UMNs signs in all four limbs (spastic quadriplegia) • Paradoxical respiratory movement if diaphgram (C4) is involved	• Sensory loss of all modalities over all four limbs	• May be present
Mid-cervical $(C_5–C_6)$	• Loss of biceps and supinator jerks, LMN paralysis (muscle wasting) involving muscle supplied these roots, e.g. C_5 and C_6 etc. • UMN paralysis below the site of compression, e.g. exaggerated triceps, finger flexion and other tendon jerks of lower limbs	• Segmental sensory loss over the arms	• May be present
Lower cervical $(C_7–C_8)$	• Normal biceps and supinator jerks • Triceps jerks are lost • UMNs signs in lower limbs (spastic paraplegia)	• Segmental sensory loss over arms and forearms	• May be present
Thoracic cord (above T_6)	• Spastic paraplegia • Loss of abdominal reflexes	• Sensory level over the chest	• Absent
Mid-thoracic $(T_6–T_9)$	• Spastic paraplegia • Loss of upper abdominal reflexes • Umbilicus is pulled downwords	• Sensory loss over abdomen	• Absent
Lower thoracic $(T_9–T_{12})$	• Spastic paraplegia • Preservation of upper abdominal and loss of lower abdominal reflexes • Umbilicus may be pulled upwards (Beevor's sign positive)	• Sensory loss over abdomen below umbilicus	• Absent
Upper lumbar $(L_2–L_4)$	• Paralysis of flexors and adductors of thighs • Weakness of leg extension • Loss of cremasteric and patellar reflexes	• Sensory loss over front of leg	• Absent
Lower lumbar $(L_5$ and $S_1)$	• Paralysis of movements of foot and plantar flexion • Plantar reflex is not elicitable • Loss of ankle jerk	• Over the calf	• Absent
Conus medularis lesion (cord plus cauda equina lesion)	• Only bilateral plantars extensor • LMN paraplegia	• Sacral loss of sensation	• Absent

few days. The abscess is common cause of compression in young. Tubercular osteitis on the other hand, has protracted illness with slow onset of paraplegia. X-ray spine will reveal an erosion, destruction of intervertebral disc and reduction of the disc space. MRI is investigation of choice. It will differentiate epidural from subdural abscess and will delineate the associated myelitis.

ii. *Prolapse of intervertebral disc:* It is a common cause of acute spinal cord compression in old age. Acute disc prolapse due to degenerative disease of the spine is more common in lumbosacral region (L_{4-5} and L_5S_1) and may cause paralysis of groups of muscles supplied by them and loss of ankle jerk (Table 54.3) but central disc protrusion at this site will compress cauda equina leading to cauda equina syndrome characterised by:

- Root pain in the legs.
- Loss of sensation over sacral dermatomes (perineum and anal region).
- Loss of bladder or anal sphincter control.

iii. *Compression of cord by tumours or metastases:* Secondaries from bronchus, breast, GI tract, prostate, kidney, etc. may metastasise in the vertebral body or spine leading to acute cord compression. The common site of involvement is thoracic region. The compression is acute or subacute in onset progresses over days to weeks. Acute cord compression occurs either due to sudden enlargement of tumour or haemorrhage into the tumour or due to sudden collapse of infiltrated vertebral body.

X-ray spine (AP and lateral) will show destruction of vertebral body or bodies with preservation of intervertebral space. CT scan/ MRI localise the lesion and define its extent.

Other tests (chest X-ray, USG abdomen) may be done to find out the primary lesion.

The primary tumours, i.e. meningioma or neurofibroma produces intradural extramedullary compression (read extramedullary compression).

Epidural hematoma: It is an uncommon but a recognised cause of extradural compression due to bleeding in the patients receiving anticoagulants or suffering from a bleeding disorder or arteriovenous malformations. Bleeding following lumbar puncture is rare cause of compression. The clinical picture is of radiculomyelopathy characterised by roots pain and paraparesis.

Management

1. **General measures:** All the general measures such as *care of skin*, *bowel and bladder*, *prevention of deep vein thrombosis* by leg exercises, *psychological support* discussed in the management of transverse myelitis are applicable here also.

2. **Specific therapy:** Nature of specific treatment depends on the underlying cause:

    i. *Traumatic paraplegia:*
    - Immobilisation and spinal traction for vertebral dislocation
    - Surgery for spine.
    - Urgent surgical decompression (laminectomy).
    - High dose methylprednisone (30 mg/kg I.V. bolus, then 5.4 mg/ kg/hr for 24 hours) if given within 8 hours of injury improves motor-sensory function in the long run.

    ii. *Nontraumatic spinal cord compression:*
    - Appropriate or broad spectrum antibiotic therapy for pyogenic infection such as acute epidural abscess.
    - Laminectomy with debridement for decompression of cord. Surgical evacuation prevents paralysis or reverse paralysis in evolution.
    - ATT for tuberculosis of the spine.
    - Vascular surgery (ligation of a feeding vessel, excision of AVM).

iii. *For neoplastic extramedullary spinal cord compression:*
   - Glucocorticoids are given in higher doses (dexamethasone 40 mg/day) to reduce cerebral oedema. The dose is reduced to 20 mg until radiotherapy is completed.
   - Local radiotherapy is initiated as early as possible. Newer techniques including intensity-medullated radiotherapy (IMRT) can deliver high doses with good response.
   - If radiotherapy fails or not tolerated, then surgery (decompression or vertebral body compression) is indicated.

iv. *Intradural tumours (meningioma/neurofibroma) require surgical resection.*

3. **Long term management**
   - *Pain:* Pain at or below the level of neurological lesion is common and sometimes distressing. Most patients responds to rehabilitation and treatment with analgesics, antidepressants or anticonvulsants. Transcutaneous nerve stimulation, acupuncture, hypnotherapy and the relaxation exercises may help. Surgical interruption of pain fibres or tract is unnecessary and not recommended.
   - *Spasticity:* It is treated by regular physiotherapy. It can be relieved by baclofen or dantrolene and in resistant cases by motor point injections, local nerve block and neurectomy.
   - *Sexual function:* In men who cannot otherwise attain erection of penis sufficient for intercourse, intracavernous papaverine, vacuum erection aids and rarely penile implants are useful. In women fertility remains normal, therefore assisted conception technique including seminal fluid enhancement, intrauterine insemination or *in vitro* fertilisation have improved the likelihood of fathering children.

Acute Inflammatory Demyelinating Polyradiculoneuropathy (Guillain-Barrè Syndrome)

Definition

Acute inflammatory demyelinating polyradiculoneuropathy (AIDP) is defined as an immune mediated demyelinating (autoimmune) disorder with an acute onset characterised by a syndrome of rapidly developing flaccid paralysis, areflexia, paraesthesias with minimal sensory loss and albuminocytological dissociation in the CSF (cerebrospinal fluid). It is also popularly known as *Guillain-Barré syndrome* after the name of French neurologist (1916).

Aetiopathogenesis

A history of preceding viral infection such as *Cytomegalovirus (CMV), Epstein-Barr virus (EBV), hepatitis virus* (B and C), *mumps* and *herpes virus* is present in about 50–60% of cases. Other infections (*Campylobacter jejuni*, typhoid, *Mycoplasma*, filarial), vaccination (for rabies, smallpox, oral polio, tetanus toxoid) and events like bee sting, surgery, MI, idiopathic glomerulonephritis and bone marrow transplantation have been implicated.

Campylobacter jejuni shares an identical immunogenic region with the ganglioside GM-I in the human peripheral nerve, and causes more severe form of the disease with axonal degeneration with or without demyelination. Two axonal variants of GB syndrome are: (1) *acute motor axonal neuropathy (AMAN)* and (ii) *acute motor sensory axonal neuropathy (AMSAN)*.

The *Miller-Fischer syndrome*, has close association with anti-GQ-lb antibody and, is specifically associated with ophthalmoplegia, areflexia without weakness and pupillary changes.

Three important pathological changes in AIDP are (i) *inflammation* (ii) *demyelination* and (iii) *remyelination*. In a minority of cases, intense axonal damage and degeneration occurs which does not recover.

Both humoral and cellular immune mechanisms contibute to the tissue damage in AIDP. Macrophages, autoreactive T lymphocytes producing cytokines and interferon-gamma cause damage to myelin sheath by penetrating the Schwann cells. The remaining Schwann cells divide and remyelinate the bare axons.

Classification

A tentative classification of Guillain-Barré syndrome subtypes has been proposed based on the various clinical expressions and different electrophysiological and pathological findings, is given in Box 1.

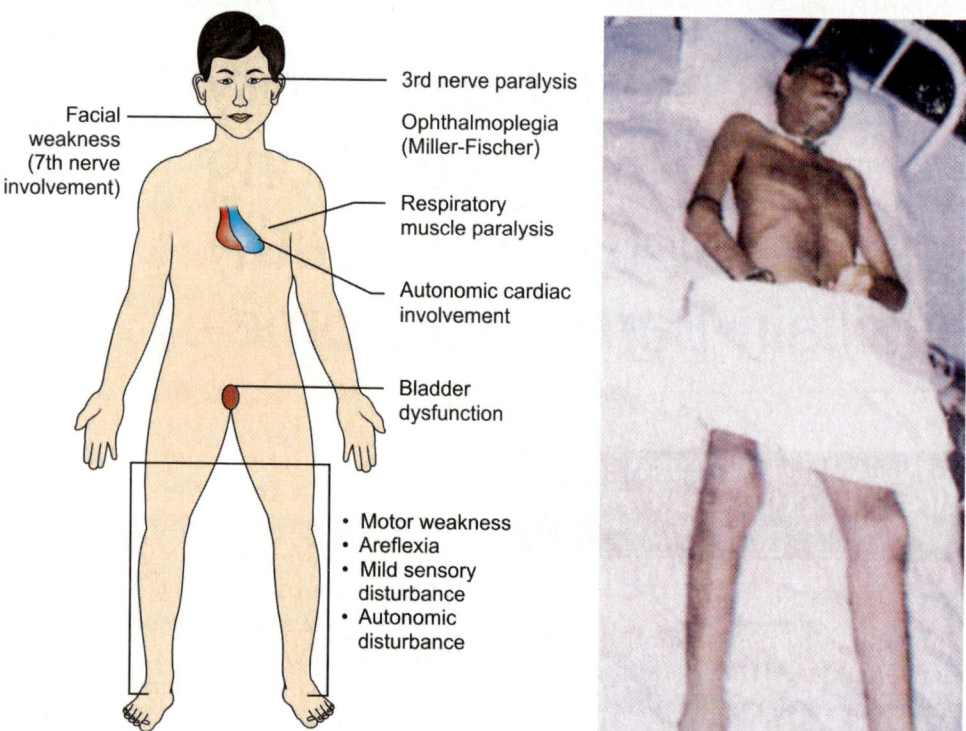

Fig. 55.1 (A): Clinical presentations of Guillain-Barré syndrome **(B)** A patient of Guillain-Barré syndrome with LMN paralysis and bilateral foot drop (feet are not shown)

Clinical Features (Fig. 55.1A and B)

Guillain-Barré syndrome (GBS) or AIDP is a nonseasonal illness, affects persons of all age groups. About two-thirds of patients report on a preceding illness or event such as upper respiratory or GI tract infection, vaccination, surgery 1–4 weeks before the onset of neurological manifestations. The agent responsible for prodromal symptoms remains unidentified. These agents have already been discussed in aetiopathogenesis.

Patients commonly present with acute onset of areflexic motor paralysis with or without sensory disturbance. Weakness begins in the legs and may be ascending (common). In some patients, there may be severe pain in lower extremities and back. The common presentation is symmetrical weakness of the lower limbs that ascends proximally over hours to several days to involve arms, facial and oropharyngeal muscles and in severe cases respiratory muscles. Less often, weakness may start in proximal groups of muscles of the limbs. The cranial nerves muscle, i.e. face (7th nerve), ocular (3rd nerve) and oropharyngeal (bulbar nerves, i.e. 9th, 10th and 12th) may be involved (cranial polyneuritis). Its severity is variable from mild illness (patient is still able to walk unassisted) to quadriplegia. Fever and constitutional symptoms are absent at onset, if present, cast doubt on the diagnosis. The diminution or loss of tendon reflexes (hyporeflexia or areflexia) is a characteristic and invariable feature. Sensory loss is uncommon, but sensory symptoms, i.e. paraesthesias and dysasthesia are common. Occasional patient may develop glove and stocking distribution of sensory loss. Sphincter disturbance may occur. Papilloedema may be present in about 1% of cases.

Autonomic disturbances (Box 2) are also common may be severe and sometimes life

Box 1 Classification of Guillain-Barré syndrome

Subtype	Characteristics
• Acute inflammatory demyelinating • polyradiculoneuropathy (AIDP)	• Demyelinating • Adults affected more than children • Anti-GM antibodies present (>50%) • Recovery rapid
• Acute motor axonal neuropathy (AMAN)	• Axonal damage • Children and young adults affected • Prevalent in China and Mexico • Anti-GDIa antibodies present • Recovery rapid
• Acute motor-sensory axonal neuropathy (AMSAN)	• Axonal damage • Uncommon, adults affected • Closely related to AMAN, recovery slow
• Miller-Fisher syndrome (MFS)	• Demyelinating, uncommon • Affects adults and children • Ophthalmoplegia, ataxia and areflexia occur • Anti GQ-lb antibodies present (>90%)

Box 2 Autonomic dysfunction in GBS

Sympathetic system		Parasympathetic system	
Decreased activity	Increased activity	Decreased activity	Increased activity
• Orthostatic hypotension • Anhidrosis (loss of sweating)	• Hypertension • Tachycardia • Tachyarrhythmias • Diaphoresis	• Urinary retention • G.I. atony • Iridoplegia	• Bradycardia • Heart blocks • Asystole

threatening. The proportion of patients developing respiratory failure and requiring assisted ventilation is about 12–23%.

Bladder dysfunction may occur in severe cases and is transient. If bladder dysfunction is a prominent feature and comes early in the course, then diagnostic possibilities other than GB syndrome should be considered.

By definition, recovery of AIDP or GBS occurs by 1 to 4 weeks of acute illness, if progression continues longer for 4 to 10 weeks; the condition is termed as *subacute inflammatory demyelinating polyradiculoneuropathy* and if progression continues beyond 12 weeks or multiple relapses occur, then it is called *chronic inflammatory demyelinating polyradiculoneuropathy (CIDP)*.

The **ECG changes** can occur due to autonomic dysfunction such as ST-T abnormalities, QRS widening, QT prolongation and heart blocks.

Clinical GBS Variants

- **Miller-Fischer syndrome** (Box 1)
- **Acute pandysautonomia** is characterised by rapid onset sympathetic and parasympathetic failure without somatic sensory and motor involvement although reflexes are lost during the course of illness. These patients develop orthostatic hypotension, dry eyes, anhidrosis, fixed pupils, fixed heart rate and bladder and bowel disturbances.
- **A pure motor variant of GBS** characterised by acute flaccid paralysis without clinical and electrophysiological involvement of sensory nerves have been described. The diagnostic criteria of AIDP or GBS syndrome are given in Table 55.1.
- **Acute motor axonal neuronopathy** (AMAN) and Acute motor sensory axonal neuronopathy (AMSAN) are two clinical severe variants of GBS (Box 1).

Table 55.1 Diagnostic criteria of AIDP or GBS (adapted from Asbury and Coblath)

1. **Features essential for diagnosis**
   - Progressive weakness in both arms and both legs
   - Areflexia
2. **Features supportive of diagnosis**
   - Progression of clinical features over days to 4 weeks
   - Mild or minimal sensory disturbance
   - Cranial nerve involvement (bilateral 7th nerve)
   - Recovery beginning 2–4 weeks after progression
   - Autonomic dysfunction
   - Absence of fever at the onset
   - Elevated CSF proteins with <10 cells/m³
   - Typically electrodiagnostic features
3. **Features making the diagnosis doubtful**
   - Sensory level
   - Asymmetry of signs and symptoms
   - Severe, persistent bowel and bladder disturbance
   - More than 50 cells/m³ of CSF

Investigations

The cerebrospinal fluid (CSF) examination and serial electrophysiological studies are critical for confirming the diagnosis of GB syndrome. Other tests are inconsequential.

1. **CSF examination:** Initially in GBS, the CSF may be normal, then becomes abnormal within 3–5 days on subsequent examinations and shows elevated proteins (100–1000 mg/dl) with normal cell count (*albuminocytological dissociation*). If the CSF cells count is greater than 20 mononuclear cells/m³, one should think of HIV infection, viral transverse myelitis, leukemia, lymphoma, neurosarcoidosis. Transient oligoclonal IgG bands and elevated myelin basic protein levels may be detected in CSF in some patients. In approximately 10% of patients, CSF proteins may remain normal throughout the period of GBS.

2. **Electrophysiological studies:** Abnormalities on electrophysiological studies have been documented in about 90% cases of GB syndrome and reflect multifocal demyelination associated with secondary, axonal degeneration. The *electrophysiological studies*, i.e. nerve conduction (Fig. 55.2) may

reveal increased *distal latency, conduction slowing, conductions block; F wave slowing* and *decreased nerve conduction velocities.* The EMG shows decreased motor unit recruitment. Subsequently, if any amount of axonal degeneration occurs, or AMAN or AMSAN develops, then there is reduced amplitude of motor action potentials, fibrillation potentials appear 2 to 4 weeks after the onset.

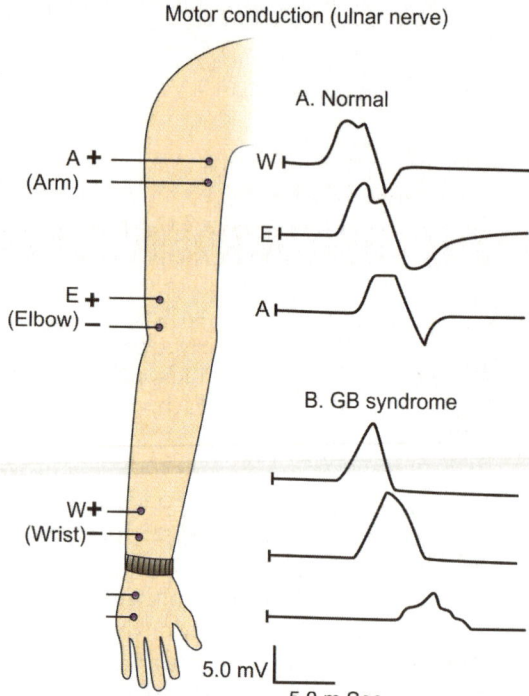

Fig. 55.2: Motor nerve conduction study in ulnar nerve. A. Normal and B. GB syndrome (read text)

Differential Diagnosis

Certain conditions that produce acute or subacute motor weakness simulating GB syndrome are given in Box 3.

Management

Ideally, all patients of GBS should be hospitalised for observation and subsequent management depending on the situation. Patients should preferably be treated in ICU.

Box 3 Clinical conditions simulating GBS
1. Acute peripheral neuropathies
• Porphyrias
• Diphtheria
• Tick paralysis
• Drug toxicity (arsenic, lead, OP compounds)
• Vasculitis
• Lyme's disease
2. Disorders of neuromuscular junction
• Botulism
• Myasthenia gravis
3. Myopathies
• Hypokalaemic periodic paralysis
• Rhabdomyolysis
4. CNS disorder
• Poliomyelitis
• Transverse myelitis
• Basilar artery syndrome

Box 4 Signs of impending respiratory paralysis
1. Signs of respiratory muscle paralysis
• An increase in respiratory rate
• Inability to count up to 20 in one breath
• Use of accessory respiratory muscles
• Suppressed cough
• Paradoxical inwards movements of abdomen during inspirations
2. Signs of impending respiratory paralysis
• Decreasing forced vital capacity
• Declining maximal respiratory pressures
• Hypoxaemia on ABG

1. **Supportive treatment:** Careful observation of cardiopulmonary function, prevention of complications (respiratory and autonomic) in ICU provides best chance for favourable outcome. Respiratory and bulbar functions, the ability to cough, heart rate and BP must be closely monitored in ICU. Look for the signs of respiratory muscle paralysis and impending respiratory failure given in Box 4. Monitor FVC and negative inspiratory pressure every 4 hourly while awake. Rapidly declining FVC ($\leq$15 ml/kg and mean inspiratory fore reaches 40 mmHg) is an indication for intubation and ventilatory support. Continuous suction may be done to remove the secretions to prevent atelectasis. The treatment includes:
   - *BP monitoring* and *frequent ECGs* may allow early detection of life-threatening situations that require prompt treatment.
   - *Nutritional support* to be provided in the form of high caloric protein diet or by beginning enteral feeding as early as possible.
   - If *hypotension* present, use *volume expanders* and *vasopressors*

   - *Subcutaneous heparin or low molecular-weight heparin* together with thromboembolic deterrent stockings may be advised routinely in patients immobilised for more than 2 weeks to lower the risk of thromboembolism.
   - *Culture of secretions,* frequent blood and urine cultures must be done for early detection of infection and prompt treatment.
   - *Chest physiotherapy* and frequent aspiration of the secretions to prevent chest infection and atelectasis.
   - *Care of skin, eyes, mouth, bowel and bladder* is an essential aspect of supportive therapy.
   - *Frequent change of posture* to be done to prevent bedsores. Physical therapy is started early because it prevents contractures, joint immoblisation and venous stasis.

2. **Specific therapy:**
   i. *High dose corticosteroids:* They were earlier recommended for their potent anti-inflammatory and immunosuppressive effects. Based on chemical trials, it is now advocated that steroids play no role in GBS management.
   ii. *Plasmapheresis:* Therapeutic plasmapheresis is recommended for few days for patients with moderate to severe GBS. The schedule entails a series of 5 exchanges (40–50 ml/kg) with a continuous flow machine over a week

Box 5 Complications of plasma exchange and IVig therapy	
Plasma exchange	*Intravenous immunoglobulin*
A. Cardiovascular	• Headache, back pain, myalgias
• Hypotension	• Fever, tachycardia
• Arrhythmias	• Rash, alopecia, eczema
• MI	• Neutropenia, haemolysis
• ARDS	• Aseptic meningitis
B. Complications due to I.V. access	• Immune complex arthritis
• Septicaemia and thrombosis	• Thromboembolism, deep vein thrombosis
C. Allergic reactions	• Transfusion hepatitis
D. Transfusion hepatitis or HIV infection	• Hypotension, acute renal failure (transient)
E. Bleeding, hemolysis and death	• CHF
	• Anaphylaxis

using saline and albumin as replacement fluid. Patients with mild disease may benefit from 2 exchanges on alternate days.

Plasmapheresis removes several factors such as antimyelin antibodies, cytokines, complement components and other inflammatory mediators of GBS.

iii. *Liquorpheresis (CSF filtration):* It is a new technique developed to purify CSF from pathological factors responsible for GBS.

iv. *Intravenous immunoglobulin:* High dose intravenous immunoglobulin (IVIG) has an equivalent benefit similar to plasmapheresis in GBS. Both treatment modalities (plasmapheresis and IVIG) being equally effective, hence, there is no added advantage to use them together. However, IVIG is often initial therapy chosen because of its ease administration and good safety record.

There is some evidence that GBS auto-antibodies are neutralised by anti-idiotypic antibodies present in IVIG accounting for beneficial effect. The dose of IVIG is 400 mg/kg/day for 5 days or 0.5 g/kg/day for 4 days (a total of 2 g/kg of body weight). The complications of both plasma exchange or plasmapheresis and IVIG are given in Box 5.

Prognosis

About 3% of patients with GBS die, mostly due to complications of ventilatory support; but some may die suddenly due to autonomic failure. Those who survive (85%) recover remarkably within several months to a year but all cases do not recover fully, i.e. areflexia may persist. Several survivors fail to achieve the previous level of activity. About 5–10% of cases may have one or more late relapses; such cases are then classified as chronic inflammatory demyelinating polyneuropathy (CIDP).

Cortical Venous and Dural Sinus Thrombosis

CORTICAL VENOUS AND DURAL SINUS THROMBOSIS

Definition

A thrombosis of cerebral (cortical) veins or dural sinus is a common complication of hypercoagulable state (following pregnancy or postpartum period (Fig. 56.1) or local infections (CNS, ear, nasal sinuses, etc.) that leads to focal and/or generalised neurological manifestations.

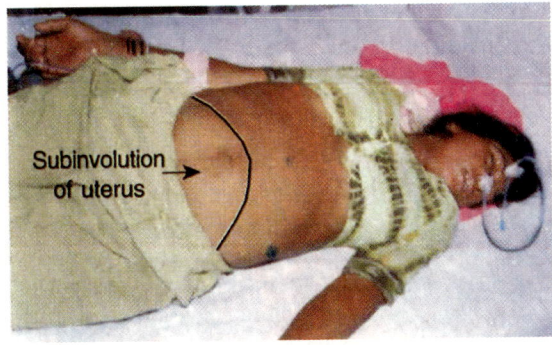

Fig. 56.1: A postpartum female with sagittal sinus thrombosis. She was unconscious, had seizures and plantars were extensors. The subinvolution of uterus is encircled

Causes

The causes may be systemic (general) or local (Box 1). All the conditions which predispose to

Box 1	Causes of cerebral venous thrombosis	
General	*Local*
• Pregnancy and postpartum state	• Sinusitis, mastoiditis, otitis
• Sepsis or septic shock	• Pyogenic meningitis
• Prolonged dehydration or hypotension	• Subdural empyema
• Oral contraceptive use	• Facial skin infection
• Polycythaemia, sickle cell anaemia, leukaemia	• Trauma, e.g. head injury
• Hyperviscosity syndrome	• Jugular vein catheterisation
• Antiphospholipid syndrome, deficiency of proteins C and S	• Skull fracture
• Debilitating states or malignancy	
• Postoperative	
• Cyanotic heart disease	

arterial thrombosis are also applicable here for venous thrombosis.

Clinical Features

Cerebral venous occlusion causes an increase in intracranial pressure and local ischaemia/infarction which is often haemorrhagic. The clinical features are divided into:

1. **Features of sepsis:** Thrombophlebitis of cortical vein or septic thrombosis of dural sinus produces fever, generalised pain, nausea, vomiting and prostration in addition to the localised signs.

2. **Features due to cortical vein thrombosis:** These are focal features depending on the area involved. These include focal cortical deficits (aphasia, hemiplegia etc.), and seizures (focal or generalised). The deficit may increase if spreading thrombophlebitis occurs.

3. **Features of cerebral venous sinus thrombosis:** The clinical features depend on the dual sinus involved (Box 2).

Investigation

1. TLC may show leucocytosis and there may be raised ESR.

2. CSF examination is not performed because it is commonly associated with raised intracranial pressure (ICP). Therefore CT scan should be done before CSF to rule out raised ICP. Otherwise, CSF may show nonspecific changes such as rise in proteins.

3. *D-dimers may be also raised*

4. CT/MRI scan shows haemorrhagic infarction underlying the occluded veins and may show thrombosis in the involved veins and sinuses (Figs 56.2 and 56.3). MR cerebral angiography confirms the diagnosis.

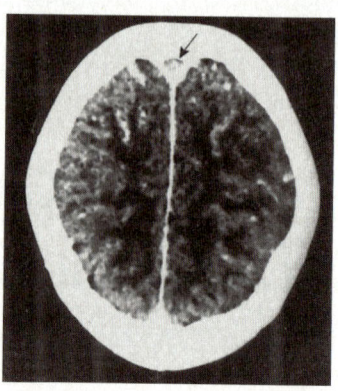

Fig. 56.3: CT scan showing a sagittal sinus thrombus (↓). Note inverse lamda (λ) sign

Box 2	Clinical features of cerebral venous sinus thrombosis
Sinus involved	*Clinical features*
1. *Cavernous sinus thrombosis*	• Chemosis, proptosis, ptosis, headache, ophthalmoplegia (internal and external), papilloedema, retinal haemorrhage and reduced sensation in trigeminal first division. 3rd, 4th and 6th cranial nerves palsy • Involvement is often bilateral, and patient is ill with fever, headache, retro-orbit pain and toxaemia
2. *Superior sagittal sinus (Figs 55.1 to 55.3)*	• Headache, papilloedema, seizures, coma • May involve veins of both hemisphere producing weakness of both legs (paraplegia) or quadriplegia with predominant lower limbs involvement and sensory focal deficits • Fever, neck stiffness or signs of meningitis if associated with bacterial meningitis
3. *Transverse sinus 6th*	• Headache, earache, hemiparesis, convulsions, papilloedema, Gradinego's syndrome (retro-orbital or facial pain, otitis media and 6th cranial nerve palsy)
4. *Jugular foramen or jugular vein*	• Commonly transverse sinus thrombosis spreads to jugular vein; hence its features may be present • 9th, 10th and 11th cranial nerve palsies

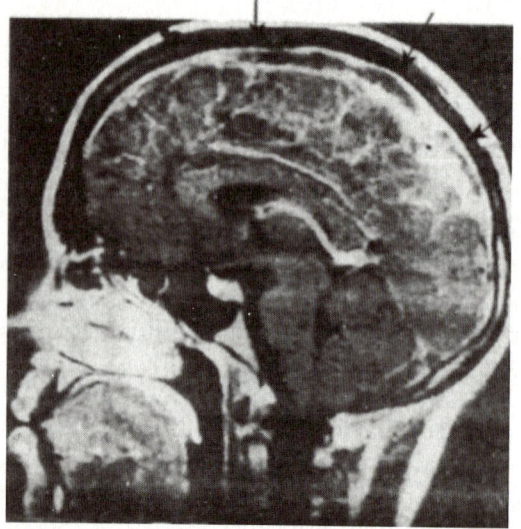

Fig. 56.2: MRI showing a sagittal sinus thrombus (indicated by arrows)

Management

1. **Supportive treatment**
   - Correction of fluid and electrolyte balance to correction dehydration.
   - Care of unconscious patient (coma). The steps have been discussed in the Chapter 44 on coma management.
   - Decongestive therapy (mannitol, glycerol, steroids, dexamethasone 4 mg 4 times a day I.V.) may be used to lower raised intracranial pressure.
   - Antibiotic therapy for infection or sepsis. Antibiotic chosen on the basis of bacteria responsible for the predisposing or associated condition is continued for 4–6 weeks or until there is radiographic resolution of thrombosis.
   - Seizures should be controlled by anti-convulsants.
   - Ventilatory support may be needed.

   - *Gynaecological examination for sepsis and postpartum status:* Retained products of conception if detected should be removed.

2. **Specific therapy with anticoagulants:** Unless there are major contraindication (e.g. septic shock), anticoagulant therapy with low molecular heparin may prove helpful provided haemorrhage is not prominent feature of infarction. Heparin therapy is followed by oral warfarin (2.5–5 mg) for 6 months monitored by INR 2–3 times.

   Successful management of aseptic venous sinus thrombosis has been reported with catheter directed urokinase therapy and with a combination of recombinant tissue plasminogen activator (rtPA) in patients refractory to heparin. Thrombectomy has to be performed sometimes in these cases.

Raised Intracranial Pressure

Definition

The normal CSF pressure measured through-lumbar route with an individual in the lateral decubitus position, ranges from 50 to 200 mm of Hg. The normal circulation of CSF is depicted in Fig. 57.1.

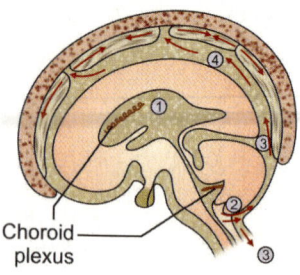

Choroid plexus

Fig. 57.1: Circulation of the CSF. (1) The CSF is synthesized in choroid plexes of the ventricles, and flows from the lateral and third ventricles through an aqueduct to 4th ventricle, (2) through foramina of Lushka and Magendie, it exits the brain flowing over the hemispheres, (3) down around the spinal cord and roots in the subarachnoid space in continuous with cerebral subarachnoid space, (4) it is absorbed into the dural venous sinuses via arachnoid villi

Now-a-days a variety of intracranial pressure (ICP) recording devices implanted in the lateral ventricle, subdural space or extradurally are in use. More recently in traparenchymal placement devices have been introduced which record ICP through an electronic pressure transducer.

This is particularly useful in measuring ICP in severe head injuries with diffuse cerebral oedema and kinked ventricles and subarachnoid spaces. In addition to pulsatile character of ICP three pressure waves are seen. The A waves are pathological and appear only in significantly raised ICP (50–100 mm water). The B and C waves are not considered pathological though these occur with increasing frequency when the ICP is increasing.

> *Normal intracranial pressure within the cranial cavity measured indirectly is 5–10 mmHg. Any ICP above 15 mmHg is taken as raised intracranial pressure.*

Pathophysiology

The volume of the intracranial contents (brain + CSF + blood) is constant regardless of the pressure generated within it.

$$V._{intracranial} = v_{brain} + v_{CSF} + v_{blood} = Constant$$

Any changes in volume of one of its contents occurs at the cost of other two (Monro-Kelly principle). This is not applicable to the pliable skull of infants.

The brain being dependent mainly on oxygen, suffer during hypotension and hypoxia the two major factors for secondary damage to the brain.

Initially when the volume of the intracranial contents increases, there is no increase in CSF pressure due to buffering mechanisms such as shift of CSF and then venous blood flow from the cranial cavity, followed by a minimal compression of the parenchyma. Once the buffering capacity is exhausted, the ICP starts rising. When the expansion of the mass lesion is slow, e.g. a tumour, the compensatory mechanisms can mask the rise in ICP. Fast expanding mass lesions shift the midline structures to opposite side (Fig. 57.2).

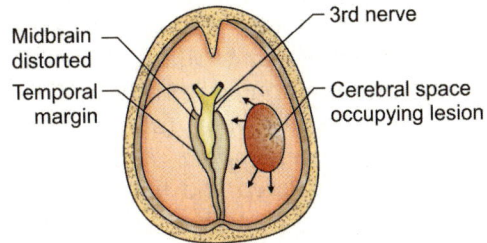

Fig. 57.2: Cerebral space occupying lesion causing displacement of mid line structures (shifting the medial temporal lobe, mid brain and 3rd cranial nerve)

The effects of raised ICP are:
   i. *Herniation syndromes* (Fig. 57.3—read clinical features).
   ii. *Fall in cerebral perfusion pressure.*

Cushing's reflex is a protective mechanism that leads to increase in blood pressure and fall in the pulse rate in an effort to increase cerebral perfusion pressure in patients with raised ICP.

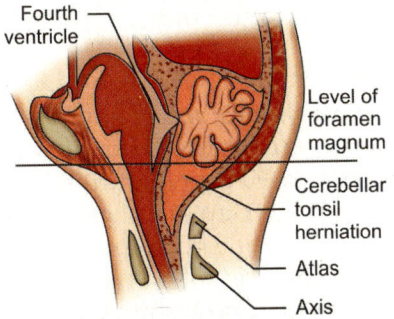

Fig. 57.3: Tonsillar cone (diagram). There is displacement of cerebellar tonsils below the level of foramen magnum due to raised intracranial pressure

Causes

Any lesion which increases the volume (and consequently pressure) of any of the cranial contents will lead to raised ICP. They are:
   i. Cerebral oedema (increased brain parenchymal).
   ii. Space-occupying lesions (extra volume).
   iii. Hydrocephalus (increased CSF volume).

MRI can now differentiate between the two types of cerebral oedema, i.e. vasogenic and cytopathic. The differences are given in Box 1. The causes of raised ICP are given in Table 57.1.

Box 1 Differences between two types of cerebral oedema	
Vasogenic	*Cytopathic*
• Produces focal signs and symptoms due to oedema	• The clinical signs are generalised, non-localising, i.e. convulsions, coma
• Blood brain barrier remains open	• Blood brain barrier is closed
• Activated diffusion coefficeint is increased	• Activated diffusion coefficient is reduced
• MRI shows increased interstitial fluid	• MRI shows swollen cells
• Responds to steroids	• Does not respond to steroids
• It is associated with tumours, haemorrhage, abscess, meningitis, cerebral infarction	• Seen in haemodialysis and ketoacidosis

Clinical Features

1. **Symptoms and signs of raised pressure itself:** The classic triad, i.e. headache, projectile vomiting and papilloedema is seen in majority of the cases with raised ICP. The headache is severe, occurs in early morning and disturbs the sleep of the patient and is generalized. This is due to decreased venous return in supine position leading to CO_2 retention, vasodilatation and increased ICP. Headache is relieved in sitting position due to improved venous return. Vomiting is projectile and often associated with nausea and it relieves the headache. The rising pressure results in

Table 57.1 Causes of raised intracranial pressure

1. **Congenital (obstructive)**
   - Arnold-Chiari malformations
   - Aqueductal stenosis
   - Dandy-Walker syndrome
   - Agenesis of arachnoid villi
2. **Head injury (traumatic)**
3. **Infections**
   - Meningitis (pyogenic, tubercular)
   - Encephalitis
   - Cerebellar abscess
4. **Space-occupying lesions**
   - Brain tumours (craniopharyngioma, medullo blastoma, astrocytoma, ependymoma, metastasis)
   - Colloid cyst of third ventricle
   - Neurocysticercosis
5. **Intracranial haemorrhage**
   - Cerebral haemorrhage
   - Subarachnoid haemorrhage
   - Hypertensive encephalopathy
6. **Venous obstruction**
   - Cortical thrombophlebitis
   - Dural sinus thrombosis
7. **Idiopathic**
   - Otitic hydrocephalus
   - Polycythaemia vera
   - Addison's disease
   - Hypoparathyroidism
   - Oral contraceptives
   - Drugs induced, e.g. tetracycline, penicillin, sulphamethoxazole, nalidixic acid
   - Hypervitaminosis A
   - Galactosaemia
   - Hypophosphatasia

papilloedema which may result in blurring of the vision, secondary optic atrophy and blindness. Severely raised ICP results in apathy, clouding of consciousness progressing to stupor and coma.

2. **Localising symptoms and signs depending on the cause and site of involvement:** Convulsions, paresis/paralysis of the limbs, cranial nerve involvement may occur due to expanding mass lesion which is the cause of raised ICP.

3. **False localising signs:** These signs occur in raised ICP but do not have any localizing value such as:

i. Bilateral plantar extensor response.
ii. Pupillary changes.
iii. Bilateral 6th nerve palsy.
iv. Bilateral mild cerebellar dysfunction.

4. **Herniation syndromes:** Two types of herniation syndrome have been described:

   i. *Central herniation syndrome* includes herniation of central structures (diencephalon and brainstem). When central herniation supervenes, there may be occipital headache with neck stiffness. Respiratory irregularities (Cheyne-Stokes respiration to tachypnoea, to irregular slow respiration), pupillary changes, decorticate posturing and bilateral extensor-plantar response, bradycardia and hypertension may follow. Eventually, apnoea appears and the pupils become dilated and fixed. Hypotension appears and brain death follows shortly after that.

   ii. *Uncus' transtentorial herniation* leads to 'Kernohan's notch' phenomenon and often produces the clinical triad of coma, contralateral decerebration and a dilated ipsilateral pupil. Occasionally posturing or hemiparesis occurs ipsilateral to the side of the herniation, due to pressure on the contralateral cerebral peduncle from the edge of tentorium cereberi. Progression of uncal syndrome caudally leads to central syndrome.

Investigations

1. **X-ray skull** may reveal sutural diastasis (separation of sutures) in infants, thinning and increased convolutional markings (silver-beaten appearance), erosion of anterior clinoid processes, widened and deep sella-turcica.

2. **CT scan of brain** shows dilatation of ventricular system (dilatation of temporal horn is an early sign), effacement of cisterns, an underlying lesion and

periventricular lucency and compression of the ventricle(s).

3. **MRI scan:** It can differentiate between vasogenic and cytopathic cerebral oedema, predicts response to shunts.

4. **Intracranial pressure monitoring (Fig. 56.4).**

Management

1. **Treatment of the underlying cause:** The ideal treatment of raised ICP is to find out the cause and treat it accordingly, for example CSF diversion for hydrocephalus, drainage of an abscess, removal of a clot or a tumour.

2. **Measures to reduce the ICP:** There are some medical and surgical measures to reduce the ICP, which may prove life-saving. Generally any ICP above 25 mmHg needs treatment.

A. *General:*
   - *Intubation and hyperventilation* are used to lower the ICP in patients with coma and unilateral pupillary changes (herniation) until definite treatment can be instituted.
   - *Airway patency* to be ensured and maintained. *Elevate the head* by 30–45°. Avoid neck flexion.
   - Symptomatic treatment with antipyretic, analgesics and anticonvulsants (if convulsions occur).
   - Adequate hydration by fluids. Avoid hypotonic fluids.
   - Catheterisation of bladder to avoid straining.

B. *Medical treatment:* The drugs that reduce the ICP are given in Box 2. Sedation and neuromuscul aparalysis, if necessary (patient will require

Box 2   Drugs used to reduce ICP
1. Mannitol (20%), e.g. 100 ml I.V. 4–6 hourly
2. Glycerol (10%) e.g. 1.2 g/kg over 4 hours
3. *Dexamethasone:* It is used in vasogenic ICP. Dose is 10–20 mg/24 hour in divided doses
4. Frusemid e, e.g. 20–40 mg I. V.

endotracheal intubation and mechanical ventilation).

C. *Surgical methods:*
   - *Ventricular drainage:* Lumbar drainage is indicated as an emergency procedure only in benign raised intracranial hypertension.
   - *Long-term measures* for reduction of elevated ICP involve shunting procedures, i.e. ventriculoperitoneal shunt (Fig. 56.5), lumbar peritoneal shunt, endoscopic third ventriculostomy and endoscopic stent placement in cerebral aqueduct.

D. *Treatment of refractory raised ICP:* High-dose barbiturates, hemicraniectomy or hypothermia are sometimes used for refractory cases of raised ICP.

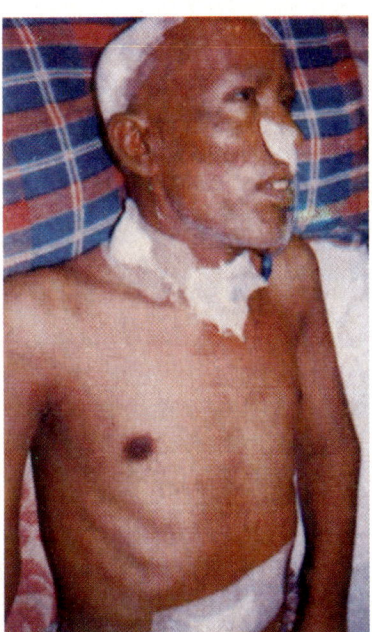

Fig. 57.5: Surgical drainage of hydrocephalus with ventriculoperitoneal shunt

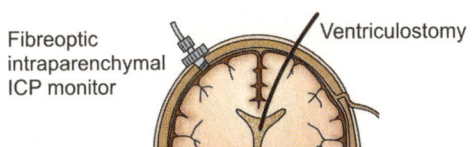

Fig. 57.4: Intracranial pressure monitoring. A ventriculostomy allows the drainage of CSF in patients with raised ICP

Emergencies in Haematology

- Acute Haemolytic Anaemia
- Thrombocytopenia and Immune Thrombocytopenic Purpura
- Thrombotic Thrombocytopenic Purpura (TTP)
- Haemophilia
- Disseminated Intravascular Coagulation (DIC)
- Agranulocytosis or Severe Neutropenia
- Aplastic Anaemia
- Acute Leukaemias
- Blood Transfusion Related Complications

Acute Haemolytic Anaemia

58

Normal lifespan of RBCs is 120 days, after which they are removed from circulation by macrophages of reticuloendothelial system (RES) present in liver, spleen and bone marrow. Normal destruction of RBCs results in release of haemoglobin which splits into *haem* (*iron*) and *globin* fractions. Iron of haem is recycled via transferrin to the marrow for reutilisation; while protoporphyrin is broken down to bilirubin, gets conjugated in the liver and excreted in the gut, where it is converted into stercobilinogen and stercobilin. Most of the stercobilinogen is excreted in the faeces (normal stool colour is due to this pigment) but some of it is partially reabsorbed and excreted as urobilinogen and urobilin in urine (present normally in urine in 1:10 concentration).

Normal serum bilirubin levels are maintained by regular destruction and synthesis of RBCs.

Globin chains are broken down and converted into amino acids which are reutilized for protein synthesis in the body.

> *Normally, there is no intravascular haemolysis*

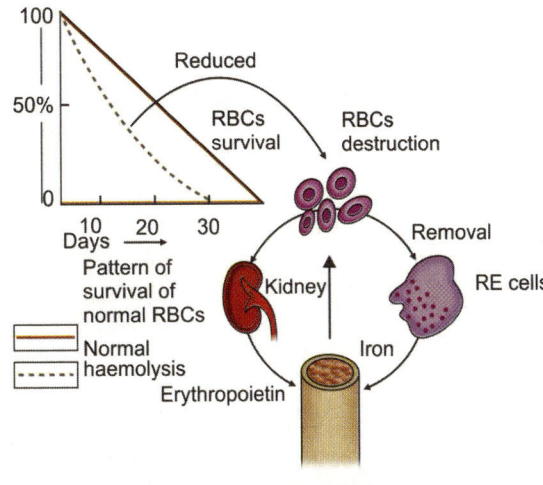

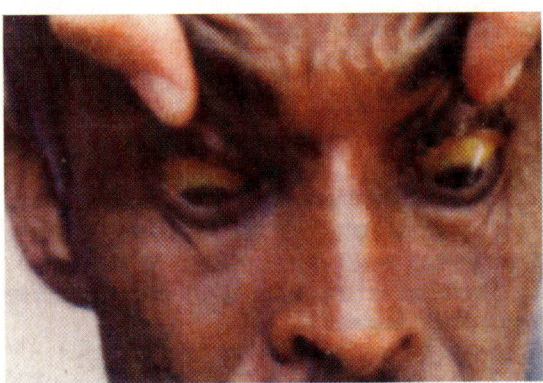

Fig. 58.1: A patient of cerebral malaria with acute haemolytic jaundice

Fig. 58.2: Components of normal erythropoiesis. Accelerated destruction of red blood cells (RBCs) by reticuloendothelial system (RE cells) which is not compensated by erythroid hyperplasia in the bone marrow results in haemolytic anaemia

ACUTE HAEMOLYTIC ANAEMIA

Definition

Anaemia resulting from rapid and increased red cell destruction is known as *haemolytic anaemia* which may be *congenital* or *acquired*. Haemolytic anemias are characterised by features of accelerated red cell destruction and a compensatory erythroid hyperplasia (reticulocytosis is the hallmark). As such the increased red cell production requires an extra amount of folic acid and Vit. B$_{12}$, hence, their deficiency may prove disastrous.

Aetiological Classification

Haemolytic anaemias may be due to intra-corpuscular defect (usually congenital) or extracorpuscular defect (usually acquired). Depending on the clinical presentation, haemolytic anaemia may be acute (usually acquired haemolytic anaemia or congenital G6PD deficiency precipitated by drugs) or chronic (usually congenital). The classification is given in Table 58.1.

Consequences of Haemolysis

Shortening of RBCs survival does not always cause anaemia as there is a compensatory increase in RBCs production in the marrow. Normal marrow has tremendous capacity to become hyperplastic and compensate for haemolysis, hence, anaemia occurs only when this compensation becomes inadequate (Fig. 58.2). The erythroid hyperplasia in the bone marrow is reflected by expansion of active marrow resulting in reticulocytosis (immature red cells) in the peripheral blood, thus, reticulocytosis is a hallmark of haemolysis. The reticulocytes are larger than red cells and stain light blue on a peripheral blood film.

Sites of Haemolysis

1. **Intravascular haemolysis (Fig. 58.3):** When RBCs are rapidly destroyed within circulation, free haemoglobin is released into the plasma. Free haemoglobin is toxic to cells and the body has evolved a binding mechanism so as to minimise its toxicity. Haptoglobin, an alpha globulin produced by the liver is first to bind free haemoglobin to form *haptoglobin-haemoglobin complex* which is too large to be excreted by the kidneys, hence, is degraded by the liver (RE cells). Haptoglobin is used for binding to Hb, hence, its levels are reduced in intravascular haemolysis. Once haptoglobins are saturated, free

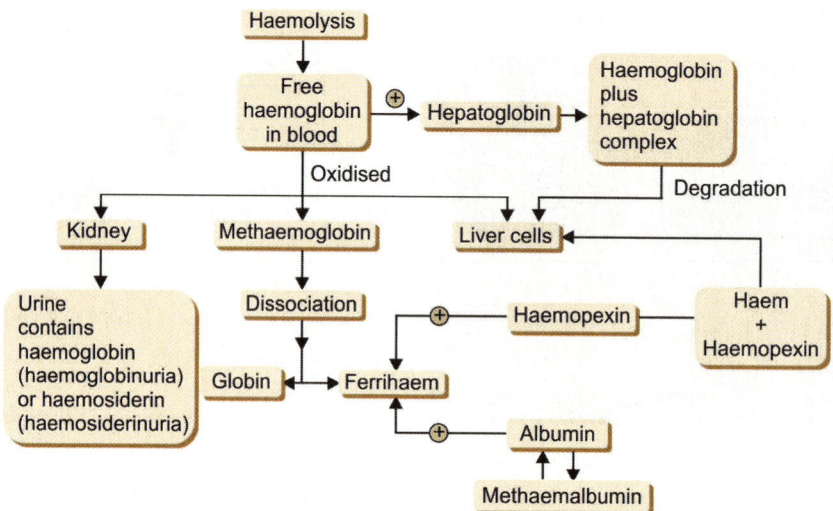

Fig. 58.3: The fate of haemoglobin in plasma during haemolysis

Table 58.1 Aetiological classification of haemolytic anaemia

Intracorpuscular defects

1. Abnormalities of RBC interior

a. Enzymatic defect
- Associated with pentose-phosphate pathway deficiency, i.e. G6PD deficiency and others
- Associated with Embeden-Meyerhof pathway deficiencies, i.e. pyruvate kinase deficiency and others

b. Haemoglobinopathies
- Thalassaemia syndrome
- Sickle cell anaemia (Hb-S)
- Other abnormal haemoglobin (Hb-C, Hb-E, Hb-D)
- Unstable haemoglobin disease

2. Membrane defect
- Hereditary spherocytosis
- Hereditary elliptocytosis
- Paroxysmal nocturnal haemoglobinuria
- Spur cell anaemia

Extracorpuscular defects

1. Antibody-mediated (immune haemolysis)
- Autoimmune haemolytic anaemia (warm and cold antibodies, drugs)
- Other immune-mediated haemolysis

2. Infections
- Malaria (falciparum) (Fig. 58.1)
- Bartonella
- Clostridium

3. Mechanical
- Microangiopathic haemolytic anaemia e.g. DIC, disseminated malignancies, vasculitis, TTP, etc.
- Mechanical valve (traumatic)
- March haemoglobinuria
- Transfusion reaction (ABO incompatibility)

4. Chemical and physical agents
- Snake bite, bee sting, spider bite, etc.
- Arsenicals

5. Hypersplenism, liver disease

haemoglobin is oxidised to form *methaemalbumin* which is detected on spectrophotometry of the plasma (Schumm's test). Methaemalbumin is degraded and free haem formed which binds to a second binding protein called *haemopexin* to form a complex.

When all the protective mechanisms are overloaded, free haemoglobin appear in the urine called *haemoglobinuria*, a characteristic feature of intravascular haemolysis. When haemolytic process is fulminant as seen in malaria, this gives rise to black urine. In smaller amounts renal tubular cells absorb the haemoglobin, degrade it and store the iron as haemosiderin. When the renal tubular cells containing haemosiderin are shed off into the urine, *haemosiderinuria* results which is always indicative of intravascular haemolysis.

2. **Extravascular haemolysis:** In most haemolytic conditions, red cells destruction is extravascular and little or no depletion of haptoglobin occurs—a differentiating feature from intravascular haemolysis. The red cells are removed from the circulation by macrophages in RE system of liver and spleen. There is no haemosiderinuria.

Evidences for Haemolysis

1. **Increased red cell destruction:** It leads to:
   - Elevated serum bilirubin predominantly indirect (unconjugated hyperbilirubinaemia).
   - Excessive urinary urobilinogen.
   - Reduced levels of haptoglobins.
   - Raised serum lactic dehydrogenase (LDH).

2. **Compensatory increased red cell production:** It leads to:
   - Reticulocytosis (characteristic).
   - Macrocytosis if folic acid and vit. B_{12} insufficient.
   - Erythroid hyperplasia of the marrow.
   - Radiological changes in the bone (skull and tubular bones).

3. **Morphological change in RBCs:** These occur in some haemolytic anaemias:
   - Spherocytosis (hereditary spherocytosis).
   - Sickle cell (sickle cell disease).
   - Elliptocytes (elliptocytosis).
   - Red cells fragments.

- Acanthocytes (spur cell anaemias or severe liver disease).
- Agglutinated cells (cold agglutinin disease due to cold IgM antibodies).
- Heinz bodies (unstable Hb disease, oxidant stress).

4. **Altered osmotic fragility and Coomb's test** (direct test detects anti-IgG and anti-C3 on RBC surface while indirect test detects IgG antibody in serum in autoimmune haemolytic anaemia).

5. **Demonstration of shortened red cell survival**
   - Red cell survival studies using 5ICr-labelled RBCs. The dominant site of destruction can be shown with external body counting over the liver and spleen.

6. **Evidences of intravascular haemolysis:** These are in addition to stated above if haemolysis is intravascular and differentiates it from extravascular haemolysis. These are:
   - Raised levels of plasma haemoglobin (haemoglobinaemia).
   - Very low or absent haptoglobins.
   - Haemoglobinuria and haemosiderinuria.
   - Presence of methaemalbumin (positive Schumm's test).

Clinical Presentations

1. **Hereditary haemolytic anaemias** may be asymptomatic or may present with anaemia, jaundice and splenomegaly or may present with complications (chronic) such as haemolytic facies, ankle ulcers, pigment gallstones, growth retardation in children, pathological fractures. They may present *acutely* with crises, i.e. aplastic crisis due to B19 parvovirus, megaloblastic crisis due to folic acid deficiency and acute haemolytic crisis due to accelerated haemolysis.

2. **Microangiopathic haemolytic anaemia:** It is an intravascular hemolysis induced by changes in the microvasculature, due to prosthetic valve (mechanical trauma), and assist intravascular devices leading to formation of *schistocytes* on PBF. The *laboratory findings* are:
   i. Negative direct antiglobin (Comb's) test.
   ii. Raised LDH levels
   iii. Indirect hyperbilirubinemia.
   iv. Reduced plasma hepatoglobin.

3. **Acquired haemolytic anaemia:** In most patients with acquired haemolytic anaemia, red cells are made normally but are prematurely destroyed in circulation. The damage is extracorpuscular, is mediated by antibodies or toxins that predispose the cells to premature destruction (haemolysis). Therefore, these anaemias are episodic, occur after some challenge, present actually with manifestations of intravascular haemolysis (antibodies, infection or toxin mediated) or extravascular haemolysis (hypersplenism). Malaria, blood transfusion, paroxysmal nocturnal haemoglobinuria, snake bite are common causes of acute acquired haemolytic anaemia (Fig. 58.1).

4. **Autoimmune haemolytic anaemia:** It is caused by either IgG antibodies that react with the antigen on the RBCs surface at body temperature (*warm antibodies*) or by IgM antibodies that react with antigen on the surface of RBC at lower core body temperature called *cold antibodies*. It can be due to infections, autoimmune diseases, malignancy and drugs.

Crises in Haemolytic Anaemia

Therefore acute haemolytic anaemia may present as a crisis, such as:
   i. **Aplastic crisis:** It is frequently seen in congenital haemolytic anaemia such as sickle cell anaemia, β-thalassaemia, hereditary spherocytosis and pyruvate kinase deficiency. The infection by B19 *parvovirus* is the most common precipitating cause. It may be sporadic or endemic. Transmission

of virus is via faeco-oral route or droplets infection.

The symptom and signs of infection such as fever, malaise, chills, upper respiratory or gastrointestinal symptoms precede the episode of aplastic crisis. The investigations reveal very low haemoglobin and hypoplasia of the bone marrow (low reticulocyte count, erythroblasto penia). Diagnosis is mainly clinical. Serology for presence of specific lgM antiviral antibodies or demonstration of parvovirus B19 particles in the blood on electron microscopy is confirmatory. Erythropoiesis ceases for 48–72 hours, though crisis may last for 1–2 weeks. Treatment is immediate red cell infusion to raise the haemoglobin. Supportive care should be instituted. The crisis is self-limiting. A single attack of parvovirus confers lifelong immunity.

ii. **Haemolytic crisis:** It is rather infrequent but early recognition is necessary to save life. The patients of unstable haemoglobin disease or enzymes deficiency (G6PD, pyruvate kinase) may develop sudden fall in haemoglobin under the effect of oxidant stress due to febrile/infective illness. The haemoglobin breaks down and gets precipitated as *Heinz bodies*—a characteristic feature. The inheritance of G6PD deficiency is sex-linked and affects approximately 1% of the Indian males. It is common in Parsees (15%), Bhansoli (11%), Khatri (9%), Punjabi (3%), Kutchi (3%) and Muslims (25%). The list of drugs that cause haemolysis in G6PD deficiency and unstable haemoglobins are listed in Box 1. Autoimmune haemolytic anaemia in which the haemolysis is mainly extravascular in the spleen due to antibodies may present with fulminant haemolytic picture sometimes. The malarial parasite (falciparum) causes acute haemolytic anaemia or crisis (Fig. 58.2) due to the reduced RBC survivals in normal healthy persons.

The clinical evaluation of acute haeolytic crisis are given in Box 2.

iii. **Megaloblastic crisis:** Haemolytic anaemia of any cause increases the demand of folic acid, therefore, concomitant folic acid deficiency may result in megaloblastic crisis. The folic acid deficiency may be

Box 1	Drugs and chemicals responsible for haemolysis in G6PD deficiency and unstable haemoglobin disease

- *Antimalarials,* e.g. primaquine, pamaquin, quinine, chloroquine
- *Sulphonamides*, e.g. sulphamethoxazole, sulphapyridine, sulphasalazine, sulphanilamide
- *Fluoroquinolones*, e.g. nitrofurantoin, nalidixic acid, norfloxacin, ciprofloxacin
- *Sulphones*, e.g. dapsone
- *Analgesic*, e.g. acetanilide
- *Miscellaneous*, e.g. vit. K, doxorubicin, methylene blue, niridazole, toludene blue, furazolidine, naphthalene (moth-balls)

Box 2	Clinical Evaluation of Acute haemolytic crisis

1. History: Ask about

- Fever
- Infection
- Drugs (read Box 1)
- Family history
- Systemic illness or predisposing illness

2. Clinical features

Symptoms
- Pallor, weakness, dyspnoea, tachycardia, fatigue, abdominal pain
- Jaundice (yellowness of eyes)
- Dark colour of urine and faeces
- Splenomegaly (recent appearance or sudden increase in pre-existing splenomegaly)
- Hepatomegaly (mild)

Signs
- Anaemia, jaundice

3. Investigations

i. *Investigations to confirm haemolysis have already been discussed*

ii. *Investigations to find out the cause*
- PBF for malarial parasite, Heinz bodies
- Serology for parvovirus B19 and other viruses
- Coomb's antiglobin tests (direct and indirect)
- Tests for underlying disorders especially the neoplasms of immune system (CLL, Hodgkin's and non-Hodgkin's lymphoma), collagen vascular disease or immunodeficiency disease

precipitated by rapid growth or pregnancy or diminished intake (anorexia) or alcoholism. The clinical features are same. In this condition, there will be macrocytosis in the peripheral blood film instead of normocytic normochromic picture of haemolytic anaemia. The bone marrow shows megaloblastosis.

iv. **Splenic sequestration crisis** is usually seen in children under the age of 2 years. It results from sudden trapping of blood in spleen leading to sudden fall in haemoglobin >2 g/dl or more. This type of crisis is common in sickle cell anaemia and its variants Hb SC disease or Hb-Sp-thalassaemia wherein splenomegaly is a characteristic feature. The precipitous fall in haemoglobin if not managed promptly, death may result. Over 10% deaths occur during first decade in children with sickle cell disease. In severe cases, splenectomy is indicated, therefore, the mothers of the child with sickle cell disease can be taught to detect the enlarging spleen in the child during acute illness and bring him to emergency.

Management

It is essentially supportive during the attack. Most of the attacks of haemolytic crisis are self-limiting.

Aims of Treatment

- To identify haemolytic process, its nature and measures to arrest it.
- To identify the type of crisis and its cause, e.g. G6PD deficiency (Heinz bodies) or infection (malarial parasite, bacterial or viral).

Steps

1. Arrangement be made for blood transfusions, therefore, immediate blood grouping and cross-matching should be ordered.
2. Send the blood sample for:
   - Complete blood count, red cell indices, reticulocyte count and PBF for type of anaemia or for malarial parasite.
   - Serum bilirubin (total and differential).
   - LDH and folate.
   - Urea and electrolyte.
   - Serology for viral infection (parvovirus B19).
3. Bone marrow examination.
4. Carry out the treatment.
   - Rest, treatment of fever and pain if present.
   - O_2 through mask.
   - Adequate hydration by fluids.
   - *Transfusions:* Packed RBCs transfusion is needed at the earliest. Each unit to be trans fused within 2–4 hours. The total requirement varies depending on the haemoglobin/haematocrit, hence, reassessment should be made after two blood transfusions.

Note: Blood or red cell transfusion may be hazardous in acquired haemolytic anaemia (having antibodies in plasma) as it may induce further haemolysis. However, it does not deter the transfusion if emergency demands it.

- Supplement folic acid 5 mg daily followed by lifelong replacement of 1 mg daily.
- No iron supplementation is warranted unless there is concomitant iron deficiency.
- Corticosteroids for autoimmune haemolytic anaemia (1 mg/kg/day) for 4–6 weeks followed by gradual reduction of the dose. Immunosuppressive drugs (cyclophosphamide, azathioprine) are other alternative to steroids.
- *Treatment of infection:* Antimalarial for falciparum infection, use artesunate/artemether for this purpose as quinine may precipitate haemolysis. Antibiotic for bacterial infection.
- Treatment of underlying primary disease responsible for haemolysis.
- Consider *splenectomy* on an individual basis weighing its hazards and benefits.

Thrombocytopenia and Immune Thrombocytopenic Purpura

CHAPTER

59

THROMBOCYTOPENIA

The platelets are one of the formed elements of blood and take part in hemostasis (Fig. 59.1). Platelets also play a role in fibrinolysis and clot retraction. Disorders of platelets manifest as bleed ing disorders. Hemostatic process requires an adequate number of platelets that are functioning normally, failing which primary hemostatic process is compromised.

Definition

Thrombocytopenia is defined as a decrease in platelet count to below $150 \times 10^9/L$ (<1,50,000/mm³). A normal platelet count is $150–350 \times 10^9/L$.

Immune thrombocytopenic purpura is also called *idiopathic thrombocytopenic purpura* (ITP) is an acquired immune-mediated disorder characterised by isolated thrombocytopenia with no explainable underlying cause.

Causes

Platelets arise from the fragmentation of mega karyocytes which are very large, polypoidal bone marrow cells produced by the process of endomitosis. They undergo 3–5 cycles of chromosomal duplication without cytoplasmic division. After leaving the bone marrow, one-third of the platelets are sequestrated in the spleen, while the other two-thirds circulate

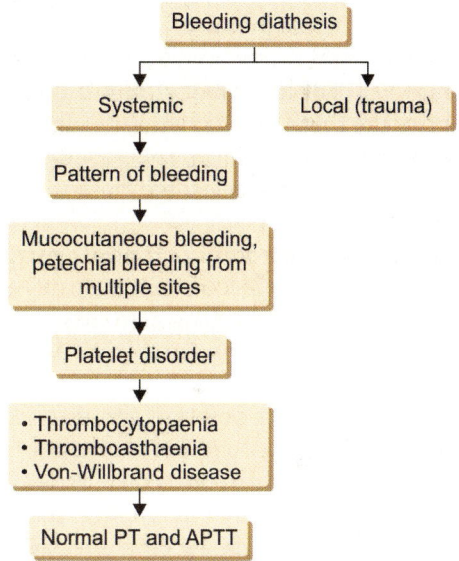

Fig. 59.1: Evaluation of patient with bleeding disorder

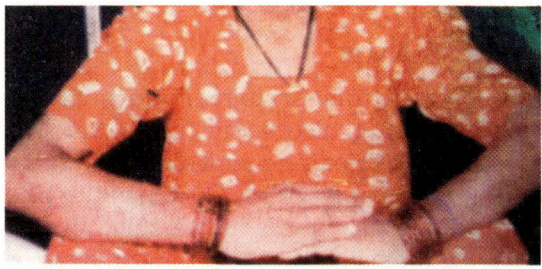

Fig. 59.2: A patient with thrombocytopenic purpura. Note the purpuric spots over the upper extremities

for platelet functions and remain for 7–10 days (normal lifespan of platelets). Normally, only a small mass of platelets is consumed in process of hemostasis; so most of the platelets circulate until they become old or senescent and are removed by phagocytic cells.

The process of thrombocytosis (platelets production) is regulated by thrombopoietin (TPO) binding to its megakaryocyte receptors. A reduction in platelet mass increases the level of TPO and thereby stimulates megakaryocytes and platelets production. Recombinant TPO is being tested for clinical use for prevention and treatment of thrombocytopenia in patients receiving cytotoxic therapy.

The causes of thrombocytopenia are given in Table 59.1. The thrombocytopenia is caused by one of the three mechanisms, i.e. decreased bone marrow production, increased splenic sequestration, and accelerated destruction of platelets.

Autoimmune thrombocytopenic purpura is the most common (acquired) cause in young subjects. Exposure to drugs, toxins, venom (snake bite), infections (malaria, dengue), gram-negative septicaemia and DIC are other common causes of thrombocytopenia encountered in clinical practice. Splenomegaly due to any cause and/or hypersplenism leads to thrombocytopenia by increasing platelets destruction, also diminishes the effectiveness of platelets transfusion in these conditions and splenectomy is the answer to these problems. The drugs causing thrombocytopenia are given in Box 1.

Clinical Features

Idiopathic Thrombocytopenic purpura is a common clinical disorder in clinical practice, presents with bleeding as a medical emergency and is associated with high morbidity and mortality if bleeding is intracranial and/or intra-abdominal.

The clinical manifestations of ITP vary from asymptomatic or mild disease to life-threatening visceral bleeding. The common sites of bleeding are:

Table 59.1 Causes of thrombocytopenia

1. Impaired production
  A. Generalised bone marrow failure
   - Aplastic anaemia
   - Megaloblastic anaemia (nutritional)
   - Leukaemia
   - Myeloma
   - Myelofibrosis
   - Marrow infiltration by solid tumours or others (myelophthisic process)
   - Fanconi anaemia
  B. Selective reduction of platelets
   - Drugs (Box 1), physical agents (irradiation)
   - Chemicals
   - Viral infections

2. Excessive destruction/consumption
  A. Immune
   - Autoimmune thrombocytopenic purpura
   - Secondary immune thrombocytopenia (SLE, CLL, viral infection, e.g. hepatitis C and HIV drugs)
   - Autoimmune neonatal thrombocytopenia
  B. Coagulation
   - Disseminated intravascular coagulation
   - Thrombotic-thrombocytopenic purpura
   - Haemolytic-uraemic syndrome
   - Heparin-induced
  C. Mechanical microangiopath y
   - Valvular disorders
  D. Increased squestration by spleen
   - Splenomegaly due to any cause, e.g. infective, congestive, infiltrative, neoplastic, etc.
  E. *Hypersplenism,* e.g. portal hypertension, myeloproliferative disease, lymphoma
  F. Dilutional loss and gestational
  G. Massive transfusionsios of stored blood (post transfusion purpura)

- *Skin,* e.g. petechiae, purpura (Fig. 59.2) ecchymosis.
- *Mucous membrane* and *gum bleeding.*
- *Nasal bleeding* (epistaxis).
- *Genitourinary tract bleeding* (haematuria, menorrhagia).
- *Intracranial* and *intra-abdominal bleeding.*

The severity of bleeding correlates with the degree of thrombocytopenia:
  i. As long as count is between $100–140 \times 10^9/L$ (1,00,000–1,40,000/mm^3), the patients are asymptomatic and bleeding time remains

normal. These are mild cases of thrombo cytopenia just detected on platelet count.

ii. Counts between 50,000 and 1,00,000 per cubic millimeter (moderate thrombocytopenia) prolong the BT and bleeding occurs following trauma, surgery or administration of drugs.

Box 1   Drugs causing thrombocytopenia

1. Suppression of platelets production
- Myelosuppressive drugs, e.g. cytosine arabinoside, daunorubicin, cyclophosphamide, busulfan, methotrexate, 6-mercaptopurine, vi nca alkaloids
- Thiazide diuretics
- Ethanol (binge drinker)
- Oestrogens

2. Immunologic platelet destruction
- Antibiotics, e.g. sulphonamide, tetracyclines, novobiocin, PAS, rifampicin, chloramphenicol
- Cinchona alkaloids, e.g. quinine, quinidine
- Sedatives, hypnotics, anticonvulsants (carbamazepine)
- Digoxin
- Alpha methyldopa
- Anti-inflammatory, e.g. aspirin, phenyl butazone
- Chloroquine , gold salts, arsenicals
- Insecticides

---

iii. Count below 50,000 (severe thrombocytopenia) leads to easy bruising, purpura or bleeding with minimal trauma.

iv. A platelet count less than 20,000 mm³ (very severe thrombocytopenia) leads to spontaneous bleeding such as petechiae, ecchymosis and internal bleeding (brain or GI tract).

Clinical Evaluation of a Case with Thrombocytopenia (Fig. 59.1)

It depends on:
1. History.
2. Clinical examination.
3. Investigations.

History

Certain elements on the history are important to determine whether bleeding is caused by underlying hemostatic disorder or by a local anatomic defect. The profuse bleeding during dental extraction, following trauma, childbirth or minor cuts or surgery indicate hemostatic defect. Following points are to be recorded on history in a patient with bleeding.

1. History suggestive of petechial spots, ecchymosis, epistaxis, gum bleeding, haematuria, menorrhagia, etc.
2. Ask for any recent drug intake or chemotherapy.
3. Antecedent viral infection (e.g. dengue fever / arbovirus).
4. Connective tissue disorders—skin rash, photosensitivity, joint and/or renal involvement.
5. Similar episode(s) in the past.
6. Family history of similar illness.
7. Pregnancy.

Certain clinical manifestations that are characteristic of primary haemostatic disorder (platelet defects) are given in Box 2. These features also differentiate it from secondary haemostatic defect (coagulation disorders).

Physical Findings on Examination

Look for the following:
- Petechiae, purpura, ecchymosis, nasal or gum bleeding.
- Facial puffiness.
- Record BP.
- Lymphadenopathy, rash, joint involvement.
- Splenomegaly.
- CNS involvement.

Investigations

They are done to confirm the diagnosis, to exclude other conditions and to determine the cause of thrombocytopenia.

i. *Bleeding time* is prolonged.
ii. *The blood count* should include WBC, RBC and platelets. Peripheral blood film for any abnormality of platelets. Reticulocyte count to be done for bone marrow response. The reduced platelet count determines the severity of thrombocytopenia and serves as a guide for blood transfusion.

Box 2	Clinical manifestations of primary and secondary hemostatic failure		
Feature	Platelet disorder (defect of primary haemostasis)	Coagulation disorders (defect of secondary haemostasis)
1. Onset of bleeding following trauma	Immediate	Delayed (hours or days)
2. Site of bleeding	Superficial, e.g. skin, mucous membrane, gums, nose, GI tract, genitourinary tract	Deep, e.g. joints, muscles, retroperitoneal
3. Physical findings	Purpura, ecchymosis	Haematomas, haemarthrosis
4. Family history	Autosomal dominant	Autosomal or X-linked recessive
5. Response to therapy	Immediately stops with local pressure	Requires sustained system therapy

iii. *Bone marrow study:* Normal or increased number of megakaryocytes are found in the bone marrow, which is otherwise normal.

iv. *Blood biochemistry and other investigations* to find out the underlying cause or primary disease.

v. *Coagulation profile* to rule out coagulation disorders as a cause of bleeding. Assay of von Willebrand's factor is also done for platelet dysfunction.

vi. *Serology* for viral and connective tissue disorders.

vii. *Detection of platelet antibodies* not only confirms the diagnosis of ITP, but also rules out other causes of excessive destruction of platelets.

viii. *Imaging studies:* Ultrasonography for splenomegaly and CT scan for any intracranial bleed.

Management

It includes general measures, hemostatic measures including platelet transfusions and measures directed against the underlying cause or primary disease.

1. **General measures:** It includes precautionary measures (Do's and Don'ts) in thrombocytopenia (Box 3).
2. **Measures to stop bleeding:** The hemostatic measures may be local or systemic:
   A. *Local measures*
      - Compression bandages.
      - Nasal packing for epistaxis.
      - Application of thrombin or other hemostatic agents.
   B. *Systemic*
      - Procure I.V. line immediately in case of bleeding.
      - Platelet transfusions.
      - Treat other hemostatic abnormalities

In the meantime, the patient is being assessed following investigations must be ordered in order to save life-threatening complications:

- Complete blood count including platelet count, reticulocyte count and blood smear.
- Blood group.
- Blood biochemistry.
- Urine for hematuria.
- Fundus examination.
- Others (screening for DIG, autoantibodies).
- Bone marrow.

Box 3	Precautionary measures in thrombocytopenia	
Do's	Don't (Avoid)
• Apply firm pressure on venepuncture site while collecting samples or I.V. administration for 10 minutes	• Avoid trauma
	• Stop use of hard toothbrushes or metal razors
• Stop drugs known to induce thrombocytopenia or bone marrow suppression	• Avoid intramuscular injection
	• Avoid use of NSAIDs
	• Avoid rectal examination, catheterization, suppositories and enemas

Platelets transfusions: Platelet transfusions are life-saving in patients with severe thrombocytopenia (count <20,000 mm³) or when there is excessive bleeding. Platelet transfusions should be given to maintain a count above $100 \times 10^9 / L$ (1,00,000/mm³) or else a target platelet count of $50 \times 10^9 / L$ is adequate.

> *Platelet transfusions are not much of value in states of accelerated destruction such as ITP; and not used in thrombotic states like haemolytic uremic syndrome or thrombotic thrombocytopenia purpura as they are likely to be consumed.*

Platelets for transfusion are derived either from random donor blood or apheresis from a single donor. It is best to use single-donor platelet apheresis in autoimmune states so as to minimize transfusion-related risks. The apheresed single-donor platelet pack raises the platelet count by $50 \times 10^9 / L$.

Certain points to be borne in mind while transfusing platelets are summarized in Box 4.

3. **Treatment of underlying cause/primary disease:** Withdrawal of an *offending drug/ toxin*. Use antisnake venom in case of snake bite poisoning.

Box 4 Points to be remembered for platelet transfusion

- Platelets have short lifespan (about 5 days), therefore, fresh platelets should be transfused.
- Platelets should be transfused rapidly within 10 minutes.
- Platelets awaiting transfusions are stored at room temperature (20°–40°C) in a gently agitated state.
- Platelet transfusion does not require cross-matching.
- Group-compatibilty of donor platelets/plasma may be ideal.
- Unnecessary platelet transfusion generates allo-immunization reducing the efficacy of further transfusions, hence, should be avoided.

4. **Treatment of immune thrombocytopenic purpura:** ITP is characterised by immune mediated destruction of platelets in spleen by IgG antibodies against glucoprotein IIb/IIIa on platelets. It is treated by steroids, intra-venous immunoglobulin, anti-RhD, danazol, colchicine, immunosuppression and/or splenectomy. IVIG (2 g/kg total in divided doses over a period of 3–5 days) or Anti-Rho D intravenous bolus dose of 50–75 mEg/kg given over 3–5 minutes raises the platelet count within 48 hours. It is preferred over IVIG. If Hb is <10 g then the dose should be reduced to half.

IVIG infusion in ITP

RES blockade after intravenous human normal immunoglobulin infusion in ITP, with saturation of FcR on splenic macrophages by free floating (un-bound) immunoglobulin molecules. This allows more antibody coated platelets to survive in the circulation

Anti-Rho D (I.V. infusion) in ITP

Anti-D lg molecules bind with Rh positive RBCs and block the FcR of the splenic macrophage due to which the platelets in the circulation survive. Stopping the destruction of platelets and already ongoing platelet-production gives a good rise in platelet count instantly.

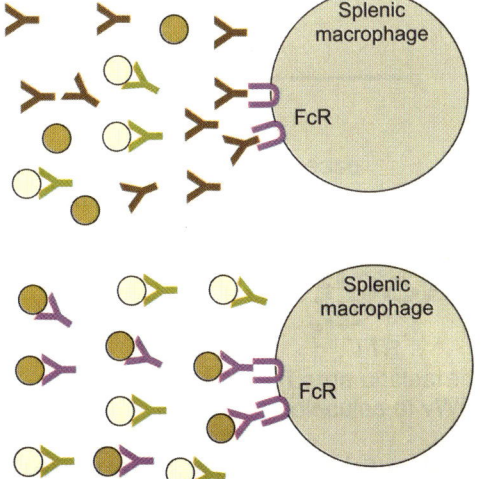

Fig. 59.3: Action of IVIG or anti-D in immune thrombocytopenic purpura

adhesion (Fig. 60.1A). The manifestations are as a result of localised platelet thrombi and fibrin deposition in micro vasculature (Fig. 60.1B). Arterioles are filled with hyaline material (fibrin and platelets) and similar material may also be seen beneath the endothelium of involved vessels. Immunofluorescence studies have shown deposition of immunoglobulins and complement in arterioles indicating an immunologic origin. Microaneurysm of arterioles may also be seen.

Causes

No specific cause is known. It is considered to be immunological in origin. It is commonly associated with pregnancy, AIDS, scleroderma and Sjögren's syndrome. Drug-related thrombotic thrombocytopenic purpura (TTP) is either due to antibody formation (ticlodipine or clopidogrel) or direct endothelial damage (cyclosporine, mitomycin, quinine).

Clinical Features

It is common in all age groups, primarily in young adults more common in females. TTP may be acute in onset but its course spans over days to weeks in most of the patients and occasionally may continue for months.

The *symptoms* and *signs* vary depending on the number and site of arteriolar lesions. The classic *pentad* of TTP consists of:

1. Microangiopathic haemolytic anaemia with fragmentation of RBCs.
2. Signs of intravascular haemolysis and fever.
3. Thrombocytopenia.
4. Neurological findings.
5. Impaired renal function.

The anaemia is mild to very severe, normocytic and normochromic. The thrombocytopenia may also be mild to severe producing bleeding tendencies. The neurological and renal abnormalities appear only when platelet count is markedly reduced (< 20 to 30 × 10³/L). Fever is often an accompaniment. The organ involvement is due to occlusion of microcirculation as

a result of fibrin thrombi and platelets leading to tissue hypoxia.

Proteinuria and mild rise in blood urea may be the presenting feature of renal involvement followed by continued rise in urea and a fall in urine output if renal failure develops.

Neurological manifestations appear in more than 90% of cases and may be a cause of death in some patients. Altered state of consciousness, confusion, delirium occur initially followed by focal neurological signs and symptoms such as seizures, hemiparesis, aphasia and visual field defects. These neurological manifestations may fluctuate and terminate in coma.

Investigations

1. **Haemoglobin** is low.
2. **Platelet count** is low.
3. **PBF** shows fragmented RBCs or schistocytes—a pathognomonic finding. Reticulocyte count is raised.
4. **Tests for haemolysis.** Serum LDH levels are raised due to intravascular haemolysis. Haemoglobinuria may be present. There is raised indirect bilirubin. Hepatoglobin levels are reduced. Direct Coombs' test is negative.
5. **Tests.for coagulation** such as PT, PTT, fibrinogen level and fibrin split products are usually normal or only mildly abnormal.
6. Reduction in vWPCP activity.
7. **Tissue biopsy:** Biopsies of skin, muscles, gingiva, lymph node may demonstrate fibrin thrombi within arterioles.
8. **Bone marrow** may be hypocellular.

Diagnosis and Differential Diagnosis

The diagnosis is based on clinical features (hemolytic anaemia with fragmented RBCs, thrombocytopenia, fever, neurologic and renal manifestation) and investigations listed above.

It has to be differentiated from a similar disorder known as *haemolytic-uraemic syndrome* which is characterised by the same arteriolar lesions which are only confined to kidneys.

This disorder is common in children. Often the patient has a prodrome of a bloody diarrhoea caused by *E. coli* 0157-H7 and the lesions are thought to be due to the elaboration of *shiga-like verotoxins* that bind to renal vascular endothelium. Patients usually infants or children present with acute haemolytic anaemia, thrombocytopenia, acute intravascular haemolysis and oliguric renal failure. There is no neurologic symptom. The peripheral blood findings and coagulation tests are usually indistinguishable from TTP. Treatment is supportive especially dialysis.

Management

1. **Plasmapheresis coupled with fresh-frozen plasma infusion:** Until recently, the disease was considered to be universally fatal but now with the availability of plasmapheresis, more than 90% of cases can survive if therapy is immediately instituted. The plasmapheresis can be done daily or even twice daily with plasma replacement. The response is judged by an increase in platelet count, fall in LDH levels and fragmented red cells. If response is obtained, plasmapheresis is continued but less frequently for several weeks to months.

2. **Role of corticosteroids and antiplatelet agents:** The efficacy of this treatment is not known.

3. **Immunomodulatory therapies with rituximab, immunosuppression by vincristine or cyclophosphamide and splenectomy:** In case of relapse following initial treatment, plasmapheresis should be reinstituted. If ineffective, or in case with primary refractoriness, second line treatment may be considered including rituximab, steroids, IVIG, vincristine, cyclophosphamide and splenectomy.

4. **Platelet transfusions** should not be given because they will act as 'fuel to fire' and can precipitate thrombotic events.

5. **Care of comatose patient:** Some patients may develop deep coma. The management of coma is same as discussed in respective chapter.

6. **General supportive measures** with I.V. fluids and oxygen must be given to treat hypoxia.

7. **Haemodialysis** should be considered for patients with significant renal impairment.

Coagulation disorders arise either due to congenital deficiency of a single factor, e.g. factor VIII in haemophilia A and factor IX in haemophilia B, or due to acquired multiple factors deficiencies secondary to liver disease or anti-coagulant therapy. Both haemophilia A and B are uncommon X-linked recessive disorders of coagulation.

HAEMOPHILIA A

Definition

It is a congenital single gene mutation (factor VIII and IX gene) disorder of coagulation resulting in deficiency of factor VIII (antihaemophilic factor) resulting from gene mutation of

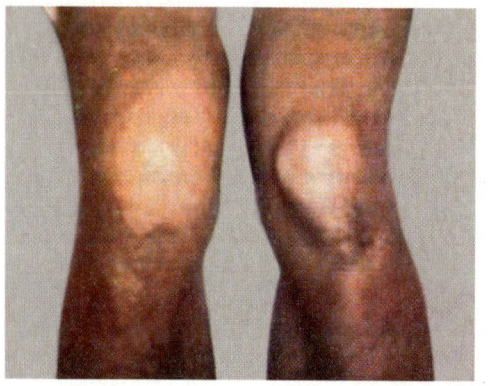

Fig. 61.1: Haemarthrosis of the right knee of a boy with haemophilia. Note the swelling of right knee as compared to left

factor VIII located on X-chromosome. It is most frequently encountered disorder of coagulation in clinical practice. It occurs in about 1 of 10,000 males. It is an X-linked disorder where the males are sufferers and females are the carriers (transmitter). About two-thirds of all patients have positive family history; while in other one-third mutation occurs *de novo*. A haermphilic person will have all his sons as normal, and all his daughters as carriers. A carrier woman has a 50% chance of having a carrier daughter or a haemophilic son in each pregnancy. Haemophilia 'breeds true' within a family thus, if one individual has severe haemophilia, all others affected will have a severe form of the disease. Female carriers of haemophilia may also have reduced factor VIII levels. A reduced factor VIII level in a carrier will result in mild bleeding disorder, therefore, all known or suspected carriers of haemophilia should have their factor VIII level measured. Inhibitors to factor VIII will develop in about 25% patients with hemophilia A and inhibitors to factor IX will develop in <5% of patients with hemophilia B.

Clinical Features

Superficial bruising or bleeding into soft tissue (*hematomas*) or joints (*haemarthrosis*) are the hallmarks of haemophilia A. Though a congenital disorder, bleeding is not noticed until babies are about 6 months old (e.g. a period of inactivity), occurs after that period because now the baby is up and about and is prone to trauma. Subcutaneous haematomas may be the earliest manifestation noted in a child as he begins to crawl; followed by bleeding into joints as he starts walking. These bleeding episodes continue throughout life.

The normal factor VIII level is 50–150% and is usually measured by a clotting assay. The severity of manifestations correlates with the degree of deficiency of factor VIII (Table 61.1).

Sites of Bleeding

The sites of bleeding are:

1. **Spontaneous mucosal bleeding** is uncommon and is visible as small swellings (haematomas).
2. **Bleeding into tight compartments** of thighs, forearms and legs lead to respective compartmental syndromes due to compression of the neighbouring and underlying structures.
3. **Bleeding into pharynx** leads to airway obstruction.
4. **Bleeding into joints [haemarthrosis (Fig. 61.1)]**, occurs spontaneously in severe haemophilia and after trauma in moderate haemophilia. The joints affected are large, i.e. knees, elbows, ankles and hips. A typical patient may have joint bleeding one or two in numbers every week. Recurrent haemarthrosis may lead to synovial hypertrophy, cartilage destruction and secondary osteoarthritis, and ultimately resulting in limitation of movements and making walking difficult.
5. **Bleeding into muscles (haematomas)** is a characteristic feature of haemophilia. It can occur in any muscle but calf and psoas muscles are commonly affected. A large psoas bleed may press on the femoral nerve. Calf haematomas are serious because calf being a tight compartment leads to compression of soleus and gastrocnemius muscles. Untreated Achilles haemorrhage causes ischaemia, necrosis, fibrosis and subsequent contraction and shortening of Achilles tendon.
6. **Bleeding into CNS** though uncommon may cause stroke and unless treated promptly may be fatal.
7. **Intra-abdominal bleeding** (intra or retroperitoneal) is uncommon and difficult to quantify and can be large producing hypotension or shock. Large retroperitoneal collection of blood may lead to mass formation (pseudotumour syndrome).
8. **Genitourinary:** Haematuria is common.

Inhibitor development to factor VIII or factor IX is characterised by new or unusual bleeding episodes that are resistant to treatment.

Diagnosis

The diagnosis is made on:

i. Clinical history of joint and soft tissue bleeding.
ii. X-linked inheritance pattern. Males suffer from the disease.
iii. Long history of bleeding with recurrent episodes leading to arthropathy in large joints.
iv. Laboratory tests or investigations to confirm the diagnosis, which will also help to determine severity and planning of future management.

Investigations

1. *A normal prothrombin time and an abnormal activated partial thromboplastin time*

Table 61.1 Severity of haemophilia and clinical features (UK criteria)		
Degree of severity	Factor VIII or IX level	Clinical features
Severe	< 1%	Spontaneous haemarthrosis and muscle haematomas, several times in a month
Moderate	1–5%	Minor trauma or surgery induces bleeding
Mild	75%	Major trauma or surgery results in excessive bleeding

indicate coagulation disorder (haemophilia A and B).

2. Demonstration of an isolated reproducibly *low factor VIII* or *factor IX activity* level in the absence of other conditions. Factor VIII and IX operate through intrinsic pathway (Fig. 61.2).

3. *Correction of abnormal partial thromboplastin time (aPTT) fully by pooled normal plasma.*

4. *Specific factor VIII coagulation assay* will confirm the diagnosis. It is also important to screen for the presence of inhibitors to factor VIII or IX at diagnosis and thereafter either by aPTT mixed with normal plasma test or by Bethesda assay.

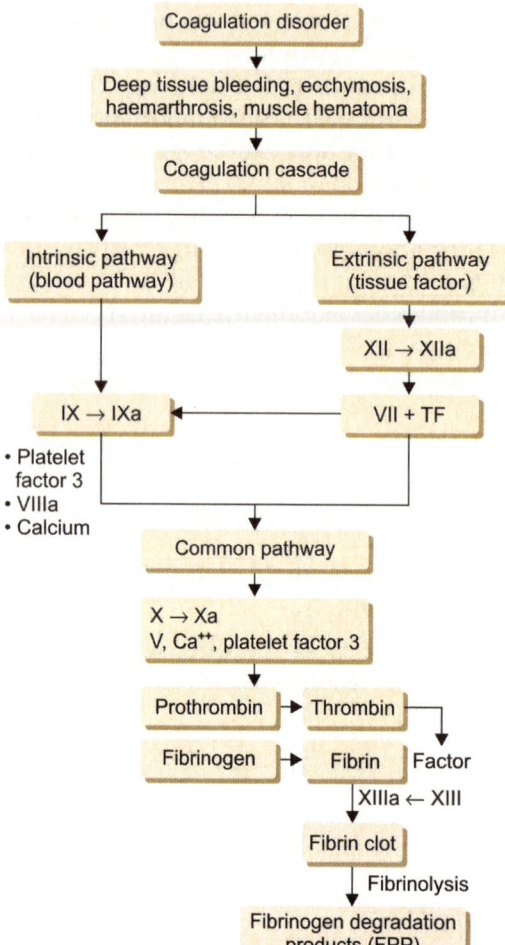

Fig. 61.2: Coagulation cascade

Management

It is an incurable disease and the males being the sufferers are likely to have bleeding in day-to-day life activities due to mild trauma (moderate disease) or spontaneously (severe disease). Recurrent bleeding into the joints or muscles may lead to contractures and crippling deformities, hence, preventive measures should be taken not to allow these complications to occur. This is only possible by making the child/adolescent and his family members understand the implications and the management of the condition. They should be able to recognise the bleeding early and be familiar with its management. It is also necessary for them to understand the genetics and mode of inheritance of haemophilia so that preventive measures can be taken if they desire so.

Moderate disease can produce bleeding with minor trauma and severe haemophilia may lead to spontaneous bleeding, which at times, may be fatal, therefore moderate to severe disease needs immediate attention and management.

The goal of therapy is to make the life of the child comfortable and normal as he grows up. This requires the family and the patient understand the treatment plans.

Treatment Plans

It includes:

1. Management of acute bleed.
2. Management of chronic complications.
3. Physical therapy and rehabilitation.
4. Management before and during minor or major surgery.
5. Carrier detection and prevention.

Management of Acute Bleed or Bleeding Episodes

Bleeding episodes should be treated early by raising the factor VIII level by replacement, additional red cell infusion if indicated (if severe anaemia) and other factor replacement measures to control the bleed. The quantity and duration of factor VIII replacement depend on the site and severity of bleeding as discussed below.

1 IU/kg of factor VIII raises the plasma levels by 2% with a half-life of 8–12 hours. The aim is to achieve plasma concentration of factor VIII above 50%, hence, a large amount of factor VIII concentrate may be needed to stop active bleeding. The rough estimate to achieve 50% level (0.5 units/ ml of plasma) in the expected plasma volume of 40 ml/kg in a 60 kg man, the dose of factor VIII will be 0.5 × 40 × 60 = 1200 IU.

Factor IX in haemophilia B is needed more than factor VIII in haemophilia A to achieve the same level. This should be born in mind while treating haemophilia B episode.

The target level of factor VIII to be achieved with duration of factor VIII replacement to control bleeding at different sites is given in Box 1. Epistaxis often stops with local measures.

Box 4	Target factor VIII level for control of acute bleed	
Site	*Level to be achieved*	*Duration*
CNS	About 50%	7–14 days
Muscles, soft tissues, GI bleed	10–20%	2–3 days

The bleeding in haemophilia is controlled with factor VIII concentrates or by other methods.

1. *Factor VIII concentrates:* Two types of factor VIII concentrates, i.e. plasma derived (prepared from pooled human plasma) and recombinant factor VIII are marketed as lyphilised factor concentrate products which can be reconstituted. Factor VIII concentrates are freeze-dried and stable at 4°C and can therefore be stored in domestic refrigerators. This facility allows the patient to treat themselves at home, thus, has revolutionized haemophilia care. Ideally plasma-derived virus-inactivated factor VIII concentrates or recombinant factor concentrate may be employed because of their good safety record and low risk of viral carriage, e.g. HIV. When factor VIII concentrates are not available, the cryoprecipitates, fresh frozen plasma or a fresh whole blood may be used. When fresh frozen plasma is thawed at 4°C, certain products remain as a precipitate cryoprecipitate. One bag of cryoprecipitate usually contains 80–100 IU of factor VIII activity and one international unit of factor VIII/IX activity is defined as "*the quantity present in one milliliter of fresh pooled plasma*". These products are cheaper and are widely available than lyophilized factor VIII concentrate. The greatest drawback of cryoprecipitate or other blood bank products is transmission of virus infection (hepatitis B and C) as they are not subjected to virus inactivation process.

Factor VIII unit/kg raises factor level by 2%, hence, a 50 kg man would need 50 × 25 = 1250 units of factor VIII to raise the level to 50%.

The other serious consequence of factor VIII infusion is the development of anti-factor VIII antibodies, which arise in about 20- 30% of severe haemophilics. Such antibodies neutralise rapidly the therapeutic infusion and making the treatment relatively ineffective. Such individuals may be treated with porcine factor VIII because antibody may have lower activity against animal factor VIII than against the human type. Alternatively, infusion of activated clotting factors, e.g. VIII or Feiba (factor VIII inhibitor bypassing activity—an activated concentrate of factors II, IX and X) may stop bleeding.

In addition to factor VIII concentrate therapy, the bleeding site should be immobilized either by splinting or bed rest.

2. *Other pharmacological agents:*
   • *Desmopressin (DDAVP)* is used in patients with mild-to-moderate haemophilia (factor VIII level 5% or more) to raise its level by three-to-fivefold. It is given intravenously (0.3 μg/kg infusion over a period of 20 minutes) or intranasally. This is often sufficient to treat a mild bleed or cover minor surgery such as dental extraction. It has no role

in management of severe haemophilia. Repeated dosing produces tachyphylaxis, hence, it becomes ineffective after 3 doses. A concentrated DDAVP intranasal spray is available for outpatient use.

- *Antifibrinolytic agents* (e.g. epsilon aminocaproic acid or tranexamic acid) are useful in management of mucosal bleeds. They are also used as an adjunct to cryoprecipitate or factor VIII concentrate for dental procedures or extraction. A single infusion of cryoprecipitate or factor VIII concentrate coupled with the administration of 4 to 6 g of epsilon aminocaproic acid 4 times daily for 72 to 96 hours is used for filling a carious tooth or dental extraction. Epsilon-aminocaproic acid is also effective when used as mouth wash. The presence of bleeding in the presence of high titer inhibitor (>5 Bethesda units) requires infusion of an activated prothrombin complex concentrate or recombinant activated factor VII. Larger doses of factor VIII I.V. for 6–18 months succeeds in eradicating the inhibitor in 70% of patients with hemophilia A.

Surgery (minor or major) or procedure in haemophilics

For major oral and periodontal surgery and extractions of permanent teeth, patient should be hospitalised and treated with factor VIII concentrate. Therapy should begin just before surgery and continued for a minimum of 48–72 hours.

Physical Rehabilitation

Physical therapy should be started after stoppage of bleeding as soon as patient is up and about.

Carrier Detection Antenatal Diagnosis and Prevention

Carriers have reduced or low normal factor VIII/IX coagulant activity. This information is utilized to assign carrier status. In families with haemophilia A, the ratio of factor VIIIc to the von Willebrand factor, which is normal in carriers, can be used with about 90% accuracy in assigning carrier status.

The use of molecular genetic techniques has revolutionised the ability to identify carriers and the antenatal diagnosis of haemophilia. Antenatal diagnosis can be undertaken in a female who has a high probability of being a carrier. This is determined by chorionic villous sampling or biopsy usually around 10 to 11 weeks of gestation, sexing the fetus and using informative factor VIII probes. Alternatively, fetus can be sexed at 16 weeks of gestation by aminocentesis and, if male, a fetal blood sample obtained at about 19–20 weeks.

Note: Prenatal diagnosis is offered when termination of pregnancy is considered if an affected foetus is identified. However, it may be done to prepare and to plan delivery.

HAEMOPHILIA B (CHRISMAS DISEASE)

Haemophilia B is due to deficiency of factor IX. It is also X-linked recessive disorder. This disorder is clinically indistinguishable from haemophilia A but is less common. The frequency of bleeding episodes depends on the severity of the deficiency of factor IX level.

Treatment is with factor IX concentrate, i.e. it is used in the same way as factor VIII is used for haemophilia A. Carrier detection and antenatal diagnosis can be accomplished if the specific mutation is known.

RECENT ADVANCES IN THE FIELD OF HAEMOPHILIA

1. Long half-life recombinant factors are being developed by various techniques, i.e. PE glycation, F_C fusion and albumin fusion.
2. Concizumab: A monoclonal antibody against tissue factor pathway inhibitor is being tried.
3. Gene therapy is being developed.

Disseminated Intravascular Coagulation (DIC)

DISSEMINATED INTRAVASCULAR COAGULATION (DIC)

Definition

It is an acquired coagulation disorder in which there is widespread generation of fibrin due to activation of the extrinsic pathway by release of tissue factor (thromboplastin), activation of intrinsic pathway by diffuse endothelial damage or generalised platelet aggregation.

There is consumption of coagulation factors and platelets (consumption coagulopathy) and secondary activation of fibrinolysis leading to production of FDPs which may further contribute to coagulation defect by inhibiting fibrin polymerization.

DIC can be either an explosive and life threatening bleeding disorder or a relatively mild or subclinical disorder diagnosed on laboratory parameters.

Pathophysiology (Fig. 62.1)

The following are the steps in pathogenesis of DIC:

1. **Thrombin generation that overpowers its controlling mechanism:** In most forms of DIC, the tissue factor—TF (thromboplastin) is released, e.g. from leukaemic cells in leukaemia and from placenta in obsteric conditions which activates the extrinsic

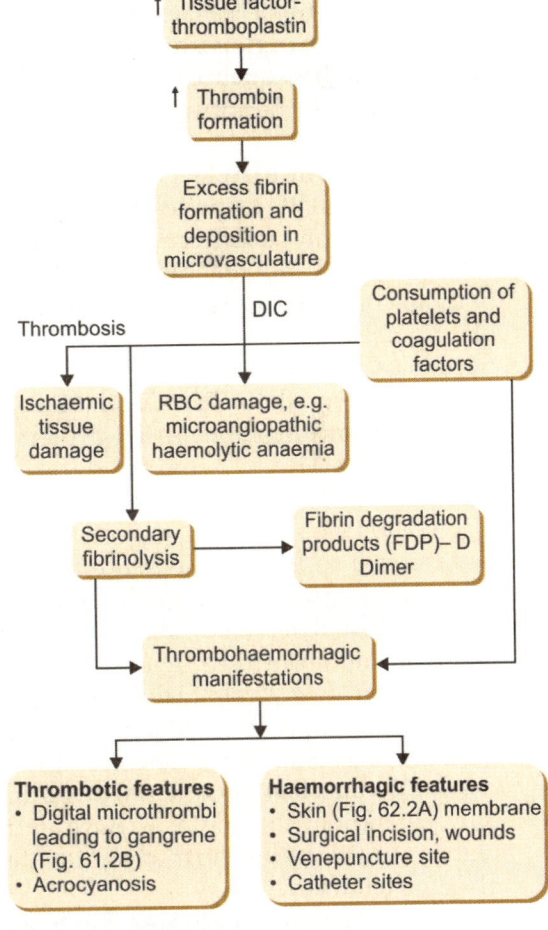

Fig. 62.1: Pathogenesis of DIC and its thrombo-haemorrhagic manifestations

pathway of coagulation by interacting with factor VII thereby initiating coagulation. The sepsis, cytokines, endotoxin, trauma, ischaemia, tumor cells can initiate DIC by release of TF. In DIC, thrombin formation is excessive, uncontrolled and overcomes the factors (antithrombin III, activated protein C) which normally inhibit thrombin formation.

2. **Fibrin deposition in microcirculation:** Large amounts of thrombin generated leads to fibrin formation from fibrinogen leading to its deposition in the microvasculature. Widespread microvascular thrombosis produces tissue ischaemia and organ damage. Microangiopathic haemolytic anaemia is a consequence of DIC as RBCs are sheared by the intravascular fibrin strands.

3. **Consumption of platelets and coagulation factors:** As DIC continues, the platelets and coagulation factors are trapped and consumed beyond the capacity of the body to compensate. This contributes to bleeding.

4. **Secondary fibrinolysis and production of fibrinogen degradation products (FDPs):** Protein C, antithrombin (AT), proteins plasmin inhibitors provide defence against fibrinolysis. A lack of these inhibitors would favour DIC and its worsening. In response to thrombosis, endothelial cells secrete plasminogen activators to initiate fibrinolysis (secondary fibrinolysis). Plasmin formed from activation of plasminogen degrades both the fibrinogen and fibrin leading to the formation of FDPs, thus, dissolves clots thereby increasing the risk of bleeding. FDPs interfere with fibrin polymerisation, thrombin activity and platelet function that further aggravate bleeding tendency.

5. **Role of chemical mediator such as cytokines:** DIC in different diseases result from release of various cytokines that act through activation of coagulation pathway. DIC occurs as chemical mediators are released from macrophages, monocytes and endothelial cells. Tissue necrosis factor (TNF) and IL-1 can cause production of TF which initiates DIC. Many of the effects of DIC such as hypotension or acute lung injury may be due to the effects of these cytokines per se.

Causes

The causes are given in Box 1.

Box 1 Causes of DIC
1. Infections
• Viral infections, e.g. arboviruses, varicella, rubella.
• Gram-negative septicaemia
• Meningococcaemia
• Malaria (falciparum), kala azar
• *Rocky mountain* spotted fever
• Histoplasmosis, Aspergillosis
2. Malignancy
• Acute promyelocytic leukaemia
• Adenocarcinomas, e.g. lung, prostate, pancreas, colon
3. Obstetric conditions
• Abruptio placentae
• Septic abortion
• Retained dead fetus
• Pre-eclampsia
• Amniotic fluid embolism
4. Haemolytic transfusion reactions, e.g. ABO incompatible blood transfusion, transplant rejection
5. Snake venom, insect venom
6. Miscellaneous
• Shock, massive transfusions, burns
• Collagen vascular disorders
• Hemolytic uremic syndrome
• Acute glomerulonephritis
• Acute pancreatitis

Clinical Features

The clinical presentation varies with the stage and severity of the syndrome. It may be asymptomatic (laboratory parameters provide the diagnosis) or may present with florid thrombo-haemorrhagic manifestations (Fig. 61.2A and B) and shock.

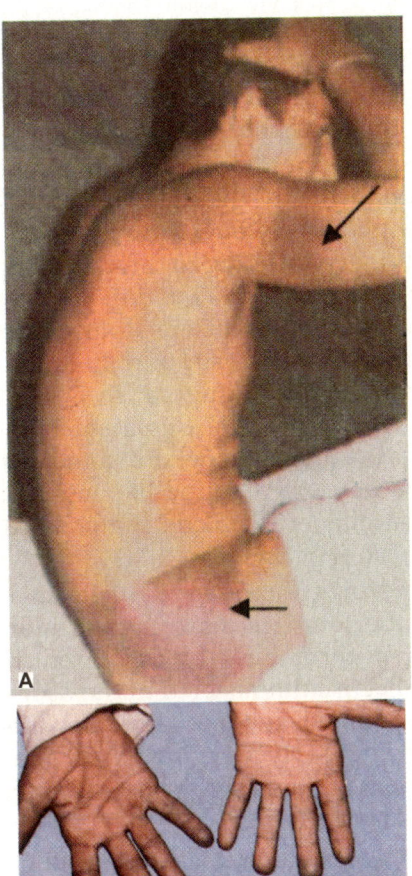

Fig. 62.2A and B: Disseminated intravascular coagulation (DIC). Note the haemorrhagic manifestations in A (arrows) and thrombotic features, i.e. gangrene of fingers in B (arrows)

Haemorrhage is the most common presentation characterised by spontaneous bruising (Fig. 62.2A) mucosal bleeding/oozing, bleeding from open wound and venepuncture or catheter sites. Usually bleeding is associated with varying degree of shock which is out of proportion to the degree of blood loss. Shock is probably due to cytokines. The major organ dysfunction leading to syndrome of DIC involving the pulmonary, renal, hepatic and CNS systems can occur.

Less often, patients present with thrombotic manifestations, i.e. acrocyanosis,

thrombosis, and pregangrenous changes in digits (Fig. 62.2B), genitalia, and nose—areas where blood flow is markedly reduced by vasospasm or microthromi.

DIC may be acute or chronic. Acute DIC is commonly seen in clinical practice, manifests with bleeding that can be rapidly progressive. Acrocyanosis is common during acute DIC due to microthrombi or vasospasms of digital vessels. On the other hand, chronic DIC occurs from a weak or intermittent activating stimulus. In this type, the production and destruction of clotting factors and platelets is balanced called compensated DIC. Patients may have episodes of mild bleeding or ecchymosis. *Trousseau*'s syndrome is a chronic form of DIC. Chronic DIC is seen in patients with intrauterine fetal death, adenocarcinomas of various organs, vasculitis, aortic aneurysm and giant haemangioma.

HELLP syndrome (hemolysis, elevated liver enzymes, low platelets) is a severe form of DIC, carries high mortality, occurs in peripartum women.

There may be renal dysfunction also due to gross hemoglobinuria.

Investigations

The pathogenesis of laboratory findings is depicted in Fig. 62.3.

1. **Peripheral blood film examination:** It may show low platelets count, and schistocytes or fragmented RBCs that arise from cell trapping and damage within fibrin thrombi/polymerization.
2. **Platelet count** is reduced due to consumption of platelets. Malignancy-related DIC may have normal platelet count.
3. **PT and aPTT and TT** (thrombin time) are prolonged due to consumption coagulopathy (Fig. 61.3).
4. **Fibrinogen levels** are reduced due to depletion of coagulation proteins.
5. **Fibrin degradation products** (FDPs). They are increased due to intense secondary fibrinolysis.

6. **D-dimers are increased:** It is done by immunoassay and is more specific FDP assay. It is both specific and sensitive test.

7. **Reduction in protein C, antithrombin (AT):** Significant reduction in levels of protein C and antithrombin corrlate with DIC severity and its adverse outcome.

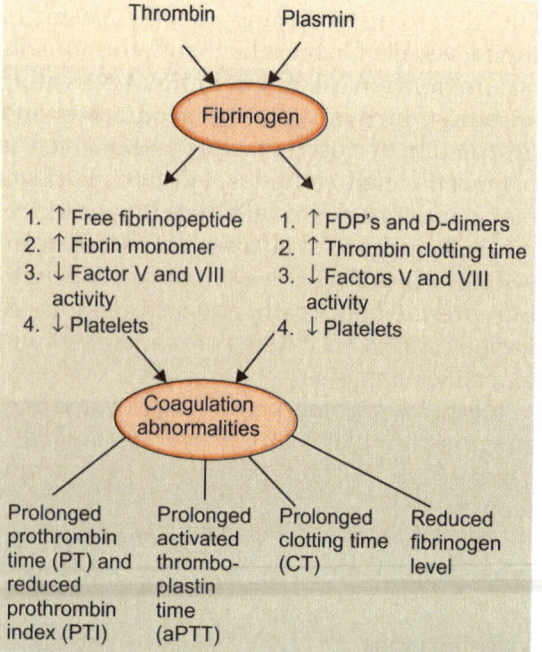

Fig. 62.3: Pathogenesis of laboratory changes in DIC. ↑ increase ↓ decrease

Management

Acute DIC is a life-threatening emergency, requires urgent treatment.

1. **General supportive care:** It means to support the circulation.
   - Tissue perfusion must be maintained by replacing intravenous fluids to combat shock.
   - Oxygen therapy to correct hypoxia.

2. **Correction of precipitating/underlying cause:** Specific measures to stop DIC will depend on its cause:
   - Appropriate antibiotic for sepsis along with supportive measures.
   - Termination of pregnancy for obstetric complications causing DIC is often necessary.
   - Anti-snake venom and other measure for snake bite.

3. **Replacement therapy (haemostatic support):** In DIC, there are low levels of platelets, coagulations factors and fibrinogen leading to thrombocytopenia, prolonged PT, APTT and TT. Replacement therapy in acute DIC aims to arrest bleeding by haemostatic support till the under lying/precipitating cause is corrected whenever possible. Replacement therapy is also indicated where some invasive procedure is required like insertion of a central line. The blood components to be transfused include:

   - *Fresh frozen plasma (FFP):* It contains all the clotting factors including fibrinogen, antithrombin III and protein C. The FFP is administered in the dose of 15–20 ml/kg and the coagulation times are checked. If correction is not adequate, repeat doses may be needed after 6–12 hours.

   - *Cryoprecipitate:* If FFP is not sufficient to replace fibrinogen and the fibrinogen levels are below 100 mg%, cryoprecipitate may be given in addition to FFP. Each unit of cryoprecipitate contains about 250 mg of fibrinogen. For an adult to 60–70 kg, with fibrinogen level <50 mg/dl, administration of 1.5 g fibrinogen (6 units of cryoprecipitate) should raise fibrinogen level to 100 mg/dl.

   - *Platelet concentrates:* 4 to 6 units (1 unit/10 kg of body weight) of platelet concentrates may be infused if platelet count is <50,000/ mm³. Coagulation time and platelet counts need to be monitored every 6–12 hours and further replacement given till there is clinical response (bleeding stops), and the haemostatic parameters (platelet count, fibrinogen levels, PT, APTT and TT) are maintained without replacement indicating recovery from DIC.

> *Monitor platelet count, PT, APTT fibrinogen level and FDPs after every few hours throughout the period of replacement therapy.*

Patients with asymptomatic DIC do not require replacement therapy unless a surgical procedure is planned.

4. **Role of heparin:** Heparin being an anti-coagulant, its use appear theoretically attractive to stop formation of thrombin in DIC, but actually it is not. For a patient who is actively bleeding, heparin would aggravate the bleeding before any potential benefits. In most of the typical situations of DIC (i.e. 95% of patients) heparin therapy has not been found useful in many controlled trials. The limited indications of heparin therapy in DIC are hypercoagu-able conditions, i.e.

   - Chronic DIC of malignancy (*Trousseau's syndrome*).
   - Hyperfibrinogenaemia with retained dead fetus prior to induction of labor.
   - In promyelocytic leukaemia (AML-M$_3$) prior to initiation of chemotherapy.
   - When patient does not demonstrate rise in platelet count and coagulation factor following replacement therapy and continues to bleed implying ongoing consumption.
   - Purpura fulminans.
   - The dose of heparin, if indicated, is 5–10 U/ kg/hour by continuous infusion or 300–500 U/hr. Low molecular heparin has been tried in chronic and acute DIC with beneficial effects.

5. **Role of antithrombin III:** In DIC, low levels of antithrombin III predict poor prognosis. High doses of antithrombin III (120–250 units/kg/day) for 2–3 days have been shown to have reversed DIC in one study; while most other studies have demonstrated improvement in coagulation profile and a shortened duration of DIC with the use of antithrombin III.

6. **Other therapies:**
   - Epsilon-amino caproic acid (EACA) and tranexamic acid are antifibrinolytic agents, are not used routinely as they may lead to serious thromboembolic complications for which concomitant heparin therapy is indicated. Occasionally, they are given along with replacement therapy and heparin in patients who continue to bleed to reduce fibrinolytic activity.
   - Protein C infusion prevents, DIC and has been used in the treatment of purpura fulminans associated with acquired protein C deficiency or meningococcaemia but this result has not been established, requires further study.
   - Gabexate mesylate (an inhibitor of serine proteases including thrombin and plasmin) has been tried in Japan with clinical and hematological improvement in DIC, but its clear advantage is yet to be reported.
   - An inhibitor of tissue factor activity, i.e. recombinant nematode anticoagulation protein C2 is being tried.
   - Currently a new therapeutic approach with recombinant human soluble thrombomodulin that binds thrombin is under-evaluation.

Agranulocytosis or Severe Neutropenia

AGRANULOCYTOSIS OR SEVERE NEUTROPENIA

Definition

Neutropenia is defined as circulatory neutrophil count below 1.5×10^9/L (<1500 cells/ L). The term *agranulocytosis* means a virtual absence of neutrophils, is used when neutropenia occurs as a reaction (immunologic) to drugs. This is an acute medical emergency characterised by high grade fever, sore throat and oral and/or perianal ulcers. Recovery is the rule if the offending drug is withdrawn and infection is prevented.

Consequences of Neutropenia

1. Neutropenia is mild when the count is between 1000 and 1500 cells/L and may have no consequence.
2. When neutrophil count falls below 1000 cells/L, the susceptibility to infections increases.
3. When the count is less than 500 cell/L, control of endogenous microflora (mouth, gut) is impaired and opportunistic infections become common.
4. When absolute count of neutrophils (band forms and mature neutrophils combined) falls below 100 cells/L, the inflammatory process is absent, needs aggressive treatment and immunisation against infection.

Causes

The causes of neutropenia are related to (i) *decreased production*, (ii) *ineffective granulocytopoiesis*, (iii) *increased destruction* and (iv) *excessive peripheral pooling*. The causes are given in Table 63.1. Hereditary neutropenias are rare, e.g. *Kostmann's syndrome* (count <100 neutrophils/L) is severe and often fatal. The *Schwachman's syndrome* is more benign associated with pancreatic insufficiency. The most common neutropenias are iatrogenic, i.e. autoimmune or drug induced (Box 1).

Box 1	Drug-induced neutropenia
Group	*Examples*
Anti-inflammatory agents	Phenylbutazone, gold, indomethacin, pencillamine, naproxen
Antithyroid drugs	Carbimazole, propylthiouracil
Antiarrhythmics	Quinidine, procainamide
Antihypertensives	Captopril, enalapril, nifedipine
Antidepressants/ psychotropics	Chlorpromazine, amitriptyline, dothiepin, mianserin
Antimalarials	Pyrimethamine, chloroquine
Anticonvulsants	Phenytoin, sodium valproate, carbamazepine
Antibiotics	Sulphonamide, penicillins, cephalosporins, chloramphenicol
Cytotoxic drugs	• Alkylating agents (nitrogen mustard, busulfan, chlorambucil, cyclophosphamide) • Antimetabolites (6-MP, methotrexate, 5-flucytosine)

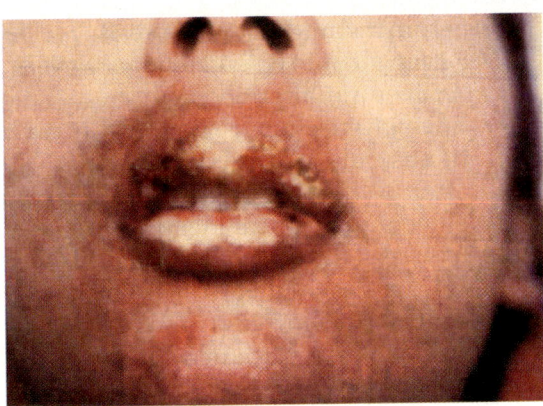

Fig. 63.1: A patient of agranulocytosis induced by drug; developed severe infection of the oral cavity with difficulty in swallowing and opening the mouth. Note redness, swelling and excoriation of lips and mucous membrane of oral cavity

Clinical Features

The manifestations depend on the degree of neutropenia. Bacterial infections are common. The onset may be acute or gradual. In acute and severe cases the conditions begin with upper respiratory tract infection, sore throat, throat and mouth ulcers (Fig. 63.1) and fever. The fever may be the only feature without any localising sign. Bacterial pneumonias, fungal infection of throat, erythroderma and GI infections are common. In severe neutropenia, septicaemia and shock may occur due to infection if immediate antibiotic therapy is not started.

Cyclic neutropenia characterised by malaise, fatigue, mouth ulcers occur in cyclic manner after every 2–3 weeks, can be diagnosed easily.

Table 62.1 Causes of neutropenia
1. Decreased production

A. Congenital
  • Kostmann's syndrome
  • Schwachmann-Diamond syndrome

B. Acquired
  • Drug induced (Box 1)
  • Chemicals, e.g. benzene
  • Infections (Box 2)
  • Acquired aplastic anaemia
  • Myelodysplastic syndrome
  • Acute leukaemia, hairy cell leukaemia
  • Malignant infiltration of marrow

2. Impaired or ineffective granulocytopoiesis
• Deficiency of folic acid and vitamin B_{12} • Drugs • Paroxysmal nocturnal haemoglobinuria
3. Peripheral destruction
• Antineutrophilic antibodies and/or splenic trapping • Autoimmune disorders, e.g. Felty's syndrome, rheumatoid arthritis, SLE • Drugs as hapten (incomplete antigen) • Hypersplenism
4. Miscellaneous
• Overwhelming bacterial infections • Haemodialysis • Cardiopulmonary bypass • Cyclic neutropenia

Evaluation of a Case with Neutropenia

- Patients with neutrophil count >1000 cells/L are mild cases without any significant abnormality on examination or laboratory testing, often recovers spontaneously within 2 weeks after stopping the offending agent and may not need further evaluation.

- Patients with neutrophil count <1000 cell/L should be investigated and treated urgently. In patients presenting with fever, sepsis, neutropenia, it is not always easy to decide whether the neutropenia is the result or the cause of infection. In such cases, a PBF examination revealing more than 20% 'band forms' indicates active bone marrow and neutropenia is the result of infection.

- History of fever, anaemia, mouth ulcers, lymphadenopathy, hepatosplenomegaly suggest acute leukaemia, could be confirmed on PBF examination.

- History of exposure to drugs and chemicals must be asked. Look for evidence of infection causing neutropenia (Box 2).

- Systemic examination for systemic disorders such as SLE, rheumatoid arthritis and Felty's syndrome must be carried out.

Box 2   Infections causing neutropenia
1. Viruses
• HIV
• Infectious mononucleosis
• Hepatitis
2. Rickettsiae
3. Gram-negative septicaemia, typhoid fever
4. Chronic infections
• Malaria
• Kala-azar
• Disseminated tuberculosis
• Visceral leishmaniasis

Investigations

The investigations are done to confirm the diagnosis, to assess its severity, to find out the cause and to differentiate *true* from pseudo-neutropenia.

1. **Peripheral blood film examination** (i.e. absolute neutrophils count) will confirm the diagnosis and determine the severity. Toxic granulation of neutrophils may be seen in neutropenia with septicaemia (Fig. 63.2).
2. **Bone marrow examination:** It is done see the bone marrow activity in patients with severe neutropenia without any cause, e.g. viral fever or drugs.
3. **Other investigations** are cause-specific:
   - Antinuclear antibodies.
   - Rheumatoid factor.

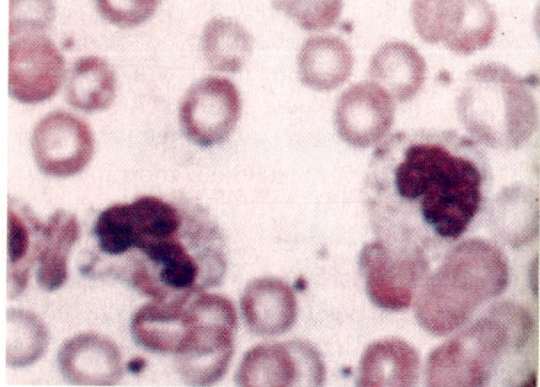

Fig. 63.2: In infection or toxic states, neutrophils have azurophilic granules (see the dark staining cytoplastic granules—toxic granules)

- Serum immunoelectrophoresis.
- Serum vitamin B_{12} and folic acid levels.
- Antineutrophil antibodies.
- Epinephrine mobilisation test [increase in absolute neutrophil count (ANC) after 30 minutes of 0.3 ml of 1:1000 epinephrine subcutaneously] is useful to assess the risk of infection. It also helps to differentiate true from pseudo-neutropenia. Increase in ANC to > 2000 cells/L is an indicator of good neutrophil reserve.

Management

1. **General measures:** Severely neutropenic patients are highly prone to endogenous and hospital-acquired infections. The patients with severe neutropenia need hospitalisation with following supportive measures, to be adopted to prevent infection:

   i. Good hand-washing practices by hospital personnel, attendants and relatives.

   ii. Isolation of patient. No attendant or personnel with an evidence of infection should be allowed to visit such patients.

   iii. Skin cleansing properly especially at orifices. Clean oral cavity and teeth frequently to avoid infection.

   iv. Avoid intramuscular injection. Aseptic technique to be adopted for I.V. access.

   v. Avoid fruits, uncooked vegetable and salads. Sterile food (irradiated or pressure cooked) should be given.

2. **Treatment of infection:** Antibiotic should not be used prophylactically because of emergence of resistant strains. Attempts should be made to localise the infection and to identify the causative organism. Therefore, culture of throat secretions, urine, sputum and blood should be sent immediately. X-ray chest may also be got done. These patients should be

given a combination of 2 or 3 broad-spectrum bactericidal antibiotics such as an aminoglycoside plus broad-spectrum penicillin *plus* cephalosporine (e.g. cefepime 2 g I.V. every 8 hourly) in case there is an evidence of infection or fever. If fever does not subside despite adequate antibiotic cover, amphotericin B or voriconazole or fluconazole is given on empirical basis. Antibiotic therapy in such patients is guided by culture and sensitivity reports. Antibiotics should be continued at least 5 days after the patient becomes afebrile.

3. **Treatment of neutropenia:** The final outcome of neutropenic patients depends on the effective management of underlying cause. The use of recombinant hematopoietic colony-stimulating factor (CSF) such as granulocyte colony-stimulating factor (filgrastin) have been successfully used to correct neutropenia associated with massive chemotherapy or radiotherapy. They may also be useful for other hypoplastic neutropenias. Other cytokines such as interleukin 3 (IL-3) and stem cell factor have been reported to act synergistically with G-CSF / GM-CSF.

Androgens are not effective in raising neutrophil counts. Prednisolone may be useful in raising the neutrophil count in autoimmune neutropenia.

4. **Treatment of underlying cause:** Transient neutropenia or agranulocytosis as a reaction to drugs is reversible if offending drug or chemical is withdrawn. If neutropenia is associated with systemic disorder, the treatment of systemic illness / disorder must be given simultaneously. In Felty syndrome with severe bacterial infection not responding to antibiotics, splenectomy may be attempted.

Aplastic Anaemia

APLASTIC ANAEMIA

Definition

Aplastic anaemia is defined as pancytopenia with hypocellularity (aplasia) of the bone marrow. **Hypocellularity** distinguishes true bone marrow failure (aplastic anaemia) from myelodysplastic syndromes where peripheral cytopenia is associated with **hypercellular marrow with dysplastic changes**. In some conditions, only one or two cell lines may be affected.

It is an uncommon condition that may be *inherited* but is more commonly *acquired*.

Mechanisms

Aplastic anaemia is due to a reduction in the number of pleuripotent stem cells pool to ≤1% of normal together with a fault in those remaining cells, or is acquired due to an immune reaction (T cell activation and cytokine production) against stem cells so that they are unable to repopulate the bone marrow. Failure of one cell line may occur resulting in isolated deficiency such as the absence of red cell precursors in **pure red cell aplasia**. An intrinsic stem cell defect exists for constitutional aplastic anaemia as cells from patients with Fanconi's anaemia exhibit chromosomal damage and death on exposure to certain chemical agents.

Causes

The cause of aplastic anaemia are given in Box 1. The exact way by which aplastic anaemia is produced by various agents is unknown. Genetic factors play a role. Immunological mechanisms play a dominant role.

Damage to haemopoietic stem cell occurs in two ways:
1. Damage to DNA (irradiation, busulphan, benzene and chloramphenicol).
2. Damage to cell membrane affecting metabolic machinery (viruses, most drugs, immune mediated). Most cases of idiopathic acquired haemolytic anaemia belong to this group. In primary (auto-immune) aplastic anaemia, there is autoimmune suppression of hematopoiesis by a T cell-mediated cellular mechanism. In some cases, defects in the stem cell telomere length have been identified.

Clinical Features

The onset of aplastic anaemia is usually insidious. The most common presenting features are due to:
- Anaemia.
- Thrombocytopenia.
- Neutropenia.
  1. **Symptoms and signs of anaemia:** The symptoms include pallor weakness, fatigue, breathlessness on exertion. There

1. Inherited

- Fanconi's anaemia
- Diamond-Blackfen syndrome
- Reticular dysgenesis (dyskeratosis congenita)

2. Acquired

A. Idiopathic (primary) probably autoimmune

B. Secondary

  i. *Diseases*, e.g. SLE

  ii. *Drugs* (direct cytotoxicity, idiosyncratic reactions)

- Cytotoxic drugs e.g. alkylating agents, antimetabolities etc.
- Antibiotics, e.g. sulphonamides, chloramphenicol
- Antirheudatic drugs, e.g. pencillamine, gold, phenylbutazone, indomethacin, ibuprofen
- Antithyroid drugs
- Anticonvulsants (hydantoins, carbamazepine etc.)
- Immunosuppressants, e.g. azathioprine, busulphan, cyclophosphamide, chlorambucil, vinblastine, 6-mercaptopurine

  iii. *Chemicals*

- Heavy metals e.g. gold, arsenic, bismuth, mercury
- Industrial solvents
- Benzene-containing solvents, e.g. kerosene, carbontetrachloride
- Insecticide, e.g. organophosphorus, carbamates, DDT (chlorinated hydrocarbon)

  iv. *Irradiation*

- Ionising radiation (radiodiagnosis, radiotherapy, nuclear power station)

  v. *Viruses*

- Hepatitis viruses (post-hepatitis)
- Epstein-Barr viruses, parvovirus B$_{19}$ (aplastic crisis)
- HIV

  vi. *Pregnancy*

  vii. *Paroxysmal nocturnal haemoglobinuria*

hepatosplenomegaly and lymphadenopathy are absent.

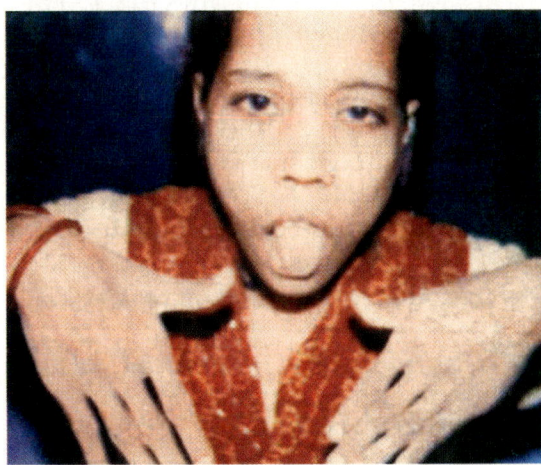

Fig. 64.1: Aplastic anaemia . The patient complained of tachycardia, fatigue and dyspnoea. Note the generalised pallor

2. **Symptoms and signs of thrombocytopenia:** Thrombocytopenia produces bleeding from the skin (petechiae, ecchymosis), nose (epistaxis), gums (gum bleeding), vagina (menorrhagia) or gastrointestinal (haematemesis or malena). There may be conjunctival haemorrhages.

3. **Symptoms and signs due to neutropenia:** Neutropenia predisposes to severe bacterial infection. Sometimes, infection may be presenting feature and fever may be the only symptom without any localising sign. Bacterial and fungal infections of the throat, pneumonias, erythroderma and gastrointestinal infections occur commonly.

4. **Café au lait spots and short stature suggest Fanconi's anaemia;** peculiar nails and leukoplakia suggest *dyskeratosis congenita*.

Investigations

i. **Pancytopenia** with normocytic normochromic blood picture is the hallmark. Often, there may be macrocytosis. However, early in the evolution of aplastic anaemia, only one or two cell lines may

is generalised pallor (Fig. 64.1). If anaemia is severe, tachycardia and murmurs associated with high flow rates (haemic munnurs) may be present. It is hereby stressed that in spite of severe anaemia,

be reduced. The presence of immature myeloid forms suggest leukaemia or myelodysplastic syndrome (MDS)

ii. **Reticulocytopenia** or virtual absence of reticulocytes.

iii. **Bone marrow (aspirate or biopsy) examination** (Fig. 64.2). There is hypocellular or aplastic bone marrow with increased fat spaces (Fig. 64.3). Sometimes, bone marrow tap may be dry.

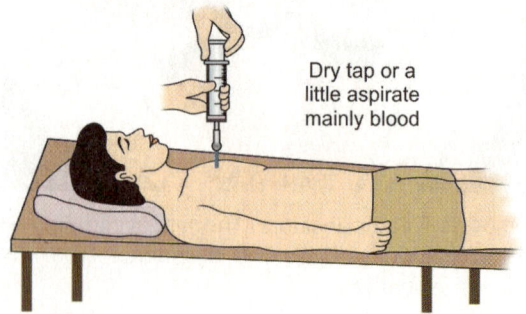

Dry tap or a little aspirate mainly blood

Fig. 64.2: Bone marrow aspiration may show dry tap

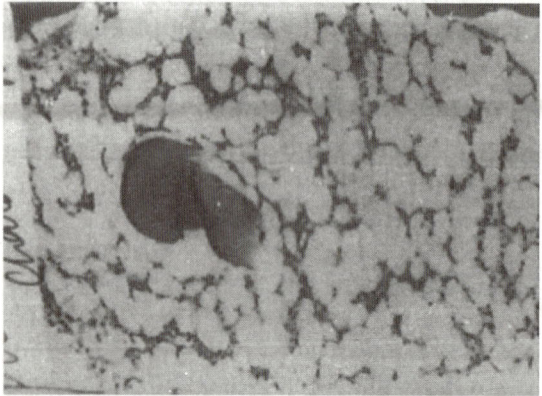

Fig. 64.3: Bone marrow examination showing only few cells and increased fat spaces (hypocellular marrow)

iv. **Marrow cytogenic studies** distinguish aplastic anaemia from myelodysplastic syndrome and Fanconi's anaemia. In acquired aplastic anaemia, no cytogenic abnormalities are seen.

v. **Screening for paroxysmal nocturnal haemoglobinuria** (haemtest, flowcytometric assays, sucrose lysis test and urinary hemosiderin) should be done at the time of diagnosis and periodically during therapy and follow up as many cases develop PNH specially after immunosuppressive therapy,

vi. **Serological screen for hepatitis virus** (A, B and C) and HLA typing for prospective bone marrow transplantation. Posthepatitis aplastic anaemia is seronegative.

vii. **MRI scan** helps to assess fat content and distinguishes aplasia from MDS.

Severe aplastic anaemia is characterised by

i. Absolute neutrophil count< 500/L
ii. Platelet count <20,000/L
iii. Reticulocyte count <1% and
iv. Bone marrow cellularity <25%

Differential Diagnosis

Aplastic anaemia should be differentiated from other conditions producing pancytopenia such as:

1. Subleukaemic or aleukaemic leukaemia.
2. Myelodysplastic syndrome (MDS).
3. Hypersplenism (e.g. portal hypertension, infiltrative splenomegaly).
4. Bone marrow infiltration (carcinoma, myelofibrosis).
5. Megaloblastic anaemia.
6. Osteopetrosis (Marble bone disease).
7. Systemic lupus erythematosus.
8. Paroxysmal nocturnal haemoglobinuria (PNH).
9. Disseminated tuberculosis .
10. Overwhelming infection.

Management

Mild aplastic anaemia improves with stoppage of an offending agent and supportive therapy. The aim of treatment for severe aplastic anaemia is to restore normal bone marrow function . To achieve this, good supportive care followed by definite therapy are essential.

l. **Withdrawal of the aetiologic agent** or treatment of underlying condition is the most direct approach to the management of aplastic anaemia. Discontinuation of a suspected drug, thymectomy in patients with thymoma, or delivery or therapeutic abortion in patients with pregnancy associated aplastic anaemia may result in recovery of the blood counts. Unfortunately, these cases are very small in number.

2. **Supportive therapy**
   - *Treatment of anaemia and bleeding:* Once the diagnosis of aplastic anaemia is made, blood transfusions are necessary to raise the haemoglobin and blood counts. Transfusions of blood products from family members should be avoided in prospective transplant candidates to prevent sensitization to minor histocompatibility antigens which increase the risk of graft rejection after transplantation. Wherever possible, only CMV negative blood products should be given to CMV—seronegative potential transplant candidates to reduce incidence of CMV infection in post-transplant period.

     Platelet transfusions should be given only when the platelet count is <10,000/ml or if there is active bleeding. If feasible single donor platelet with HLA matched platelets are preferred to minimise the risk of sensitization especially in prospective bone marrow transplant candidates. Antiplatelets and NSAIDs should be avoided. Menstruation may be suppressed either by oral oestrogens or FSH/LH and antagonists given nasally.

     Packed red cells also should be transfused when the haemoglobin level is <7 g/dl. Packed red cells should be filtered to remove leukocytes and platelets to reduce sensitization. Chronic administration of red cell transfusions results in secondary haemochromatosis, as each unit has approximately 200 to 250 mg of iron. Serum ferritin levels should be monitored, and chelation therapy with desferoxamine should be given to reduce iron overload.

   - *Treatment of infection/sepsis:* Patients with aplastic anaemia who develop sepsis or any other severe bacterial infections require intensive parenteral antibiotic therapy. Hence in febrile neutropenia (absolute neutrophil count <0.5 per 10^9/L), prompt institution of appropriate antibiotic cover is of paramount importance. Usually, a third generation cephalo sporins or a newer penicillin along with an aminoglycoside is the initial therapy. When indwelling catheters become contaminated vancomycin may be added. However, if fever persists, antifungals are added as *aspergillosis* and *candidiasis* are common in these patients. Herpetic lesions need intravenous acyclovir. Prophylactic use of antibiotics in a febrile neutropenic patients has no benefit and predisposes to the emergence of resistant strains.

2. **Immunosuppressive agent:** In most of the cases the possible aetiological mechanism could be autoimmune. In the absence of a compatible donor, immunosuppressive therapy offers a 50 to 75% chance of long term survival. Two important drugs used in combination or sequentially are antilymphocyte globulin (ALG) or antithymocyte globulin (ATG) and cyclosporine. It is preferred mode of therapy in patients of severe aplastic anaemia (i.e. pancytopenia with neutrophils < 0.5 per 10^9/L, platelets < 20 per 10^9/L) who are older than 20 years of age and also in patients with very severe aplastic anaemia (neutrophil count <0.2 per/10^9/L) and who are less than 20 years of age but have no bone marrow donor. The effects of ALG/ATG manifests within 2–3 months after administration. The dose of equine ATG is 40 mg/kg/day I.V. for 4 days. Rabbit ATG is more immunosuppressive than equine ATG. Steroids (prednisolone 1–2 mg/kg/day) are given for 7–10 days along with ATG as prophylaxis for serum sickness. Platelet transfusions are required during ATG infusion as

they can produce thrombocytopenia with bleeding.

Side-effects of ATG therapy include, anaphylaxis, serum sickness, haemolysis, thrombocytopenia, leucopenia, infections, etc.

Combined therapy with ATG and cyclosporine induces higher and earlier response as compared to ALG/ATG alone, particularly in patients with very severe aplastic anaemia. The dose of cyclosporine initially is 12 mg/kg/day orally in adults with subsequent adjustment according to blood levels (150–200 mg/ml). Side-effects include hypertension, gum hypertrophy, hepatotoxicity, hyperkalaemia, hypertrichosis, seizures, infections and malignancies.

Role of androgens. There is no role of *glucocorticoids* and *androgens* as primary form of therapy in aplastic anaemia. However, in mild aplastic anaemia, androgens, i.e. oxymetholone 2–3 mg/kg orally daily may be useful in improving cytopenias. However, short courses of steroids are employed as a prophylaxis against serum sickness during ATG therapy.

4. **Haematopoietic growth factors (HGF):** Recombinant haematopoietic growth factors, i.e. erythropoietin, granulocyte-colony stimulating factor (G-CSF), granulocyte macrophage colony stimulating factor (GM-CSF), interleukins (ILS) 1, 3 and 6 and stem cell factor can improve the blood counts, in only a small number of patients. In patients who respond, blood count drops to pretreatment values following discontinuation of growth factors. Therefore, their use particularly G-CSF (filgrastim) following intensive immunosuppression with ATG and cyclosporine has been controversial. It does not clearly speed up granulocyte recovery and perhaps increases the risk of progression later to myelodysplastic syndrome or to AML.

5. **Bone marrow transplantation (haemopoietic stem cell transplantation):** Transplantation from an HLA compatible sibling donor is a definite first line and curative treatment for aplastic anaemia. The recommendations for bone marrow transplantation are clear for children, adolescents and young. However, opinion is divided regarding BMT in older adults even if a sibling donor is available as results of immunosuppressive therapy (IST) and BMT are comparable. Current survival rates achievable with allogeneic BMT (70–90%) reflect improvement in post-transplant management. High dose cyclophosphamide with ATG for pretransplant immunosuppression and cyclosporine prophylaxis for graft versus host disease (GVHD) after transplantation has markedly reduced the incidence of graft failure and GVHD and has significantly improved long-term survival (90% at 2 years after transplantation). Most patients do not have a suitable sibling donor. Occasionally, a full phenotypic match found within the family may serve as well. Alternate donors are either unrelated but HLA-matched volunteers or closely but not perfectly matched family members. Survival with alternative donor is about half that of conventional sibling donor. In transplant candidate, blood transfusion from a family member should be avoided.

Newer Therapeutic Options

Alemtuzumab is an anti-CD52 monoclonal antibody act against the antigen present on the lymphocytes and other hemopoietic stem cells. This has been tried in patients refractory to immunosuppressive therapy in certain clinical trials and found it useful in prolonging the survival.

Acute Leukaemias

ACUTE LEUKAEMIAS

Definition

Acute leukaemias are malignant proliferation of lymphoid or myeloid precursor cells resulting in accumulation of blast cells (>25% of the marrow cells are blast cells) in the bone marrow with subsequent replacement of normal haematopoiesis. Extra-marrow infiltration involves lymph nodes (lymphadenopathy), spleen (splenomegaly), liver (hepatomegaly) or other organs. Acute lympho blastic leukaemia is a disease of childhood whereas acute myeloid leukaemia (AML) is most frequently seen in adults.

Aetiology

The exact aetiology is unknown. No single cause can be pinpointed in acute leukaemia. The factors that predispose to leukaemias are given in the Box 1.

Terminology and Classification

The terms 'acute' and 'chronic' reflect the speed of evolution of the disease. In acute leukaemia, the history is usually short and life expectancy without treatment is also short. In chronic leukaemia, the patient remains unwell for months and survival usually extends over years.

Acute leukaemias are classified into:

1. Acute lymphoblastic leukaemia (ALL).
2. Acute myeloblastic leukaemia (AML).

Subclassification of acute lymphoblastic and acute myeloblastic leukaemia is given in Tables 65.1 and 65.2. The WHO has modified FAB classification of acute myeloid leukaemia by reducing the number of blasts required for diagnosis from 30 to 20% and incorporated

Box 1	Factors associated with leukaemias

1. Genetic predisposition
- Increased incidence of leukaemia in identical twins of patients with leukaemia
- Increased incidence occurs in Down's syndrome, Bloom's syndrome, ataxia telengiectasia and others.

2. Retrovirus
- Adults T cell leukaemia/lymphoma (HTLV-1)

3. Cytotoxic drugs
- Chlorambucil, cyclophosphamide, melphalan
- Procarbazine, etoposide

4. Ionising radiation
- A significant exposure to atomic radiation
- Following therapeutic radiotherapy and diagnostic radiographs of the fetus in pregnancy

5. Exposure to benzene and aromatic hydrocarbons in industry

6. Immune deficiency states
- Hypogammaglobulinaemia

Table 65.1	Subclassification of acute lymphoblastic leukaemia	
Immunological	*% of cases*	*FAB subtype*
Pre-B ALL	75 (most common)	L1, L2
T cell ALL	20 (uncommon)	L1, L2
B cell ALL	5 (rare)	L3

molecular, morphologic and clinical features (Table 65.3).

Pathogenesis and Clinical Features

Acute leukaemia (Fig. 85.1) presents with symptoms and signs of short duration (days to months). The symptoms and signs result from:

1. **Expansion of leukaemic cells at the expense of normal haematopoietic cells** leading to anaemia; thrombocytopenia and granulocytopenia in various combinations.
2. **Infiltration of leukaemic cells** into other organs i.e. liver, spleen, mediastinum, CNS, soft tissue and testis.
3. **Expansion of the leukaemic mass within marrow** of bones leads to bone pain and sternal tenderness.

4. **DIC with bleeding** may occur with acute promyelocytic leukaemia (AML-M3).
5. **Gum hypertrophy and leukaemia cutis** are characteristic of acute monocytic leukaemia (AML-M$_4$/M$_5$).

The symptoms and signs of acute leukaemia are depicted in Box 2.

Investigations

1. **Total WBC** count is elevated, can be as high as 1,00,000/mm³ or more. It can be normal or low (pancytopenia) in about

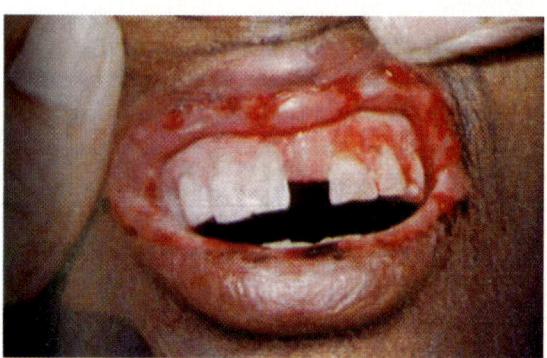

Fig. 65.1: Gum bleeding due to acute leukaemia

Table 65.2	FAB classification of acute myeloid leukaemia (AML)			Cytochemistry *(staining)*		
Subtype	*FAB type*	*Frequency(%)*	*Morphology*	*MPO*	*SB*	*NSE*
AML minimally differentiated	M 0	3–5	No azurophil granules	(–)	(–)	(–)
AML without maturation	M 1	15–20	A few azurophilic granules or Auer rods	(±)	(±)	(–)
AML with maturation	M 2	25–30	Azurophilic granules, Auer rods are often present	(++)	(++)	(–)
Acute premyelocytic leukaemia	M 3	5	Hypergranular promyelocytes, Auer rods	(+++)	(+++)	(–)
Acute myelo-monocytic leukaemia	M 4	20–25	≥20% monocytic blasts and granulocytic blasts	(++)	(++)	(++)
Acute monocytic leukaemia	M 5	5	• Monoblastic (M5A) • Promonocytic (M5B)	(±)	(–)	(++)
Acute erythro-leukaemia	M 6	5	• Erythroblasts >50% of nucleated cells • Myeloblasts >30% of non-erythroid cells	(±)	(–)	(–)
Acute megakaryocytic leukaemia	M 7	10	• Megakaryoblasts >30% of all nucleated cells • 'Dry' aspirate; biopsy is done	(–)	(–)	(–)

50% of cases. The peripheral blood film shows blast cells and other primitive cells (Fig. 65.2). Blast cells may be absent in 10% cases (*aleukemic leukemia*).

Table 65.3 WHO classification of AML

i. AML with recurrent cytogenetic translocations
AML with t(8;21) (q22;q22); *AML1 (CBFα)/ETO*
Acute promyelocytic leukemia [AML with t(15;17) (q22;q12) and variants; PML/RARα]
AML with abnormal bone marrow eosinophils [inv (16) (p13;q22) or t(16;16) (p13;q22) CBFβ/MYH1]
AML with 11q23 (*MLL*) abnormalities
ii. AML with multilineage dysplasia
With prior myelodysplastic syndrome
Without prior myelodysplastic syndrome
iii. AML and myelodysplastic syndrome, therapy-related
Alkylating agent-related
Topoisomerase type II-related
Other types
iv. AML not otherwise categorized
AML minimally differentiated
AML without maturation
AML with maturation
Acute myelomonocytic leukaemia
Acute monocytic leukaemia
Acute erythroid leukaemia
Acute megakaryocytic leukaemia
Acute basophilic leukaemia
Acute panmyelosis with myelofibrosis
Myeloid sarcoma

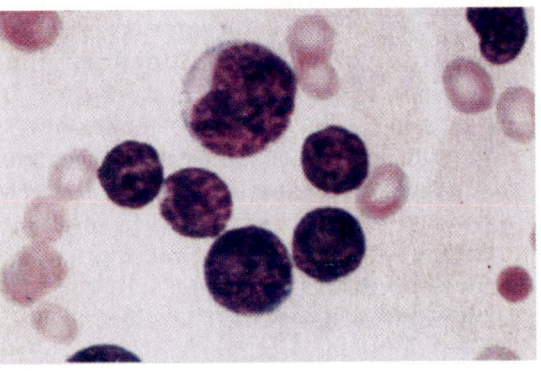

Fig. 65.2: Leukaemic cells in acute lymphoblastic leukaemia characterised by round or convoluted nuclei, high nuclear/cytoplasmic ratio and absence of cytoplasmic granules in peripheral blood

2. **The haemoglobin is low (anaemia)** and the platelet count is decreased (thrombo cytopenia).

3. **Bone marrow** aspiration is done to confirm the diagnosis. The marrow is hypercellular with replacement of marrow elements by leukaemic blast cells in varying numbers. For diagnosis of acute leukaemia, bone marrow must show 25 to 30% blasts cells (>25%). It is also essential to confirm the complete remission and relapse following treatment. In addition to morphological evaluation (presence of auer nodes is pathognomonic of AML), the cells are also

Box 2	Symptoms and signs of acute leukaemia	
Presentation	*Symptoms*	*Signs*
Anaemia	Tiredness, weakness, exertional dyspnoea, anorexia, weight loss	Pallor, tachycardia, tachypnoea, murmurs, good volume pulse
Thrombo-cytopenia	Easy bruising, gum bleeding (Fig. 64.1) epistaxis, malena (GI haemorrhage), visual disturbance	Ecchymosis, purpura, mucosal bleeding, retinal haemorrhage
Granulo-cytopenia	Fever, sore throat, respiratory infection (pneumonia), cellulitis, stomatitis	Signs of infection (sore throat or mouth ulcers) Signs of respiratory infection (pneumonia) Peri-rectal abscess, fungal infections
Leukaemic infiltration	Dragging pain in abdomen due to masses Infiltration in skin, soft tissue	Lymph node enlargement, gum hypertrophy Liver and/or spleen enlargement Sternal tenderness, bone pain The mass lesion present as a tumour of leukaemic cells (granulocytic sarcoma or chloromas)
CNS involve-ment	Headache, vomiting, convulsions	Papilloedema Intracranial bleed with localising or diffuse signs

subjected to flow cytochemistry, electron microscopy, immunophenotyping, cytogenetics and molecular studies. In general, ALL blasts cells are smaller, have a thin rim of cytoplasm and are Tdt-positive. AML blast cells are larger, have discrete chromatin granules, multiple nucleoli and auer rods. They are Sudan black and myeloperoxidase positive.

4. **Immunophenotyping:** The recent development of monoclonal antibodies as well as advances in flow cytometry has made immunophenotyping readily available (Table 65.4). It is useful in:

Table 65.4	Immunophenotyping in acute leukaemia
Subtype	Flow cytometry/monoclonal antibodies
ALL	
T cell	CD4 (helper)/CD8 (suppressor)
B cell	CD 19 (B4)/CD 20 (B1)/CD 22 (surface)
Pre-B	CD9
CALLA	CD 10
AML	
M1, M2, M3	CD13 or CD33
M4, M5	CD11 or 13 or 14 or 15 or CD33
M6	Glycoprotein, spectrin
M7	CD41 (glycoprotein IIb/IIIa)/CD43

- Definite lineage (B cell versus T cell) and stages of differentiation of ALL and identifying characteristic features of AML.
- Aiding in lineage determination of acute leukaemias that are morphologically undifferentiated.
- In differentiating acute leukaemia from other non-hematological disorders.
- Recognizing mixed lineage/biphenotypic acute leukaemia (ALL with myeloid markers or AML with lymphoid markers).

5. **Chromosomal abnormalities:** Three major techniques of molecular analysis such as southern blot analysis (commonly used), the PCR and fluorescent *in situ* hybridization demonstrate chromosomal abnormalities inherent in leukaemic cells (Table 65.5).

6. **LDH, uric acid and alkaline phosphatase:** Levels in the blood are elevated in acute leukaemia due to rapid turnover of the cells.

Table 65.5	Chromosomal abnormalities and onco-genes in acute leukaemia involved	
Type	Chromosomal aberration	Involved
1. **ALL**		?MLL
• Early B type	t (4: 11)	BCR-ABL
• Common ALL type	t (4: 19)	
• Pre-B	t (I: 19)	IGH-IL3
• B-ALL	t (8:14)	IGH-MYC
2. **AML**		
• M2	t (8:21)	
• M3	t (15:17)	PML-RAR a.
• M4	inv 16	
• M5	t(9:II), IIq23	
• M6	del (7q) and del (5q)	
• M7	t(I2:21)	
	trisomy 21	

7. **Coagulation profile** may show features of thrombocytopenia or DIG in AML-M3.

8. **CSF examination:** It is mandatory in all patients of ALL to evaluate CNS involvement at presentation and during follow-up.

9. **X-ray chest:** It may show a mediastinal mass in T cell ALL.

10. **Renal function,** e.g. urea and creatinine.

11. **Viral serology** (CMV, HSV-1, varicella).

12. **HLA typing** of the patient, siblings and parents for potential allogenic BMT.

Management

I. Specific combination chemotherapy.

II. Supportive therapy.

The first decision in management of acute leukaemia must be whether or not to give specific therapy because it is generally aggressive and has many side-effects. It may not be appropriate for the very elderly or patients with other disorders to use aggressive chemo-therapy. In these patients, only supportive therapy is sufficient. The general strategy for acute leukaemia is given in Fig. 65.3.

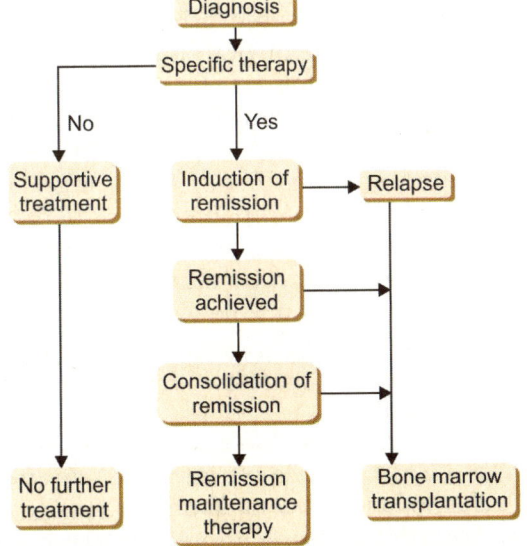

Fig. 65.3: Treatment plan in acute leukaemia

I. Specific Combination Chemotherapy

The aim of treatment is to achieve complete remission by destroying the leukaemic clones of cells without destroying the residual normal stem cell components from which repopula-tion of hemopoietic tissues will occur to restore normal hemopoiesis.

Complete remission is defined as blood neurophils ≥1500/L and platelets count ≥1,00,000/L with no blasts in peripheral blood film. Bone marrow cellularity should be >20% with trilineage maturation and should contain <5% blasts.

Once decision to give it has been taken, the patient should be prepared for it as follows:

1. Existing infections identified and treated such as UTI, oral candidiasis, dental, gingival and skin infections.
2. Anaemia corrected by blood transfusions or red cells concentrate infusions.
3. Thrombocytopenia controlled with platelet transfusions.

4. If possible, insert central venous line for delivery of chemotherapy.
5. Therapeutic regimen should be explained to the patient for compliance.

Steps of therapy

1. *Remission induction phase:* It means to reduce the leukaemic cells below the level of morphologic detection. This is achieved by combination chemotherapy. During this phase, patient goes through a period of severe bone marrow hypoplasia requiring intensive support, and in-hospital care.
2. *Remission consolidation phase:* If remission has been achieved by induction therapy, residual leukaemic tissue is destroyed by therapy during the consolidation phase. This consists of a number of courses of combination chemotherapy again resulting in periods of marrow hypoplasia.
3. *Remission maintenance phase:* Maintenance therapy generally not indicated in AML. If the patient of ALL remains in remission after consolidation phase, then low dose oral therapy is given for 18 months to 2 years as maintenance therapy. If relapse does not occur, then it is discontinued thereafter and patient is observed.

Cranial irradiation and intrathecal methotrexate is necessary for CNS prophylaxis in ALL to prevent CNS relapse. The drugs most commonly employed for two main varieties of acute leukaemia are listed in Box 3.

If a patient fails to go into remission with induction treatment, alternative drug combinations can be tried but outlook of such patients is poor unless they undergo allogeneic stem cell transplant.

The most commonly used intensive treatment protocol (MCP-841) for ALL in children is given in Table 65.6.

II. Supportive Therapy

Adequate supportive therapy is needed during or following aggressive chemotherapy:

Box 3	Drugs regimes in different phases of acute leukaemias	
Phase	**ALL**	**AML**
Induction	• Vincristine (I.V.)	Daunoru-bicin (I.V.)
	• Prednisolone (oral)	Cytarabin (I.V.)
	• L-asparaginase (I.V.)	Etoposide (I.V.) or oral)
	• Daunorubicin (I.V.)	Thioguanine (oral)
	• Methotrexate (intrathecal)	
Consolidation	Daunorubicin (I.V.)	Cytarabin (I.V.)
	Cytarabin (I.V.)	Amsacrine (I.V.)
	Etoposide (I.V.)	Mitozantrone (I.V.)
	Methotrexate (I.V.)	
Maintenance	Prednisolone (oral)	Not reco-mmended
	Vincristine (I.V.)	
	Mercaptopurine (oral)	
	Methotrexate (oral)	

i. *Anaemia* is treated with red cell concentrate to raise haemoglobin above 10 g/dl.

ii. *Thrombocytopenia:* Bleeding due to thrombocytopenia is treated by platelet transfusions to maintain the count above $10 \times 10^9/L$. Coagulation abnormalities, if occur, should be appropriately treated.

iii. *Infection:* Fever (>38°C) lasting over 1 hour in a neutropenic patient (neutrophil count <1 × $10^9/L$) indicates possible septicaemia. Parenteral antibiotic (broad-spectrum) therapy including a combination of an aminoglycoside (e.g. gentamicin) with a broad-spectrum penicillin (e.g. piperacillin/tazobactum) or a fourth generation cephalosporine having antipseudomonas activity, (e.g. cefepime) is used on empirical basis. This combination is best bactericidal and should be continued for 5 days after fever has subsided. This therapy covers both gram-positive (*Staph. aureus* and *Staph. epidermidis*) and gram-negative (*E. coli*, Pseudomonas, Klebsiella) organisms

that are likely to be involved in infection in a neutro penic patient. Patients with lymphoblastic leukaemia are prone to develop pneumonia due to *Pneumocystis carinii* which responds to cotrimoxazole.

Fluconazole is used for both prophylaxis and treatment of oral and pharyngeal monilial infection.

For systemic fungal infection (candi-diasis or aspergillosis), intravenous amphotericin is used (0.5–1 mg/day for 3 weeks) . Amphotericin is hepatic and renal toxic, hence, renal and hepatic functions should be monitored during therapy. Voriconozole is less toxic than amphotericin.

Herpes simplex infection is treated with acyclovir.

Clinical trials have used both G-CSF and GM-CSF to lower infection rate after chemotherapy but not found successful.

iv. *Adequate hydration* with oral or intravenous fluids must be maintained because most of these patients are severely anorexia.

v. *Administration of allopurinol* (a xanthine oxidase inhibitor) to treat and prevent hyperuricaemia.

vi. *Metabolic abnormalities:* In certain types of leukaemias where the rate of cell division is rapid, e.g. B type ALL, T type ALL, patients may develop *tumour lysis syndrome char acterised by hypercalcaemia, high level of phosphates and hyperkalaemia* resulting from a high rate of cellular breakdown. This is a potential life-threatening situation and difficult to treat once it develops. It can be prevented by adequate hydration during chemotherapy if uric acid levels are high. Dialysis may be required in certain cases. Therefore, during chemotherapy to leukaemia, electrolytes and uric acid should be monitored.

Bone Marrow Transplantation (BMT)/Stem Cell Transplantation

The bone marrow or stem cell transplantation is done with a hope of 'cure' in acute leukaemia.

Table 65.6 MCP-841 protocol for ALL in children		
Drug	*Dose*	*Days*
L-asparaginase	6000 U/m²	2, 4, 6, 8, 10, 12, 14, 16, 18, 20 (alternate day therapy)
Vincristine	1.4 mg/m²	1, 8, 15, 22, 28 (weekly therapy)
Daunomycin (dauno-rubicin)	30 mg/m²	8, 15, 28
Prednisolone	40 mg/m²	1 to 28 (daily)
Intrathecal methotrexate	12 mg	1, 8, 15, 22, 28
Induction-2 (month 2)		
Cyclophosphamide	750 mg/m²	1, 15
6-mercaptopurine	75 mg/m²	Days 1 to 7, 15 to 22
Intrathecal methotrexate	12 mg	1, 8, 15, 22
Cranial radiotherapy	1200 cGy	Days 5 to 15
Consolidation combination chemotherapy phase (month 4)		
Vincristine	1.4 mg/m²	1, 15
Cyclophosphamide	750 mg/m²	1
Daunomycin (Daunorubicin)	30 mg/m²	15
Cytosar (cytosine-arabinoside)	100 mg/m²	1, 2, 3 and 15, 16, 17
6-mercaptopurine	750 mg/m²	1 to 8 and 15 to 22
Maintenance chemotherapy phase (3 monthly cyclic therapy for 6 cycles)		
L-asparaginase	6000 U/m²	1, 3, 5, 7
Vincristine	1.4 mg/m²	1
Daunorubicin (Daunomycin)	30 mg/m²	1
Prednisolone	40 mg/m²	Day 1 to 7
6-mercaptopurine	75 mg/m²	Days 15 to 90 (5 days a week)
Methotrexate	15 mg/m²	Days 15, 22, 29, i.e. weekly therapy up to 90 days

1. **Allogeneic bone marrow transplantation:** Bone marrow transplantation from a suitable syngeneic (identical twin) or allogeneic (nonidentical) donor (HLA and mixed lymphocyte culture matched) is increasingly being tried as the only therapeutic measure with the hope of 'cure' in young leukaemic patients (<20 years of age). The basic principle of marrow transplantation is to reconstitute the patient's hemopoietic system after total body irradiation and intensive chemotherapy (called conditioning therapy) to aplate the recipient's hemopoietic and immunological tissue. The indications of bone marrow transplantation in acute leukaemia are given in Box 4.

Box 4	Indications of bone marrow transplantation in acute leukaemia

- AML in first remission
- ALL (common pre-B type) in second remission
- T and B cell lymphoblastic leukaemia in first remission

After conditioning, healthy marrow (matched for HLA) from a suitable donor is injected intravenously. The injected cells 'home' to the marrow start hemopoiesis (production of RBCs, WBCs and platelets) within 3–4 weeks. It takes longer time (1–2 years) to have good lymphocyte function. Therefore, during this period after transplantation, patients are at increased risk of infections.

The main complications of allogeneic BMT are given in Box 5. The long-term survival for patients undergoing allogeneic BMT in acute leukaemia is around 50%. Up to 30% succumb to procedure-related morbidity (e.g. graft versus host disease, etc.) and in rest 20%, the disease relapses.

Graft versus host disease (GVHD): The GVHD and interstitial pneumonitis are

Box 5	Complications of allogeneic BMT

- Mucositis
- Infection (viral, bacterial and fungal)
- Acute graft versus host disease
- Pneumonitis
- Cataract formation
- Chronic graft versus host disease
- Secondary malignant disease
- Infertility

causes of concern in BMT because they may cause serious morbidity and mortality. GVHD is due to cytotoxic activity of donor T lymphocytes which become sensitized to their new host considering it as foreign. The GVHD may be acute or chronic.

Acute GVHD: It occurs usually after 2–3 weeks of transplantation but may be delayed (up to 60 days). It may involve skin, liver and gut, may vary from mild to lethal disease. It appears to be associated with infection, but the cause of association is unknown. Various agents used to prevent it include methotrexate, cyclosporine, ATG, high doses of steroids and T cell depletion of donor marrow. The more severe disease is very difficult to control but high doses of corticosteroids may be useful.

Chronic GVHD: This may occur independently or may follow acute disease described above. It has late onset (few weeks to few months). Its manifestations resemble a connective tissue disorder, although in mild cases, a rash may be the only presenting feature. Chronic GVHD is treated with steroids. Cyclosporine can be used in association with steroids.

2. **Autologous bone marrow (stem cell) transplantation—peripheral blood stem cell transplantation:** In autologous bone marrow transplantation, the patient's own marrow is harvested and frozen, to be given back again after achieving a good remission with intensive chemotherapy. It is indicated in patients of acute leukaemia in whom good or complete remission has been achieved with chemotherapy and acceptable HLA-matched donor is not available for allogeneic BMT. This procedure carries a lower-mortality rate than the allogeneic BMT but the greatest disadvantage of this procedure is high relapse rate (50%). Autologous bone marrow transplantation in acute leukaemia is better than chemotherapy alone.

Stem cells for transplantation were originally obtained by harvesting them from the bone marrow. Recently, they have been collected from the peripheral blood during recovery phase following a period of chemotherapy induced marrow hypoplasia. The dose of stem cell collected from the peripheral blood is much greater than that of harvested from the marrow, hence, making *stem cell transplantation* easier and a reduction in transplant-related mortality to less than 10% in patients under 55 years of age.

Prognosis: Without treatment, the median survival rate of patients with acute leukaemia is about 5 weeks. Median survival for ALL patients is about 2 years and for AML patients about 1 year if remission is achieved. The poor prognostic features in acute leukaemia are given in Box 6.

Box 6 Poor prognostic factors in acute leukaemia	
• Increasing age	• Male sex
• High leucocyte count at the time of diagnosis	• Cytogenetic abnormalities
• CNS involvement in ALL at diagnosis	• Presence of Philadelphia chromosome in ALL

Blood Transfusion Related Complications

BLOOD TRANSFUSIONS

Red Blood Cell Transfusions

Red blood cell transfusions are given to raise the hematocrit level in patients with anaemia or to replace losses after acute bleeding episodes.

Preparations of Red Cells for Transfusion

Several types of preparations containing red blood cells are available.

A. Fresh Whole Blood

The advantage of O⁺ whole blood for transfusion is the simultaneous presence of red blood cells, plasma, and fresh platelets. Fresh whole blood is never absolutely necessary since all the above components are available separately. The major indications for use of whole blood are cardiac surgery or massive hemorrhage when more than 10 units of blood is required in a 24-hour period.

B. Packed Red Blood Cells

Packed red cells are the component most commonly used to raise the hematocrit. Each unit has a volume of about 300 ml, of which approximately 200 ml consists of red blood cells. One unit of packed red cells will usually raise the hematocrit by approximately 4%. The expected rise in hematocrit can be calculated using an estimated red blood cell volume of 200 ml/unit and a total blood volume of about 70 ml/kg. For example, a 70 kg man will have a total blood volume of 4900 ml, and each unit of packed red blood cells will raise the hematocrit by 4%.

C. Leukocyte Poor Blood

Patients with severe leukoagglutination reactions to packed red blood cells may require depletion of white blood cells and platelets from transfused units. White blood cells can be removed either by centrifugation or by washing. Preparation of leukocyte poor blood is expensive and lead s to some loss of red cells. Most blood products now are leukoreduced in-line during acquisition and are thus prospectively leukocyte-poor.

D. Frozen Packed Red Blood Cells

Packed red blood cells can be frozen and stored for up to 3 years, but the technique is cumbersome and expensive and frozen blood should be used sparingly. The major application is for the purpose of maintaining a supply of rare blood types. Patients with such requirements may donate units for autologous transfusion should the need arise. Frozen red cells are also occasionally needed for patients with severe leukoagglutination reactions or anaphylactic reactions to plasma proteins, since frozen blood has essentially all white blood cells and plasma components removed.

E. *Autologous Packed Red Blood Cells*

Patients scheduled for elective surgery may donate blood for autologous transfusion. These units may be stored for up to 22 days before freezing is necessary.

F. *Compatibility Testing*

Before transfusion, the recipient's and the donor's blood are typed and cross-matched to avoid hemolytic transfusion reactions. Although many antigen systems are present on red blood cells, only the ABO and Rh systems are specifically tested prior to all transfusions. The A and B antigens are the most important, because everyone who lacks one or both red cell antigens has IgM isoantibodies (called isoagglutinins) against the missing antigen or antigens in his or her plasma. The isoagglutinins activate complement and can cause rapid intravascular lysis of the incompatible red blood cells. In emergencies, type O/Rh-negative blood can be given to any recipient, but only packed cells should be given to avoid transfusion of donor plasma containing anti-A or anti-B antibodies.

The other important antigen routinely tested for the D antigen of the Rh system. Approximately 15% of the population lack this antigen. In patients lacking the antigen, anti-D antibodies are not naturally present, but the antigen is highly immunogenic. A recipient whose red cells lack D and who receives D-positive blood may develop anti-D antibodies that can cause severe lysis of subsequent transfusions of D-positive red cells.

Blood typing includes a cross-match assay of recipient serum for unusual alloantibodies directed against donor red blood cells by mixing recipient serum with panels of red blood cells representing commonly occurring minor antigens. The screening is particularly important if the receipient has had previous transfusions or pregnancy.

BLOOD TRANSFUSION RELATED COMPLICATIONS

The study of red blood cells (RBCs) antigens and antibodies directed against them forms the basis of transfusion medicine. The cells and proteins in the blood express antigens which are controlled by polymorphic genes, i.e. a specific antigen may be present in one individual but not in others. A blood transfusion may immunise the recipient against the donor antigens as the recipient does not have that antigen called alloimmunisation. Repeated blood transfusions increase the risk of alloimmunisation.

Antibodies directed against RBCs antigens may result from natural exposure (food and bacteria), called autoantibodies; are of IgM type. These antibodies are often insignificant clinically due to the low affinity for antigens at body temperature. However, these IgM antibodies can activated complement cascade and result in haemolysis. On the other hand, antibodies that result from allogenic exposure such as transfusion or pregnancy are usually of IgG type. The IgG antibodies commonly bind to antigens at warmer temperature and may haemolyse RBCs. Unlike IgM, the IgG antibodies can cross placenta and bind fetal RBCs having the corresponding antigen, resulting in haemolytic disease of the newborn or hydrops fetalis.

Alloimmunisation to leucocytes, platelets and plasma proteins may also result in transfusion complications such as fever and urticaria but generally do not cause haemolysis.

Therefore, complications resulting from the blood transfusion may be immunological (alloimmunisation, incompatibility) and nonimmunological such as transmission of infection, volume overload, iron overload, bleeding and electrolyte changes, etc. (Table 66.1)

Blood Croups

The blood groups are determined by antigens on the surface of RBCs. The ABO and Rh systems are important blood groups but incompatibilities involving many other blood groups (such as Lewis, Kell, Duffy, Kidd), may cause haemolytic transfusion reactions and/or haemolytic disease of newborn (Box 1).

ABO System

This is the most important system because naturally occurring IgM anti-A and anti-B antibodies are capable of producing rapid and severe haemolysis of incompatible RBCs.

The ABO system is under the control of a pair of allelic genes H and h, and also three allelic genes, A, B and ≡, producing the genotype and phenotypes given in Table 66.2. The A, B and H antigens are very similar in structure. The H gene codes for enzyme H which attaches

Table 66.1 Complications of blood transfusion

1. Immunological
    i. Alloimmunisation
   ii. Incompatibility
      a. *Red cells*
         • Immediate haemolytic and serological transfusion reactions
         • Delayed haemolytic and serological transfusion reactions
      b. *Leucocytes and platelets*
         • Nonhaemolytic (febrile) transfusion reactions
         • Post-transfusion purpura
         • Poor survival of transfused platelets and granulocytes
         • Graft vs host disease
         • Transfusion related acute lung injury
      c. *Plasma proteins—allergic reactions*
         • Urticaria and anaphylactic reactions

2. Nonimmunological
    i. *Transmission of infection*
         • Transmission of infection, e.g. hepatitis (B, C, D), HIV, other viruses (CMV, EBY, HTLV-1, Parvovirus B-19)
         • Parasites, e.g. malaria, trypanosomiasis, toxoplasmosis
         • Transfusion of blood contaminated with bacteria
   ii. *Volume overload (hypervolaemia)*
  iii. *Iron overload due to multiple transfusions*
   iv. *Bleeding and electrolyte changes:* Massive transfusion of stored blood may cause bleeding and electrolyte changes
    v. *Thrombophlebitis*
   vi. *Air embolism*
  vii. *Hypotensive reactions in patients receiving ACE inhibitors*

Box 1 RBC blood group systems and alloantigens

Group	Antigens	Alloanti-body	Reactions
Rh (D, C/c, E/e)	REC protein	IgG	HTR,HDN
Lewis (Leᵃ, Leᵇ)	Oligo-saccharide	IgM/IgG	Rare HTR
Kell (K/k)	RBC protein	IgG	HTR, HDN
Duffy	-do-	-do-	-do-
Kidd	-do-	-do-	HTR (often delayed) HDN (mild)

HTR: Haemolytic transfusion reaction,
HDN: Haemolytic disease of newborn

fructose to the basic glycoprotein backbone to form H substance which is precursor for A and B antigens.

The A and B genes control specific enzymes responsible for the addition of H substance for group A and B. The O gene is amorphic and does not transform H substance and therefore O is not antigenic. The A, B and H antigens are present on most body cells, tissue fluids (saliva and gastric juice).

Rh System

The Rh system is the second most important blood group system in pretransfusion setting because of the high frequency of development of IgG RhD antibodies in Rh-negative individuals after exposure to RhD-positive red cells following blood transfusions or during pregnancy.

The antibodies (anti-D alloantibody) formed are of major importance in causing HDN and HTR. About 85% people are Rh-positive in a population. The system is coded by two allelic antigen pairs E/e and C/c while the third pair is D (called RhD positive) and no D (RhD-negative). The three Rh genes E/e, D and C/c are arranged in tendem on chromosome I and inherited as a halotype cDE or Cde.

Complications of Blood Transfusion

The adverse effects of blood transfusion or complications of blood transfusion are

Table 66.2	Antigen and antibodies in ABO system in order of frequency		
Phenotype	Genotype	Antigens	Antibodies
O (46%)	OO	None	Anti-A and Anti-B
A (42%)	AA or AO	A	Anti-B
B (90%)	BB or BO	B	Anti-A
AB (3%)	AB	A and B	None

tabulated in Table 66.1. These reactions though rare but can be fatal. About 50% of the fatalities associated with blood transfusion are due to immediate haemolytic transfusion reactions; the remainder are mainly due to post-transfusion hepatitis.

Diagnosis and Management

I. Immunological Reactions

Transfusion reactions may result from immune and nonimmune mechanisms. Immune reactions (immediate or delayed) are often due to preformed donor or recipients antibodies. However, cellular elements (RBC, platelets and leucocytes) and plasma proteins may also cause adverse reactions. These are:

A. *Alloimmunisation:* All transfusions carry a risk of immunisation to the many antigens present on RBCs, leucocytes, platelets and plasma proteins. Alloimmunisation does not cause clinical problems with first transfusion, but subsequent transfusions may result in transfusion reactions such as HDN and rejection of tissue transplants (graft vs host disease). Matching for D antigen is the pretransfusion selection test to prevent it.

B. *Acute haemolytic transfusion reactions:* These occur when the recipient has preformed antibodies that lyse the donor RBCs. These are due to incompatible blood transfusions (ABO isoagglutinins) that result in poor survival RBCs. This is the most serious acute complication of blood transfusion. There is complement activation by antigen and antibody reaction usually due to IgM antibodies.
- *Clinical Features*
  - Rigors, chills, fever (Fig. 66.1).

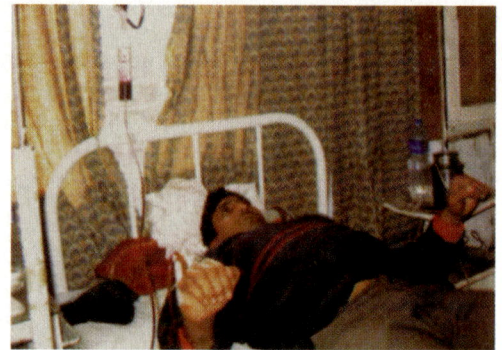

Fig. 66.1: Blood transfusion reaction. Patient developed chills and rigors following blood transfusion

- Acute lumbar pain or chest pain.
- Tachypnoea, tachycardia, hypotension.
- Haemoglobinuria, haemoglobinemia.
- Acute renal failure.
- Activation of coagulation may occur; bleeding due to DIC is bad prognostic sign.
- *Diagnosis:* The diagnosis is confirmed by finding an evidence of haemolysis (e.g. haemoglobinuria) and incompatibility between donor and recipient. All documentations should be checked to locate the error such as:
  - Sample taken from a wrong patient.
  - Mislabelling of the blood sample (patient's name on the sample is not correct).
  - Labelling or handling error in the laboratory.
  - Failure to perform proper identity check before the blood is transfused, i.e. blood transfused to a wrong patient. The blood grouping of the patient's sample (sent for compatibility test), a new sample taken from the patient after reaction and the donor units should be checked to confirm whether error has taken place. This is a serious matter, needs meticulous checks at all stages in the procedure of blood transfusion. The laboratory tests for haemolysis are

raised indirect bilirubin, LDH levels and low serum hepatoglobin and haemoglobinuria.

- *Treatment*
  - At the first instance of any suspicion, the transfusion should be stopped and the donor unit returned to the blood bank laboratory with a new blood sample from the patient to exclude a haemolytic transfusion reaction (HTR).
  - The immune complexes that result in RBCs lysis can precipitate acute renal failure. Diuresis should be induced using fursemide or mannitol with intravenous fluids.
  - Tissue factor released from the lysed erythrocytes can initiate DIC. Coagulation profile such as PT, APTT, fibrinogen and platelet count should be monitored in patients with haemolytic reaction, if develops, treated accordingly (read chapter on DIC).
  - Monitoring the patient's vital signs before and during transfusion reaction is important to identify these reactions properly.
  - Additional RBCs transfusion may be necessary to treat falling hematocrit.

C. *Delayed haemolytic reactions:* This may occur in patients alloimmunised by previous transfusion or pregnancies. The antibody level is too low to be detected by pre-transfusion compatibility testing but a secondary immune response occurs after transfusion, resulting in delayed haemolysis usually by IgG antibody.

- *Clinical features*
  - Patient develops anaemia and jaundice about a week after transfusion due to an extravascular haemolysis.
  - Most patients are clinically silent.
  - The blood film shows spherocytosis and reticulocytosis.
  - Direct antiglobulin test is positive.

- *Treatment*
  - No specific therapy is usually required, although additional RBCs transfusion may be necessary to treat falling haematocrit.
  - A good transfusion history by the clinician can lower the risk. If the patient has had past transfusion or cross-matching difficulties, the blood bank may be able to locate the problem.

D. *Febrile nonhaemolytic transfusion reaction:* Febrile reactions are a common complication of blood transfusion in patients who have previously been transfused or pregnant. The usual cause is the presence of leucocytes antibodies in the recipient against the transfused leucocytes leading to release of pyrogens and cytokines. These reactions are characterised by mild fever (>38°C), chills and rigors, flushing and tachycardia. Analgesic may be needed to reduce fever, and blood transfusion should be stopped. Febrile reactions may be prevented further by the use of leucocyte depleted blood in such patients.

E. *Transfusion-related acute lung injury:* Potent leucocyte antibody (anti-HLA-antibodies) in the plasma of donors who are usually multiparous women, may cause severe pulmonary reactions called *transfusion-related acute lung injury* characterised by fever, cough, dyspnoea, hemoptysis and shadowing in perihilar and lower lung fields on the chest X-ray (non-cardiogenic pulmonary oedema). Treatment is supportive. Patient usually recovers without sequelae. Testing the donor's plasma for anti-HLA antibodies can support the diagnosis.

F. *Post-transfusion purpura:* This reaction presents as thrombocytopenia 7 to 10 days after platelet transfusion and occurs predominantly in females and is related to presence of platelet specific antibody in the recipient's serum, and the most frequently recognised antigen in HPA-1a found on the glucoprotein IIIa receptor. This delayed thrombocytopenia is due to production of antibodies that react to both donor and recipient platelets. Additional platelet transfusions may worsen the thrombocytopenia and should be avoided. Treatment with I.V. immunoglobulin may neutralise the offending antibodies, or plasmapheresis can be used to remove the antibodies if needed.

Allergic (Urticaria) and Anaphylactic (Systemic Anaphylaxis) Reactions

a. *Urticarial (allergic) reactions* characterised by pruritic rash, oedema, headache, dizziness are often attributed to plasma proteins incompatibility, but in most cases, they are unexplained. They are common but rarely severe.

Mild reactions may be treated symptomatically by temporarily stopping the transfusion and administration of chlorpheniramine 10 mg I.V. The transfusion may be completed after the signs and/or symptoms resolve. Patients with history of allergic reactions to blood should be premedicated with an antihistamine. Cellular components can be washed to remove residual plasma for extremely sensitized patient.

b. *Anaphylaxis* is a severe reaction, presents after transfusion of only a few milliliters of blood component. Symptoms and signs include difficulty in breathing, acute bronchospasm (wheezing), hypotension, shock, loss of consciousness and respiratory arrest.

Treatment of anaphylaxis include:
- The transfusion should be stopped.
- Adrenaline (0.5 mg I.M. or S.C. 1:1000 dilution) with chlorpheniramine 10 mg I.V. stat. Steroids may be used in severe cases.
- Endotracheal intubation and maintain vascular access in severe cases.

Prevention: Prevention of allergic reactions include patients who are IgA deficient may be sensitized to this Ig class and are at risk of developing this reaction associated with plasma transfusion. Individuals with severe IgA-deficient should receive only IgA deficient plasma and washed cellular blood components. Therefore, patients who have anaphylactic or repeated allergic reactions to blood components should be tested for IgA-deficiency.

II. Nonimmunological Reactions

a. *Volume overload:* Blood components are volume expanders, can lead to volume overload on rapid transfusion. Monitoring the rate and volume of transfusion along with the administration of a diuretic can reduce this complication.

b. *Iron overload:* Each unit of RBC contains 200–250 mg of iron. Iron overloading is rare, affects various organ systems. i.e. endocrine, hepatic and heart commonly after 100 units of transfusion. Alternative therapy to blood transfusion, i.e. erythropoietin is preferable if large amount is needed to be transfused.

c. *Hypothermia:* Blood components stored in refrigeration (4°C) or frozen (–18°C or below) can result in hypothermia when rapidly transfused. Cardiac arrhythmias can result due to exposure of SA node to cold fluid. Use of an in-line warmer will prevent this complication.

d. *Hyperkalaemia and hypocalcaemia:* RBCs leakage during storage increases the plasma concentration of K^+ in the unit. Neonates and patients of renal failure are at high risk of hyperkalaemia. Citrated blood transfusions can lead to hypocalcaemia because citrate chelates the calcium. It is transient, does not require calcium infusion.

e. *Infections* include transmission of hepatitis. HIV, syphilis, malaria, etc. Screening of the blood by nucleic acid amplification testing (NAT) for HIV and hepatitis C RNA has reduced the incidence.

Emergencies in Endocrinology and Metabolism

- Diabetic Ketoacidosis (Diabetic Coma)
- Hyperosmolar Hyperglycaemic Non-Ketotic Coma
- Hypoglycaemia
- Thyroid Crisis or Storm
- Myxoedema Coma
- Acute Adrenal Crisis/Insufficiency
- Pituitary Apoplexy
- Hypocalcaemia (Tetany)
- Hypercalcaemia (Hypercalcaemic Crisis)

Diabetic Ketoacidosis (Diabetic Coma)

DIABETIC KETOACIDOSIS (DIABETIC COMA)

Definition

It is an acute metabolic complication of diabetes in which hyperglycaemia is associated with metabolic acidosis due to markedly raised (>5 mmol/L) ketone levels. It is a dire medical emergency and remains a serious cause of morbidity and mortality if left untreated principally in type 1 diabetics. It can occur in both types of diabetes mellitus but commoner in type 1 and rare in type 2.

Pathophysiology (Figs 67.1 and 67.2)

The concept of pathogenesis of diabetic keto acidosis is depicted in Fig. 67.1.

It is often caused by relative or absolute deficiency of insulin in established type 1 diabetics combined with counter regulatory hormones (e.g. glucagan, GH, cortisole and catechlomine) excess. Both insulin deficiency and excess glucagon are necessary for development of DKA as follows:

1. The decreased ratio of insulin to glucagon induces hepatic neoglucogenesis, glycogenolysis and impair peripheral utilisation of glucose leading to severe hyperglycaemia (Fig. 67.2), also activate the ketogenic process in liver and thus initiate the development of metabolic

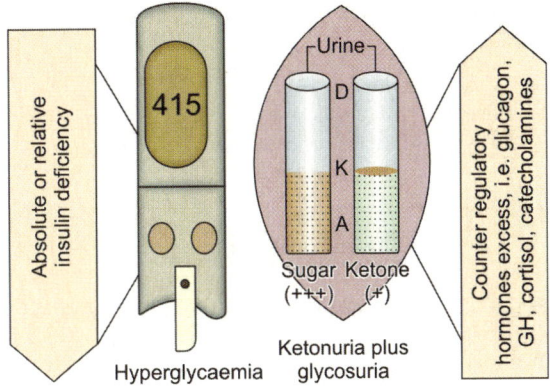

Fig. 67.1: Concepts of pathogenesis of diabetic ketoacidosis (DKA)

ketoacidosis. For ketosis to occur, there is increased levels of free fatty acids in the plasma which are transported to liver for oxidation and conversion to ketones bodies (Fig. 67.2). Normally these FFA are converted into triglycerides and lipoproteins.

The overproduction of ketones by the liver is the primary event of ketoacidosis in addition to hyperglycaemia. Dehydration results due to osmotic diuresis. Hyperkalaemia results due to shift of K^+ from intracellular to extracellular spaces.

Precipitating Factors

As diabetic ketoacidosis results primarily due to deficiency of insulin, hence, patient may

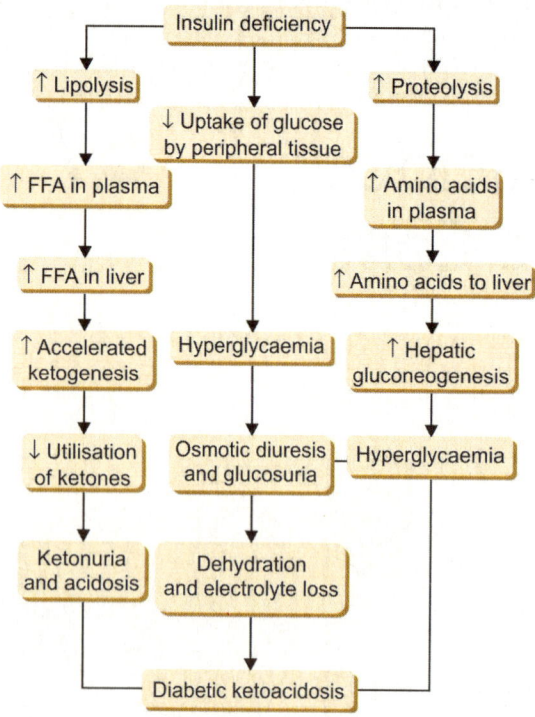

Fig. 67.2: Pathophysiology of diabetic ketoacidosis

present with diabetic ketoacidosis straightway without any knowledge of being diabetic. Otherwise, in patients of type 1 diabetics, it results either due to cessation of insulin dose or inadequate dosage of insulin. The precipitating factors are given in Box 1.

Clinical Features

Diabetic ketoacidosis (DKA) is the presenting feature in about 10% of undiagnosed cases.

Box 1	Precipitating factors for diabetic Ketoacidosis
• Infections (pneumonia, UTI, gastroenteritis, sepsis)	• Drugs, e.g. steriods, thiazides
• Alcohol intake	• Surgery
• Acute vascular episodes (cerebral, coronary, peripheral)	• Emotional stress
	• Pancreatitis
• Acute MI	• Ignorance about the disease
• Trauma	• Poverty, unemployment

They are brought in the state of disturbed consciousness or coma to the hospital where the diagnosis is confirmed. A similar proportion of cases may also develop it spontaneously without any precipitating illness / cause. The onset of DKA is insidious occurring over hours or days. *The triad of type 1 diabetes 'polyuria, polydipsia, polyphagia'* is characteristic due to hyperglycaemia and osmotic diuresis. Unique feature of DKA is that patient is dehydrated in the presence of excessive thirst. Weakness, lethargy, headache, myalgia are nonspecific symptoms. *GI symptoms* such as nausea, vomiting (coffee ground in appearance) and abdominal pain are characteristic features, the pain even may be mistaken for *acute abdomen* (*acute appendicitis*) and even operated upon. No patient is to be subjected to surgery without urine examination. The pain in abdomen is related to acidosis, is due to pooling of fluid in the intestinal tract. Ileus is due to temporary autonomic neuropathy, electrolyte disturbance and hyperglucagonaemia. Vomiting in DKA is an ominous sign. The *respiratory symptoms* include dyspnoea and deep rapid respiration. The *CNS symptoms* include weakness, lethargy altered mental status, drowsiness cerebral oedema and eventually coma. This is due to dehydration, hypotension and increased plasma osmolarity.

Physical Signs

1. There is *tachypnoea, tachycardia, hypotension* and *low body temperature* (*hypothermia*). These are due to fluid and electrolyte disturbance (acidosis) which stimulates the respiratory centre (tachypnoea) and causes vasodilatation (tachycardia) and hypothermia (low body temperature).
2. **Signs of dehydration** (e.g. dry tongue, mucous membrane and skin, soft eyeballs, sunken cheeks) and hypotension or shock (cold clammy skin, oliguria and obtunded consciousness).
3. **Kussmaul breathing,** a deep and rapid respiration is due to metabolic acidosis.

4. **Acetone smell** (like 'pear drops' or nail varnish remover) is due to hyperketonaemia.
5. There may be *hypotonia, hyperreflexia* and incoordinated ocular movements.
6. Abdominal tenderness (may resemble acute pancreatitis or surgical abdomen).
7. **Obtunded consciousness, cerebral oedema stupor or coma.** The deterioration of consciousness is proportional to fall in pH and plasma osmolarity. Plasma osmolarity is calculated as

Calculated osmolarity (CO) =

$$2Na^+ + \frac{Glu}{18} + \frac{BUN}{2.8}$$

The normal osmolality is 280–300 mOsm/kg

The level of consciousness depending on plasma osmolality and pH is as follows:

Osmolality	pH	Level of consciousness
At 324 mOsm/kg	7–7.24	Produces drowsiness
At 340 mOsm/kg	-do-	Produces semicoma
At 370 mOsm/kg	<7.0	Produces coma

Investigations

The characteristic metabolic abnormalities diagnostic of DKA are depicted in Box 2. There is hyproglycaemia, ketonaemia, hyperkalacemia, hyperphosphatemir, acidosis and elevated blood urea and serum creatinine.

Diagnosis and Differential Diagnosis

The diagnosis of DKA in a patient known to have type 1 diabetes is not difficult, but has to be differentiated in a patient who is not known to be diabetic.

The DKA has to be differentiated from CVA, hypoglycaemia and hyperosmolar coma due to altered mental status (coma). Uraemia and alcohol poisoning have to be differentiated because of presence of metabolic acidosis.

Gastroenteritis has to be differentiated because of nausea, vomiting and signs of dehydration in DKA.

Box 2	Biochemical features of DKA
Increased (↑)	*Decreased (↓) or normal*
• Blood glucose (250–600 mg%)	• Serum sodium (125–135 mEq/L)
• Plasma ketone	• Serum magnesium
• Plasma osmolality (300–320 mOsm/ml)	• Serum potassium initially increase, later decreased
• Haematocrit	• Bicarbonate (<15 mEq/L)
• WBC count (>11,000/L)	• PCO_2 (20–30 mmHg)
• Blood urea, creatinine	• pH 6.8 to 7.3
• Serum FFA and triglycerides	
• Anion gap	
• Serum amylase and lipase (20–25% cases)	

The first step in diagnosis is to test the urine for glucose and ketones (Fig. 67.1). If urine is negative for ketone, another cause for the acidosis is likely. If it is positive, plasma glucose examination is required to be certain. Hyperglycaemia and ketonuria confirm the diagnosis of DKA (a strongly positive urine dipstick for glucose and ketone—Fig. 67.1).

The ketones may be tested by semiquantitative nitroprusside methods (Ace test and keto rix) in serial dilutions of the plasma. Undiluted plasma may give a strongly positive result when starvation alone is the problem while a strong reaction in dilution exceeding 1:1 is a presumptive evidence of ketoacidosis. The causes and diagnosis of ketonuria are given in Box 3.

Complications of DKA

1. Cerebral oedema.
2. Acute respiratory distress syndrome.

Box 3	Differential diagnosis of ketonuria	
Causes of ketonuria	*Diagnosis*	
• Diabetic ketoacidosis	Hyperglycaemia with ketonaemia/ketonuria	
• Starvation	Low glucose, normal bicarbonate	
• Alcoholic ketoacidosis	Normal to low blood glucose and bicarbonate	
• Salicylate poisoning	Elevated serums alicylate levels. Normal to low blood glucose	

3. Thromboembolism.
4. Disseminated intravascular coagulation.
5. Acute circulatory failure.

Management

Principles of Treatment

1. *Replacement of fluid loss* to correct dehydration and hyperosmolality.
2. *Correction of electrolytes* (Na⁺ and K⁺) and acidosis.
3. *Identification and correction of a precipitating cause.*
4. *Correction of hyperglycaemia with insulin.* Bed side glucometer should be used to titrate the insulin therapy.
5. *Close monitoring* of the patient by laboratory parameters (e.g. plasma glucose, urea, electro lytes, arterial pH and bicarbonate) at an interval of 1–2 hours initially until the patient's condition stabilizes.

A. Management of DKA in Adults

- *General Measures*
  - Continuous gastric aspiration if patient is in coma or have vomiting.
  - If no urine is passed within 4 hours, then catheterize and put an indwelling catheter.
  - Give an antibiotic early in case of infection or if an invasive procedure is used.
  - Give oxygen.

- *Fluids and Electrolyte*

The average loss of fluid loss in moderately severe diabetic ketoacidosis in an adult is about 3–6 litres.

Initially normal saline 0.9% should be administered I.V. and about 2–3 L saline may be infused over 2–3 hours, subsequently 0.45% normal saline may be given depending on the calculated volume deficit. Subsequently change to glucose saline (0.45%) as soon as blood glucose approaches to 200–250 mg%. Excessive fluid replacement (>5 L in 8 hours may lead to ARDS or cerebral oedema).

- *Insulin*

Rapid acting (soluble) insulin is used either intravenously or intramuscularly (Table 67.1).

An initial bolus dose of 0.15 unit/kg of insulin is given I.V. followed by 0.1 unit/kg/hour continuous infusion, if no response within 2–4 hrs, dose of insulin may be doubled. If used intra muscular, then given 20 U insulin stat than 6 U/hour. Insulin I.V. continued until acidosis resolves and patient becomes metabolically stable.

- *Response to treatment*

Two points must be emphasised while monitoring the response to treatment:

1. The plasma glucose level invariably falls more rapidly than the plasma ketone level; it may be possible that plasma glucose is approaching normal but ketone bodies are still present. Therefore, insulin administration should not be stopped because glucose concentration is approaching normal; rather, as mentioned above, glucose should be started with insulin replacing normal saline until the ketosis has disappeared which may take few days.
2. The key parameters of accurate assessment to response is the pH and the calculated anion gap.

All patients should be followed by maintaining a chart outlining the amount and timing of insulin and fluids together with a record of vital signs, urine output and blood biochemistry. Without such a record, therapy tends to become chaotic.

Continue with regimen until fluid deficit replaced, ketonuria abolished and adequate oral intake of carbohydrate feasible. Now the patient can be shifted to his old regimen of insulin again by monitoring of glucose and adjustment of meals.

Potassium therapy. The average total body potassium deficit resulting from osmotic diuresis, acidosis and G.I. loss is about 3–5 mEq/kg (i.e. 200 mEg in 60 kg person). Initially K⁺ levels may be elevated, hence K⁺ replacement should not be started before insulin therapy. During treatment with insulin and fluids, hypokalemia develops. Thus potassium repletion should start as soon as good urine output and low serum potassium is documented (<3.5 mEq/L).

Administer 20–40 mEq/L of potassium in each litre of I.V. fluid to maintain the serum K^+ at >3.5 mEq/L. Food rich in potassium should be prescribed when the patient starts taking orally.

Bicarbonate therapy. In the presence of severe acidosis (pH <7.0). ADA advises 50 mEq/L of $NaHCO_3$ in 200 ml of sterile water with 10 mEq/L KCL per hour for 2 hours until pH is >7.0, the phosphate supplement should be considered. Hypomagnesemia may develop during DKA, may require supplementation.

Phosphate replacement: It is seldom required. If severe hypophosphatemia of less than 1 mg/dl develops during insulin therapy, a small amount of phosphate can be replaced as potassium salt.

• *Treatment of precipitating factors*

Precipitating causes of DKA should be searched for in each and every case and appropriate measures must be taken to treat them. Education of the patient is an important aspect for insulin therapy. Since infection is the most common precipitating cause, routine antibiotic therapy is sufficient. Treatment of underlying illness such as CVA, AMI, trauma or stress, if present.

• *Treatment of complications*

Cerebral oedema is common cause of death, can be treated by bolus infusion of 1 g mannitol/kg of body weight in the form of 20% solution or intravenous dexamethasone 8 to 12 mg initially, then 4 mg every 6 hours.

Table 67.1 Diabetic petacidosis management in an adult
1. Confirm diagnosis (↑ plasma glucose, positive serum ketones, metabolic kitosis)
2. Admit to hospital; intensive care setting may be necessary for frequent monitoring or if pH <7.00 or unconscious.
3. Assess serum, electrolytes (K^+, Na^+, Mg^+, Cl^-, bicarbonate, phosphate)   • Acid-base status—pH, HCO_3^-, PCO_2, b-hydrobutyrate   • Renal function (creatinine, urine output)
4. Replace fluids 2–3 L of 0.9% saline over first 1–3 h (10–20 mL/kg per hour); subsequently, 0.45% saline at 250–500 mL/h change to 5% glucose and 0.45% saline at 150–250 mL/h when plasma glucose reaches 250 mg/dL (13.9 mmol/L)
5. Administer short-acting insulin: I.V. (0.1 kg), then 0.1 units/kg per hour by continuous IV infusion; increase two-to threefold if no response by 2–4 hours. If the initial serum potassium is <3.3 mmol/L (3.3 meq/L), do not administer insulin until the potassium is corrected.
6. Assess patient. What precipitated the episode (noncompliance, infection, trauma, pregnancy, infarction, cocaine)? Initiate appropriate workup for precipitating event (cultures, CXR, ECG).
7. Measure capillary glucose every 1–2 hours; measure electrolytes (especially K^+ bicarbonate, phosphate) and anion gap every 4 hours for first 24 hours.
8. Monitor blood pressure, pulse, respirations, mental status, fluid intake and output every 1–4 hours.
9. Replace K^+: 10 mEq/h when plasma K^+ <5.0–5.2 mEq/L (or 20–30 mEq/L of infusion fluid). ECG normal, urine flow and normal creatinine documented; administer 40–80 mEq/h when plasma K^+ <3.5 mEq/L or if bicarbonate is given. If inital serum potassium is >5.2 mmol/L (5.2 mEq/L), do not supplement K^+ until the potassium is corrected.
10. See text about bi-carbonate or phosphate supplementation.
11. Continue above until patient is stable, glucose goal is 8.3–13.9 mmoL/L (150–250 mg/dL), and acidosis is resolved. Insulin infusion may be decreased to 0.05–0.1 units/kg per hour.
12. Administer long-acting insulin as soon as patient is eating. Allow for a 2–4 hours overlap in insulin infusion and SC insulin injection.
Abbreviation: CXR, chest X-ray; ECG, electrocardiogram
Adapted from M Sperling, in *Therapy for Diabetes Mellitus and Related Disorders* American Diabetes Association, Alexandria, VA, 1998; and AE Kitabchi et al. Diabetes Care, ... 2009

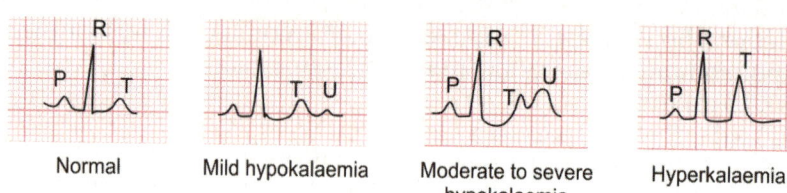

Normal   Mild hypokalaemia   Moderate to severe hypokalaemia   Hyperkalaemia

Fig. 67.3: ECG changes in K$^+$ disturbance. High peaked T waves are sign of hyperkalemia. Flattened T waves with U waves indicate hypokalemia

Monitoring

- ECG (Fig. 67.3) can be monitored as a guide to therapy.
- Check glucose and electrolytes 2–4 hourly until patient becomes stable.

Prevention

Diabetic ketoacidosis can be an initial presentation in a child, therefore, physician should be alert if a child presents with dehydration, fever, hyperventilation or drowsiness or polyuria and polydypsia.

- Type 1 diabetic during sick period should be managed properly with periodic review of glucose and ketones.

- Use supplemental short-acting insulin during stress.
- Treat infection with antibiotic cover. Adjust the dose of the insulin during infection as insulin requirement rises during infection.
- Insulin should not be stopped even if the child refuses to take usual diet. A palatable liquid diet containing carbohydrates and salt may be given along with insulin and adequate fluid intake. If child does not retain fluid, it is advisable to shift the child to a hospital.
- Check urine ketone whenever blood glucose is >300 mg/dl.

Hyperosmolar Hyperglycaemic Non-Ketotic Coma

Definition

Hyperosmolar hyperglycaemic non-ketotic coma (HHNKC) is an acute metabolic decompensation of the diabetic state in type 2 diabetics, characterised by extreme hyperglycaemia (blood glucose> 600 mg/dl) and increased osmolality (> 320 mOsm/kg) with dehydration without significant ketosis or acidosis.

Aetiology: The patients of type 2 DM prone to develop it include:

1. Type 2 diabetes detected for the first time (undiagnosed diabetics).
2. Middle aged or older diabetics (> 50 years of age).
3. Those living alone.
4. Those with no access to medical treatment.
5. Those with associated infection or stroke.

Precipitating illness/factors: Certain precipitating illnesses/factors are:

- Acute infections, burns, trauma.
- Vascular episode (CVA or AMI).
- Alcohol excess or excessive consumption of beverages.
- Hyperalimentation.
- Drugs, e.g. thiazides, steroids, phenytoin, chlorpromazine, diazoxide, immuno-

suppressive, sympathomimetics, beta-blockers, calcium channel blockers, etc.
- Recurrent vomiting.
- Dialysis (peritoneal or hemodialysis) in a patient with uraemia.
- Use of osmotic agents (e.g. mannitol).
- Recent surgery.
- Heart failure.

Pathogenesis (Fig. 68.1)

A partial or relative deficiency/insufficiency of insulin may initiate the process by reducing glucose utilisation of muscle, fat and liver while inducing hypergluconaemia and increasing hepatic glucose output. It is a syndrome of profound dehydration produced by persistent sustained hyperglycemia which is more than DKA, results in profuse osmotic diuresis which the patient is not able to compensate by drinking enough water to keep up with urinary fluid losses. The dehydration results in further rise in blood sugar. The patients who are prone to develop the syndrome are elderly diabetics living either alone or in a nursing home or develop a stroke or infection that worsens further hyperglycaemia and prevents adequate water intake. The full blown picture usually develops when urine output falls considerably. Loss of total body water relative to total body sodium is greater resulting in hyperosmolality.

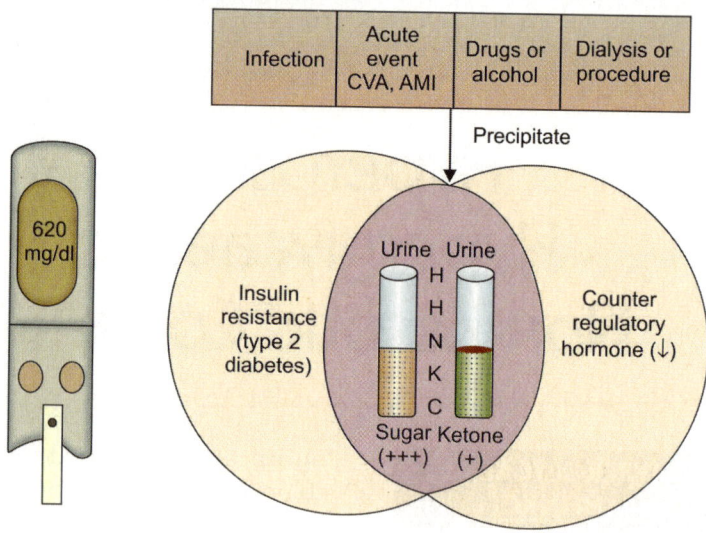

Fig. 68.1: Pathogenesis and diagnosis of HHNKC (high osmolality, i.e. > 350 mOSm/kg, very high blood sugar ≥ 600 mg%, minimal or no ketosis)

Absence of ketosis is due to higher levels of endogenous insulin reserve (type 2 diabetics have insulin resistance with some insulin reserve), inhibition of lipolysis by the hyperosmolar state, lower levels of counter-regulatory hormones and free fatty acids than in DKA and there is an associated glucagon resistance.

Coma is due to hyperosmolar state induced by severe dehydration and hyperglycaemia. Plasma osmolality > 340 mOsm / kg is associated with obtunded consciousness progressing to coma.

Clinical Features

The features of HHNKC evolve slowly over several days to weeks. The patient may have *polyuria, polydipsia* and *polyphagia* for days and weeks with *dehydration, lethargy* and *weakness* prior to development of *drowsiness* or *coma*. Notably absent are symptoms of nausea, vomiting, abdominal pain and Kussmaul breathing characteristics of DKA. As the syndrome progresses, the important protective measure, i.e. thirst is impaired due to depression of thirst centre in hypothalamus by hyperosmolality or hyperglycaemia. Other **CNS features** include seizural activity—some time

Jacksonian in type, myoclonic jerks, transient hemiplegia and transient visual symptoms (hemianopia). Infections, particularly pneumonia and gram-negative septicaemia are common and indicative of grave prognosis. Bleeding probably caused by disseminated intravascular coagulation (DIC) and acute pancreatitis may occur.

The **physical findings** include:

Tachycardia, signs of dehydration, rapid shallow respiration (in contrast to Kussmoul breathing in DKA), hypotension or shock, altered mental status (drowsiness or coma).

Investigations

They are given in Box 1.

Diagnosis and Differential Diagnosis

The diagnosis of HHNKC should be suspected in any elderly diabetic who presents with acute or subacute deterioration of CNS functions with profound dehydration. There may be an evidence of infection. Diagnosis is made by hyperglycaemia, hyperosmolality and mild acidosis without ketonuria or ketonaemia (Fig. 68.1). Prerenal azotaemia is present. The acidosis is mild without ketosis, is due

Box 1 Laboratory parameters in hyperosmolar hyperglycaemic non-ketotic coma

- Plasma glucose (mg/dl)   > 600 (600–1200)
- Arterial pH   osmolality > 7.30
- Serum bicarbonate (mEq/L)   > 15
- Effective serum osmolality   > 350 (350–380)
  (mOsm/kg)

Note: The effective serum osmolarity is calculated by = $2 \times Na\,(mEq/L) + glucose\,divided\,by\,18\,(mg/dl) + BUN/2.8$

- Aninon gap (Na$^+$+ K$^+$)– (Cl$^-$ – 20 HCO$_3$)
- Urine or serum ketone   Small or absent
- Blood urea/creatinine   May be high (pre renal azotemia)
- Serum sodium (mEq/L)   135–145

Table 68.1 Differentiating features between OKA (diabetic ketoacidosis) and HHNKC (hyperosmolar hyperglycaemic non-ketotic coma)

Feature	DKA	HHNKC
Age	Younger patients	Older patients
Type of DM	Common in type 1	Common in type 2
Dehydration	Mild to moderate	Marked
Respiration	Kussmaul breathing	Shallow, rapid respiration
Consciousness	Diminished	Comatosed
Temperature	Normal or low	May be high
Blood glucose	> 250 mg/dl	> 600 mg/dl
Blood urea	Normal or slightly raised	Markedly raised
Sodium	Low to normal (125–140 mmol/L)	Normal to high (130–160 mmol/L)
Potassium	Low to normal (3–5.0 mEq/L)	Normal to high (4–6.0 mEq/L)
Bicarbonate	<15 mmol/L	16–30 mmol/L
Ketones in blood	Marked (++ to +++)	Absent to minimal (+)
Osmolality	High and variable (350–380 mOsm/kg)	Very high (350–450 mOsm/kg)
Anion gap	40	20

to a combination of starvation, retention of inorganic acids secondary to renal hypoperfusion and elevation of plasma lactate (due to hypotension or shock).

The differences between two common types of comam, i.e. DKA and HHNKC are tabulated in Table 68.1.

Management

As mortality rate in HHNKC is high (>50%), hence immediate treatment is necessary. Protocol for the management of adult patients with HHNKC is depicted in Fig. 67.2.

Principles

1. Fluid replacement to correct dehydration.
2. Low or small doses of insulin to correct hyperglycemia.
3. Correction of electrolytes (e.g. Na$^+$ and K$^+$).
4. Identification and correction of precipitating cause. Above all, frequent monitoring for glucose, pH, electrolytes, urea, creatinine is necessary.
1. **Correction of dehydration:** The most important measure is initial rapid infusion of large amounts of intravenous fluids to reestablish circulation and urine flow. The average fluid deficit is more (10–11 L) as compared to DKA (6 L only). While free water is ultimately needed because of hyperosmolar state, initial therapy still should be with isotonic (0.9%) saline and 2 to 3 litres should be given during first 1–2 hours. Subsequently, half-strength (0.45%) saline should be used. As the glucose level approaches normal, 5% dextrose can be given as a vehicle for free water. Hydration alone will often result in reversal of hyperosmolar coma and decreases plasma glucose and serum osmolarity. Fluid replacement should correct estimated deficits within first 24 hours. In patients with renal or cardiac compromise, monitoring of serum osmolality, and CVP monitoring must be performed during fluid replacement and to avoid unnecessary fluid overload. The end point of fluid therapy is to restore urinary output to 50 ml/hr or more.
2. **Insulin therapy:** Many authors recommend small doses of insulin as many

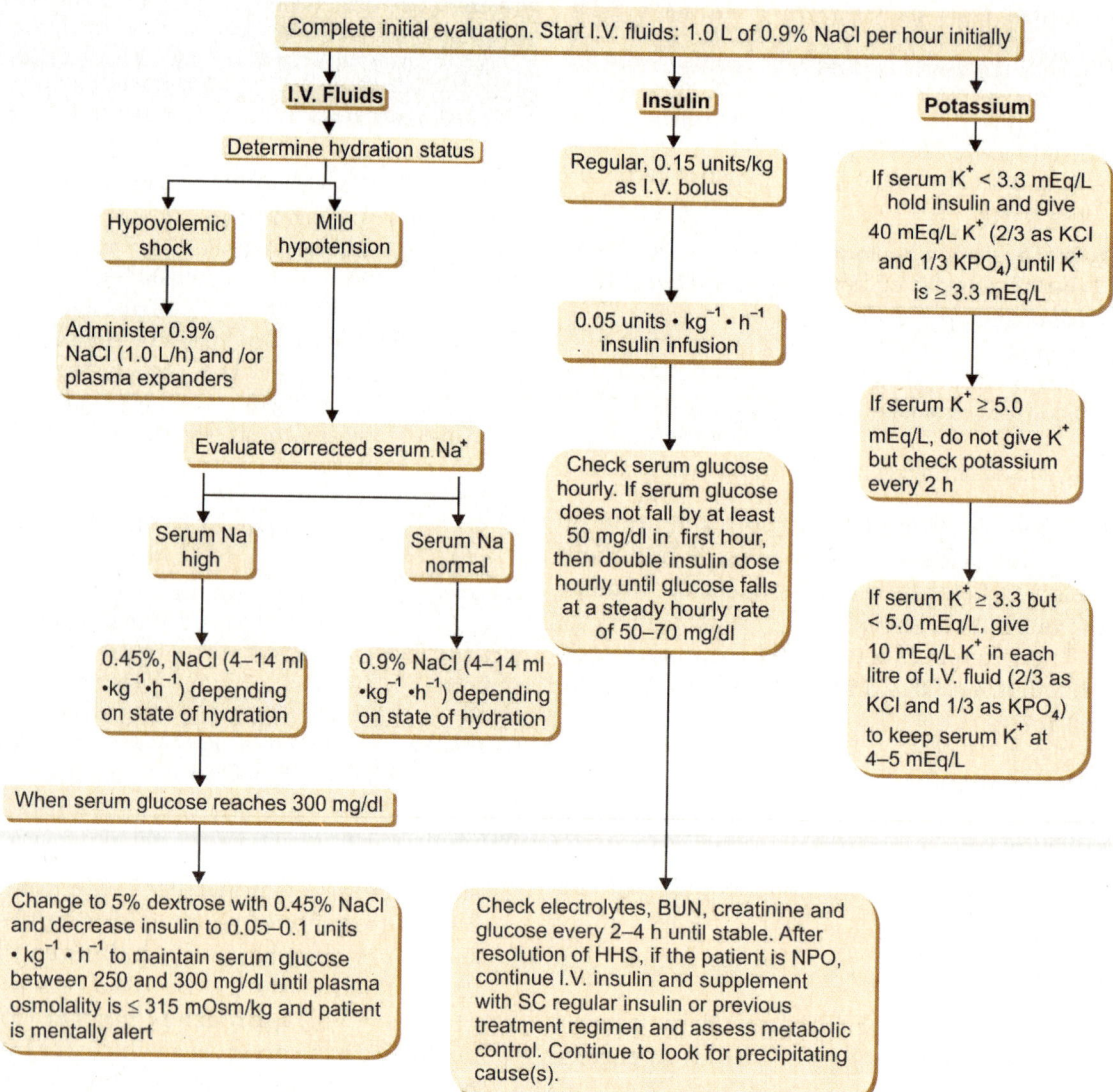

Complete initial evaluation. Start I.V. fluids: 1.0 L of 0.9% NaCl per hour initially

I.V. Fluids

Determine hydration status

Hypovolemic shock | Mild hypotension

Administer 0.9% NaCl (1.0 L/h) and /or plasma expanders

Evaluate corrected serum Na$^+$

Serum Na high | Serum Na normal

0.45%, NaCl (4–14 ml $\cdot$kg^{-1} $\cdot$h^{-1}) depending on state of hydration | 0.9% NaCl (4–14 ml $\cdot$kg^{-1} $\cdot$h^{-1}) depending on state of hydration

When serum glucose reaches 300 mg/dl

Change to 5% dextrose with 0.45% NaCl and decrease insulin to 0.05–0.1 units $\cdot$ kg^{-1} $\cdot$ h^{-1} to maintain serum glucose between 250 and 300 mg/dl until plasma osmolality is ≤ 315 mOsm/kg and patient is mentally alert

Insulin

Regular, 0.15 units/kg as I.V. bolus

0.05 units $\cdot$ kg^{-1} $\cdot$ h^{-1} insulin infusion

Check serum glucose hourly. If serum glucose does not fall by at least 50 mg/dl in first hour, then double insulin dose hourly until glucose falls at a steady hourly rate of 50–70 mg/dl

Check electrolytes, BUN, creatinine and glucose every 2–4 h until stable. After resolution of HHS, if the patient is NPO, continue I.V. insulin and supplement with SC regular insulin or previous treatment regimen and assess metabolic control. Continue to look for precipitating cause(s).

Potassium

If serum K$^+$ < 3.3 mEq/L hold insulin and give 40 mEq/L K$^+$ (2/3 as KCl and 1/3 KPO$_4$) until K$^+$ is ≥ 3.3 mEq/L

If serum K$^+$ ≥ 5.0 mEq/L, do not give K$^+$ but check potassium every 2 h

If serum K$^+$ ≥ 3.3 but < 5.0 mEq/L, give 10 mEq/L K$^+$ in each litre of I.V. fluid (2/3 as KCl and 1/3 as KPO$_4$) to keep serum K$^+$ at 4–5 mEq/L

Fig. 68.2: Protocol for the management of adult patients with HHNKC

patients are extremely hypersensitive to insulin and the glucose concentration may fall suddenly. If significant ketonemia is not present, just replacement of fluid alone (0.9% saline) without insulin may result in significant fall in blood glucose. Otherwise also insulin should not be started immediately, it should be used after adequate fluid replacement, However, insulin administration is similar to management of DKA. Regular insulin by continuous intravenous infusion is the treatment of choice. Once hypokalemia is excluded, an intravenous bolus dose of regular insulin (0.1 U/kg) may be given followed by 0.05 U/kg/hour in adults until blood glucose comes to 250 mg%). When glucose concentration approaches 250 mg%, and remain stabilised then maintenance state of glucose (around 250 mg%) is achieved by neutralization of glucose with insulin until patient become conscious and starts accepting orally. Now patient can be shifted to subcutaneous insulin.

3. **Potassium replacement:** With the absence of acidosis/ketosis, there may be no initial hyperkalaemia as seen in DKA. Insulin therapy and volume expansion decrease the K^+ concentration, hence, K^+ replacement is required early in the management than DKA. Once renal function is restored, K^+ may be given to prevent hypokalaemia. Potassium supplementation (10 mEq/L) may be initiated after serum levels fall below 5.0 mEq/L and urine output is good. This potassium supplementation is sufficient to maintain serum K^+ of 4–5 mEq/L.

4. **Other supportive measures:** These are similar to DKA (read DKA). Seizures in HHNKC syndrome should not be taken as a manifestation of primary cortical pathology and unnecessary phenytoin may not be given. Treatment with phenytoin not only fails to relieve seizures which are due to hyperosmolality but worsen hyperglycaemia by impairing endogenous insulin release.

5. **Identify the precipitating factors** and efforts should be made to correct them to avoid future episodes.

6. **Complications:** All the complications are preventable.
   - *Hypoglycaemia:* This is the most common complication of HHNKC due to overzealous administration of insulin as well as hypersensitivity to insulin.
   - *Hypokalaemia:* Potassium levels fall rapidly with fluid replacement and initiation of insulin; if not prevented or corrected early, may result in hypokalaemia which may induce cardiac arrhythmias.
   - *Hyperglycaemia:* It occurs secondary to interruption/discontinuance of intravenous insulin therapy after recovery without subsequent coverage with subcutaneous insulin.
   - *Cerebral oedema:* It is rare but frequently fatal. The exact pathogenesis is unknown but is attributed to sudden movement of water into CNS when plasma osmolality declines too rapidly with treatment. It is, therefore, necessary to replace Na^+ and water deficits gradually and to add dextrose to infusion fluid as soon as blood glucose reaches between 250–300 mg%. These measures reduce the incidence of cerebral oedema.
   - *Control pontine myelinosis:* Rapid reversal of serum osmolarity and blood glucose in HHNKC results in central pontine myelinosis which can be corrected by slow infusion of fluids.
   - *Arterial and venous thrombosis:* These are preventable due to early correction of dehydration and shock.

Hypoglycaemia

HYPOGLYCAEMIA

Definition

Normal lower limit of fasting plasma glucose is 70 mg/dl. *Hypoglycaemia* is defined as low blood sugar (<70 mg%) or relatively low plasma glucose (<55 mg/dl) are usually associated with symptoms of sympathetic overactivity and neuroglycopenia. According to Diabetic Control and Complication Trial (DCCT), hypoglycaemia is defined as an event or state resulting in seizures, confusion, coma and other neurological symptoms consistent with hypoglycaemia (e.g. sweating palpitation, hunger or blurred vision) and finger-prick blood glucose less than 50 mg% and its amelioration by treatment that raises the blood glucose.

Hypoglycaemia is major hazard of insulin treatment and is also common with oral hypoglycaemia agents (OHA) especially in elderly. Neonatal hypoglycaemia in infants born to diabetic mothers is well-known.

Hypoglycaemia is a medical emergency requiring urgent management. Today, with advances in the management of diabetes and its complications, cases of hypoglycaemia progressing to coma and death are being seen rarely.

Occasionally, hypoglycaemia may be the presenting feature of an acute illness and is called spontaneous hypoglycaemia.

Fasting hypoglycaemia in an otherwise healthy, well-nourished adult is rare and is mostly due to insulinoma or adenoma of islets of Langerhans'. Adenoma may be single, familial but multiple adenomas are found in MEN-I type syndrome.

Aetiology

The most common cause of hypoglycaemia in diabetes is *iatrogenic*, e.g. drug-induced; whereas spontaneous hypoglycaemia in non-diabetic population is due to multiple causes.

Alcohol induced hypoglycaemia due to alcohol-mediated inhibition of neoglucogenis, common in malnourished individuals, occurs due to excessive intake of alcohol or alcohol induced gastritis and vomiting.

Immunopathologic hypoglycaemia. It is extremely rare conduction in which antiinsulin antibodies or antibodies to insulin develop spontaneously.

The causes of hypo glycaemia in diabetics are summarized in Box 1 and illustrated in Fig. 69.1.

Spontaneous hypoglycaemia: Spontaneous hypoglycaemia occurring in nondiabetic population is classified into (i) fasting and

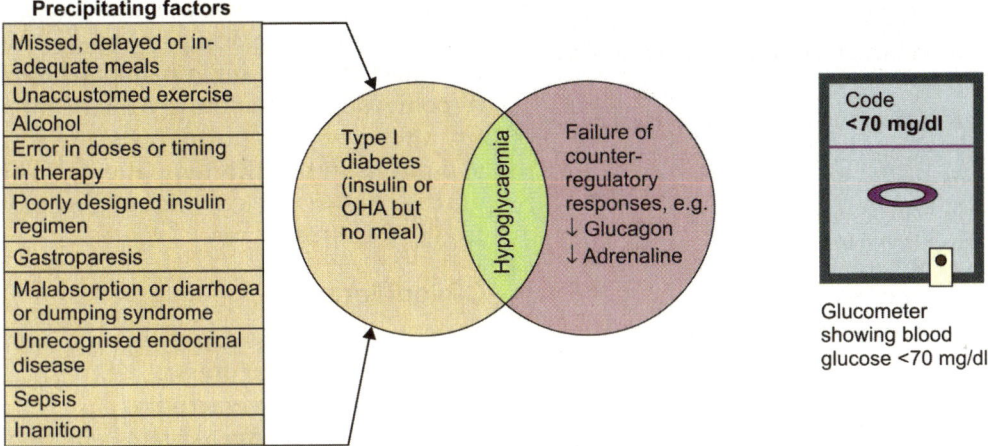

Precipitating factors

Missed, delayed or in-adequate meals
Unaccustomed exercise
Alcohol
Error in doses or timing in therapy
Poorly designed insulin regimen
Gastroparesis
Malabsorption or diarrhoea or dumping syndrome
Unrecognised endocrinal disease
Sepsis
Inanition

Type I diabetes (insulin or OHA but no meal)

Hypoglycaemia

Failure of counter-regulatory responses, e.g. ↓ Glucagon ↓ Adrenaline

Code <70 mg/dl

Glucometer showing blood glucose <70 mg/dl

Fig. 69.1: Aetiopathogenesis and diagnosis of hypoglycaemia

(ii) postprandial (reactive). The differences are summarised in Box 2.

The causes of fasting as well as postprandial hypoglycaemia are given in Table 69.1.

Box 1	Causes of iatrogenic hypoglycaemia in diabetics
• Missed or delayed meals	• Change in drug therapy or insulin
• Excess of insulin	• Error in doses and its timing
• Sudden reduction in diet or more fasts	• Poorly planned treatment regimen
• Unaccustomed exercise	• Endocrinal causes, e.g. Addison's disease, hypothyroidism
• Alcohol use	
• Alimentary causes, e.g. diarrhoea, mal-absorption, diabetic gastroparesis	• Patient's causes, e.g. unintelligent, unco-operative, poor, uneducated, etc.
• Renal failure	

Box 2	Differential diagnosis of spontaneous hypoglycaemia	
	Fasting	*Postprandial (reactive)*
	• Low blood sugar occurs after hours of fasting	• Low blood sugar occurs in response to meals, hence, called reactive.
	• It occurs usually in the presence of a disease (*see* the long list of causes in Table 69.1)	• It usually occurs in the absence of disease, i.e. normal population or associated with anxiety.
	• It occurs due to an imbalance between glucose production and utilisation in peripheral tissue (e.g. hyperinsulinism extrapancreatic tumors, drugs and insulin)	• The most common cause is alimentary hyperinsulinism (GI surgery, dumping syndrome, bariatric surgery, etc.)

Pathophysiology

Counter-regulatory mechanisms: In response to a falling blood sugar, there is normally increased secretion of counter-regulatory hormones which antagonize the blood-glucose lowering effects of insulin. *Glucagon, cortisol, GH* and *adrenaline* are the counter-regulatory hormones which fail over time;

hypoglycaemia-induced secretion of glucagon becomes impaired within 5 years of developing type 1 diabetes. Similarly after several years, the adrenaline response to hypoglycaemia also becomes defective; so that if hypoglycaemia develops, glucose recovery may be seriously compromised. Autonomic neuropathy may also contribute to defective adrenaline response. Those who develop deficient counter-regulatory responses may

Table 69.1 Causes of fasting and postprandial hypoglycaemia in non-diabetics

Fasting hypoglycaemia

I. Primarily due to underproduction of glucose

A. Hormones deficiencies
- Hypopituitarism
- Adrenal insufficiency
- Glucagon insufficiency
- Catecholamine insufficiency

B. Enzymatic defect
- Glucose-6-phosphatase
- Liver phosphorylase
- Pyruvate carboxylase
- Fructose 1–6 biphosphatase

C. Substrate deficiency
- Ketotic hypoglycaemia of infancy
- Severe malnutrition
- Late pregnancy

D. Liver disease
- Severe hepatitis or cirrhosis

E. Drugs and toxins
- Alcohol
- Propranolol, salicylates

II. Primarily due to overutilisation of gluocose

A. Hyperinsulinism
- Insulinoma
- Exogenous insulin or sulphonylureas
- Insulin-autoimmunity

B. Inappropriate insulin levels
- Extrapancreatic tumours
- Systemic carnitine deficiency
- Cachexia with fat depletion, e.g. cancer

Postprandial hypoglycaemia

A. Alimentary hyperinsulinism
- Post-gastrectomy
- Bariatric surgery
- Post-gastrojejunostomy
- Post-pyloroplasty
- Post-vagotomy (dumping syndrome)

B. Hereditary fructose intolerance. It is a cause in children

C. Galactosaemia—a cause in children

D. Leucine sensitivity—a cause in infants.

E. Idiopathic (immunopathological)
- Antibodies to insulin or insulin receptors.

F. Pseudohypoglycaemia—occurs during stress or anxiety. It is also seen in certain chronic leukaemias when leucocytes count are markedly elevated, which utilise the glucose. This is usually asymptomatic.

also have impaired central activation of neuro-endocrine secretion. Failure of counter-regulatory mechanisms with impaired awareness of hypoglycaemia alter the glycaemic threshold for the onset of hormone secretion and symptoms in the affected patients, i.e. blood glucose has to fall to a critical lower level to trigger these responses.

Clinical Features

The symptoms and signs of hypoglycaemia are given in Box 3, occur due to:

1. **Sympathetic overactivity.**
2. **Neuroglycopenia** as brain being the main utiliser of glucose.

Box 3 Symptoms and signs of hypoglycaemia

Sympathetic overactivity	*Neuroglycopenia*
• Palpitation	• Headache
• Sweating	• Fatigue
• Anxiety	• Impaired consciousness
• Tremors	• Dizziness
• Shivering	• Inappropriate behaviour
• Pallor	• Difficulty in speech
• Vomiting	• Confusion, drowsiness
	• Seizures
	• Focal neurological signs such as hemiplegia, amnesia
	• Coma

In most instances, the patient has no difficulty in recognizing the symptoms of hypoglycaemia and can take appropriate timely measures. However, in certain circumstances (e.g. during sleep or during periods of strict glycaemic control) and in patients with long duration of diabetes, warning symptoms are not always perceived by the patient even when awake, so that appropriate action is not taken and neuroglycopenia with reduced consciousness ensues. Occasionally, sudden death occurs during sleep in an otherwise healthy young type 1 diabetic ('dead-in-bed' syndrome), hypoglycaemia-induced cardiac arrhythmias or acute respiratory arrest with impaired baroreflex sensitivity has been proposed as the cause.

When blood sugar falls rapidly, adrenergic (sympathetic) symptoms predominate, but if the fall of blood sugar is gradual neuroglyco-penic symptoms dominate.

Patients who have frequent episodes of hypo glycaemia may not experience the symptoms of hypoglycaemia until blood glucose is well below the 50 mg/dl level and they may usually present with serious neurological deficits. This phenomenon is termed as *hypoglycaemic unawareness*, seen in type 1 diabetics with long duration of diabetes, is reversible in the initial stages.

Reactive (postprandial) spontaneous hypogly-caemia as discussed earlier occurs in response to food (3–5 hours ingestion of food). True reactive hypoglycaemia occurs in non-di-abetic patients who have undergone some sort of gastrointestinal surgery or suffer from some gastrointestinal disorders. Rapid gastric emptying with inappropriate insulin release is the proposed mechanism of hypoglycaemia in such patients.

Fasting hypoglycaemia, e.g. during fasting state, indicates some underlying disease which results in either underproduction or overuti-lisation of glucose under the effect of insulin.

Physical Signs

Common signs include *diaphoresis, pollar, tachy-cardia, systolic hypertension* and *bilateral plantar extensors*. These may not occur in patients with reputed episodes.

Diagnosis

The documentation of hypoglycaemia is done by **Whipple triad**, i.e. (i) symptoms consistent with hypoglycaemia, (ii) low plasma glucose level < 55 mg and (iii) relief of symptoms after intake of glucose.

If a non-diabetic develops similar symptoms particularly confusion, loss of consciousness or convulsions, then a diagnostic work-up is required as follows:

1. **Document hypoglycaemia** from finger-prick by glucometer or dextrostix and draw samples for glucose, insulin levels, C-peptide, ketones, liver function tests, etc. Diagnosis of hypoglycaemia is made on a finger stick blood glucose <50 mg/dl concommitantly elevated plasma insulin, proinsulin and C-peptide levels and a negative sulphonyl urea screen.

2. **Tests for spontaneous hypoglycaemia (post prandial):** The only test is to document hypoglycaemia (< 50 mg%) during sponta-neously developed symptoms.
   - A 5-hour oral glucose tolerance test showing a plasma glucose of 50 mg% or less is suggestive.

3. **Diagnostic tests for insulinoma**
   (i) An insulin level of 20 U/ml or more in the presence of blood glucose value below 40 mg/dl. is diagnostic.
   (ii) Elevated circulating proinsulin levels (C-peptide) differentiates between insulinoma and factitious hyperinsu-linism (Box 4).

Box 4 Factition hypoglycemia vs insulinoma	
Fractitious Hypoglycaemia	*Insulinoma*
1. Low blood sugar	Low blood sugar
2. High insulin levels	High insulin level
3. Low C-peptide level	High C-peptide level

   (iii) *C-peptide suppression test:* Absence of suppression of C-peptide during hypoglycaemia induced by 0.1 ml of insulin/kg/hr is diagnostic of insulin-emia. A normal person would suppress the peptide level to 50% or more during hypo glycaemia.
   (iv) Insulin/glucose ratio >0.4 suggest insulinoma. Normally this ratio is less than 0.4.
   (v) After recovery from the emergency situation, appropriate tests such as ultrasound, CT scan and MRI are done to arrive at the diagnosis and to locate the tumour (insulinoma) preopera-tively.

Differential Diagnosis

The differences between hypoglycaemic coma and hyperglycaemic coma are given in Table 69.2.

Management

Domiciliary treatment

Oral treatment with glucose tablets or glucose containing fluids, candy is appropriate if patient is able and willing to take it. An initial dose is 20 g of glucose.

Emergency treatment

Severe hypoglycaemia means 'hypoglycaemia requiring the assistance of another person for recovery', can result in serious morbidity and has a recognised mortality of 2–4% in insulin-treated patients. The unrecognized mortality may be still higher. Therefore, hypoglycaemia associated with unconsciousness or stupor should be treated on emergency basis. The treatment should not be withheld for want of a biochemical confirmation of diagnosis. The steps of treatment include:

1. Stop the drug if it is the cause. Most of these cases are either due to OHA or insulin-induced hypoglycaemia.

2. Start intravenous administration of 25–50 ml of 50% glucose through a big vein over a period of 2–3 minutes followed by an infusion of 5 to 10% glucose guided by serial plasma glucose measurements. An unconscious patient may improve within 15–20 minutes to permit ingestion of sugar. Sulphonylurea-induced hypoglycaemia lasts longer (>48 hours), hence, requires continuous monitoring and prolonged infusion of glucose. In patients who do not regain consciousness within 1–2 hours, cerebral oedema should be suspected for which I.V. dexamethasone may be administered along with mannitol.

3. If I.V. therapy is not practical due to collapsed veins then glucagon (1 mg SC or I.M.) is preferable. It is more useful in patients with type 1 DM than type 2 DM. Glucagon is not useful in alcohol-induced hypoglycaemia.

   The *somatostatin analogue octreotide* can be used to suppress insulin secretion in sulphonylurea-induced hypoglycaemia. After episode, patient is asked to eat to replete the glycogen stores.

4. Treatment of the underlying cause of hypoglycaemia would be essential to prevent relapses:

   - The treatment of postprandial hypoglycaemia following surgery is just alteration in dietary habits. Frequent small feeds are advised in nonspecific reactive hypoglycaemia, the diet should contain some slowly absorbable carbohydrates and more proteins. Alpha glucosidase therapy may be useful adjunct to a low carbohydrate diet. Octreotide 50 mcg S.C. 2 or 3 times a day 30 min before each meal has been reported to

Table 69.2	Salient features of hypoglycaemic and hyperglycaemic coma	
Feature	Hypoglycaemic coma	Hyperglycaemic coma
Pulse rate	Increased	Increased
Pulse volume	Good	Weak (low)
Temperature	May be low or normal	May be low
Respiration	Shallow or Normal	Rapid and deep
BP	Normal, may be increased	Decreased
Skin and tongue	Moist	Dry
Breath	No acetone smell	Acetone smell may be present
Reflexes	Brisk (plantars extensors)	Diminished (plantars flexor)
Urine glucose	Negative	Positive
Plasma glucose	<50 mg/dl	> 200mg/dl
Plasma acetone	Negative	Usually present
Plasma HCO$_3$	Normal	<20 mEq/L
PCO$_2$	Normal	Diminished
Blood pH	Normal	<7.3

improve symptoms due to late dumping syndrome. Treatment with GLP-1 receptor agonist may prevent postgastric bypass hypoglycaemia.

- Anticholinergics may be useful in reducing rapid gastric emptying.
- Avoidance of leucine containing diet in leucine sensitivity.
- Avoid use of alcohol. Prevention of alcohol-induced hypoglycaemia in addition to stoppage of alcohol include adequate food intake and avoidance of sugar mixers while ingesting alcohol.
- Avoid food containing sugar or fructose, if there is hereditary fructose intolerance.

- Treat the critical or other illness if found to be the cause, e.g.
  - *Treatment of insulinoma* by medical therapy (diazoxide or octreotide) or surgery for cure (resection of adenoma)
  - *Treatment of autoimmune* disorders by steroids and immunosuppressive drugs. Treat the causative factors for autoimmune hypoglycaemia, i.e. stop the offending drug, i.e. methimazole, pencillamine, isoniazide, procainamide etc. and most consistent therapeutic benefit is achieved by dietary management with small, frequent low carbohydrate meals.

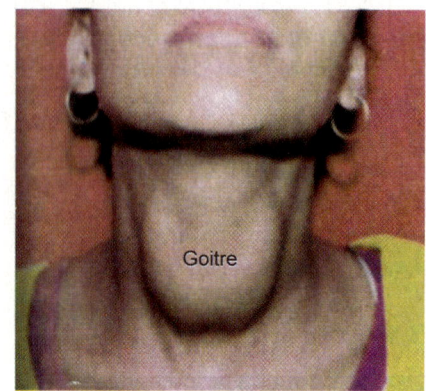

Fig. 70.1: Graves' disease

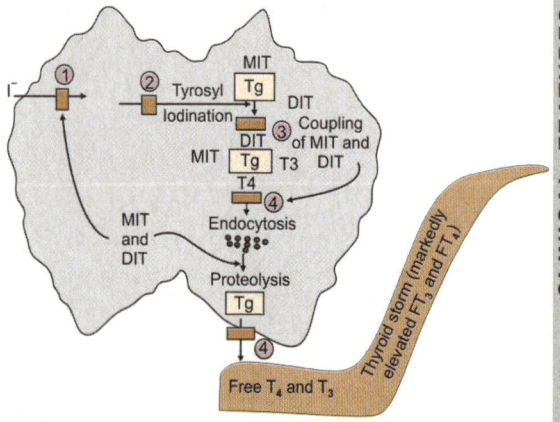

Step in hormone synthesis
(1) Iodine uptake (2) Iodination of tyrosyl thyroglobuli (Tg)
(3) coupling reaction (4) endocytosis (5) release of free T_4 and T_3
MIT: monoidotyrosin DIT: dl-iodotyrosin T_3: triodothyronine
T_4: tetraidothyronin

CLINICAL FEATURES

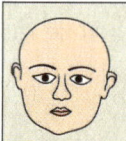
- Diffuse or multinodular goitre
- Staring look or frightening face
- Wide palpebral fissures
- Exophthalmos
- Lid lag or lid retraction
- Excessive watering of eyes
- Diplopia

- Tachycardia/palpitation
- Good volume or water-hammer pulse
- Exertional dyspnoea
- CHF
- Hypotension instead of hypertension
- Cardiac arrhythmias (AF is common)

- Diarrhoea or steatorrhoea
- Vomiting
- Weight loss

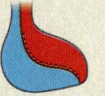
- Nervousness, irritability
- Restlessness, psychosis
- Tremors
- Muscular weakness (proximal myopathy)
- Exaggerated tendon reflexes
- Confusion, stupor, coma

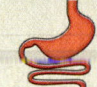
- Perspiration
- Loss of hairs
- Pretibial myxoedema
- Redness of palms
- Hot skin (hyperpyrexia)

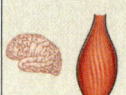
- Menstrual irregularity
- Abortions
- Infertility
- Loss of libido or impotence

Miscellaneous
- Hyperpyrexia (>104°F)
- Excessive thirst
- Dehydration
- Undue excitability/anger
- Gynaecomastia

Fig. 70.2: Features of thyroid storm (markedly elevated FT3 and FT4 hormones)

THYROID CRISIS OR STORM

Definition

Thyrotoxic crisis or storm is a life-threatening situation due to fulminant increase in the signs and symptoms of thyrotoxicosis. This rare condition with a mortality of about 10% is rapid deterioration of thyrotoxicosis with hyperpyrexia (>104°F), severe tachycardia (or new onset arrhythmia) and altered mental status with extreme restlessness, nausea, vomiting and jaundice.

Causes

The causes of thyrotoxicosis and thyrotoxic crisis are same because the latter condition just presents with an exaggerated form of the former. The most common cause of thyroid storm is Graves' disease. The other causes are listed in Box 1.

Box 1	Causes of thyrotoxicosis and thyroid crisis

- Graves' disease (Fig. 70.1)
- Multinodular toxic goitre
- Solitary toxic adenoma
- Factitious thyrotoxicosis (self-administration of excessive thyroid hormone)
- Iodine-induced hyperthyroidism (*Jodbasedow's* disease)

Note: Precipitation of underlying thyrotoxicosis due to the causes mentioned above lead to thyroid crisis, hence, they are the primary events.

Precipitating Factors

The primary event is thyrotoxicosis. The secondary events leading to thyroid storm are not quite clear. The basic precipitating event is either an increase in free hormone level due to a shift from protein bound state to free-hormone state secondary to circulating inhibitors to binding, or there is an exaggerated response to a given level of thyroid hormones or both. The exaggerated sympathetic response or hyperadrenergic response seen in thyroid storm is due to increase in the number of baroreceptors on the target cells and post-receptor events.

Box 2	Precipitating factors responsible for thyroid storm/crisis
Thyroidal factors (acute rise in thyroid hormone)	Nonthyroidal illness
• Surgery on thyroid	• Surgery of any type CVA, sepsis
• Withdrawal of antithyroidal drugs	• Diabetic ketoacidosis
• Radio-iodine therapy	• Trauma
• Iodinated contrast media use	• Stress, e.g. emotional
• Vigorous thyroid palpation	• Pulmonary embolism

A large number of factors both thyroidal and non-thyroidal can precipitate thyroid crisis in a patient with thyrotoxicosis (Box 2).

In the past, this syndrome occurred postoperatively in patients poorly prepared for surgery, but now it is less common. Now, so called medical storm occurs commonly in untreated or inadequately treated patients. It is precipitated by surgery or a complicating illness usually sepsis.

Clinical Features (Fig. 70.2)

Most patients presenting with thyroid storm/crisis have received either under-treatment (inadequately treated) or no treatment or have recently developed the disease (fresh case). However, thyrotoxic crisis may occur in a patient previously unrecognised to have thyrotoxicosis especially in an elderly with a nodular goitre.

There are no specific diagnostic criteria but high grade fever (>104°F) out of proportion than infection, severe tachycardia and CNS symptoms (irritability, restlessness, seizures, delirium or coma) with vomiting diarrhoea, dehydration and hypotension in setting of thyrotoxicosis should raise the possibility of thyroid crisis (Fig. 70.2). The elderly usually go into congestive heart failure and develop cardiac arrhythmias (atrial fibrillation). Atypical presentation (apathetic thyrotoxicosis with thyroid storm characterised by apathy, prostration and coma but with minimal elevation of temperature) can occur in elderly. A scoring system used for diagnosis of thyroid storm is given in Table 70.1.

Table 70.1 Scoring system for diagnosis of thyroid storm (Burch et al.) in a patient with thyrotoxicosis

Dysfunction	Score
1. **Thermoregulatory dysfunction**	5
• 100° – 100.9°F	10
• 101° – 101.9°F	15
• 102° – 102.9°F	20
• 103° –103.9°F	25
• >104°	30
2. **CNS effects**	
• Agitation (mild)	10
• Delirium, lethargy, psychosis	20
• Severe seizure, coma	30
3. **GI tract and hepatic dysfunction**	
• No dysfunction	0
• Moderate dysfunction (vomiting, diarrhoea, pain abdomen)	10
• Jaundice (severe)	20
4. **CVS dysfunction**	
• Heart rate 90–109/min	5
110–119/min	10
120–129/min	15
130–139/min	20
> 140/min	25
5. **Others**	
• Atrial fibrillation	10
• Congestive heart failure	
Mild—pedal oedema	5
Moderate—Basal crepts	10
Severe—Pulmonary oedema	15
• History of precipitating cause	10
• With total score >45, thyroid storm is highly likely	
• Score between 25–44 suggests impending storm	
• Score <25, thyroid storm is unlikely	

Investigations

1. **Thyroid hormones:** The FT_3 and FT_4 are markedly elevated and TSH is markedly depressed. The levels of the hormones can not differentiate a patient with thyrotoxicosis from thyroid storm because there is no cut off limit of elevated hormones in the two conditions and secondly hormone levels are not directly related to the clinical picture. The diagnosis of thyrotoxicosis is purely clinical. Measurement of TPO antibodies or RTAb may be useful if diagnosis is unclear.

2. **Blood examination:** Microcytic anaemia and thrombocytopenia can occur.

3. Renal, hepatic profile to see their dysfunction under the effect of thyroid hormones.

4. **Blood sugar:** Both hyperglycaemia and hypocalcaemia can occur in thyroid storm.

5. **Serum calcium:** There may be hypercalcaemia under the effects of thyroid hormones.

6. **X-ray chest (PA view)** may show enlargement of cardiac silhouette.

7. **ECG:** This may show good voltage of QRS complexes, severe tachycardia, cardiac arrhythmia (AF is common).

8. Investigations done to find out the cause, e.g. **USG, radioactive iodine uptake** and **thyroid scanning** to plan definite treatment.

Management

Since the diagnosis of thyroid crisis/storm is made clinically, therefore, treatment should begin after sending the samples for thyroid hormones assay.

Aims of Treatment

• Supportive therapy.
• To undertake measures to alleviate thyrotoxicosis as early as possible.

Supportive measures

A. *Correction of dehydration:*
   • Adequate amount of fluids (glucose and saline) to correct dehydration as early as possible. Vitamins should be supplemented.
   • *Glucocorticoids:* Dexamethasone 2 mg 6 hourly is given because of increased glucocorticoid requirements and decreased adrenal reserve in thyrotoxicosis. It also inhibits peripheral conversion of T_4 to T_3 as discussed below.

B. *Treatment of pyrexia*
- Patient should be preferably placed in a cooled, humified, oxygen tent, if possible.
- To bring down fever with external cooling and acetaminophen. Avoid salicylates as they increase free thyroid hormone levels.
- Antibiotics to be given if infection present.

C. *Treatment of congestive heart failure or arrhythmias:*
- Digitalisation is required to control ventricular rate in those with atrial fibrillation.
- Diuretics are added to digoxin for treatment of CHF.

D. *Treatment of infection by appropriate anti biotics if there is an evidence of sepsis.*

Specific therapy

It is aimed at to bring down the elevated thyroid hormones and to block their systemic effects. The measures include:

i. *Inhibition of thyroid hormone synthesis by antithyroid drugs:* As injectable preparation of antithyroid drugs is not available, therefore, oral therapy with neomercazole (20–30 mg after every 6 hours) or methimazole (15–25 mg orally every 6 hours) or propyl thiouracil (600 mg stat and 200–300 mg after 6 hours with a total dose of 1000–1500 mg/day) is started orally followed by a maintenance dose of 60 mg neomercazole or methimazole or 600 mg of propylthiouracil (PTU). PTU has an added effect of reducing conversion of T_4 to T_3, hence is considered as drug of choice.

ii. *Inhibition of hormone release:* Large doses of iodine, e.g. Lugol's iodine (10 drops t.d.s.), saturated solution of KI (8 drops 3 times daily) or sodium iodide 1 g I.V. or sodium ipodate 500 mg to 1 g oral prevents the release of preformed hormone in circulation. Iodine should be given only after about an hour of antithyroid drug therapy (it blocks the thyroid hormone synthesis via Wolff-Chaikoff effect) otherwise iodine will facilitate hormone biosynthesis. Improvement is seen within 24 hours and hormones level come down to normal or near normal within 5 to 7 days. After this, iodine can be withdrawn and antithyroid drugs therapy continued for thyrotoxicosis.

iii. *Blockade of conversion of T_4 to T_3:* Hydrocortisome 300 mg I.V. bolus and then 100 mg and hourly or dexamethasone 2–4 mg I.V. every 6–8 hourly inhibits peripheral conversion of T_4 to T_3, then it is gradually tapered off. It also provides protection against relative deficiency of steroids during thyroid storm as discussed under supportive measures. PTU, beta-blockers and sodium ipodate also decrease peripheral conversion of T_4 to T_3.

iv. *Removal of thyroid hormone from circulation:* Plasmapheresis has been used for this purpose in few studies. This mode of therapy is routinely not available.

v. *Blockade of peripheral effects of hormones:* Propranolol in dose of 20–80 mg every 6 hourly is drug of choice to counter the peri pheral effects of thyroid hormones especially on CVS and CNS. Treatment can be given initially with I.V. propranolol (0.5–1 mg every 4 hourly). Esmolol—an ultrashort acting beta-blocker is preferred in patients with CHF in dose of 250–500 mg/kg I.V. stat followed by infusion at a rate of 50–100 mg/kg/min.

vi. *The precipitating cause* should be found out and treated simultaneously.

vii. Definite treatment with ^{131}I or surgery is delayed until the patient becomes euthyroid.

Myxoedema Coma

MYXOEDEMA COMA

Definition

It is an advanced stage of long-standing hypothyroidism (Fig. 71.1) characterised by florid symptoms and signs of hypothyroidism with hypothermia and stuporous or comatose state provoked by a precipitating factor.

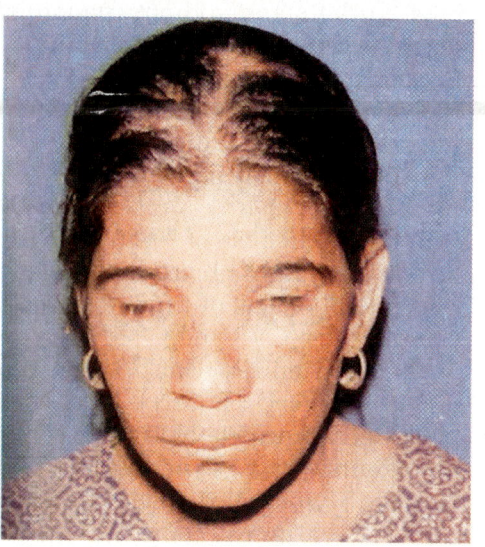

Fig. 71.1: Long-standing hypothyroidism in a 65 years female. Note the gross features of hypothyroidism (e.g. periorbital oedema, thick lips, wrinkles, swollen face, dry skin). Such a patient is prone to develop myxoedema coma under the effect of a precipitating factor but it is a rare phenomenon

Myxoedema coma is a medical emergency, seen in older persons, occurs commonly during winter months and carries a high mortality rate (about 50%), if left untreated.

Precipitating Factors

The factors that push the patient of hypothyroidism into myxoedema coma are given in Box 1.

Box 1	Precipating factors for myxoedema coma
• Infection, e.g. pneumonia	• Stroke (CVA)
• Exposure to cold	• CNS depressants, e.g. tranquillisers, sedatives and antidepressants
• Hypoventilation	
• Hypoglycaemia	
• Dilutional of hyponataemia	
• Trauma	• Cardiovascular disease (e.g. CHF), MI
• GI bleeding	• Respiratory disease (infection, COPD)

Hypoventilation leading to hypoxia and hypercapnia plays a major role in pathogenesis. Hypoglycaemia and dilutional hyponatraemia also contribute to the development of myxoedema coma.

Clinical Features

1. **Altered mental status or coma:** The mental deterioration is gradual. To start with, patient may have confusion or disorientation before lapsing into coma.

2. **Hypothermia:** Myxoedema coma is usually but not always accompanied by a subnormal body temperature (as low as 25°C). Because the ordinary clinical thermometers do not record such low temperatures as they are not graduated below 33° or 35°C, the true severity of hypo thermia may not be appreciated. The body is cold and dry. Hypothermia may precede the development of coma.

3. **Other features:** In addition to character-istic features of hypothyroidism such as weight gain, cold intolerance, hoarseness of voice, bradycardia, dry toad skin, sparse hair, nonpitting oedema, menstrual irreg-ularity, impotence and constipation, etc. there may be some other features or some altered features:
   - The patient may display areflexia (loss of tendon reflexes) instead of delayed tendon jerks.
   - Patient may have hypotension instead of hypertension of hypothyroidism.
   - Seizures may accompany the comatose state.
   - Hypoventilation (hypoxaemia, hyper-capnia) with depressed shallow respira-tion may be caused by respiratory muscle weakness, upper airway obstruction by large tongue (macroglossia) or depres-sion of respiratory centre.
   - Hypoglycaemia may occur due to hypothyroidism combined with cortisol deficiency.

Investigations

They are done to confirm the diagnosis and to find out the precipitating cause.

1. **T_3, T_4, TSH:** The T_3 and T_4 levels are low and TSH levels are high.
2. **Plasma cortisol:** This is done to find out cortisol insufficiency which is commonly associated with it.
3. **Random blood sugar:** Hypoglycaemia can occur.
4. **Blood gas analysis** to find out hypoxaemia and hypercapnia.

5. **Serum sodium and plasma osmolarity:** Dilutional hyponatraemia is common in 50% of patients due to inappropriate secretion of ADH.
6. **EKG:** For low voltage graph or cardiac involvement (conduct defects, pericardial effusion).
7. **Chest X-ray:** May show cardiomegaly due to pericardial effusion or features of congestive cardiac failure.

Differential Diagnosis

The conditions which are associated with coma and hypothermia may mimic myxoedema coma. These include:

1. **Brainstem infarction** in older persons may lead to both coma and hypothermia.
2. Hypothermia due to any cause and renal failure may itself induce physiological changes simulating myxoedema such as delayed relaxation of deep tendon reflexes. Coma is due to hypothermia and renal failure.

Management

Myxoedema coma is an medical emergency, carries a high mortality, hence, treatment must begin before the biochemical confirmation of the diagnosis.

1. **Replacement thyroxine therapy:** The treatment ideally recommended is intrave-nous thyroxine 500–600 µg stat then 100 µg I.V. daily till patient comes out of coma but intravenous preparation of thyroxine is not available in India, therefore, oral therapy with 500 µg is begun followed by 100 µg 6 hourly through Ryle's tube. Alternatively liothyronine (T_3) I.V. or via Ryle's tube in doses ranging from 10 to 25 µg/every 8–12 hours is given. This treatment has been advocated because conversion of T_4 into T_3 is impaired in myxoedema. Another option is to use a combination of T_4 (200 µg) and T_3 (25 µg) as a single I.V. dose followed by daily treatment with T_4 (50–100 µg/day) and T_3 10 µg 8 hourly).

2. **Concomitant hydrocortisone therapy:** As there is commonly associated adrenal insufficiency or reduced adrenal reserve, hydrocortisone intravenous infusion (5–10 mg/hour) or 100 mg I.V. stat followed by 25–50 mg 8 hourly may be administered after collecting the blood sample for basal cortisol level. If plasma cortisol is normal, this can be stopped.

3. **Supportive therapy**
   - *Endotracheal intubation and ventilatory support*: If hypercapnia present and needs ventilation. Monitor blood gas analysis.
   - *Fluid replacement:*
     - Avoid hypotonic fluids because of risk of water intoxication due to SIADH. Hyponatremia ($Na^+<120$–130 mEq/L) is treated with I.V. normal saline. Severe hyponatraemia is treated with bolus doses of NaCl with monitoring of sodium level.
     - Fluid restriction (<1 litre) or hypertonic saline for severe dilutional hyponatraemia, if present.

   - *External/rewarming of the body with blankets* if temperature is 30°C to prevent heat loss. Avoid active rewarming as this may lead to vascular collapse due to vasodilatation.
     - *In case of hypoglycaemia,* 25–50% glucose solution may be given.
     - *General care of coma patient:* It consists of frequent turning or change of posture, prevention of aspiration by suction, care of bowel and bladder, etc.
     - *Vitals should be monitored.*
     - *Treatment of coexisting diseases* such as infection by antibiotics. Management of other associated disease appropriately.

Mortality

The mortality is very high (60–70%): Severe hypothermia, delay in initiating therapy, inadequate doses of thyroxine, failure to recognize and treat the precipitating factors are responsible for it.

Acute Adrenal Crisis/ Insufficiency

Definition

Acute adrenal crisis or insufficiency is sudden deterioration of adrenocortical functions leading to insufficient cortisol. It occurs commonly due to rapid and overwhelming intensification of chronic adrenal insufficiency (*Addison's disease*), but occurs uncommonly due to acute adrenal destruction secondary to haemorrhage, sepsis or sudden withdrawal of steroids, etc.

Adrenal crisis is a medical emergency, needs immediate attention and treatment. If diagnosis is missed, the patient will probably die of it.

Causes

They are given in Table 72.1.

1. **Precipitation of chronic adrenal insufficiency** by hyperthyroidism, sepsis, surgical stress or intercurrent infection, prolonged fasting, etc.
2. **Acute bilateral destruction of adrenal glands** by haemorrhage (anticoagulation or a coagulation disorder), embolisation or sepsis in previously healthy subjects.
3. **In children, it may be associated with septicaemia** (pseudomonas infection or meningococaemia—called *Waterhouse-Friderichsen syndrome*).
4. **Sudden withdrawal of steroids** from patients with adrenal atrophy due to chronic steroid use.
5. It may occur in patients with *congenital adrenal hyperplasia or those with poor adrenal reserve* when they receive drugs causing further suppression of steroid synthesis such as phenytoin, rifampicin and ketoconazole, etc.

Table 72.1 Aetiology of adrenal crisis/acute adrenal insufficiency

Adrenal causes	Pituitary causes
• Sudden precipitation of Addison's disease of adrenal origin	• Postpartum pituitary necrosis (Sheehan's syn...
• Bilateral adrenal haemorrhage (anticoagulant therapy or a coagulation disorder)	• Necrosis or bleeding into pituitary microa...
• Bilateral adrenal thrombosis, e.g. antiphospholipid syndrome	• Head trauma • Lesions of pituitary stalk
• Adrenal necrosis due to sepsis or septicaemia (Waterhouse-Friderichsen syndrome)	• Pituitary or adrenal surgery for Cush...

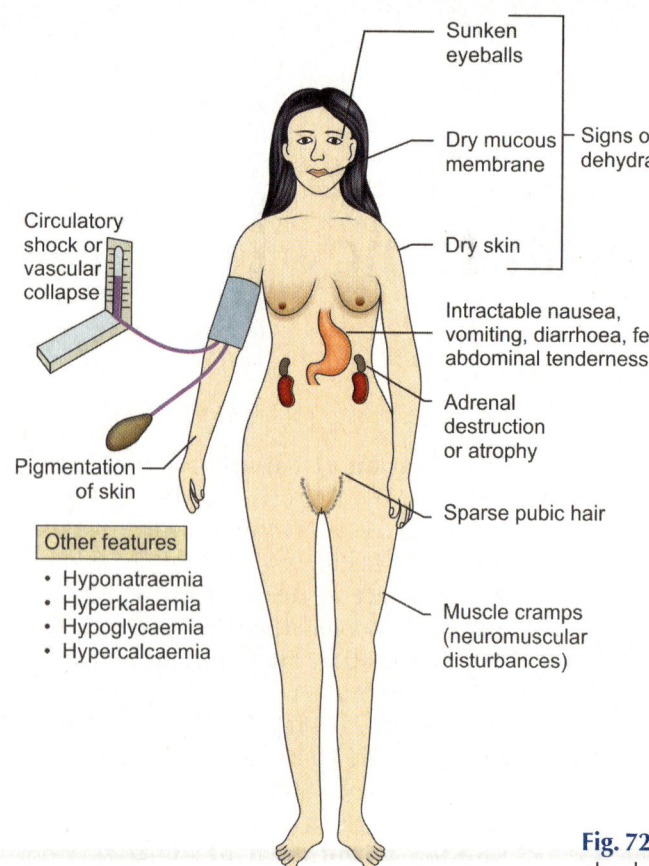

Fig. 72.1: Clinical features of acute adrenal insufficiency (acute precipitation of Addison's disease)

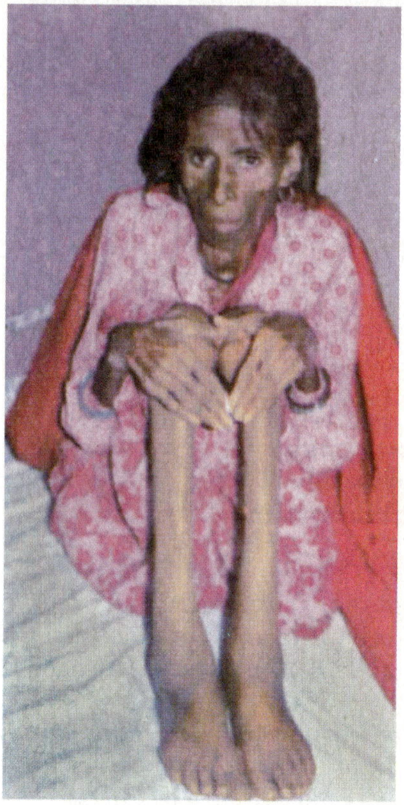

Fig. 72.2: A patient of Addison's disease. Note sunken cheeks and eyeballs, dry pigmented skin and mucous membrane. Patient had long duration of diarrhoea and developed pedal oedema. Such a patient is likely to develop acute crisis during sepsis or surgery

6. Following administration of etormdate which is used intravenously for rapid anesthesia induction or intubation.

...ical Features

...es of acute adrenal insufficiency are ...Fig. 72.1. The features result from ...oids and mineralocorticoids and ...eficiency with ACTH excess ...t, acute adrenal crisis include ...symptoms and signs of ...se (Fig. 72.2) such as acute ...e or shock with severe ...dration, hyponatraemia, ...some instances hypogly- ...aemia. Muscle cramps,

intractable nausea, vomiting and diarrhoea, and unexplained fever may be present. The crisis is often precipitated by surgery or sepsis.

Investigations

1. **Eosinophil count** may be high.
2. **Plasma cortisol (morning and evening):** It will be low (<3 mcg/dl at 8 am). A plasma cortisol in normal range in acutely ill patient does not rule out adrenal insufficiency.
3. **Short one hour ACTH (cosyntropin) stimulation test:** In adrenal insufficiency, serum cortisol does not rise in response to ACTH. (i.e. cortisol level remains

Box 1 Symptoms and signs of adrenal insufficiency	
Glucocorticoid deficiency	*Mineralocorticoid insufficiency*
• Weight loss, weakness, lack of energy, fatigue • Anorexia, nausea, vomiting • Diarrhoea or constipation	• Hypotension (postural), low BP • Shock • Hyponatraemia • Salt craving and abdominal pain
• Postural hypotension, syncope, shock • Joint pain, myalgia • Hypoglycaemia, hyponatraemia and hypercalcaemia • Anaemia, lymphocytosis, eosinophilia	• Hyperkalemia
ACTH excess	*Adrenal androgen insufficiency*
• Pigmentation on sun-exposed areas, pressure sores, e.g. elbow, knee and mucous membrane, conjunctivae, palmar creases and recent scars	• Decreased body hair (e.g. pubic, axillary) and loss of libido especially in females • Lack of energy • Dry and itchy skin

below the cut off limit of 500–550 nmol/L sampled one hour after ACTH stimulation).

4. **ACTH levels** will help to diagnose whether adrenal insufficiency is primary (high level) or *secondary* (low level). Low plasma cortisol with high level ACTH simultaneously suggests primary adrenal insufficiency/crisis.

5. **Serum DHEA levels** <1000 ng/ml in all patients with Addison's disease.

6. **Serum Na⁺ and K⁺ level.** Serum Na$^+$ is normal to low and K$^+$ is high. Blood sugar levels low. Serum calcium level may be high.

7. **Screening for steroid auto antibodies for autoimmune adrenalitis.** They are positive in 50% cases with autoimmune Addison's disease/crisis. Antibodies to 21-hydroxylase help confirm the diagnosis of autoimmune adrenal disease/crisis. Antibodies to thyroid may be present in 45% cases.

8. **CT scan** of adrenal glands may reveal the underlying cause (hemorrhage, infliltration or masses).

9. **Blood, sputum, or urine culture** may be positive of bacterial infection is the precipitating cause of the crisis.

Management

Aims

- Rapid elevation of glucocorticoids levels.
- Replacement of sodium and water deficits. The hyponatraemia (Na$^+$ <120 mmol/L) is in itself an emergency. This may lead to delirium, coma and seizures.
- There is little time to consider specific laboratory confirmation of the diagnosis in an adrenal crisis which is a life-threatening emergency, hence, the management is often instituted immediately when the diagnosis is made.

Treatment

1. **Fluid replacement:** Large volume of 5% dextrose in saline or 0.9% normal saline (1L/hr)should be infused immediately with continuous cardiac monitoring.

2. **Steroid replacement therapy:** Intravenous hydrocortisone 100 mg IV as a bolus or dexamethasone 4 mg IV stat, followed by a continuous infusion of hydrocortisone at a rate of 10 mg/hour. An alternative approach is to give 100 mg I.V. hydrocortisone as a bolus, then 100 mg I.V. after every 6 hours for first day, then same dose is given 8 hourly for second day until gastrointestinal symptoms abate and patient starts accepting orally.

Dexamethasone is preferred because its effect lasts for 12–24 hours and it does not interfere with measurement of plasma or urinary steroids during subsequent ACTH stimulation test.

3. **Treatment of hypotension or shock:** Effective treatment of hypotension or shock requires glucocorticoid replacement and repletion of sodium and water deficits. Vasoactive agents (e.g. dopamine) may be indicated in severe hypotension as an adjuvant to fluid therapy.

4. **No need for mineralocorticoid replacement:** With large doses of steroids, e.g. 100 to 200 mg hydrocortisone, the patient receives a maximal mineralocorticoid effect, hence, supplementation of mineralocorticoid will be superfluous.

5. **Identification of precipitating cause and its treatment:** Since bacterial infection frequently precipitates acute adrenal crisis, broad-spectrum antibiotic should be administered empirically while waiting for culture reports. The patient must also be treated for electrolyte abnormalities, hypoglycaemia and dehydration.

Following improvement, the steroid dosage is tapered over next few days to maintenance levels, and mineralocorticosteroid therapy is reinstituted. Most patients who present with acute adrenal insufficiency have deficiency of both glucocorticoids and mineralocorticoids, hence, in addition to maintenance dose of glucocorticoids (7.5 to 10 mg/day), a lifelong replacement of mineralocorticoid (fludrocortisone 0.05 to 0.1 mg/day) orally can be started as soon as saline drip is stopped and patient accepts orally.

Prevention of Further Episodes

1. **Concurrent illness:** The patient is advised to add salt to the diet during the period of excessive exercise with sweating, hot weather/season and during vomiting or diarrhoea. During an episode of febrile illness, patient should double the dose of steroids for 3–5 days and consult his/her physician if the illness persists longer. Acute gastroenteritis needs immediate hospitalization for fluid and steroids therapy to prevent dehydration and shock.

2. **Surgery:** *Minor procedures* under local anaesthesia (e.g. dental extraction) do not need any change in steroid regimen. *Moderate stressful procedures* (e.g. endoscopy, bronchoscopy, arteriography), need to be covered with an additional dose of 100 mg of hydrocortisone I.V. just before surgery, another 100 mg is given just before anaesthesia and then 100 mg I.V. every 8 hourly till the patient stabilizes. The steroid dose is then tapered rapidly to maintenance dosage.

Pituitary Apoplexy

Definition

Pituitary insufficiency—a rare endocrinopathy characterised clinically by acute symptoms such as *sudden headache, visual disturbances, ophthalmoplegia, signs of meningeal irritation* and *altered mental status* caused by sudden or abrupt haemorrhage or infarction of the pituitary gland.

Pituitaty apoplexy is an endocrine emergency that may result in severe hypoglycaemia, hypotension and shock, CNS hemorrhage and death.

Although haemorrhage occurs in 10–15% cases of pituitary adenomas but most of them are clinically silent. Pituitary apoplexy may be diagnosed only in 2–10% of adenomas on development of typical features or on resolution of hypersecretory states. Pituitary apoplexy may occur spontaneous in a pre-existing pituitary tumour, postpartum hemorrhage (Sheehan's syndrome) or in association with diabetes, hypertension, sickle cell anaemia or acute shock.

Pathophysiology

Haemorrhage and necrosis of the pituitary adenoma are the cardinal pathological features of pituitary apoplexy and occur due to:

i. Pituitary adenomas are more vulnerable to bleeding than other tumours.
ii. A rapidly growing adenoma outstripes its blood supply and produces ischaemia followed by necrosis and secondary hemorrhage.
iii. Compression of a large pituitary stalk carrying blood vessels by an expanding tumour mass may render the entire anterior lobe ischaemic followed by secondary haemorrhage.
iv. Fragility of the tumour blood vessels predispose to bleeding.
v. *Sheehan syndrome (pituitary necrosis following postpartum uterine hemorrhage) is characterised by amenorrhea* and inability to

Box 1 Predisposing factors for pituitary apoplexy	
• Radiation	• Following severe coughing and sneezing
• Drugs e.g. bromocriptine, anticoagulants and oestrogens	• Head trauma
• Following cardiac surgery	• Pregnancy
• Following procedures, e.g. angiography	• Diabetes
	• Following dynamic tests for pituitary function, e.g. pituitary stimulation tests

Table 73.1 Clinical presentations of pituitary apoplexy

Structure involved/compressed	Symptoms and signs
• Sudden enlargement of tumour mass	• Headache, sudden and severe retro-orbital and frontal pain
• Optic nerve	• Decreased visual acquity and visual field defects
• The III, IV and VI cranial nerve compression	• Ophthalmoplegia, ptosis and pupillary defects
• Meningeal irritation (disruption of dura or leakage of blood into subarachnoid space)	• Nausea, vomiting, headache, alteration in the level of consciousness, e.g. lethargy, stupor and coma
• Internal carotid artery	• Hemiplegia
• Compression of corticotrophs (loss of ACTH)	• Acute adrenal insufficiency
• Compression of gonadotrophs (loss of LH, FSH)	• Gonadal dysfunction
• Compression of pituitary stalk	• Diabetes insipidus
• Compression of thyrotrophs	• Hypofunction of thyroid
• Nonspecific, noncompressive	• Fever, anosmia, CSF rhinorrhoea and facial pain. Respiratory and cardiac rhythm disturbances

lactate. Hypopituitarism develops acutely usually with severe secondary adrenal insufficiency).

Causes and Predisposing Factors

The predisposing factors are given in Box 1.

Clinical Features

The clinical features are due to tumour mass and its pressure effects within sella turcica and outside sella turcica (Table 73.1).

Presentation can be acute characterised by rapid onset of neurological symptoms, hypoglycaemia, hypotension and coma. Death can occur. In subacute presentation, symptoms evolve over days to weeks and may present with evidence of hormone deficiency at a later date.

Course

The clinical course of pituitary apoplexy varies hence, difficult to predict the outcome. In mild benign form, the symptoms (headache and visual disturbances) develop slowly and persist over days to weeks and then improve; in fulminant form, the sudden onset of blindness, coma and hemodynamic disturbances (respiratory and cardiac) may lead to death.

Recovery of functions may occur with or without surgical intervention. Residual endocrine disturbance is the rule and panhypopituitarism invariably persists in most of the cases. In some cases, there may be selective loss of one or two trophic hormones.

Differential Diagnosis

Because of its diverse clinical presentation, pituitary apoplexy has to be differentiated on clinical and investigative grounds from the following conditions:
1. Subarachnoid haemorrhage.
2. Bacterial meningitis.

Investigations

- **Plain X-ray skull:** It may show enlargement of sella turcica and destruction of clinoid processes (Fig. 73.1). It can be normal also.
- **Pituitary CT/MRI scan:** The CT scan of the head may show a high density or inhomogeneous gland with or without evidence of blood in subarachnoid space and MRI scan is more useful than CT scan in identifying pituitary haemorrhage or haemorrhage in a tumour with pituitary stalk deviation and compression of pituitary tissue (Fig. 73.2).
- **Angiography:** It is done to differentiate pituitary apoplexy from subarachnoid haemorrhage due to aneurysmal rupture.
- **Other hormone levels:** Initially they may be normal except cortisol whose deficiency may develop acutely. Thyroid hormones (T_3, T_4, TSH) and gonadal hormone fall over weeks.

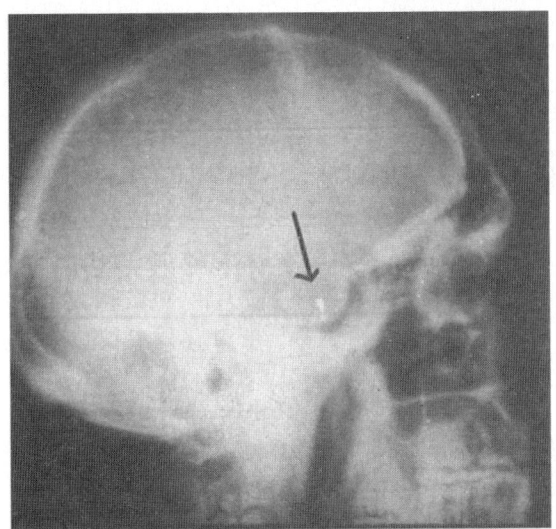

Fig. 73.1: X-ray skull (lateral view). There is widening and deepening of pituitary fossa (↓) with destruction of clinoid processes suggestive of a pituitary tumour

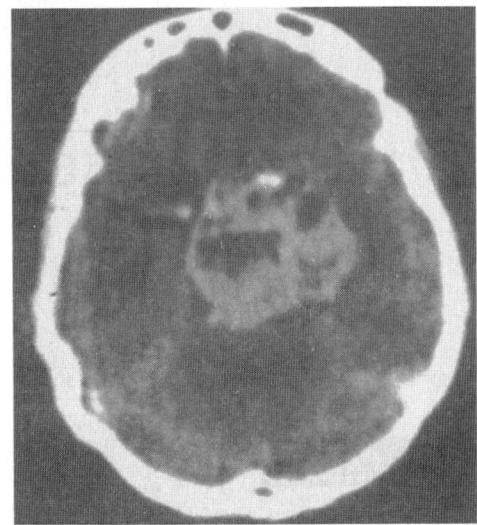

Fig. 73.2: CT scan showing a pituitary tumour with haemorrhage (hyperdense area)

Management

1. **Medical treatment of hypopituitarism:** It invariably relieves pituitary apoplexy. Hydrocortisone 100 mg I.V. initially, then every 6 to 8 hourly until surgery is done. Acute adrenal insufficiency is common and an early finding in pituitary apoplexy. Electrolytes and fluids should be administered carefully to correct hydration and electrolyte balance. Patient should be watched closely for diabetes insipidus. In acute setting, other hormone replacement may not be required but subsequently steroids, thyroid hormone and gonadal hormones (testosterone in males, oestrogen and progesterone in females) may be required as replacement therapy for hypopituitarism on long-term basis.

2. **Surgical treatment:** Neurosurgical decompression via transsphenoidal approach is definite therapy for pituitary apoplexy. Rapid down-hill course and severe visual loss are indications for surgery. Recent evidence suggests that early decompression may partially or completely restore the pituitary functions and lessen the need for hormonal replacement therapy.

Hypocalcaemia (Tetany)

HYPOCALCAEMIA

Normal calcium homeostasis is maintained within normal range (8.5 to 10.5 mg/dl or 2.1 to 2.5 mmol/dl) by parathyroid hormone (PTH), vitamin D and calcitonin (Fig. 74.1). About 50% of calcium is unbound and is responsible for physiological actions. Rest 50% is bound to albumin (40%) and anions (10%). Changes in pH influence the binding of calcium. Alkalosis produces hypocalcaemia by increasing the binding of calcium to albumin while acidosis has the reverse effect.

Definition

Hypocalcaemia is defined as a state in which calcium concentration in serum falls below the lower limit of normal, i.e. 8.5 mg/dl (after correction for serum albumin).

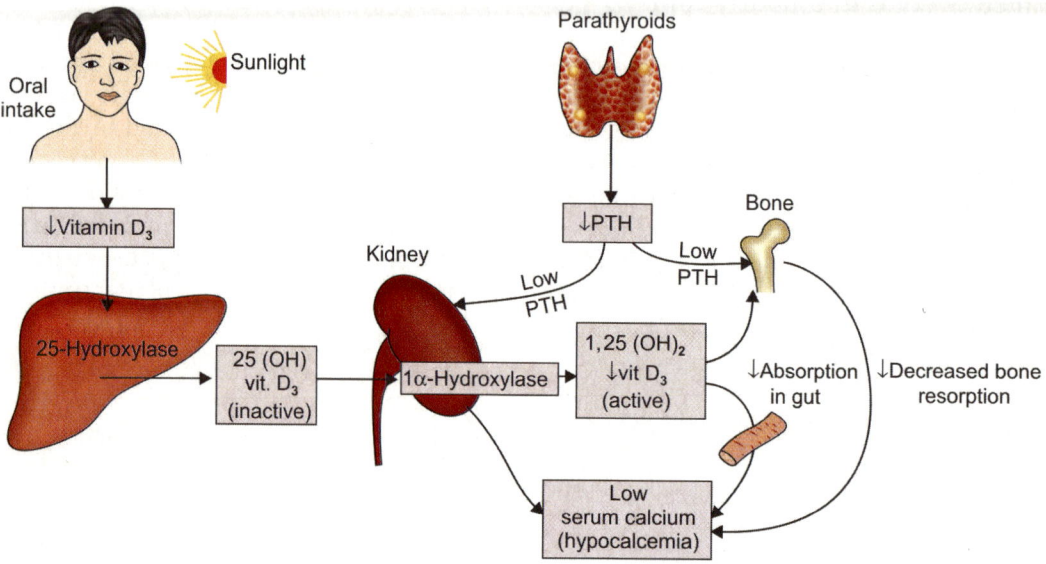

Fig. 74.1: Pathogenesis of hypocalcaemia—low or decreased interaction of PTH and vitamin D producing hypocalcaemia

Correction formula: Add 0.8 mg/dl to serum calcium level with every 1 g/dl fall in serum albumin level below 4 g/dl. Hypoalbuminaemia is most common cause of hypocalcaemia, hence most accurate measurement of serum calcium is the ionised calcium concentration

Causes

Hypocalcaemia may occur in acute, subacute and chronic forms. Acute hypocalcaemia is usually transient and asymptomatic, occurs in intensive care setting and severe sepsis, burns, acute renal failure and following extensive blood transfusions with citrated blood (Box 1). **Acute hypocalcaemia** with certain illness or medications (protamine, heparin and

Box 1 Causes of acute hypocalcaemia	
• Sepsis	• Toxic-shock syndrome
• Burns	• Hypomagnesaemia
• Acute pancreatitis	• Extensive transfusions
• Acute renal failure	• Plasmapheresis
• Alkalosis	• Malignancy
• Drugs, e.g. diuretics, protamine , heparin and glucagon	• Alcohol excess
	• Old age
	• Parathyroid surgery

glucagon) is also transient, does not produce tetany and resolves with treatment of medical conditions or stoppage of drug. Acute pancreatitis also causes hypocalcaemia by precipitation of Ca^{++}, does not require treatment except the underlying cause.

Chronic hypocalcaemia, however, is usually symptomatic and requires treatment. The most common causes of chronic hypocalcaemia is chronic kidney disease (decreased production of 1,25-dehydroxyvitamin D_3) and hypoparathyroidism (PTH deficiency). Vitamin D deficiency leads to hypocalcaemia in children than in adults. In advanced osteomalacia, adults may also manifest with hypocalcaemia. The causes of chronic hypocalcaemia are given in Table 74.1, is based on the PTH level and its ineffectiveness due to the fact that PTH is responsible for minute to minute regulation in serum calcium concentration.

Table 74.1   Causes of hypocalcaemia
1. **Physiological**
• Hypoalbuminemia
2. **Reduced intake or absorption**
• Malabsorption, short bowel and small bowel bypass
• Vitamin D deficit (decreased absorption, decreased production of 25-hydroxyvitamin D or 1,25- dihydroxyvitamin D)
3. **Increased loss**
• Alcoholism
• Chronic kidney disease and diuretic therapy
4. **Endocrine diseases (low parathyroid hormone)**
• Hypoparathyroidism (genetic or acquired)
• Postparathyroidectomy
• Pseudohypoparathyroidism
• Medullary carcinoma of thyroid (calcitonin secretion)
5. **Conditions associated with secondary hyperparathyroidism**
• Septic shock, pancreatitis
• Rhabdomyolysis
• Induced by drugs (antibiotics plicamycin)
• Vitamin D resistance, renal insufficiency
• Hyperphosphatemia
• Osteoblastic metastases from cancer prostate

Clinical Features

The clinical manifestations vary from asymptomatic state to life-threatening features like convulsions, tetany (Fig. 74.2), laryngeal spasm, depending on the level of ionized calcium. The neuromuscular and neurological manifestations of hypocalcaemia are due to enhanced neuromuscular excitability

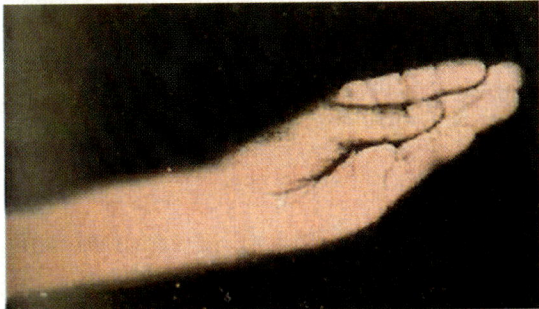

Fig. 74.2: Manifest tetany characterised by spontaneous carpal spasms (main d' accoucheur hand)

due to lowered threshold; and common features include tetany, perioral paraesthesias, numbness, muscle cramps and fasciculations. The symptoms and signs of hypocalcaemia and tetany are given in Boxes 2 and 3.

Box 2	Clinical features of hypocalcaemia
Mental	Irritability, depression, psychosis, convulsions
Neurological	Tetany (the features are given in Box 3), paraesthesias, seizures
Cardiac	Precipitation of CHF by beta-blockers, arrhythmias, prolonged QTc on ECG
Eye	Cataracts, optic neuritis, papilloedema

Severe hypocalcaemia can cause mental features (irritability, depression , psychosis), seizures, myopathy and heart failure. The QT interval is prolonged on ECG and arrhythmia can occur. In some cases, there may be increased intracranial pressure including papilloedema. Respiratory arrest can occur.

Latent tetany (absence of signs and symptoms of tetany) is diagnosed by provocative tests:

Box 3	Symptoms and signs of tetany

Children

A characteristic triad of carpopedal spasm, stridor and convulsions may occur in various combinations. The hands in carpopedal spasm, carpel spasm adopt a peculiar posture in which there is flexion at metacarpophalangeal joint and extension at the interphalangeal joints and there is apposition of thumb (main d' accoucheur hand) is given in Fig. 73.2. Pedal spasms are less frequent. The stridor (loud sound) is produced by closure of the glottis.

Adults

Tingling sensations in the peripheral parts of limbs or around the mouth. Less often painful carpopedal spasms, muscle cramps, facial grimacing may occur. Stridor and convulsions are rare.

1. **Trousseau's sign (Fig. 74.3):** Raising the BP above systolic level by inflating the sphygmomanometer cuff, produces typical carpopedal spasms within 3–5 minutes.

2. **Chvostek's sign:** A tap at the facial nerve in front of tragus at the angle of jaw produces facial twitchings within 3 minutes.

Diagnosis and Differential Diagnosis

Hypocalcaemia is suspected in a patient with tetany and other features described above. Tetany can occur due to alkalosis and magnesium deficiency. The differential diagnosis of hypocalcaemia is given in Table 74.2.

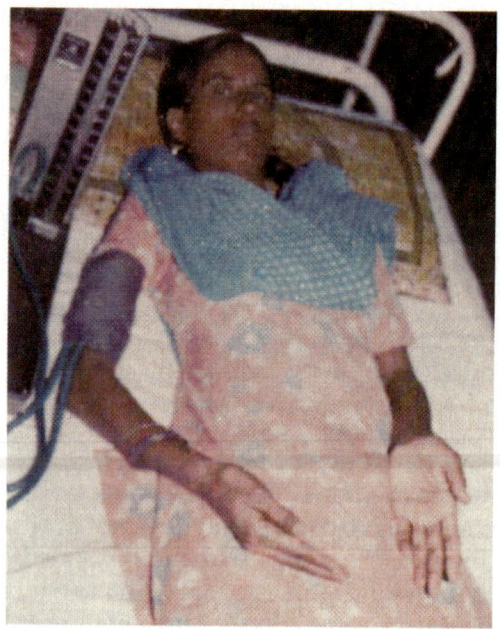

Fig. 74.3: Latent tetany converted into manifest tetany by Trousseau's sign

Investigations

1. Total serum calcium is low (< 8.5 mg/dl)
2. In true hypocalcemia, ionised serum calcium is also low (<4.6 mg/dl)
3. Serum phosphate is usually elevated in hypoparathyroidism or in advanced chronic kidney disease (CKD)
4. Serum magnesium levels are low
5. In respiratory alkalosis, total serum calcium is normal but ionised serium calcium is low
6. The ECG shows a prolonged QTc interval.

Table 74.2 Differential diagnosis of hypocalcaemia

Conditions	Total serum calcium concen-tration	Ionised serum calcium concen-tration	Serum phosphate concen-tration	Serum PTH concen-tration	Comments
1. Hypoalbuminaemia	↓	N	N	N	Adjust calcium by correc-tion formula
2. Alkalosis • Respiratory (e.g. hyper-ventilation) • Metabolic (e.g. Conn's syndrome)	N	↓	N	N or ↑	Read the textbook
3. Vit. D deficiency	↓	↓	↓	↑	Read text
4. Chronic renal failure	↓	↓	↑	↑	It is due to depressed hydroxylation
5. Hypoparathyroidism • Post-surgical • Idiopathic • Infants	↓	↓	↑	↓	Read textbook
6. Pseudohypoparathyroidism	↓	↓	↓	↓	Characteristic phenotype
7. Acute pancreatitis	↓	↓	N or ↓	↑	• Usually clinically evident • Serum amylase ↑

↑ : Increase   ↓ : Decrease   N : Normal

Management

Treatment for hypocalcaemia depends on severity and its progression. The low serum calcium associated with hypoalbuminaemia does not require treatement. Mild hypocal-caemia needs only observation and oral supple-mentation of calcium and vitamin D. Severe symptomatic hypocalcaemia in the presence of tetany seizures or arthythmias, should be treated as an emergency with 10% calcium gluconate (90 mg elemental calcium in 10 ml); 2 ampoules (20 ml) infused I.V. over 10 minutes followed by infusion of 60 ml (5–6 ampoules) in 500 ml of glucose (1 mg/ml) at a rate of 0.5–2.0 mg/kg/hour. Serum calcium should be monitored every 4–6 hours and infusion rate adjusted to keep the serum calcium between 8–9 mg/dl. This is followed by oral calcium and vitamin D supplementation. Hypomagnesemia, if present, may be corrected by magnesium administration simultaneously. If tetany is not relieved by giving calcium, magnesium may be tried.

Hypocalcaemia due to hyperventilation (alkalosis) can be overcome by rebreathing expired air in a paper bag or administering 5% CO_2 in oxygen.

Treatment of chronic hypocalcaemia due to hypoparathyroidism, pseudohypoparathy-roidism and CRF is with oral calcium (2–4 g of elemental calcium every day) and vitamin D (0.5–2 μg calcitrol/day) for life-long. Vitamin D metabolite or calcium is given prophylactically to patients receiving chronic anticonvulsant therapy. Commercial preparations of PTH for hypoparathyroidism are unsatisfactory as its administration needs frequent injections and hormone therapy becomes ineffective due to antibody formation.

A check of urinary calcium execretion is recommended after the initiation of therapy because hypercalciuria (urine calcium excretion >300 mg or 7.5 mmol/day) or urine calcium-creatinine ratio greater than 0.3 may impair kidney function in these patients.

Hypercalcaemia (Hypercalcaemic Crisis)

HYPERCALCAEMIA

Definition

It is defined as a state in which serum calcium level is above the upper limit of the normal, i.e. above 10.5 mg/dl in the presence of normal serum protein. It may be *mild asymptomatic* (10.5–12.0 mg/dl), *moderate symptomatic* (12–15 mg/dl) and *severe medical emergency* (>15 mg/dl).

Causes

Hypercalcaemia results either from an increased entry of calcium into the extracellular fluid (from bone resorption or intestinal absorption) or a decreased renal calcium clearance (Fig. 75.1). More than 90% of cases are due to hyperparathyroidism or associated with malignancy. The common causes of hypercalcaemia are given in Table 75.1.

Clinical Features

The clinical features depend on the severity of hypercalcaemia. Its presentation varies from asymptomatic state (recognised only on routine calcium measurement) to severe symptomatic hypercalcaemia associated

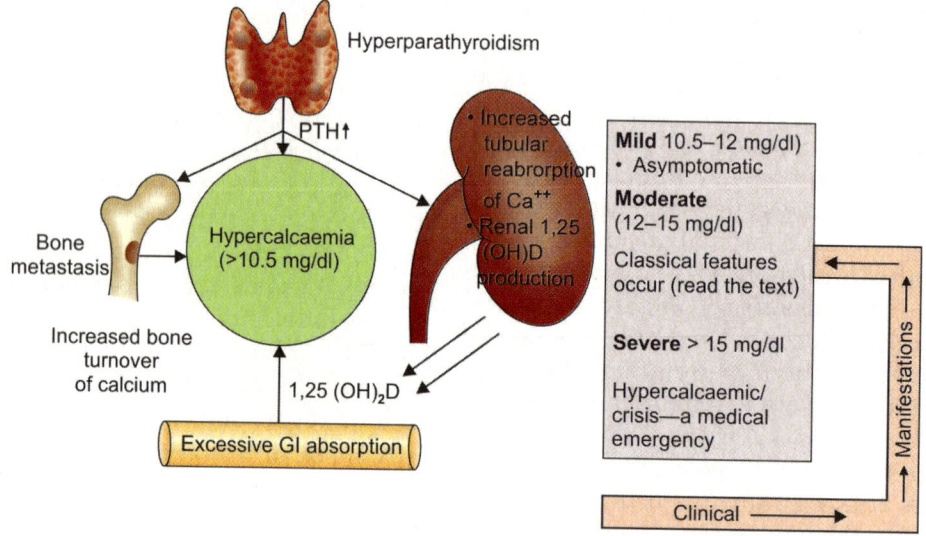

Fig. 75.1: Pathogenesis and severity of hypercalcaemia

Table 75.1 Causes of hypercalcaemia

1. Increased intake or absorption

- Milk alkali syndrome, total parenteral nutrition
- Vitamin D or A excess

2. Endocrinal disorders

- Primary hyperparathyroidism (adenoma)
- Secondary and tertiary hyperparathyroidism
- Acromegaly
- Adrenal insufficiency
- Thyrotoxicosis
- Phaeochromocytomas

3. Neoplastic diseases

- Tumor metastases (excessive production of PTH)
- Solid tumor with secretion of PTH like protein
- Hematological malignancies, i.e. multiple myeloma, leukemia, lymphoma (elaboration of osteoclast activating factor)

4. Miscellaneous

- Thiazide diuretics, lithium intake
- Paget disease of bone
- Hypophosphatasia
- Immobilisation
- Familial hypocalciuric hypercalcemia
- Complication of kidney transplant
- Aluminium intoxication

Box 1 Symptoms and signs of hypercalcaemia

CNS	Mental confusion, depression, lethargy, irritability, insomnia, inability to concentration, fatigue, stupor and coma
Neuro-muscular	Paraeasthesia, muscle cramps, weakness, diminished tendon reflexes.
GIT	Nausea, vomiting, anorexia, constipation, peptic ulcer disease, pancreatitis.
Renal	Polyuria, nocturia, polydipsia due to tubular defects, dehydration, renal colic due to stones, nephrocalcinosis, hematuria
Cardiac	Bradycardia, AV blocks, arrhythmias, palpitations, hypertension, short QTc interval on ECG, sensitivity to digitalis.
Eye	Band keratopathy, calcification of lens
Skin	Pruritus, skin necrosis (small vessel thrombosis)
Bone	Bone and Joint pain

Investigations

Investigations are done to confirm the diagnosis, to find out the cause and to exclude other disorders associated with hypercalcaemia.

1. **Raised serum calcium on initial estimation:** It must be confirmed on two or three occasions along with phosphorus and serum alkaline phosphatase. Urinary calcium excretion also helps in the diagnosis.

Clue: A patient with raised total serum calcium (adjusted total calcium level >10.5 mg/dl) or ionised calcium >4.6–5.3 mg/dl, low phosphorus <2.5 mg/dl and normal to increased urinary calcium is likely to have hyperparathyroidism because of increased PTH or PTH reactive protein secretion.

2. **Measure PTH levels:** Elevated PTH (parathormone) levels in the presence of hypercalcaemia suggest:
   - Hyperparathyroidism (primary secondary).
   - Lithium toxicity
   - Familial hypocalciuric, hypercalcaemia (a calcium/creatinine ratio <0.01 is suggestive of this condition).

with altered sensorium and coma. Generally symptoms (Box 1) appear when serum calcium is more than 12.0 mg/dl, but some patients even at this level are asymptomatic. When calcium exceeds 13 mg/dl (3.2 mmol/L), calcification in kidneys, skin, vessels, lungs, heart and stomach and renal insufficiency may develop, particularly if blood phosphate levels are normal or elevated due to impaired renal function. *Severe hypercalcaemia* is usually defined as serum calcium levels of 15 mg/dl (3.7 mmol/L) or above, is a medical emergency. When serum calcium is in between 15 mg/dl and 18 mg/dl, coma and cardiac arrest can occur. Fluid loss secondary to hypercalcaemia-induced polyuria and vomiting produces dehydration and reduction in GFR. This leads to a further rise in serum calcium setting up a vicious cycle and ends in a hypercalcaemic crisis.

3. **Measurement of 1,25-dihydroxyvitamin D3:** The levels of 1,25-$(OH)_2$D levels are high in many (but not in all) patients of primary hyperparathyroidism, sarcoidois, tuberculosis and vit. D intoxication. In other causes (CKD, dialysis) associated with hypercalcaemia, its levels are low.

4. **Localisation of parathyroid adenoma if hyperparathyroidism is the cause:** High resolution ultrasonography, CT scan, thallium technetium substraction scan, scintigraphy with 99 mTc sestamibi and single photon computed tomography (SPECT) in isolation or in combination help in the diagnosis (Fig. 75.2). and most useful for localisation of parathyroid adenomas.

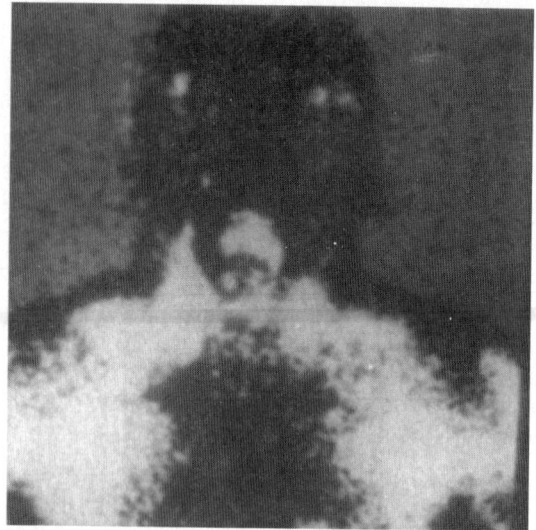

Fig. 75.2: Thallium technetium substraction scan revealed a parathyroid adenoma in a patient with hyperparathyroidism

5. **If PTH levels are low,** then it indicates non parathyroidal hypercalcaemia and should be investigated accordingly:
   - Increased Ca^{++} and increased phosphate with high urinary calcium indicate vitamin D intoxication, excessive absorption of Ca^{++} from GI tract, excessive release of phosphate from bones in malignancy, renal diseases and granulomatous disease.

6. **Investigations for malignancy (chest X-ray and CT scan) and multiple myeloma (protein electrophoresis and bone scan)** in older people should be carried out. The ECG should be done for QTc.

7. A sequential analysis of **CaSR gene** is commonly performed for diagnosis of FHH (familial hypocalciuric hypercalcaemia).

8. **Bone radiographs** for demineralisation, subperiosteal absorption of bone, mottling of skull or pathological fractures chondro-calcinosis is sometimes found.

Diagnosis and Differential Diagnosis

The diagnosis of hypercalcaemia is based on clinical features with raised serum calcium on two to three occasions. Further investigations are done to find out the cause. Differential diagnosis rests between its differential causes.

Hypercalcaemia in an adult who is asymptomatic is usually due to primary hyperparathyroidism.

In malignancy—associated hypercalcaemia, symptoms of malignancy bring the patient to the clinician and hypercalcaemia is detected on biochemical investigations. In such patients, the interval between detection of hypercalcaemia and death is often less than 6 months.

Long duration of symptoms of hypercalcaemia (i.e. 1 to 2 years) along with renal stones, primary hyperparathyroidism is likely the cause rather than malignancy.

Management

Mild hypercalcaemia does not require immediate therapy. The type of treatment is based on the severity of hypercalcaemia and nature of associated symptoms. Except in malignancy-associated hypercalcaemia, acute management of hypercalcaemia through aggressive hydration and forced diuresis is usually successful prior to definite therapy. The serum calcium can be decreased significantly within first 24–48 hours to relieve acute symptoms and prevent death. Treatment of chronic hypercalcaemia by medical therapies

Table 75.2 Therapies for severe hypercalcaemia

Therapy	Dose and route	Onset of action	Comments/monitor
A. Most useful therapies			
• Hydration with saline	250–1000 ml/hour (4–6 L in 24 hours)	Hours during infusion	Look for fluid overload, cardiac compensation
• Forced diuresis (Saline + frusemide)	20–80 mg of frusemide, 4–6 hourly I.V.	Hours during treatment	Look for electrolytes, monitor K^+
B. Bisphosphonates			
• First generation, e.g. etidronate	7.5 mg/kg/day I.V.	1–2 days	• Infuse over 4–24 hours, half the dose in renal failure
• Second generation, e.g. pamidronate	30–90 mg/week as I.V.	1–2 days	• Hyperphosphataemia may occur
• Third generation, e.g. zolendronate	4 or 8 mg/5 min infusion	1–2 days	• Infuse over 4–24 hours, half the dose in renal failure • May casue fever (20%), hypo-phosphataemia, hypocalcaemia
C. Calcitonin	4–8 U/kg every 6–12 hourly, I.V. I.M. or S C	Within few hours	• Allergic reactions, give test dose • Tachyphylaxis
D. Other therapies			
• Plicamycin • Prednisolone	25 g/kg/day I.V. 20 mg b.i.d. or t.i.d. orally (40–100 mg/day)	Days, weeks	Monitor blood count, LFT • Useful in certain malignancies • Produces glucocorticoids side-effects
• EDTA	50 mg/kg/day I.V.	During use	• Hypercalcaemia crisis • Avoid in renal failure
• Dialysis	Low or no calcium dialysate haemodialysis/peritoneal dialysis	Days	• Useful in hypercalcaemia crisis in renal failure
• Cinacalcet	15–30 mg orally once or twice daily	Days	• May cause nausea, vomiting • Hypocalcaemia may occur, hence weekly monitoring of calcium is advised

is less satisfactory unless underlying cause can be corrected. The various therapies for hypercalcaemia are given in Table 75.2.

The calcimimetic agent cinacalcet hydrochloride suppresses PTH secretion and decreases serum calcium concentration and holds promise in the treatment of hypercalcemia as an initial therapy for hyperporathyroidism.

The most effective way to reduce calcium in emergency situation (hypercalcaemic crisis) is rehydration with isotonic saline 4–6 L in 24 hours (except cardiac patients or patients with CRF). However loop diuritics should not be initiated unless the volume status has been restored to normal. Intravenous bisphosphonates should be given to patients with severe hypercalcaernia along with saline. They are powerful inhibitors of bone resorption, are commonly used for treatment of hypercalcolmia of malignancy in adults. The onset of action of bisphosphonates is delayed by 24–48 hours. *Pamidronate* having a long duration of action (weeks to months) is a preferred drug; is given in a dose of 30–90 mg as an I.V. infusion over 2–4 hrs or *zoledronate* 5 mg I.V. over 15–20 min. They normalize the calcium in most of the patients. *Calcitonin* is another drug which has a short duration of action, can bring down the calcium rapidly in few cases. It blocks the bone resorption and increases urinary calcium excretion. Tachyphylaxis is a problem with calcitonin, hence, simultaneous use of bisphosphonates is needed.

For patients with Vit. D deficiency, vit. D replacement may be beneficial to patients with hyperparathyroidism. Serum PTH level may fall.

Secondary and *tertiary hyperparathyroidism* associated with azotemia are treated with calcitriol oral or I.V. after dialysis, suppresses parathyroid hyperplasia of kidney-disease. During this therapy serum calcium and phosphorous must be monitored. Alternatively vit. D analogue (paricalcitol, doxer calciferol) can be used to suppress PTH, but are less effective.

Oestrogen replacement therapy reduces hypercalcaemia in postmenopausal women with hyperparathyroidism. Similarly oral raloxifene (60 mg/day) may be given to postmenopausal women with hyperparathyroidism. It reduces serum calcium while having anti-oestrogen effect on breast tissue.

A monoclonal antibody *denosumab* 120 μg subcutaneous monthly may be effective. However, larger doses may increase the risk of jaw osteonecrosis and serious infections. It inhibits osteoclasts, thus reduces bone resorbtion and serum calcium level. It is approved for use in malignancy-induced hypercalaemia.

Steroids are used for treatment of hypercalcaemia due to sarcoidosis, vitamin D intoxication, lymphoma and hematological malignancies. Intravenous phosphate has calcium lowering effect but there is associated risk of precipitation of calcium as calcium phosphate complex with its use (fatal hypocalcaemia). Fatal hypotension and ARF have been reported with its use. Dialysis removes the calcium rapidly and dramatically and is used to lower calcium in presence of renal failure or volume overload.

Surgical parathyroidectomy. It is recommended for patients with hyperparathyroidism who care symptomatic or who have nephrolithiasis or bone disease. During pregnancy, parathyroidectomy is performed in the second trimester in women who are symptomatic or have serum calcium above 11 mg/dl.

Emergencies in Nephrology

- Acute Nephritic Syndrome
- Acute Kidney Injury or Acute Renal Failure, Oliguria and Anuria

Acute Nephritic Syndrome

ACUTE NEPHRITIC SYNDROME

Definition

The acute nephritic syndrome (Fig. 76.1) is the clinical correlate of acute glomerulonephritis and is characterised by:

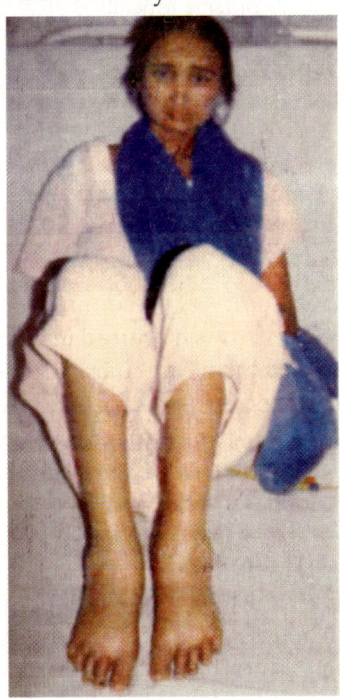

Fig. 76.1: An 18-year-old female presented with hypertension, oedema, puffiness of face with haematuria—acute nephritic syndrome

- **Haematuria** (macroscopic or microscopic and red cell casts are typically present in urine).
- **Proteinuria** (<3 g/day—not in nephrotic range; usual is 1–2 g/day).
- **Hypertension and oedema:** Owing to salt and H_2O retention.
- **Oliguria (urine output < 400 ml/day).** It is due to depressed GFR.
- **Uraemia**—acute renal failure (reduced GFR rise in serum creatinine).

Pathology

The hallmark of acute nephritic syndrome is glomerular inflammation (hypercellularity) and the classic pathologic correlate of the nephritic syndrome is proliferative glomerulonephritis. The proliferation of glomerular cells is due initially to infiltration of the glomerular tuft by neutrophils and monocytes with subsequent proliferation of endothelial and mesangial cells (endocapillary proliferation). In *most severe* form, nephritic syndrome is associated with acute inflammation of most of glomeruli, e.g. acute diffuse proliferative glomerulonephritis. In *less severe form* fewer than 50% of the glomeruli may be involved, i.e. focal proliferative glomerulonephritis. In its *mildest form*, cellular proliferation is just confined to the mesangium, i.e. mesangioproliferative glomerulonephritis.

Rapidly Progressive Glomerulonephritis (RPGN)

It is a clinical correlate of nephritic syndrome but is of subacute onset characterised by development of renal failure over days to weeks, in association with a nephritic urinary sediments, subnephrotic protein-uria, oliguria, hypervolaemia, oedema and hypertension . The classic pathologic finding is severe extracapillary proliferation leading to crescents formation in more than 50% of glomeruli (crescentic glomerulonephritis). In practice, the clinical term rapidly proliferative glomerulonephritis (RPGN) and the patho-logical term crescentic glomerulonephritis are interchangeably used.

The association of acute nephritic syndrome with haemoptysis (Goodpasture's syndrome), antineutrophil cytoplasmic antibodies (ANCA) small vessel vasculitis, SLE or cryoglobuli-naemia is called *pulmonary-renal syndrome*.

Causes of Acute Nephritic Syndrome

The causes of acute nephritic syndrome and RPGN are more or less same and both can result from renal-limited primary glomer-ulonephritis or secondary glomerulopathy complicating systemic disease.

Most common causes include post-strepto-coccal glomerulonephritis, bacterial endocar-ditis, immune-complex nephritis as in SLE and effect of circulating autoantibodies against glomerular basement membrane (GBM) in Goodpasture's syndrome. The causes are given in Box 1.

Clinical Features (Fig. 76.2)

1. **Oedema or puffiness of** face in the early hours of the morning with or without oedema feet. It is due to proteinuria, salt and water retention, hypertension and reduced GFR.
2. **Oliguria:** Urine output is less than 400 ml/day. It is due to depressed GFR.
3. **Subnephrotic proteinuria <3 g/day:** It leads to oedema, occurs due to leakage

---

Box 1 Diseases associated with acute nephritic syndrome

A. Primary glomerular diseases
- Membranoproliferative glomerulonephritis (GN)
- Mesangial proliferative GN
- Pauci-immune GN (rapidly progressive crescentic)

B. Secondary to systemic diseases
- Post-infectious GN
  ❖ Bacterial, e.g. post-streptococcal, SABE
  ❖ Viral, e.g. HBV
- Systemic collagen vascular diseases
  ❖ Systemic lupus erythematosus
  ❖ Systemic vasculitis, e.g. PAN, Wegener's granulomatosis (ANCA small vessel vasculitis)
- Haematological diseases
  ❖ Henoch-Schönlein purpura
  ❖ Haemolytic-uraemic syndrome
  ❖ Thrombotic thrombocytopenic purpura
  ❖ Cryoglobulinaemia
  ❖ Serum sickness
- Glomerular basement membrane (GBM) diseases
  ❖ Goodpasture's syndrome

C. Miscellaneous
- Guillain-Barré syndrome
- DPT vaccination, IgA nephropathy

---

of proteins into Bowman's capsule due to glomerular injury and subsequently into the urine. About 20% adults even may have nephrotic range of proteinuria.

4. **Smoky or brown coloured urine:** Oliguria with smoky urine is a characteristic feature of acute nephritic syndrome. The change in colour of the urine is due to gross or micro-scopic haematuria. There may be pyuria due to leakage of degenerated WBCs in the urine.

5. **Hypertension:** The headache, giddiness, malaise and weakness in acute nephritic syndrome is associated with hypertension which is due to salt and water retention. Occasionally hypertension may be associ-ated with mental features called hyperten-sive encephalopathy.

6. **Systemic symptoms:** Headache, nausea, malaise, anorexia, flank pain are reported in 50% cases.

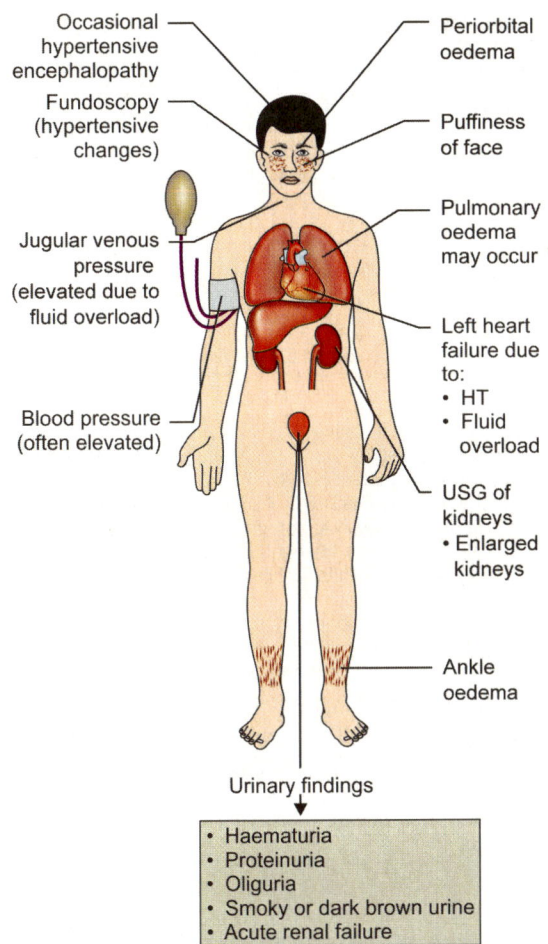

Fig. 76.2: Clinical manifestations of acute nephritic syndrome

Labels in figure:
- Occasional hypertensive encephalopathy
- Fundoscopy (hypertensive changes)
- Jugular venous pressure (elevated due to fluid overload)
- Blood pressure (often elevated)
- Periorbital oedema
- Puffiness of face
- Pulmonary oedema may occur
- Left heart failure due to:
  • HT
  • Fluid overload
- USG of kidneys
  • Enlarged kidneys
- Ankle oedema
- Urinary findings
  • Haematuria
  • Proteinuria
  • Oliguria
  • Smoky or dark brown urine
  • Acute renal failure

Streptococcal tonsillitis or pharyngitis, otitis media, or cellulitis may be responsible. The latent period of 1–3 weeks is for formation of immune complexes and their deposition into glomeruli. The features of underlying cause or systemic illness, or causative agent may be present at the time of acute nephritic syndrome.

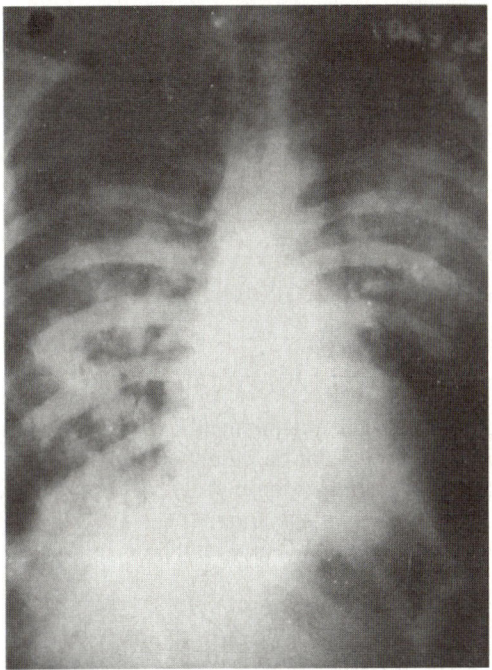

Fig. 76.3: Pulmonary oedema in a patient with acute nephritic syndrome

7. **Circulatory congestion or left heart failure:** It occurs due to capillaritis, increased cardiac output, and shortened circulation time, complicated further by acute left heart failure (pulmonary oedema Fig. 76.3.) due to salt and water retention and hypertension, producing cough, breathlessness, end-inspiratory crackles and rales. Haemoptysis may occur.

8. **Associated features:** In classical post-streptococcal GN causing acute nephritic syndrome, the patient is usually a child, will have history of sore throat 1–3 weeks prior to the onset of syndrome.

Investigations

A list of investigations is given in Table 75.1. If the clinical diagnosis of acute nephritic syndrome is clear cut, e.g. in post-streptococcal glomerulonephritis, renal imaging or renal biopsy is usually unnecessary. A biopsy is required if the diagnosis is uncertain, i.e. clinical features are unusual, or if renal failure is rapidly progressive suggesting the diagnosis of RPGN (crescentic glomerulonephritis).

Differential Diagnosis

The differential diagnosis is depicted in Fig. 76.4.

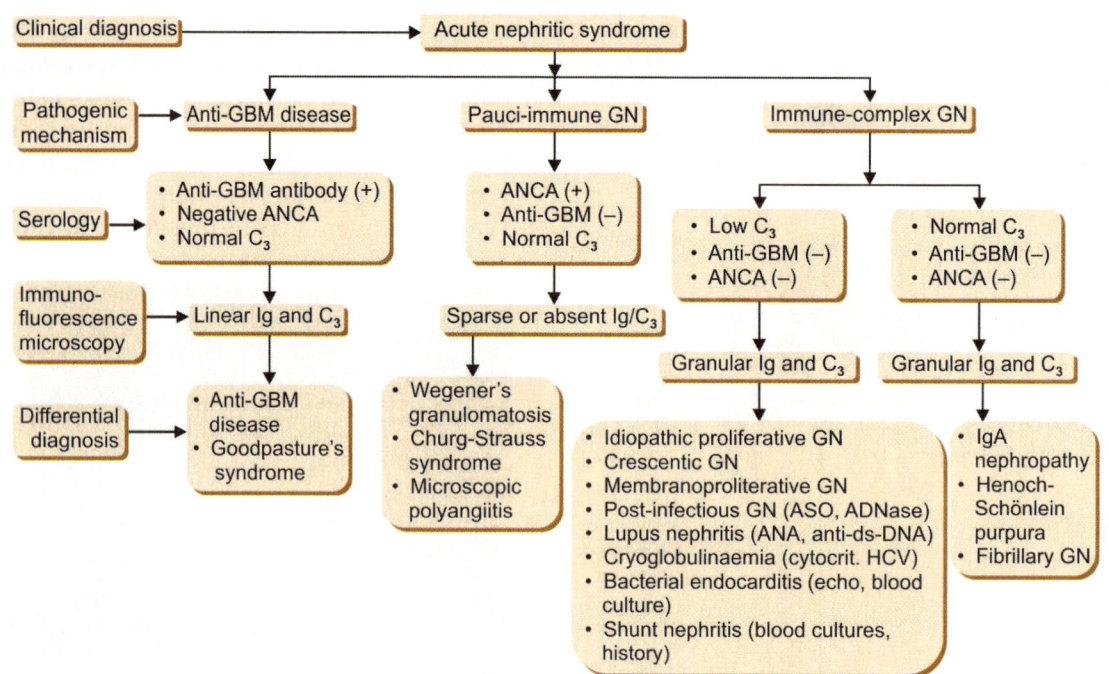

Fig. 76.4: Flowchart depicting the differential diagnosis of acute nephritic syndrome based on complement (C3), anti-glomerular basement membrane (anti-GBM) antibody and ANCA (antineutrophil cytoplasmic antibody). Ig, Immunoglobulin; C 3, third component of complement; ANA, antinuclear anitbody; anti-ds DNA, anti-double stranded DNA antibody; HGV, hepatitis C virus; Echo, echocardiogram; ASO, anti-streptolysin-O antibody titre; ADNase, anti-deoxyribonuclease antibody titre

Table 76.1 Investigations of acute nephritic syndrome

Tests	Results
• Complete urine examination	Proteinuria and high specific gravity
• Microscopic urine examination	RBCs (dysmorphic) and red cells casts, pyuria
• Blood urea and serum creatinine	May be elevated
• Culture (throat swab, ear discharge swab or swab, from inflamed skin)	Nephrogenic strains of group A β-haemolyticus streptococci not always
• ASO-titre	Elevated in poststreptococcal nephritis (30%)
• C_3 level	May be reduced, C_4 levels are normal
• Antinuclear antibody	Present in significant titre in SLE
• Rheumatoid factor, cryoglobulins and circulating immune complex	Positive in 60–70% cases
• Creatinine clearance	Reduced
• 24 hours urinary protein	Subnephrotic proteinuria (< 3 g/day)
• Chest X-ray	Cardiomegaly, pulmonary oedema—not always
• Renal imaging	Usually normal
• USG of kidneys	May show mildly enlarged kidneys with normal echogenicity
• Renal biopsy considered if there is no contra-indication.	Glomerulonephritis

Management

The management is directed to control the symptoms and signs till the illness is resolved in post-streptococcal GN which is usually a self-limiting illness; otherwise cause has to be found out and properly treated.

1. **Rest:** Hospitalization of the patient for observation and assessment is necessary. Strict bed rest is advised to patients with severe hypertension or pulmonary oedema.

2. **Monitoring:** Most patients require daily recording of fluid intake and output, daily weighing and measurement of BP.

3. **Infection:** Antibiotics are used to eradicate the infection in case of post-streptococcal GN. Sore throat may be treated with penicillins. Long-term prophylaxis after the development of streptococcal glomerulo nephritis is not recommended.

4. **Diet, salt and fluid control:** Salt restricted diet is necessary. Proteins are restricted only if severe uraemia is present. In oliguric patients, fluid restriction is necessary to maintain body weight and to avoid fluid overload. During diuretic phase, liberal fluids with salt and potassium become necessary. Sodium and potassium are to be monitored.

5. **Diuretics:** They are used to control oedema, fluid overload and hypertension. Frusemide 40 mg I.V. daily for few days may be necessary initially because of renal failure, followed by oral substitution.

6. **Hypertension:** It is controlled by diuretics, salt restriction, fluid adjustment and anti-hypertensive drugs such as angiotensin converting enzyme inhibitors (ACE inhibitors), i.e. enalapril 2.5–10 mg daily or angiotensin receptors antagonists, e.g. Losartan 25–50 mg/day either alone or in combination may be used depending on the severity of hypertension.

7. **Immunosuppression:** Glucocorticoids and immunosuppressive drugs are mainstay of treatment for anti-GBM disease, Pauci-immune GN and immune-complex GN complicating SLE and RPGN.

8. **Plasmapheresis:** It is useful adjunct to immunosuppression in patients with severe immune-complex nephritis (Goodpasture's syndrome)

9. **Dialysis:** Peritoneal dialysis, hemodialysis or haemofiltration will be required in cases with severe renal failure.

10. **Treatment of complications:** Such as hypertensive encephalopathy and pulmonary oedema is on the same lines as discussed individually in respective sections as full chapters.

Acute Kidney Injury or Acute Renal Failure, Oliguria and Anuria

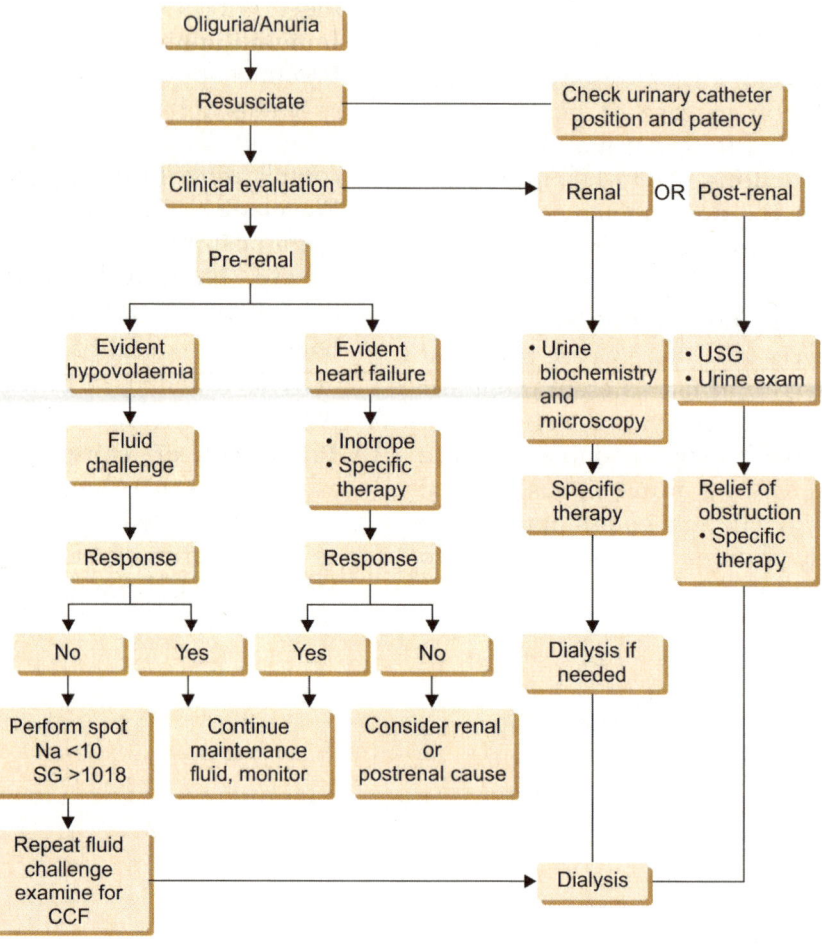

Fig. 77.1: Flowchart for evaluation and management of oliguric renal failure (ARF)

ACUTE RENAL FAILURE/ACUTE RENAL INJURY/OLIGURIA/ANURIA

Definition

Acute renal failure (ARF) or *acute kidney injury (AKI)* is defined as sudden and most often reversible loss of renal functions, which develops over a period of day or weeks, leads to retention of waste products of metabolism such as urea and creatinine. An increase in plasma creatinine concentration to >200 mol/L (>2 mg%) is often taken as the biochemical definition of renal failure. A reduction in urine output (oliguria) occurs usually but not always.

Oliguria is defined as urine output <400 ml/day while anuria is defined as either no urine passed or just not more than 50 ml passed in 24 hours.

Acute on chronic renal failure: Sudden deterioration of renal functions with rapid rise in blood urea and creatinine with fall in GFR (urine output) in a patient of established chronic renal failure is called *acute on chronic renal failure*.

Stages of AKI

- **Stage 1:** It is a 1.0 to 1.5 fold increase in serum creatinine or a decline in urinary output to 0.5 ml/kg/hr over 6–12 hours.
- **Stage 2:** It is 2.0 to 2.9 fold increase in serum creatinine or decline in urinary output to 0.5 ml/kg/hr over 12 hours or longer.
- **Stage 3:** It is a 3-fold or greater increase in serum creatinine or decline in urinary output to less than 0.3 ml/kg/hr for 24 hours or longer or anuria for 12 hours or longer.

Causes

Depending on the cause, acute renal failure is classified into three groups:

1. **Pre-renal:** Cause lies outside the kidney, is commonly due to contraction of blood volume.
2. **Renal:** Cause lies inside the kidney (intrinsic renal disease).
3. **Post-renal:** Cause lies below the kidney in its excretory passage, i.e. pelvis, ureter, bladder and urethra.

The causes are given in Table 77.1.

The most common causes of ARF are blood loss, fluid and electrolyte depletion, diarrhoea, non-diarrhoeal G.I. infections, glomerulonephritis, poisoning (drugs, snake venom, heavy metals) and G6PD deficiency associated with intravascular hemolysis. Fluid depletion is the major cause of ARF in tropics due to infectious diarrhoea leading to hypovolaemia. Heat stroke is another cause in tropics. Infectious diarrhoea is also a common cause in children.

Table 77.1 Aetiological classification of acute renal failure

1. Pre-renal (most common)

Renal hypoperfusion/underperfusion
- Fluid loss (vomiting, diarrhoea)
- Blood loss (haemorrhage)
- Diuretics
- Sepsis (decreased vascular resistance)
- Anaphylaxis (vasodilation and blood pooling)
- Burns (loss of fluid, plasma, blood, etc.)
- Cardiac failure (low cardiac output)
- Heat stroke (perspiration)
- Hypoproteinaemia (retention of extracellular fluid)
- Renal vascular disease, e.g. renal artery stenosis/occlusion, vasculitis
- Hepatorenal syndrome

2. Renal (Common)
- Acute glomerulonephritis
- Interstitial nephritis, e.g. due to drugs, pyelonephritis (infection), and idiopathic
- Acute tubular necrosis, e.g. ischaemic, toxic (radio contrast media, antibiotics), rhabdomyolysis, haemoglobinuria
- Renovascular hypertension, pre-eclampsia
- Diseases of renal microvasculature, e.g. disseminated intravascular coagulation, thrombotic thrombocytopenic purpura, haemolytic-uraemic syndrome

3. Post-renal (Least common)
- Ureteric, e.g. calculi, blood clot
- Bladder neck obstruction, e.g. benign prostatic hypertrophy, calculi, cancer
- Urethra, e.g. stricture, congenital valves

Acute glomerulonephritis and RPGN together account for large number of cases of ARF in children.

Malaria is a common cause of ARF in tropical countries. Falciparum infection causes most of these cases due to intravascular haemolysis or heavy parasitaemia. Intravascular haemolysis in malaria could also be drug-induced in patients with G6PD deficiency. Leptospirosis can also lead to ARF but is rare in India.

Acute interstitial nephritis due to drugs (β-lactams, sulfonamides, NSAIDs, rifampicin), herbal indigenous medicine and certain bacterial and viral infections are emerging as important causes of ARF.

Septic abortions, pre-eclampsia, abruptio placentae, placenta previa and postpartum ARF are important obstetric causes of ARF.

Obstructive uropathy (stone, tumour retroperitoneal fibrosis) is also an important but least common group leading to ARF. Benign hypertrophy of prostate is another important cause of reversible ARF.

Pathogenesis

In pre-renal reversible ARF, renal hypoperfusion is the most important underlying mechanism, systemic hypotension is present in most of these cases. When perfusion pressure falls as in shock, hypovolaemia, heart failure or narrowing of the renal arteries; two compensatory mechanisms come into action, i.e. vasodilatation under the effect of prostaglandins and vasoconstriction under the effect of catecholamines, angiotensin and/or vasopressin; the net effect being vasoconstriction resulting in fall in GFR.

In post-renal reversible failure, the intratubular and ureteral pressure rises with progression of disease and this leads to rise in intravascular resistance and fall in GFR subsequently. Intratubular obstruction due to uric acid and oxalate crystals, calcium and myeloma proteins leads to ARF.

Acute renal failure due to intrinsic renal disease is complex in pathogenesis. There may be one or more of the following abnormalities, i.e. haemodynamic changes, tubular back-leakage of filtrate or decrease in glomerular permeability.

Pathology

The pathological changes in ARF may be seen in glomeruli, interstitium, tubules and small vessels of the kidney and these are variable. **Acute tubular necrosis (ATN)** is probably the most common pathological lesion in established ARF. ATN may result from ischaemia or nephrotoxicity caused by chemicals and bacterial toxins and frequent use of nephrotoxic antibiotics (Box 1). Renal ischaemia is due to sepsis, hypovolaemia, hemorrhage and shock.

In nephrotoxic ATN, a similar sequence is observed as described above, but it is initiated by direct toxicity to tubular cells. It is due to oxygen free radicals, binding of toxins or drugs to inhibit cell protein synthesis.

Fortunately, tubular cells can regenerate and reform the basement membrane. If the patient is supported during the regeneration phase, kidney functions return.

ARF may be caused by acute glomerulonephritis (post-streptococcal) and RPGN. These

Box 1 Common nephrotoxins causing ATN and ARF
1. Antimicrobial
• Aminoglycosides (gentamicin)
• Amphotericin B
• Vancomycin
• Sulphonamides
2. Anti-inflammatory drugs
• NSAIDs
3. Cytotoxic drugs/agents
• Cyclosporine
• Cisplatin
• Radiographic contrast media
4. Organic solvents
• Ethylene glycol
5. Endogenous nephrotoxins
• Myoglobinuria, hemoglobinuria
• Hyperuricaemia, Bence-Jones proteinuria
6. Bacterial toxins
7. Herbomineral indigenous drugs

are characterized by marked proliferation of glomerular cells and frequently epithelial crescents formation (crescentic GN). Similarly in acute interstitial nephritis causing ARF, the pathological changes include peritubular and interstitial infiltration with polymorphs and eosinophils.

Clinical Features of ATN/ARF (Intrinsic)

The clinical features depend on the type of ARF and the causative factor (Table 77.2). ARF is usually asymptomatic and is diagnosed by biochemical parameters such as recent rise in blood urea or serum creatinine. Oliguria (urine output <400 ml/day) is frequent but not an invariable feature because non-oliguric acute renal failure is also known and clinically recognised entity.

Patients of *pre-renal azotaemia* complain of *thirst*, and have *postural hypotension* and tachycardia. There will be signs of dehydration.

The patients of *renal azotaemia* present with symptoms and signs of the underlying disease/cause (Table 77.1). Oedema feet and hypertension may occur due to salt and water retention.

Occurrence of gross haematuria with or without flank pain and a distended bladder points to *post-renal cause* such as benign prostate hypertrophy in >50 years old male.

Investigations

1. **Urinalysis**
   A. *Specific gravity and osmolarity:* Volume depletion in pre-renal azotaemia stimulates sodium and water reabsorption producing urine of high specific gravity >1.018. Measurement of urine osmolarity and ratio of urine to plasma osmolarity are other renal indices of diagnostic value. The great majority of patients with oliguric pre-renal ARF have urine osmolarity above 350 mOsm. The ratio of urine to plasma osmolarity less than 1.1 suggests ATN (Table 77.3).
   B. *Chemical composition:* Mild proteinuria is consistent with pre-renal and obstructive disorders, but can also be seen in most cases of acute interstitial nephritis. Massive proteinuria occurs in renal vein thrombosis. Positive reaction for blood indicates heme pigment, may be seen in conditions associated with microscopic or gross haematuria, hemoglobinuria and myoglobinuria.
   C. *Urinary sediment:* The urinary sediment is scanty in pre-renal and post-renal ARF. Pre sence of crystals and RBCs in urine point towards post-renal ARF. In ATN, epithelial cells, casts and coarse granular pigment casts are diagnostic. The urine sediments in pre-renal and renal azotaemia are given in Table 77.3.
   D. *Urinary sodium:* The assessment of urinary sodium in oliguric patients differentiates pre-renal and renal ARF (Table 77.3). Urinary concentration of sodium below 20 mEq/L in oliguric renal failure suggests pre-renal ARF.
   E. *Creatinine and urea:* The ratio of urinary to plasma creatinine is a useful parameter for classifying ARF. Ratios greater than 40 strongly suggests pre-renal ARF; while values less than 40 (even <20) can occur in both renal and post-renal ARF.

2. **Blood biochemistry:** In ARF, the urinary waste products excretion is inadequate, hence, both the blood urea and serum creatinine rise in ARF depending on its severity. Serial measurements of urea and creatinine in blood are helpful in planning the management of ARF as these parameters do not differentiate between various causes of renal failure. In severe ARF, blood urea may rise by 20–40 mg% and serum creatinine by 1–2 mg% daily.

Hyponatremia and hyperkalemia are important electrolyte disturbance in ARF. Patients with moderate to severe ARF may

Table 77.2 Clinical features based on cause of ARF

Cause	Clinical features	Urinalysis/Serum
I. Pre-renal ARF		
	• Symptoms and signs of dehydration (e.g. thirst, postural hypotension, tachycardia, low JVP, dryness of mouth, skin, mucous membrane, weight loss and oliguria).	• Hyaline casts • High specific gavity >1.018, urine osmolality >500 mOsm/kg • $FE_{Na}(\%)<1\%$
	• Decreased 'effective' circulatory volume, e.g. heart failure, cardiac tamponade, hepato-renal syndrome • Treatment with NSAIDs or ACE inhibitors	• $U_{Na+} < 20$ mEq/L • Serum BUN: Cr ratio > 20:1
II. Intrinsic renal ARF		
A. Renal vessel disease • Renal artery thrombosis embolism	• History of atrial fibrillation or recent MI • Flank or abdominal pain	• Proteinuria • RBCs in urine (occasional)
• Renal vein thrombosis	• Haematuria and/or oliguria • Evidence of nephrotic syndrome or pulmonary embolism, flank pain, oedema feet	• Proteinuria, haematuria
B. Glomerular disease • Glomerulonephritis/ vasculitis	• Compatible clinical history (e.g. recent sore throat, skin infection), sinusitis, lung haemorrhage, skin rash, or ulcers, arthralgias, new cardiac murmurs, history of hepatitis B or C infection)	• Red cell and granular casts • Mild proteinuria • Dysmorphic RBCs, and WBCs in urine
• Haemolytic uraemic syndrome or thrombotic thrombocytopenic purpura	• Compatible clinical history (e.g. recent GI infection, cyclosporine), fever, pallor, ecchymoses, neurological abnormalities	• May be normal • Mild proteinuria • Red cells/granular casts
• Malignant hypertension	• Severe hypertension with headache, cardiac failure retinopathy, neurologic dysfunction, papilloedema	• Proteinuria and/or haematuria may be present
C. Acute tubular necrosis • Ischaemic ATN	• Recent haemorrhage, hypotension, e.g. cardiac arrest, surgery	• Muddy brown granular casts or tubular epithelial casts is pathognomonic. • $FE_{Na} >1\%$ • $U_{Na+} >20$ mmol/L • Specific gravity <1.015, urine osmolality 250–300 mOsm/kg • Serum BUN: Cr ratio <20:1
• Toxins-induced ATN • Exogenous	• Recent radiocontrast study, nephrotoxic antibiotics or cytotoxic drugs, sepsis, chronic renal failure (acute on chronic renal failure)	• Same as above
• Endogenous	• History suggestive of rhabdomyolysis (seizures, coma, ethanol abuse, trauma)	• Urine supernatant positive for heme

Contd.

Table 77.2 Clinical features based on cause of ARF (*Contd.*)

Cause	Clinical features	Urinalysis/Serum
	• History suggestive of haemolysis (malarial infection, G6PD deficiency, blood transfusion)	• Urine supernatant pink and positive for heme
	• History suggestive of tumour lysis (chemotherapy), myeloma (bone pain) or ethylene glycol ingestion	• Urate crystals, dipstick negative, proteinuria, oxalate crystal respectively
D. Acute tubulointerstitial renal diseases		
• Allergic interstitial nephritis	• Recent ingestion of drug, fever, rash or arthralgias	• WBCs and RBCs casts with or without eosinophils • U_{Na} (mEq/L) is variable FE_{Na}(%) < 1 to > 1.1% serum BUN: Cr ratio <20:1
• Acute pyelonephritis	• Fever, dysuria, flank pain and tenderness, pyuria, toxic look	• Leucocytes, red cells • Proteinuria • Urine culture may be positive.
III. Post-renal ARF		
	• Abdominal or flank pain, haematuria palpable distended bladder	• Usually normal, haematuria, WBC if renal stone disease is suspected • Urine osmolality <400 mOsm/kg • FE_{Na} variable • Serum BUN: Cr ratio > 20:1
FE_{Na} (%)—fractional excretion of sodium		

Table 77.3 Urinary abnormalities in pre-renal and renal ARF

Abnormality	Pre-renal	Renal (ATN)
• Specific gravity	>1.020	<1.010
• Urinary osmolality (mOsm/kg)	>500	<350
• Urine to plasma osmolarity (ratio)	>1.1	<1.1
• Urine Na+ (mEq/L)	<20	>20
• FeNa (%)	<1	>1
• Urine to plasma creatinine ratio	>40	<40 (may be even <20)
• Renal failure index	<1	>2
• Urinary sediment	Scanty	Active
• Urinary proteins	Minimal	Moderate to severe

show evidence of metabolic acidosis (low plasma bicarbonate concentration).

3. **Radiological examination**
   • *Ultrasound of kidneys:* It is most commonly employed investigation of choice, determines the size and echogenicity of the kidneys, helps to differentiate between acute and chronic renal failure and Doppler ultrasound helps to assess the patency of renal artery and veins. Presence of normal sized or slightly enlarged kidneys points towards intrinsic ARF. Small contracted kidneys (<9 cm) raise the possibility of chronic renal failure. Dilated pelvicalyceal system indicates obstructive uropathy.
   • *Plain X-ray abdomen:* It is used to determine kidney size, shape and to identify radio-opaque calculi.
   • *Intravenous pyelography:* It is best avoided in ARF because of contrast induced deterioration of renal function. USG and CT scan provide more valuable informations.

- *Contrast enhanced CT scan:* It provides reli able information regarding size of the kidneys and presence of hydrone-phrosis. It is also required to confirm acute bilateral cortical necrosis if patient remains oliguric for more than 3 weeks.
- *Arteriography and venography:* Renal arteriography has a role in ARF secondary to sudden interruption of renal blood flow as occurs in renal artery thrombosis/embolism. Venography is useful for confirming renal vein thrombosis.
- *Renal biopsy:* Renal biopsy may be considered in those patients in whom the cause of ARF is uncertain or in cases where disease specific therapy is needed, e.g. glomerulonephritis, vasculitis or acute interstitial nephritis.

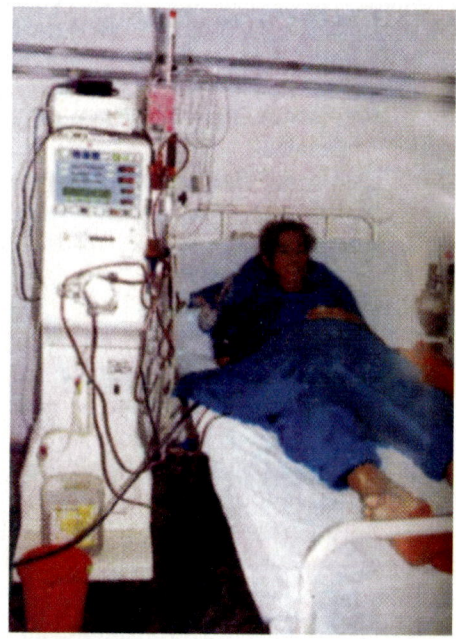

Fig. 77.2: A patient of acute renal failure being dialysed in haemodialysis section

Management

General principles: The initial treatment of ARF is focussed on reversing the underlying cause and correcting fluid and electrolyte balance. By definition, pre-renal azotaemia is rapidly reversible upon correction of the primary hemodynamic abnormality and post-renal azotaemia resolves upon relief of obstruction. Therefore, every effort should be made to prevent further injury and provide supportive measures until recovery of renal functions has occurred. Renal functions recover spontaneously in patients with ATN, but other causes of ARF require specific therapies.

Monitoring: The decision to give fluid or to remove fluid is most difficult, requires careful physical exami nation and CVP monitoring. Fluid challenge (Fig. 77.3) is of value in patients suspected to have pre-renal azotaemia or early ATN and should be tried in patients without clinical evidence of fluid overload. Restoration of renal blood flow with intravenous volume expansion is ineffective in restoring renal functions once ATN is established.

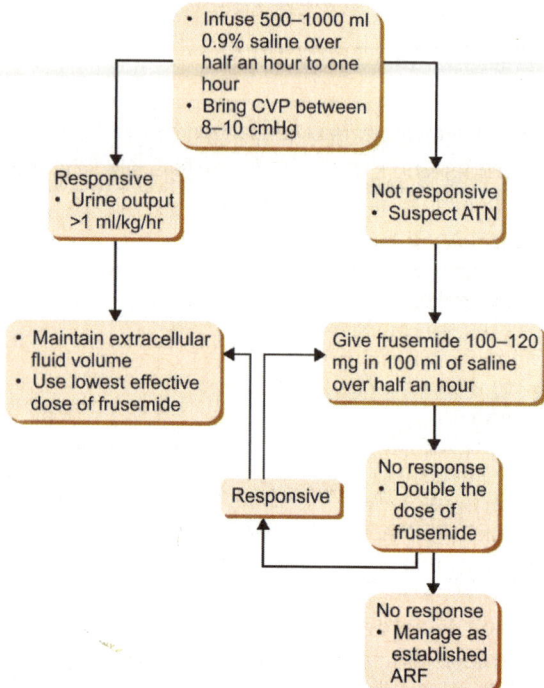

Fig. 77.3: Fluid challange as a guide for differentiation and management of the pre-renal azotaemia and ATN

Management of Acute Tubular Necrosis (ATN)

Established ARF develops following severe and prolonged pre-renal ARF. In such cases, the histological pattern of acute tubular necrosis is usually seen. Alternatively, patients may present *de novo* with established ARF due to intrinsic disease of the kidneys, e.g. RPGN or obstructive uropathy.

Aims of Emergency Resuscitation

- Treatment of hyperkalaemia ($K^+ > 6$ mEq/L).
- Control of hypertension, left heart failure or volume overload, if associated.
- Correction of metabolic acidosis.
- To find out the underlying cause and treat it accordingly.
- Measure urine output, weight, BP, blood urea and creatinine daily.
- In case of deterioration of clinical condition, falling GFR (persistent oliguria), rising urea, creatinine, an emergency dialysis may be instituted (Fig. 77.2).

The steps of management are:
1. *Fluid therapy:* In patients with established ARF, the fluid intake should be restricted to sum of previous day urine output plus 500 ml for insensible loss. Replace other fluid losses (gastric aspirate, diarrhoea, etc.), with equal amounts of saline. In febrile patients, add 100–150 ml/day of fluid for each degree rise in body temperature over 37°C.
2. *Diuretic therapy:* Diuretics have been tried in patients with ATN to decrease its severity. They are useful in early course of ATN (e.g. immediately after hypotension, mismatch transfusion, crush injury, burns, etc.), can convert oliguric state to non-oliguric state. Although non-oliguric state has better outcome than oliguric state, but there is no convincing evidence till date that conversion from an oliguric to non-oliguric state decreases either the mortality or the need for dialysis. At present, there is no convincing evidence to confirm usefulness of high dose diuretics. Diuretics are used as continuous infusion (frusemide 0.1 to 3 mg/kg/hr) in normal saline rather than intermittent infusion.

   Intravenous chlorthiazide 250–500 mg every 8–12 hours or metolazone 2.5–5 mg oral once or twice is also a resonable choice. Diuretics are detrimental in ARF induced by radio contrast agent and rhabomyolysis.
3. *Vasopressor therapy:* If fluid challenge fails to achieve the desired mean arterial pressure, then noradrenaline or dopamine is the next crucial step. In cardiogenic shock with ARF, ionotropes dobutamine/dopamine can be used.

   Low-dose dopamine: Low dose dopamine (1–3 g/kg/min) used earlier as reno-vaso-dilator and renoprotective have failed to demonstrate its effectiveness either in prevention or treatment of established ARF. It is best avoided.
4. *Nutrition:* Protein intake needs to be restricted in patients with ARF. In mild to moderate cases, about 30 g (0.6 g/kg) of proteins can be given per day. Adequate calories should be given with vitamins and mineral supplementation. In critically ill patients, nutrition is provided through nasogastric tube or parenterally.
5. *Potassium and calcium balance:* Hyperkalaemia (serum $K^+ > 5.5$ mEq/L) is a serious biochemical abnormality and is the leading cause of death in ARF. Acidosis, uraemia and hypercatabolic state contribute to hyperkalaemia and hypermagnesemia. Several modes of therapy for hyperkalaernia are available. Mild to moderate hyperkalaemia can be treated by medical means (e.g. insulin with glucose, use of calcium gluconate and cation exchange resins), but in severe hyperkalaemia (serum $K^+ > 7$ mEq/L) dialysis is desirable. Patient should be advised to restrict intake of potassium containing foodstuffs, i.e. fruits, and dry fruits to avoid hyperkalaemia. For treatment (read chapter on hyperkalaemia).

Hypocalcemia and hyperphosphataemia can be improved with diet and phosphate-binding agents such as aluminium hydroxide (500 mg orally) over the short term and calcium supplements, i.e. calcium carbonate (500–1500 mg orally) and acetate orally over longer periods.

Hypermagnesaemia can occur because of reduced magnesium excretion by renal tubules, so magnesium containing antacids and laxatives should be avoided.

6. *Acid-base balance:* Mild to moderate metabolic acidosis is common in ARF, does not require treatment. However, the advanced cases of ARF need 50–100 ml of 7.5% $NaHCO_3$ every 8 to 12 hourly to maintain serum bicarbonate >15 mEq/L. Avoid sodium bicarbonate in patients with fluid overload.

7. *Nephrotoxic drugs:* They should be discontinued or avoided. The doses of medications that require kidneys for their elimination should be adjusted.

8. *Platelet dysfunction:* Platelet dysfunctions (aggregation, adhesiveness) occur in uraemia *per se* and predispose to bleeding. Patients with prolonged bleeding time or with active bleeding can be treated by cryoprecipitate or desmopressin or oestrogen.

H_2-receptor antagonists or proton-pump inhibitors can be given prophylactically to prevent an upper GI bleeding.

9. *Treatment of infection:* Sepsis is most common cause of death in ARF. The rate of infectious complications is very high (80%). Infections can occur via indwelling catheter or venous catheters. Pulmonary, urinary and wound infections occur frequently in post-traumatic and postoperative cases, need energetic treatment. Prophylactic antibiotics have no role. If infection is suspected clinically and patient's condition is deteriorating, antibiotics (gentamicin or amikacin *plus* a third generation cephalosporin) should be started pending cultures reports. Full doses may be given initially followed by adjustment doses subsequently.

10. *Dialysis* (Figs 77.1 and 77.2): This should be considered as an adjunct to the conservative therapy for ARF. Indications for dialysis in ARF are not specific but have to be individualized. Some guidelines for dialysis are:

   a. *Biochemical:*
   - Blood urea >200 mg/dl.
   - Serum creatinine >10 mg/dl.
   - Serum K^+ >6 mEq/L (an evidence of hyperkalaemia).
   - Serum HCO_3 <10 mEq/L (metabolic acidosis).
   - pH< 7.2 (metabolic acidosis).

   b. *Clinical:*
   - Oliguria < 400 ml/day for 5 days.
   - Anuria (urine output <50 ml/day) for 3 days.
   - Fluid overload or pulmonary oedema.
   - Symptomatic uraemia, i.e. uraemic encephalopathy, uraemic pericarditis, uraemic bleeding diathesis, resistant heart failure. A review of experience with early and daily dialysis in hypercatabolic states reveals marked improvement in patient's survival. Good dialytic therapy simplifies management of ARF. Diet and fluid can be liberalized and most uraemic symptoms are ameliorated.

Modes of dialysis

   i. *Intermittent hemodialyses:* It is standard form of renal replacement therapy for patients with ARF.

   ii. *Intermittent peritoneal dialysis:* It is preferred over hemodialysis in patients who are either hemodynamically unstable or have active bleeding. It is not to be used in patients with peritonitis or who have undergone abdominal surgery.

   iii. *Continuous renal replacement therapy:* It includes continuous arteriovenous or venovenous haemofiltration, dialysis or haemodiafiltration. In critically ill patients, the continuously administered therapies are preferred now-a-days. Their advantages over intermittent dialysis include more strict fluid and metabolic control, decreased haemodynamic instability and an enhanced possibility of removing cytokines in patients with sepsis or multiorgan failure. Another advantage is to administer unlimited nutritional support parenterally. The disadvantage of this therapy is that it needs prolonged anticoagulation and constant monitoring.

Recovery Phase (Diuretic Phase of ATN)

Recovery in ARF is usually associated with diuresis. There is step-wise increase in urine flow, but, sometimes a large amount of urine (5–8 L) may be passed, which should be taken care of. Excessive loss of water, sodium, potassium occurs. Fluid losses are better managed with half-isotonic saline. Patients should be encouraged to drink water to satisfy their thirst; remaining fluid deficit is corrected by parenteral fluid therapy. Electrolytes should be monitored during this period and appropriate replacement done whenever needed.

Renal Disease (Renal ARF)

Specific treatment of intrinsic renal disease, i.e. acute GN, vasculitis by steroids, alkylating agents and/or plasmapheresis depending on primary pathology.

Post-renal ARF: It is treated by relieving obstruction (stenting) or by suprapubic catheterisation or nephrostomy.

Poisonings as Emergencies

Management of a Case with Poisoning

MANAGEMENT OF A CASE WITH POISONING

Any substance which produces adverse reactions/effects in a living organism is called poison. Acute poisoning is the common cause of morbidity and mortality throughout the world and is the most common cause of non-traumatic coma in young persons (<35 years of age). Hospital-based data suggests that about 10% of all acute medical admissions are due to poisoning.

Types of Poisoning

1. **Self-poisoning:** It refers to the deliberate ingestion of an overdose substance/drug not meant for consumption. It is also called suicidal or intentional poisoning. Aluminium phosphide, OP compound poisoning are its examples.

2. **Accidental poisoning:** It occurs in children below 5 years of age, but can occur in adults, is either due to accidental exposure (inhalation of gases) or ingestion of fluid or substance from a wrongly labelled bottle, and also includes stings, bites or eating poisoned foods/plants (e.g. mushroom poisoning).

3. **Non-accidental poisoning:** It is a deliberate administration of a poison to a child.

4. **Homicidal poisoning:** It means to kill someone by poisoning.

Diagnosis

Although acute poisoning can mimic any acute illness, but the correct diagnosis is based on high degree of suspicion on history, is established on the physical examination, response to an antidote and clinical course.

History

Although accurate history is an important clinical weapon for diagnosis, but at times, is difficult to obtain from patients who are confused or obtunded and information obtained from the relatives and friends may not be dependable. The points to be noted on the history are given in Box 1.

Poisoning is likely to be missed if it is not suspected. The suspicious circumstances include:

1. Unexplained illness in a previously healthy person.
2. A history of underlying psychiatric illness such as depression.
3. Recent changes in health, economic status or social relationships.
4. Chemical exposure or illness following ingestion of food, drink or medication. The onset of illness in industrial workers or occupational workers may indicate chemical poisoning.
5. Patients falling ill immediately after landing from a foreign country or after arrest for criminal activity should be suspected of

- Time
- Route of administration
- Duration
- Name and amount of the poison, chemical ingredients involved (summon the bottle/container/wrapper of poison to verify it)
- The print code on the pills or label may be used to identify the ingredients and potential toxicity of suspected poison by consulting a reference text, a computerised database, the manufacturer or a regional poisoning centre
- Family, friends, police, pharmacists, physicians and employes should be asked regarding the habits, hobbies, behaviour, available medications and clinical grounds for suspicion of poisoning
- Circumstances of exposure (location, surrounding, intent)
- Symptomatology, e.g. time of onset, nature and severity of symptoms
- Time and type of first-aid given
- Medical history for any acute illness
- Psychiatric history
- History of alcohol or drug overdose

having an illicit drug concealed in body cavity (the GI tract).

Physical Examination

A search for the clothes, belongings and place of discovery may help to recover a suicidal note, or a container which may have the remaining tablets or chemical.

The physical examination should focus initially on the vital signs and cardiopulmonary and neurological status. Before proceeding for detailed clinical examination. First ensure A, B, C of cardiopulmonary resuscitation:

- The airway (A) is clear.
- The patient is breathing (B) properly and adequately.
- The circulation (C) is adequate and is not compromised. If the patient is alert and is hemodynamically stable, proceed to examination as follows:
  1. **Level of consciousness:**The Glassgow Coma Scale (given in chapter on coma in neurological emergencies) may be

employed to assess the degree of unconsciousness though it has never been validated for use in poisoned patients.
2. Look for respiratory effort and cyanosis, presence or absence of cough and gag reflex.
3. Record pulse rate and blood pressure.
4. Examination of eyes (for nystagmus, size of the pupil, and its reaction), abdomen (for bowel activity and bladder size) and skin (for bums, bullae, colour, warmth, moisture, pressure sores, puncture marks) to narrow down the diagnosis to a particular poison.
5. Look for an evidence of trauma or physical illness.
6. Temperature—measure with a low reading rectal thermometer.
7. When history is unclear, all orifices should be examined for presence of chemical burns, and drug packets.
8. The odour of breath or vomitus and the colour of the skin, nails or urine may give valuable informations for diagnosis.

The physical signs of the poisoning are given in Fig. 78.1. Diagnosis and differential diagnosis of the poisoning based on biochemical analysis is given in Box 2.

Laboratory Tests

In most patients, the diagnosis is made on the history and clinical signs alone. As these cases are medicolegal, hence, urine, serum and vomitus (or gastric lavage may be preserved for analysis especially where there is fatality. They may be useful to confirm or rule out suspected poisoning. Otherwise also, subsequent management of poisoned patients depends on the measurement of amount of toxin/poison and severity of the poisoning. Grading of severity is useful for clinical course and response to treatment.

In unconscious patients, a qualitative screen of the urine (e.g. urine immunofluorescence for drugs of misuse screening test) is an effective way to confirm recent use of drugs such as benzodiazepines, cocaine, opioids, ecstasy,

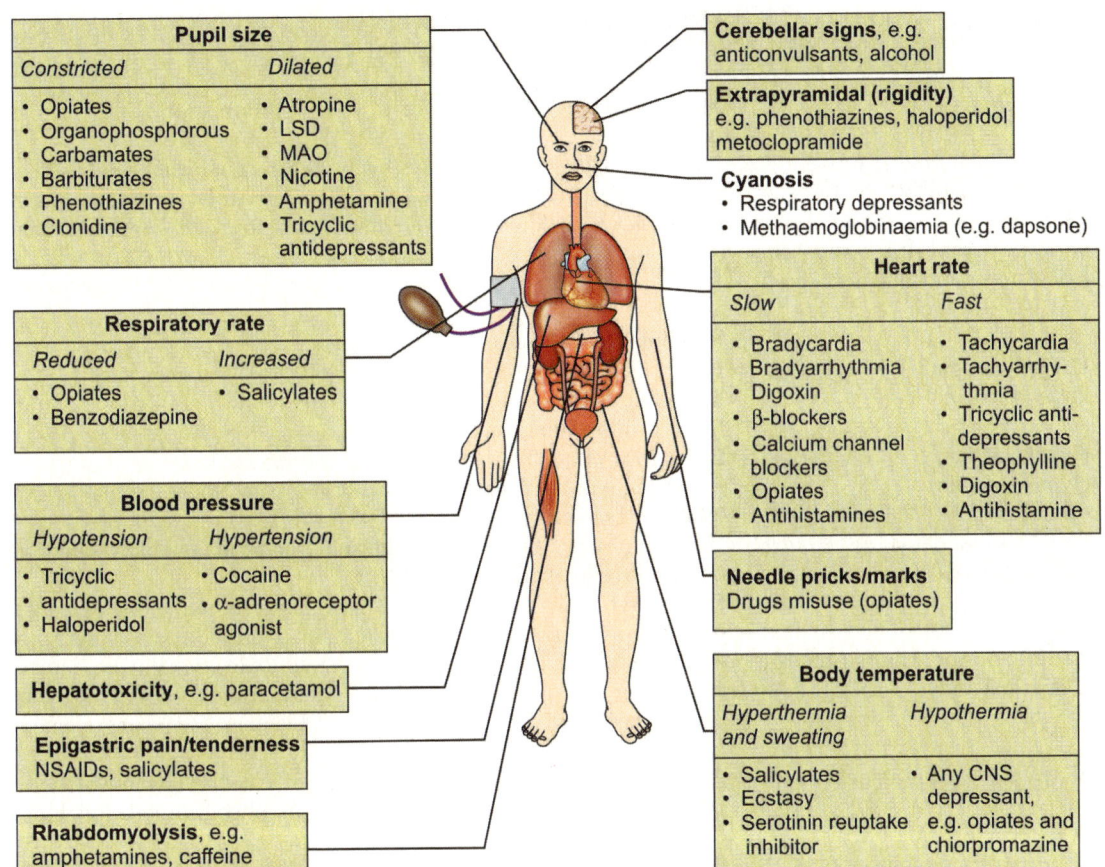

Fig. 78.1: Clinical manifestations (signs) in a case with poisoning

and cannabis. Routine screens may not, however detect fentanyl derivatives, tramadol and other synthetic opioids. Occasionally measuring drugs of misuse and their metabolites in blood by gas chromatography-mass spectroscopy (GC-MS) may be required for medico-legal purposes. Personal communication with the laboratory is essential. A negative result on a screen may mean the poison is not detectable by the test used or its concentration is too low for detection at the time of sampling. In the latter situation, repeating the test at later time may give a positive result.

Response to Antidotes

The response to an antidote may be taken as a clue to diagnosis. Resolution of symptoms of hypoglycaemia with dextrose confirms

hypoglycaemia. Resolution of altered mental status and abnormal vital signs within minutes of I.V. administration naloxone or flumazenil is virtually diagnostic of opiates and benzodiazepine poisoning respectively. The prompt reversal of dystonia with I.V. benzotropine or diphenhydramine confirms drug-induced dystonia. Vin rose urine colour following a diagnostic use of desferoxamine confirms iron intoxication when measurements of serum iron and iron binding capacity test are not available immediately. Reversal of central and peripheral manifestations by physostigmine confirms anticholinergic poisoning.

Time Course of Events

It is also helpful in making a diagnosis of poisoning. Signs and symptoms developing

Box 2	Diagnosis and differential diagnosis based on laboratory assessment
Parameter	Differential diagnosis
• Metabolic acidosis	• Methanol, ethylene glycol, salicylate, carbon monoxide, ethanol poisoning.
• An abnormally low anion gap	• Bromide, iodine, lithium, nitrate, hypocalcaemia or hypemagnesaemia.
• An osmolal gap >10 mmol/L (i.e. difference between measured serum osmolality and the calculated osmolality from serum Na$^+$, glucose, urea)	• Alcohol, glycol or ketone or an unmeasured electrolyte or sugar. It can be due to DKA or lactic acidosis from which poisoning has been differentiated.
• Ketosis	• Isopropyl alcohol and salicylate poisoning.
• Hypoglycaemia	• Poisoning by β-blockers, quinine, ethanol, OHA, and salicylates.
• Hyperglycaemia	• Poisoning by acetone, a beta-adrenergic agonist, a calcium channel blocker, iron or theophylline.
• Hypokalaemia	• Poisoning by barium, a beta-adrenergic agonist, a diuretic, theophylline.
• Hyperkalaemia	• Poisoning with an α-adrenergic agonist, a beta blocker, digitalis, ACE inhibitors or fluoride.
• Pulmonary oedema (ARDS) e.g. low PaO$_2$, low PaCO$_2$	• Poisoning with carbon monoxide, cyanide, an opoid, paraquat, salicylate or a sedative-hypnotic. • Poisoning by inhaled gases, fumes or vapors (ammonia, metal oxides, mercury, phosphine (PH$_3$ due to aluminium phosphide poisoning).
• Radio-opaque densities on abdominal X-rays	• Ingestion of calcium salts, chloral hydrate, chlorinated hydrocarbon, heavy metals, illic t drug packets, iodinated compounds, K$^+$ salts, psychotherapeutic agents, lithium, phenothiazines, salicylates or enteric coated tablets.
• Bradycardia and AV block	• Poisoning by antiarrhythmics, beta-blockers, calcium channel blockers, cholinergic agents (carbamate and organophosphorus insecticide), digitalis, lithium or tricyclic antidepressants.
• QRS and QTc prolongation	• Poisoning by antiarrhythmics, tricyclic antidepressants, heavy metals, lithium, local anaesthetic, meperidine and quinine and related antimalarial.
• Tachyarrhythmias	• Poisoning with digitalis, sympathomimetics, chloral hydrate, aliphatic or halogenated hydrocarbons and aluminium phosphide.

acutely, peaking within several hours and subsequent resolution over hours or days in an otherwise healthy person suggest an acute poisoning.

Management

Principles

I. General management:
  • To support the vital functions (circulatory and respiratory).
II. Specific management (Table 78.1):
  • To delay or prevent further absorption of poison.
  • To enhance excretion of poison (through faeces or urine).

  • To administer specific antidote, wherever applicable to prevent re-exposure.

I. Supportive Therapy

The supportive therapy may be needed to maintain physiological homeostasis until detoxification process is completed, and to prevent and treat secondary complications such as aspiration, bedsores, cerebral and pulmonary oedema, renal failure, rhabdomyolysis and generalised organ dysfunction due to prolonged hypoxia or shock.

A. *Respiratory support*
  • If respiratory depression is minimal, 60% O$_2$ via a mask may be sufficient.

A nasopharyngeal or oropharyngeal airway should be inserted for constant monitoring for ventilation.

- Loss of gag or cough reflex is an indication for intubation (a gag reflex is assessed by positioning the patients on their side and making them gag using a sucker).
- Patients with severe excitation may also require intubation for airway protection.
- If ventilation remains inadequate, intermittent positive pressure ventilation (IPPV) should be instituted. Blood gas analysis is useful to confirm the need for IPPV.
- Hypoxaemia is common in unconscious patient, may go undetected after ingestion of poisoning (e.g. opiates, barbiturates, etc.), hence, monitoring by oximetry or arterial blood gas analysis is mandatory for severely poisoned patients with depressed ventilation.
- Pulmonary arterial or capillary wedge pressure measurement is indicated in patients with pulmonary oedema to determine its nature. Drug-induced pulmonary oedema is usually non cardiogenic (normal or low capillary wedge pressure). A Swan-Ganz catheter may be put to measure the pressure and to monitor the fluid and diuretics therapy.
- Extracorporeal membrane oxygenation may be appropriate for severe but reversible respiratory failure.

B. *Cardiovascular Support*
- Hypotension (BP <90 mmHg) is a common feature of drug overdosage, is caused by vasodilatation, hypovolaemia, myocardial depression, hypoxia, etc. should be treated appropriately.
- Shocked patients (tachycardia, cold clammy skin, oliguria) should be managed accordingly with vasopressor (dobutamine) and I.V. fluids under CVP monitoring.

- Arrhythmia are common. Find out the cause and treat it accordingly. Known arrhythmogenic factors such as hypoxia, acidosis and hypokalaemia should be corrected. Lidocaine and phenytoin are safe for drug-induced ventricular arrhythmias.
- Bradyarrhythmias and hypotension due to beta-blockers and calcium channel blockers may respond to glucagon (5–10 mg I.V.) and calcium chloride (1–2 g I.V.) respectively. Antibody (Fab antibody) to digoxin is indicated in digitalis-induced arrhythmias. Hypotension commonly accompanies bradyarrhythmia, should be managed simultaneously.

Hypertension (diastolic BP > 105 mmHg) if there is no previous history, should be treated with lorazepam in anxious and agitated patients. For

Box 3	Commonly employed antidotes
Poison	*Antidote*
Paracetamol	N-acetylcysteine, methionine
Organophosporous and carbamates	Atropine (muscarine effects) pralidoxime (nicotinin effects)
Amanita phylloids	Benzylpenicillin
Calcium channel blockers	Calcium chloride/ gluconate
Methanol and ethylene glycol	Ethanol, fomepizole (4-methylpyrazole)
Iron	Desferrioxamine
Opiates	Naloxone, nalmefene
Cyanide	Sodium nitrate, sodium thiosulphate
Anticholinergics	Physostigmine
Isoniazid	Pyridoxine
Sulphonylureas	Octreotide
Lead, mercury, copper	BAL, calcium EDTA, D-penicillamine
Anticoagulants	Vitamin K
Beta blockers	Glucagon, adrenaline
Digitalis	Fab antibody
Carbon monoxide	Oxygen, hyperbaric oxygen
Snake venom	Specific antivenin

Table 78.1 Steps to delay or prevent further absorption of poison

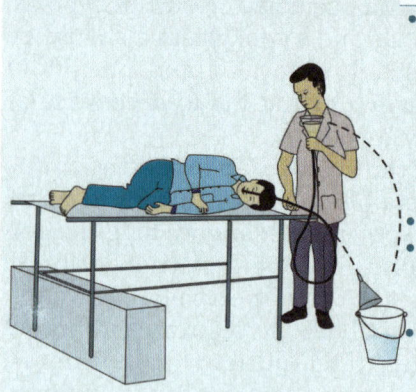

Fig. 78.2: Specific management of poisoning

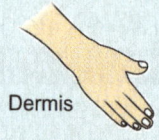

Dermis

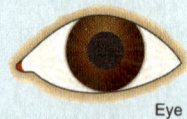

Eye

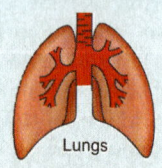

Lungs

Blood

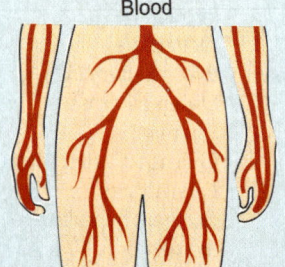

I. Decontamination of gastrointestinal tract

- **Gastric lavage:** Only if a potentially life-threatening amount of toxic substance has been ingested within the last hour. Not to be used for acids, alkalis or petroleum distillates. It is useful for liquid poison and poisoning by small pill fragments. It should be done within an hour of poisoning. It also helps to collect the gastric sample for analysis. It should not be attempted in comatosed patients with absent gag reflex unless they are intubated before hand.
- **Induced emesis** by syrup of ipecac.
- **Activated charcoal:** 50 g can be given to an adult orally if a potentially toxic amount of poison has been ingested the last hour, useful only if the toxin or drug can be bound to charcoal.
- Multiple doses of charcoal are given (50 g every 4 hours) in poisoning by carbamazepine, dapsone, quinine and theophylline. It is contraindicated in patients with ileus, or intestinal obstruction or those who have ingested corrosives in which endoscopy is planned.
- **Catharsis:** It is induced by cathartic salts (disodium phosphate, magnesium citrate, sodium sulphate) or saccharide (mannitol or sorbitol) to promote fecal excretion of poison. Contraindicated in corrosive poisoning diarrhoea, and intestinal obstruction
- **Whole bowel irrigation:** Polyethylene glycol solution is given for potentially toxic ingestion of iron, lithium and theophylline and to clear packets of drugs from body packers. Do not use it in patients with suspected intestinal obstruction

II. Decontamination of other sites

- **Removal of clothing/skin washing:** Wash the skin with copious amounts of soap and water for chemical or pesticide exposures.
- **Irrigation of eyes:** Wash eyes thoroughly for at least 15 minutes with normal saline or water.
  - Remove particles from palpebral fissures. If pain persists, fluorescein drops and slit-lamp examination for corneal damage are essential.

III. Exhalation of poison

- **Oxygen and bronchodilator:** Give high-flow oxygen, e.g. 12 L/min. Nebulised β2-adrenoceptor agonists if patient has wheezing.

STEPS TO ENHANCE POISON EXCRETION

Urinary alkalinisation: It enhances elimination of acidic drugs (e.g. salicylates phenobarbitone and some pesticides, e.g. 2–4 D. Give 1 litre of 1.26% sodium bicarbonate I.V. over 3 hours. Check urine pH, remains between 7.5 and 8.5. Avoid use of large volumes, i.e. forced diuresis, and watch for hypokalaemia.

Extracorporeal methods of an elimination, e.g. haemodialysis or haemoperfusion: It is useful for serious poisoning with salicylates, theophylline, ethylene glycol, methanol, carbamazepine. It is also useful for poisoning in patients with renal, cardiac or hepatic disease who will not be able to eliminate poison by useful mechanisms.

Contd.

Table 78.1 Steps to delay or prevent further absorption of poison (*Contd.*)

NEUTRALISATION OF POISON BY SPECIFIC ANTIDOTE

Antidotes counteract the effects of poisons by neutralising them (e.g. antigen-antibody reaction), by chelation (chemical binding) or by antagonising their physiological effects (activation of opposing nervous system activity, competitive inhibition). Antidotes can reduce both morbidity and mortality, but most antidotes are toxic too. The antidotes to various poisons are given Box 3.

PREVENTION OF RE-EXPOSURE

The methods of poisoning prevention are depicted in Box 4

Box 4 Methods of poisoning prevention

Method	*Mode of action*
• Addition of 'Bitrex' and other bittering agents to household products	• Prevent consumption of large quantities as it tastes bitter
• Addition of antidote to the toxin, e.g. combination tablets of methionine and paracetamol	• As antidote is incorporated, glutathione remains repleted and hepatocellular injury is prevented
• Child-resistant containers	• Reduces chances of poisoning in children
• Secure preservation (almirah, locked cupboard)	• Inaccessibility reduces chances of poisoning
• Hazard warning signals	• Warning by label to potential toxicity, route of administration and protective measures
• Education	• Warning on safe storage and handling of chemicals and drugs reduces poisoning incidence
• Supervision	• Careful supervision reduces chances of poisoning in children
• Legislation, e.g. health and safety regulations	• Make a safe work place with safeguards in the use of dangerous chemicals

persistent hypertension, I.V. nitroprusside (0.25–8 g/kg/min) may be used. If tachycardia is present, use I.V. beta-blocker esmolol (25–100 g/kg/min). I.V. or labetalol I.V. may be used.

C. *Care of Unconscious Patient (read Chapter on Coma in neurological emergencies)*
  • For coma management, remember mnemonic ABCD.
  • In all cases, the patient should be nursed in the lateral position with lower leg straight and the upper leg flexed. In this position, risk of aspiration is minimized.
  • Remove any obstructing object, vomitus or dentures. Maintain patent airway.
  • Nursing care of mouth and measures to avoid pressure sore should be instituted.
  • Unnecessary catheterization of bladder should be avoided. Condom drainage is best to avoid bed-wetting. Bladder

in poisoned patients can be emptied by gentle suprapubic pressure.
  • I.V. access and intravenous fluid to be started immediately and correct dehydration by I.V. fluids at least for 24 hours.
  • Rest of the management is same as for any other unconscious patient including the monitoring of vital parameters (pulse, BP, temp, respiration, etc.).
      Hypoglycemia in unconscious patient can be managed with 50–100 ml of 25–50% dextrose. In alcoholic intoxicaion, thiamine is useful.
  • Use the antidote in unconscious patient to reverse the coma as early as possible.

D. *Treatment of Specific Problems*
  • *Convulsions/seizures:* These may occur in serious tricyclic antidepressants, antihistamine, phenothiazine and

strychnine poisoing or may occur following drug withdrawal. Diazepam 10 mg I.V. is the standard treatment for fits of any cause. The patient should receive a loading dose of phenytoin (lg I.V. over 4 hours) followed by 100 mg 8 hourly if fits do not get immediately controlled with diazepam. Persistent fits must be controlled rapidly as they may otherwise result in hypoxia, brain damage and laryngeal trauma. The underlying cause should be cor rected. Propofol infusion has been reported to be effective in resistant drug induced arrhythmias.

- *Hypothermia* (rectal temperature (35°C) is a problem in elderly or in those poisoned with chlorpromazine or another neuroleptic. Hypo thyroidism must be excluded. The patient should be covered with a space blanket and given intravenous and intragastric fluids at normal body temperature. Inspired gases should also be wanned to 37°C.

- *Stress bleeding:* Measures to prevent stress ulcers in poisoned patients include adminis tration of antacids through Ryle's tube or I.V. H2 antagonists.

- *Hyperthermia:* Remove all the clothings and do sponging with taped water and fanning (read management of hyperpy-rexia as an emergency)

- *Metabolic, renal and hepatic abnormalities:* and secondary complications should be treated by standard measures.

II. Specific Management

It depends on the route of exposure, i.e. direct contact (eye, skin), ingestion (GI tract), inhala-tion (lungs) and inoculation (blood). The steps of management are depicted in Table 78.1 and Fig. 78.2.

Corrosive (Acid and Alkali) Poisoning

The term corrosive poisoning include acid and alkali poisoning which cause tissue destruction when they come in contact with mucous membrane.

CORROSIVE ACID POISONING

Acute corrosive acid poisoning is common due to suicidal ingestion of an acid (sulphuric acid, HCl, nitric acid) present in many products of household use (toilet cleaning agents).

Laboratory workers (hydrochloric acid, nitric acid, sulphuric acid) and goldsmith (aqua ragia) ingest acids accidently in recent years, button cell battery ingestion in children is being increasingly recognised.

These poisons corrode and destroy the local tissues commonly of mouth, pharynx and upper GI tract with which they immediately-come in contact after ingestion (Fig. 79.1).

Mode of Action

Corrosive acids act locally and usually do not produce systemic effects. They produce coagulative necrosis by precipitation of tissue proteins which retards injury and limits the penetration into the tissue. Sloughing and expulsion of large areas of surface lining of stomach and oesophagus may result in perforation and peritonitis. With process of healing stricture formation results.

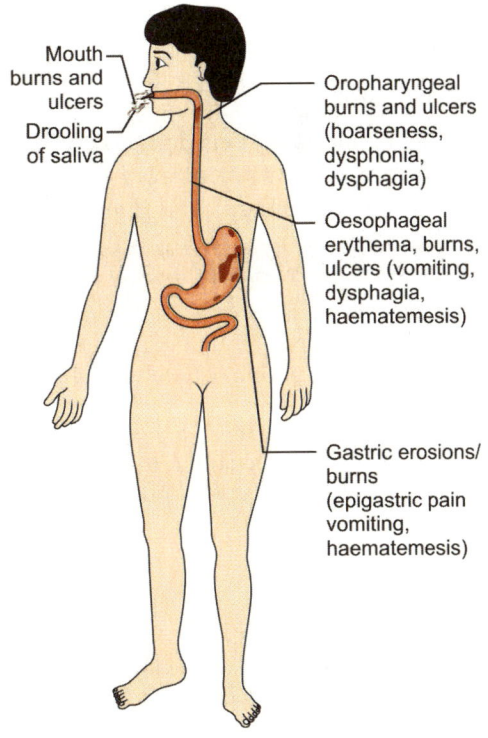

Mouth burns and ulcers

Drooling of saliva

Oropharyngeal burns and ulcers (hoarseness, dysphonia, dysphagia)

Oesophageal erythema, burns, ulcers (vomiting, dysphagia, haematemesis)

Gastric erosions/burns (epigastric pain vomiting, haematemesis)

Fig. 79.1: Corrosive poisoning

Note: The term corrosive poisoning include both acid and alkali poisonings which cause tissue destruction when they come in contact with mucous membrane

Types

- **Accidental:** It is common in children.

- **Suicidal:** It is common in adults.
- **Inhalational:** It is due to inhalation of acid fumes.

Common Acid Poisons

- **Sulphuric acid:** It is present in toilet cleaner, battery acid, laboratory, etc.
- **Hydrochloric acid:** It is present in toilet-cleaner, soldering fluxes, laboratory, etc.
- **Oxalic acid** (anti-rust).
- **Nitric acid** is used by goldsmiths, stone-cleaners
- **Hydrofluoric acid** (present in toilet bowl cleaners, anti-rust compound and stone-cleaners).

Clinical Features

The clinical manifestations depend on the con centration and quantity of acid consumed. The symptoms and signs are given in Box 1.

They include GI symptoms, destruction and discolouration of skin and mucous membrane. The acids being liquid pass easily through the mouth into oesophagus. Injury pattern depends on the state of stomach whether full or empty. If stomach is full, acid is easily diluted and gastric mucosa is spared, acid flows towards pyloric antrum where maximum effect occurs.

In severe cases of acid poisoning following complications may occur:

1. **Hypotension and circulatory shock** due to vomiting and dehydration. The patient feels excessive thirst and tongue is dry. There is tachypnoea and tachycardia. There may be features of metabolic acidosis.

2. **Mediastinitis** due to rupture of oesoph-agus producing collection of air in the mediastinum (mediastinal emphysema). The mediastinal crunch (crunching sound on sternal compression) may be felt. There

Box 1 Symptoms and signs of corrosive acid poisoning		
Site of injury	*Symptoms*	*Signs*
A. Ingestinal Poisoning		
1. Mouth and oropharynx	• Pain in mouth, throat and drooling of saliva	• Skin and oropharyngeal burns, ulcers, oedema, necrosis, discolouration of mouth
	• Difficulty in speech (hoarseness or dysphonia) due to oedema of glottis	• Deep mucosal burns may produce anaesthesia
	• Choking and stridor	• Drooling of saliva over lips produces charring of skin over angles of mouth, chin and chest
	• Constant cough, dyspnoea	• In severe cases, the tongue is shapeless, a pulpy mass
		• Teeth may become chalky white and loose shine in severe poisoning (corrosion of teeth)
2. Oesophagus	• Painful swallowing, retrosternal pain, neck pain/tenderness	• Oesophageal burns and ulcers. The mucosa is red and swollen
	• Haematemesis (vomiting with altered blood and mucus)	
3. Stomach	• Epigastric pain, burning and tenderness	• Gastric burns
	• Vomiting. It is strongly acidic, will cause effervescence on coming in contact with earth and will stain clothes	
4. Respiratory tract (due to aspiration)	• Cough and dyspnoea • Hoarseness and dysphonia • Labored breathing	• Tracheitis and pneumonia • Pleural effusion may develop
B. Inhalational poisoning (inhalation of gases i.e. chlorine, fluorine, bromine, iodine, etc.)		
	• Upper respiratory obstruction, cough, dyspnoea	• Non-cardiogenic pulmonary oedema, (rales, crackles)

may be fever, increase in respiratory rate, constant cough and laboured breathing.

3. **Stricture of oesophagus:** It develops on healing (chronic phase) of acid burns in oesophagus producing oesophageal narrowing.

Inhalation of volatile acids, fumes or gases such as chlorine, fluorine, bromine or iodine cause upper airway obstruction and *non cardiogenic pulmonary oedema*.

Investigations

1. **Routine laboratory tests**
   - Complete hemogram, haematocrit.
   - Liver function tests.
   - Renal function tests (blood urea, serum creatinine).
   - Serum electrolytes.
2. **Arterial blood gas analysis**
3. **Radiology**
   - Chest X-ray. It may show diffuse mottling or ARDS like picture in inhalational poisoning or due to aspiration of gastric contents after ingestion. In case of oesophageal perforation, air may be present in mediastinum (*mediastinal emphysema*).
   - Plain X-ray abdomen in case perforation is suspected.
4. **Endoscopy:** Laryngoscopy and upper GI endoscopy are done using a small-bore, flexible endoscope as soon as the patient is hemodynamically stable and perforation is excluded. It documents the anatomical site and often severity of the injury (Box 2).

Box 2	Endoscopic classification of corrosive injury
Grade	Extent of injury
0	Normal mucosa
I	Oedema and hyperaemia only
IIa	Friability, erosions and superfical ulcerations
IIb	IIa (described above) plus discrete and deep ulcers
IIIa	In addition to grade II changes, there are multiple ulcers and scattered areas of necrosis
IIIb	Extensive confluent necrosis

Management

It depends on the extent of injury (Box 3).

Box 3	Extent of injury, management and complications
Endoscopic grading	Management
I	• Oral fluids for 24–48 hours. Discharge the patient with advice of oral toilet with antiseptics and a soft diet
II (a and b)	• I.V. fluids for 24–48 hours, then start oral fluids • Begin with soft diet after 48 hours if patient can swallow
III (a and b)	• In presence of dysphagia, nutritional supplementation intravenously or by a feeding jejunostomy • Antibiotics (a combination of an aminoglycoside and a cephalosporin) • Controversial use of steroids. A recent study in children has shown no benefit; while a meta-analysis published recently suggest beneficial effect of steroids • Resuscitate the patient for dehydration, shock, etc.

A. *Immediate resuscitation therapy*

1. Dilute the poison immediately by giving a glass of water to drink.
2. *Fluid therapy:* Mild injury (grade I) can be managed with oral fluids. Moderate (grade II) injury requires I.V. fluids for 48 hours followed by small oral feeds of fluid. Severe injury initially may be treated by I.V. fluids, and may require feeding jejunostomy.
3. Maintain patent airway and supportive treatment.
4. The important "Do's" and "Don'ts" are given in Box 4.

For inhalation poisoning remove the patient from further exposure to fumes and gas. Treat non-cardiogenic pulmonary oedema.

Treatment of eye contact: It is similar to alkali poisoning (read alkali poisoning next).

Box 4	Immediate "do's" and "don'ts" in corrosive acid poisoning
Don'ts	*Do's*
• Do not panic • Do not induce vomiting • Do not put Ryle's tube as it may cause perforation of thinned mucosa of oesophagus or stomach. Now some gastroenterologists recommend immediate cautious placement of a small flexible gastric tube and removal of gastric contents followed by gastric lavage. • Do not try to neutralise the acid with alkali or with water	• Immediate liberal use of water or milk mixed with milk of magnesia, aluminium hydroxide and magnesium oxide to neutralise the acid. The best antidote is 5% magnesium oxide. Lime water, any vegetable oil or ghee, egg-white are other alternatives to neutralise the acid • Make arrangements to transfer the patient to a hospital. Look at the oral cavity and remove any caustic granules and flakes gently • Correct hypotension with isotonic fluids and blood products. Suction of ice may reduce thirst • If the patient has respiratory distress, do immediate tracheal intubation or tracheostomy • Give oxygen • Intravenous H_2 receptors blockers may be used for symptomatic relief and may help in early healing • Use antibiotics if infection supervenes • Relief of pain by morphine or pethidine • Skin, oral and eye lesions may be irrigated with plenty of water

Treatment of skin contact: Wash the skin with water for 15 minutes. Do not use any chemical antidote or alkali.

For hydrofluoric acid burns, soak the affected area in benzalonium chloride solution or apply 2.5 calcium gluconate gel, then consult plastic surgeon or skin specialist.

Do not use calcium chloride. Use of a Bier-block technique or intra-arterial infusion of calcium gluconate is required for extensive burns.

B. *Post-resuscitation management:* Next step is to rule out an oesophageal and gastric perforation by:

- Symptoms and signs.
- Chest X-ray and plain X-ray abdomen (film to be taken in erect position). If there is no perfo ration, a cautious upperGI endoscopy by a small calibre flexible endoscope may be done by trained endoscopist. The endoscopy is safe and will delineate the injury and extent of mucosal damage. Depending on the classification of injury on endoscopy, proceed as given in Box 3.

  - Airway maintenance may require tracheostomy
  - In the event of perforation, thoracotomy and/or laparotomy is done at the earliest and oesophageal or gastric resection with appropriate bypass procedure may be required.

Long-term complications include oesophageal and gastric stenosis/stricture (Fig. 79.2) requiring endoscopic dilatation and corrective surgery.

CORROSIVE ALKALI POISONING

Acute corrosive poisoning with alkali occurs due to ingestion of common household products containing alkali. Common alkaline products include industrial bleach, drain cleaners (sodium hydroxide), surface cleaners (ammonia, phosphates), laundry and dishwasher detergents (phosphates, carbonates), disk batteries, denture cleaners (borates, phosphates) and clinitest tablets (sodium hydroxide).

In India acids are more frequently implicated in poisoning than alkalis.

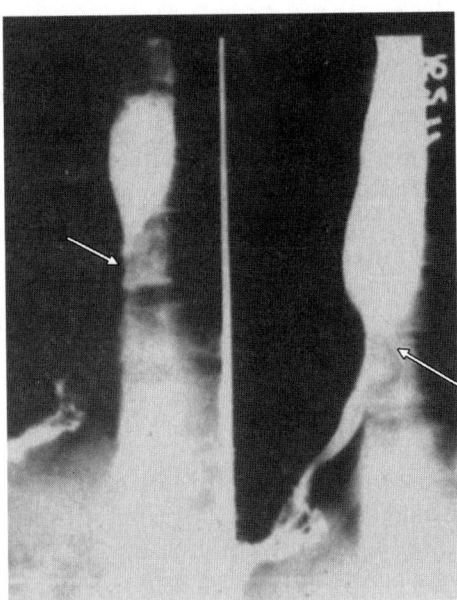

Fig. 79.2: Oesophageal stricture (↓) following corrosive (acid) poisoning

Mode of Action

Alkalis penetrate the tissues rapidly, produce corrosive effects by extracting water from the tissues causing tissue dehydration. They produce liquefactive necrosis of the tissues with which they come in contact with, therefore, there is higher risk of perforation of the oesophagus and stomach than acids do. Their action is bit slow but sustained one.

Types of Poisoning

- **Accidental ingestion:** It is common in children.
- **Suicidal:** It is common in adults especially females.

Clinical Features

1. Burning and severe pain extending from the mouth to the stomach erythema, burns and ulceration. The pain radiates all over the abdomen.
2. Sudden caustic, soapy, nauseous taste in the mouth.
3. Vomiting soon follows which is strongly alkaline and contains frothy material with shreds of mucus and altered blood (haematemesis). The vomit will not effervescence when it comes in contact with the earth.
4. Dysphagia and dyspnoea may occur. Purging which is not seen in acidic poisoning is almost always present in alkali poisoning. There may be pain and tenesmus. Stools are mixed with blood and mucus.
5. Gastric and oesophageal perforation is common than acidic poisoning. It is a delayed sequelae. Complications include stricture of oesophagus or pylorus.
6. Alkali coming in contact with eyes cause oedema of conjunctivae, corneal ulceration and blindness.

Examination

It reveals destruction and oedema of the affected skin and mucous membranes, and blood in vomitus and stools.

Investigations

They are more or less same as discussed in acid poisoning. Radiographs may reveal evidence of perforation or the presence of radiopaque disk bateries in the oesphogus or lower GI tract.

Management

Management is same as that of acid poisoning because both produce corrosive injury to GI tract.

  i. **Neutralization of alkali** with weak acid should not be attempted as it may lead to further injury by liberating heat due to reaction with acids. Dilute the effects with a glass of water immediately. Do not induce vomiting. Some gasteoenterologists recommend removal of residual material with a small flexible gastric tube.
 ii. **Treatment of skin contact:** Wash the skin with running water until the skin no longer feels soapy. Relive pain and treat shock.
iii. **Treatment of eye contact:** Anaesthetise the conjunctival and corneal surfaces

with topical anaesthetic. Irrigate the eye with water or saline continuously for 20–30 minutes, holding the lids open. Check pH with pH paper and repeat irrigation with normal saline for another 20–30 minutes until pH is near 7.0. Check for corneal damage with fluorescein and slit-lamp examination. Consult an ophthalmologist for further treatment, if necessary.

iv. **General supportive measures,** treatment of shock, parenteral nutrition may berequired.

v. The various **Don'ts and Do's** discussed in acid poisoning are also applicable here.

vi. **Prompt endoscopy** is recommended in symptomatic patients to evaluate the extent of damage. CT scan also aids in the diagnosis. If radiography reveals the location of ingested button/disc battery in the oesophagus, immediate endoscopic removal is necessary.

vii. **Glucocorticoids and silastic oesophageal stents** have traditionally been used for alkali burns to prevent oesophageal stricture formation, but their efficacy is not proven. Animal studies suggest use of steroids. Prednisolone is used in the dose of 1–2 mg/kg every 4–6 hourly for at least 2 weeks.

vii. **Prophylactic use of antibiotics is also recommended.**

ix. **Oesophageal stricture or gastric outlet obstruction** may require subsequent dilatation and bougienage or surgical reconstruction.

Methylalcohol (Methanol) and Ethylene Glycol Poisoning

Methanol (methylalcohol, wood alcohol) is used as a detergent, is a component of varnishes, paint removers, wind-shield washer solutions, copy machine fluid, anti-freeze solutions and solvents. It is also a denaturant used to make ethanol unfit forconsumption.

Mode of Poisoning

Methanol poisoning occurs commonly due to intentional use of cheap illicit liquor (hooch) in alcoholics as a substitute for ethanol. It may also be a contaminant in bootleg whisky. The poisoning may occur in isolation or in an epidemic proportion *(hooch tragedy).* People of lower socio-economic status are vulnerable to this poisoning.

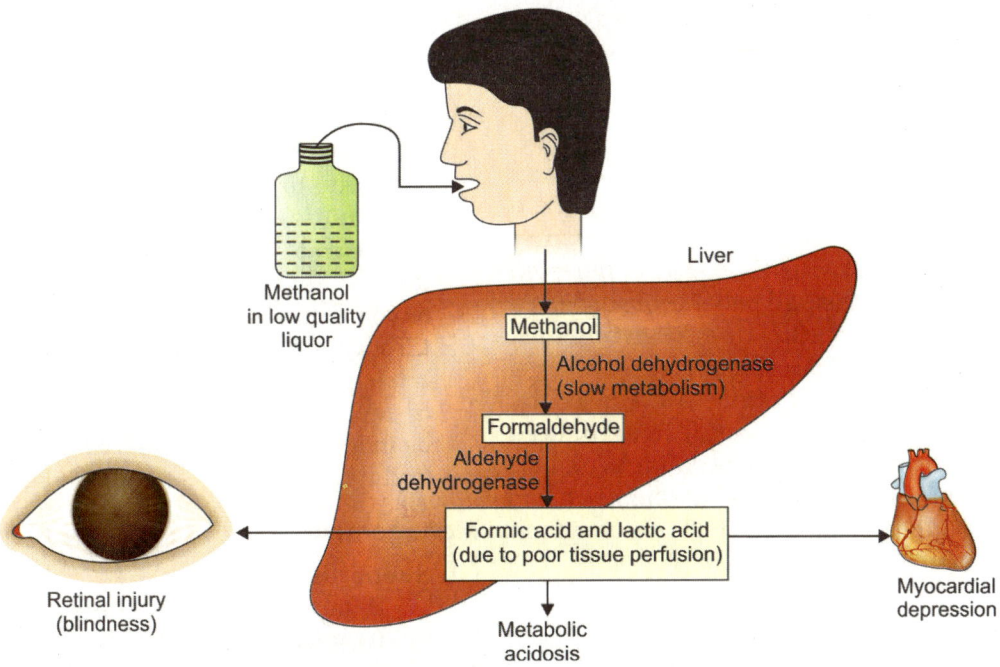

Fig. 80.1: Methylalcohol (methanol) poisoning—mechanisms and tissue toxicity

Mechanisms of Action

After ingestion, it is rapidly absorbed and concentrated in the liver, GI tract, eyes and kidneys. Its level peaks within 1–2 hours of ingestion. Its binding is negligible. It is mainly metabolised in the liver (Fig. 80.1) but up to 10% is excreted unchanged by the lungs and kidneys. In the liver, methanol is converted into formaldehyde and then into formic acid by the enzyme *alcohol dehydrogenase.* Both methanol and its metabolites are toxic, the latter causing more serious side-effects.

The half-life of elimination at low serum levels is 14–20 hours and at high serum level is 24–30 hours. Ethanol (ethylalcohol) competes with methanol for enzyme alcohol dehydrogenase for metabolism. Ethyl alcohol has more affinity for this enzyme hence, has found place in its treatment by increasing the elimination half-life of methanol to 30–36 hours (in the absence of enzyme, methanol is not metabolised further).

The fatal oral dose of methanol is 30–240 ml (20–150 g), but 30 ml of a 40% solution can be fatal.

Clinical Features

The clinical features depend on the amount ingested. The time of onset of symptoms and signs after ingestion is variable and features are late in onset when ethanol is ingested concurrently. Hence, all patients of suspected methanol poisoning should be closely observed for an extended period of time before discharge.

The early manifestations are caused by methanol itself; while late features are produced by its toxic metabolites (formaldehyde and fooric acid). Shortly after the ingestion, patients usually appear drunk. The features are given in Box 1.

Diagnosis

The diagnosis is usually suggested by history of ingestion, ethanol-like intoxication, clinical features and an elevated serum osmolarity. It is confirmed by measurement of the serum methanol level (usually >6 mnol/L or >20 mg/dl). Later, the diagnosis is suggested by increased anion gap, metabolic acidosis and elevated serum methanol and formate levels. Calculation of the osmolal gap and anion gap helps to assess the severity of intoxication because most centres do not have facility for methanol estimation.

Serum methanol level (mg/dl) = Osmolal gap × 2.6

Investigation

1. **Serum methanol level:** More than 20 mg/dl levels are considered toxic; and more than 40mg/dl indicate severe intoxication. A low or absent serum methanol level does not rule out serious intoxication in symptomatic patients because the whole methanol might have been metabolised to formic acid, hence, formate levels are elevated in such a situation.

2. **Serum formate levels** are elevated. Raised formate levels confirms the intoxication even if methanol levels are normal. Unfortunately, this investigation is not readily available.

3. **Arterial blood gas analysis, serum osmolarity and anion gap** must be done if there is suspicion of methanol poisoning. This helps to assess the severity also where methanol levels cannot be estimated.

4. **Renal and liver function tests** must be done if there is history of concurrent ethanol ingestion.

5. **CTscan:** CT scan of the brain may show bilateral putamen necrosis. A diagnosis of methanol poisoning can sometimes be made in retrospect on the basis of this finding.

Management

1. **Supportive measures**
   1. Removal of unabsorbed methanol by gastric aspiration and by administration of 50 g of activated charcoal to adsorb the poison. This measure is helpful if poisoning is <4 hours duration.

Box 1	Symptoms and signs of methanol poisoning
Early	*Late (after 24 hours)*

1. At low concentration (> 20 mg/dl)

• Nausea, vomiting and abdominal pain	• Seizures
	• Severe metabolic acidosis
• Headache, vertigo, dizziness	• Increased osmolal gap (>10 mOsm/L)
• Ethanol-like intoxication	

2. At high concentration (>40 mg/dl)

• Alteration in consciousness	• Visual disturbances, e.g. clouding and diminished vision, dancing and flashing spots, fixed or dilated pupils, disc hyperaemia and blindness due to retinal injury
• Convulsions	
• Coma	
• Metabolic acidosis	
• An increased osmolal gap (>5 mOsm/L)	• Coma
	• Severe intoxication may produce myocardial depression, bradycardia, shock, etc.
	• Death may occur

ii. *Alkalinization of the urine* to enhance the elimination of formic acid.

iii. *Treatment of metabolic acidosis by sodium bicarbonate.* A large amount of sodium bicarbonate may be needed. If blood pH is <7.2 or serum HCO_3^- is <15 mmol/L then I.V. $NaHCO_3$ is given after calculation as follows:
HCO_3^- = Body weight (kg) × 0.4 × (difference between desired and measured bicarbonate level).

One half of the calculated deficit should be replaced within 4 hours for which 10–15 ampoules of 10 ml 7.5% $NaHCO_3$ are added to 1 litre glucose bottle and infused. Once the pH is >7.2 or serum HCO_3^- level is >18 mmol/L, no further bicarbonate administration is needed and patient is observed and monitored.

iv. *To correct volume deficit* by administration of fluids and parenteral nutrition supplementation with 10 to 25% dextrose to be given through a large vein via a cannula.

v. *Control of seizures* by I.V. diazepam (5–10 mg doses slowly at a rate of 1–2 mg/mm) or I.V. phenytoin infusion in normal saline starting with a loading dose (18–20 mg/kg) followed by a maintenance dose of 100 mg 8 hourly.

2. Specific measures

i. *Saturation of enzyme alcohol dehydrogenase by administration of ethanol:* Ethanol has stronger affinity for this enzyme and saturation of this enzyme by ethanol will prevent metabolism of methanol to toxic formaldehyde and formic acid metabolites.
The indications of ethanol are:
   • When methanol measurement cannot be done but there is strong history and symptomatology to suggest the poisoning and osmolal gap is >5mOsm/L.
   • Presence of metabolic acidosis and osmolal gap is 5–10 mOsm/L.
   • Serum methanol level >20 mg/dl. The dose of ethanol to be given to achieve its desired level of 100 mg/dl are depicted in Box 2. It is given in a loading dose followed by maintenance dose. Therapy should'continue till methanol levels fall below 10 mg/dl and all signs of toxicity disappear.

ii. *Supplement thiamine and folate:* Large doses of intravenous folate (50 mg or 1 mg/kg after every 4 hours) and thiamine 100 mg qid should be given. They enhance the metabolism of formic acid to CO_2 and H_2O.

iii. *Haemodialysis:* It enhances the elimination of methanol and formic acid. Its indications are:
   • Serum methanol levels >50 mg/dl (15 mmol/L).
   • Suspected methanol poisoning with significant metabolic acidosis or osmolal gap >10 mOsrn/L.

Box 2 Dosage of ethanol in methanol poisoning

Dose	Intravenous		Oral
	5%	10%	50%
Loading	15 ml/kg	7.5 ml/kg	1.5 ml/kg
Maintenance	2–3 (ml/kg/hr)	1 to 1.5 (ml/kg/hr)	0.2–0.3 (ml/kg/hr)
During dialysis	3–5 (ml/kg/hr)	1.5 to 2 (ml/kg/hr)	0.3 to 0.5 (ml/kg/hr)

Box 3 Summary of methanol poisoning treatment

Parameter	Supportive treatment	Ethanol therapy	Haemodialysis
Osmolal gap	<5 mmol/L	5–10 mmol/L	>10 mOsm/L
Methanol level	<20 mg/dl	>20 mg/dl	>50 mg/dl

- When clinical and metabolic abnormalities are resistant to preceding treatment.

iv. *A newer agent: 4-methylpyrazole (fomepizole)* inhibits the enzyme alcohol dehydrogenase and thus prevents metabolism of methanol to its toxic metabolites. It is given as 10 mg/kg I.V. infusion over 1 hour before dialysis and repeated once or twice at 12 hours intervals. During dialysis, a dose of 1.5 mg/kg/hour is given. In fact, it is proposed as an alternative to ethanol as an initial therapy.

Treatment of methanol poisoning is summarised in Box 3.

ETHYLENE GLYCOL POISONING

Ethylene glycol is the major constituent in most anti-freeze compounds . The toxicity is due to its metabolism to highly toxic organic acids, i.e. glycolic and oxalic acids. Diethylene glycol is nephrotoxic solvent that has been improperly substituted for glycerine in various liquid medications (cough syrup, teething medicine, acetaminophen) causing deaths.

Clinical Features

These are more or less similar to methanol poisoning, i.e. confusion, severe anion gap, metabolic acidosis, tachypnoea, convulsions and coma. As it is nephrotoxic, hence, produces oxalate crystalluria and acute renal failure.

Treatment

- Nasogastric aspiration and activated charcoal to remove the poison.
- Correction of fluid deficit by I.V. fluids.
- **Treatment of metabolic acidosis** (saline or osmotic diuresis, thiamine and pyridoxine supplementation, and fomepizole) similar to methanol poisoning. Dialysis can be used in severe acidosis (pH <7.3 or osmolar gap exceeds 20 mOsm/kg).

Both ethyl alcohol and fomepizole compete for alcohol dehydrogenase with ethylene glycol. Both fomepizole and ethyl alcohol reduce the toxicity, hence ethanol I.V. should be infused to achieve blood level of 22 mmol/L (100 mg/dl) followed by infusion of fomepizole.

Carbon Monoxide Poisoning

CARBON MONOXIDE POISONING

Carbon monoxide, a colourless, odourless and tasteless gas, is produced on combustion of any fuel gas in the absence of adequate oxygen and ventilation and may lead to domestic carbon monoxide poisoning. The most common source of carbon monoxide poisoning is smoke inhalation (Fig. 81.1). Accidental poisoning include heating systems in rooms that are not properly ventilated (e.g. gas, wood, kerosene heaters and stoves and brick ovens), industrial exposure, and exhaust fumes of petrol engine. The poisoning is mostly accidental exposure but can also be suicidal. The motor vehicle is the most common cause of intentional poisoning.

Mechanism of Toxicity

Carbon monoxide readily combines with haemoglobin (has an affinity of 200–250 times than that of oxygen) to form carboxyhaemoglobin, prevents the formation of oxyhaemoglobin, thus, leads to decrease in oxygen carrying capacity of blood. It also shifts the oxygen dissociation curve to the left, further reducing the oxygen delivery to the tissues.

Carbon monoxide acts as a cellular poison, competes with oxygen for other haematoproteins such as myoglobin, and enzymes (peroxidases, catalases and cytochromes). In the initial stage, it is transported to the tissues via plasma, and not via haemoglobin. Therefore, blood carboxyhaemoglobin levels may be normal in early stages of poisoning.

Clinical Features

The clinical features of carbon monoxide poisoning are due to formation of carboxyhaemoglobin, the formation of which depends on the concentration, duration of exposure and activity of the person at the time of exposure. The clinical features depending on the level of toxicity are given in Box 1.

The subacute manifestations occurring within a few days of exposure include peripheral neuropathies, skin lesions (bullae, purpura), muscle necrosis (rhabdomyolysis, myoglobinuria) and renal damage (albuminuria, glycosuria).

Delayed manifestations which occur after 7–10 days of poisoning include headache, nausea, vomiting, aphasia, disorientation, gait abnormalities and incontinence.

Levels of carboxyhaemoglobin are not reliable indicators of severity of poisoning, therefore, mild, moderate and severe intoxication given in Box 1 are rough estimates of the levels.

Diagnosis

Carbon-monoxide poisoning should be suspected in any person with severe headache or acutely altered sensorium, especially

457

Box 1	Symptoms and signs of carbon monoxide poisoning	
Severity	*Carboxy-haemoglobin*	*Symptoms and signs*
Mild	<25%	• Cherry-red or pink colour of skin • Dyspnoea on exertion, tachypnoea • Headache, lack of concentration, psychomotor retardation, fatigue, vertigo • Nausea, vomiting, abdominal pain • Visual disturbances • Angina may be precipitated in patients with coronary artery disease
Moderate	25–50%	• In addition to above, there may be confusion, seizures, collapse and cerebral oedema
Severe	>50%	• Hypotension, slowing of pulse rate, respiratory depression, pulmonary oedema, coma • ECG abnormalities (ST-T changes, atrial fibrillation, ventricular ectopics and conduction defects). Angina may develop
Very severe	>70%	• Rapidly fatal

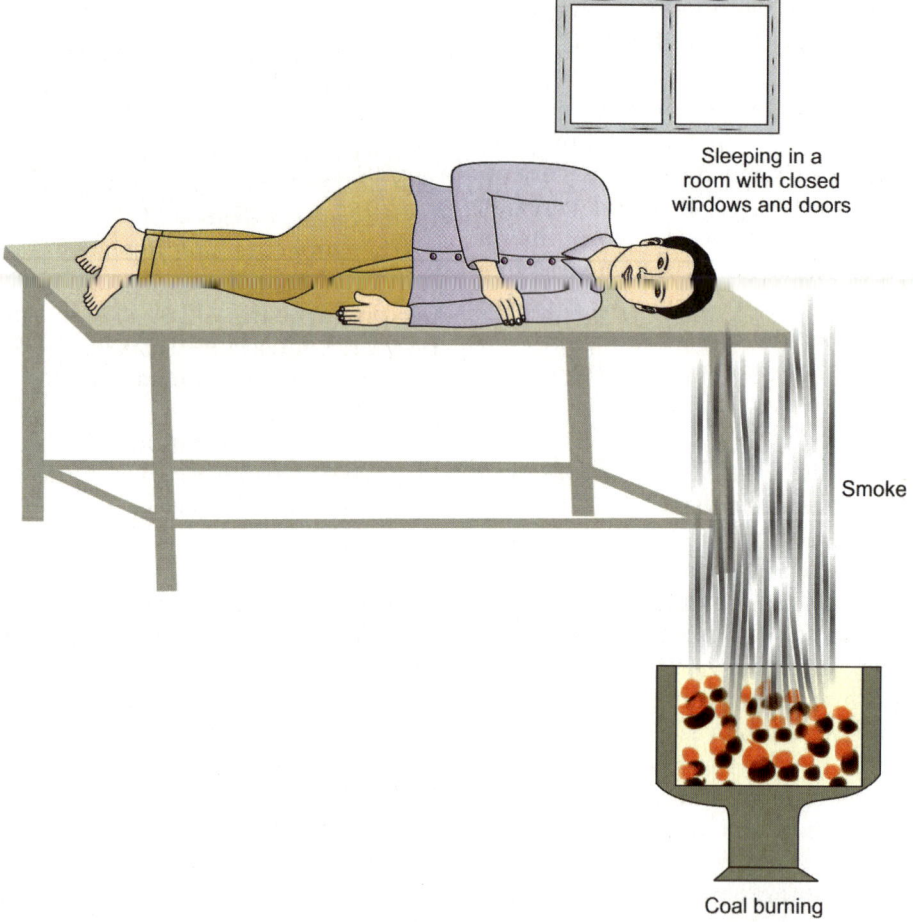

Sleeping in a room with closed windows and doors

Smoke

Coal burning

Fig. 81.1: Carbon monoxide poisoning

during cold weather, when improperly vented heating system may have been used. Diagnosis depends on specific measurement of arterial or venous carboxyhemoglobin saturation.

Investigations

- Raised arterial or venous carboxyhaemoglobin saturation on blood gas analysis.
- Metabolic acidosis on blood gas analysis.
- Partial pressure of O_2 and calculated oxygen saturation by pulse oximeter may be normal as it cannot distinguish oxyhaemoglobin from carboxyhaemoglobin. Actual oxygen saturation is decreased.

Now-a-days a newer pulse oximetry device, i.e. the pulse co-oximeter is capable of distinguishing oxyhaemoglobin from carboxy haemoglobin.

Management

The main steps in the management of carbon monoxide poisoning are:

1. **Supplement oxygen:** The patient should be removed immediately from the source of exposure and 100% oxygen be administered by tight fitting high flow reservior face mask or endotracheal intubation. The half-life of carboxyhaemoglobin is 5 hours at room air which can be reduced to half by supplemental 100% O_2. Patients with mild symptoms require O_2 for just 4–6 hours to bring the carboxyhaemoglobin concentration to less than 5% which is safe.

2. **Ventilatory support:** Endotracheal intubation and mechanical ventilation with 100% oxygen are indicated in patients with coma, significant CNS dysfunction or cardiovascular instability.

3. **ECG monitoring for cardiac arrhythmia:** Patients with severe intoxication can develop hypotension, arrhythmias, ischaemic, chestpain and CHF. The arrhythmias and hypotension should be treated appropriately.

4. **Role of hyperbaric oxygen (HBO$_2$) therapy:** The role of hyperbaric oxygen in the treatment of carbon monoxide poisoning is controversial but most of studies support its use. It is indicated in patients with coma, syncope and seizures and in patients with less severe symptoms and signs of CNS and CVS dysfunction that do not resolve with O_2 and supportive therapy. Hyperbaric oxygen therapy reduces the duration of toxicity by shortening the half life of carboxyhemoglobin and prevents the development of delayed neuropsychiatry sequelae.

Carbon mono-oxide is rapidly eliminated via the lungs on application of HBO$_2$ therapy. The typical course of HBO$_2$ therapy consists of 2–3 compressions to 2–28 ATA for me one and half to 2 hours each session. It is common for the first two compressions to be delivered within 24 hours of the exposure.

Copper Sulphate Poisoning

COPPER SULPHATE POISONING

Copper as a metal is not poisonous but copper salts such as sulphate, carbonate and subacetate are poisonous in large amounts. Out of all salts, copper sulphate is usually encountered in poisoning due to its easy accessibility as *blue vitriol or neela thotha* which is a widely used compound. Accidental cases of poisoning out numbers the suicidal cases but homicidal cases are rare. Copper sulphate is used in leather industry, ink-making industry and white-washing. It is also added to impart a rich green colouration to preserved and tinned peas, vegetables and pickles, but the quantity used is so small to cause any toxic effect and the salt is rapidly converted to a harmless albuminate of copper. It is used in agriculture to control bacterial and fungal diseases and as an algaecide and herbicide. It is also used to kill slugs and snails in irrigation and municipal water treatment system.

Mode of Action

It is available as a dust, wetable powder or liquid concentrate. The lowest toxic ingested dose is 11 mg/kg.

It produces toxicity mainly by generating the free radicals (superoxide radicals) from molecular oxygen which disrupt the cellular membranes. It causes haemolysis by disrupting the RBCs membrane, denatures the haemoglobin and leads to formation of Heinz bodies. Even at low concentration, it interferes with cellular enzymes such as glucose-6 phosphate dehydrogenase, glutathione reductase and catalase (a free radical-scavenger).

Clinical Features (Fig. 82.1)

After ingestion, it diffuses into the mucosal cells and then into blood producing systemic effects. It is largely caustic in nature. The toxicity is largely:

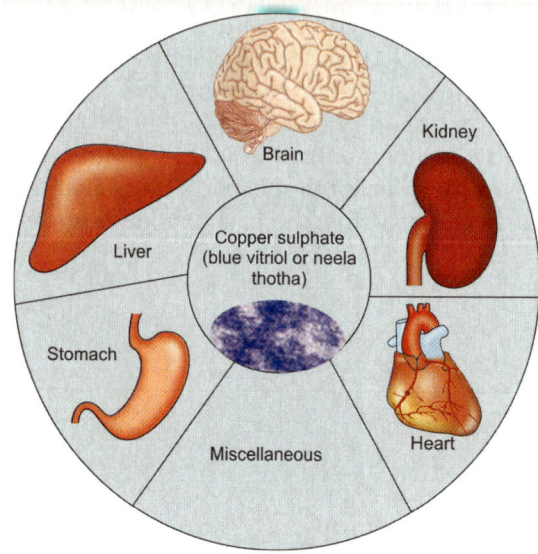

Fig. 82.1: Toxic effects of copper sulphate on various organ systems

1. **Gastrointestinal:** Early symptoms pertain to its local effects on the G.I. tract. It produces burning pain in epigastrium, nausea, thirst, eructations and repeated violent vomiting and metallic taste. Vomiting reduces its toxic effects, but however, it may be retained in the stomach in an depressed consciousness state or in an unconscious victim. Vomitus is blue-green in colour and can be distinguished from bile by adding ammonium hydroxide to the vomitus, which turns deep blue (colour does not change with bile). Diarrhoea (rarely bloody), colic, ulceration and haemorrhagic gastritis can occur.

2. **Liver toxicity:** Jaundice may occur on 2nd to 5th day due to liver injury. Liver biopsy shows centrilobular necrosis with bile stasis.

3. **Renal toxicity:** It occurs on 3rd or 4th day of poisoning, manifests as proteinuria, haematuria (microscopic or macroscopic), oliguria and acute renal failure due to acute tubular necrosis. Diarrhoea, vomiting and dehydration promote renal toxicity.

4. **Neurological:** Manifestations include headache, muscle cramps and convulsions. In some cases, there may be complete paralysis of the limbs followed by drowsiness and coma.

5. **Cardiovascular manifestations:** They include headache, cold sweats, weak pulse, hypotension etc. Acute circulatory collapse develops as a complication due to consumption of a large dose and carries poor prognosis. It commonly occurs in those patients who do not have sufficient vomiting following ingestion leading to profound toxicity.

6. **Skin:** Copper sulphate is readily absorbed through the skin and can produce burning pain, itching and allergic dermatitis.

7. **Eye involvement:** Leads to conjunctivitis and keratitis.

8. **Others:** Diffuse myalgias, rhabdomyolysis, myoglobinuria, acute pancreatitis, acidosis, methemoglobinemia can occur.

Death is due to shock or hepatorenal failure.

Chronic Copper Sulphate Poisoning

It occurs due to chronic exposure to copper sulphate, seen among miners due to inhalation of copper dust or fumes and also seen in welders. It may also occur following consumption of food contaminated with *vedigris* obtained from dirty copper vessels. Repeated ingestion of copper salts produces:

1. Haemolytic anaemia.
2. Metallic taste in mouth, nausea, vomiting, dyspepsia, abdominal pain and sometimes diarrhoea. Green and purple lining of the gums may be seen.
3. Impaired immune response.
4. Hepatic and renal damage.
5. Peripheral neuritis and atrophy of the muscles.
6. Conjunctivitis and corneal ulceration.
7. Skin, hair, urine and sweat become yellow-green.

Investigations

Copper sulphate produces intravascular-haemolysis which is responsible for various complications. There is no correlation between haemolysis and serum copper levels. The various tests performed are:

1. **Blood tests:** There may be anaemia of normocytic normochromic type due to blood loss (haematemesis and malena) and haemolysis. Peripheral blood film may show small, crenated, fragmented RBCs and spherocytes. Reticulocytosis is seen due to haemolysis.

2. **Renal profile:** Urine may show proteinuria, haematuria and haemoglobinuria. Blood urea and serum creatinine levels get elevated in presence of renal failure.

3. **Liver function tests:** Due to intravascular haemolysis, there may be unconjugated hyperbilirubinaemia. The enzymes are normal.

4. Hyperkalaemia may occur.

Box 1	Drugs and dosage of chelating agents in copper sulphate poisoning	
Drugs	Dosage	Side effects
Calcium EDTA	15–25 mg/kg in 250–500 ml of 5% dextrose I.V. over a period of 1–2 hours twice a day for 5 days (Max. dose is 50 mg/kg/day)	Raised intracranial pressure
BAL (dimercaprol)	100 mg 8 hourly intramuscular for 2 days then 150 mg I.M. 12 hourly for 5 days	Nausea, vomiting, febrile reactions. Antihistamines given 30 minutes before the injection reduces these side effects
Penicillamine	2 g/day orally in divided doses for 1 week	Skin rashes, fever, anaemia, agranulocytosis, proteinuria and nephrotic syndrome

Management

1. **General measures**

   i. To remove the poison from the stomach by gastric lavage or nasogastric tube aspiration.

   ii. Stomach wash with 1% potassium ferrocyanide to form cupric ferrocyanide which is nonabsorbable and can be removed.

   iii. Administer white of egg or milk to form albuminate of copper which is insoluble and can be removed.

   iv. Catharsis by giving castor oil to promote excretion of unabsorbed copper sulphate through the intestine.

   v. I.V. fluids to maintain proper hydration. Blood transfusions may be needed for anaemia.

   vi. Symptomatic relief of gastric symptoms by antacids and H_2-antagonists.

2. **Chelating agents:** Calcium EDTA, BAL and D-penicillamine are commonly employed chelating agents given in 5 days courses separated by 2–3 days of rest. The doses and side effects of these drugs are given in Box 1.

3. **Management of complications:**
   - Forced alkaline diuresis (50–100 mEq of $NaHCO_3$ in 100 ml of half saline) is indicated in case of intravascular haemolysis.
   - Circulatory support by adequate fluid replacement to prevent renal failure.
   - Peritoneal/haemodialysis if acute renal failure develops. The evidences also suggest that removal of copper by dialysis is also indicated in the early stages of poisoning when free copper is present in the circulation.
   - To prevent haemolysis, vit. C, E and riboflavin can be given.

Epidemic Dropsy

EPIDEMIC DROPSY

Definition

It is defined as oedema (dropsy) occurring in epidemic form due to consumption of contaminated edible oil (mustard oil) with argemone oil—a toxic ingredient.

It is known to occur in epidemics in India, and recent epidemic of this poisoning has been reported from Delhi and the adjoining areas in 1990.

Mode of Poisoning

It is ingestional. Mustard oil is used as a cooking oil in certain parts of India especially West Bengal from where first epidemic broke. Mustard, sometimes gets contaminated with Mexican poppy (*Argemone mexicana*) seeds (in India, it is known as Sialkanta, Daurdy, Satyanashi, Brahmdandi or Pila datura). Consumption of this contaminated oil (Fig. 83.1A) leads to poisoning called *epidemic dropsy*. The toxic ingredients of argemone oil are *sanguinarine* and *disanguinarine.*

Mechanism of Action

The active ingredients present in argemone oil (sanguinarine and disanguinarine) are vasodilators, cause widespread vasodilatation in the deeper layer of skin, subcutaneous tissue, subperitoneal and subpericardial regions, and capillaries dilatation occurs also in viscera, i.e. ovaries, uterus, liver, intestines and eyes (uvea and iris). There also occurs increased capillary permeability leading to exudation into subcutaneous tissue causing pitting oedema of legs and feet.

The extensive vascular dilatation combined with increased capillary permeability leads to hyperkinetic circulation, high cardiac output failure (collapsing pulse, wide pulse pressure) and progressively oedema. Theft occurs generalised anasarca similar to wet beriberi.

Clinical Features (Fig. 83.1B)

The most characteristic early feature is oedema of the extremities extending upwards and may become generalised. The extremities are warm erythematous and tender on pressure. There may be fever. Nausea, vomiting and abdominal pain are also common, may even precede the onset of oedema and ascites. In addition, there may occur exanthematous eruptions on face, trunk and limbs. Telangiectatic and nodular eruptions may also be observed. Ecchymotic patches and bleeding has also been observed. There are signs of high cardiac output (warm extremities, bounding pulses, wide pulse pressure).

In severe cases, there is development of progressive cardiac failure leading to dyspnoea, tachypnoea, tachycardia and hypotension. The pulse is regular and

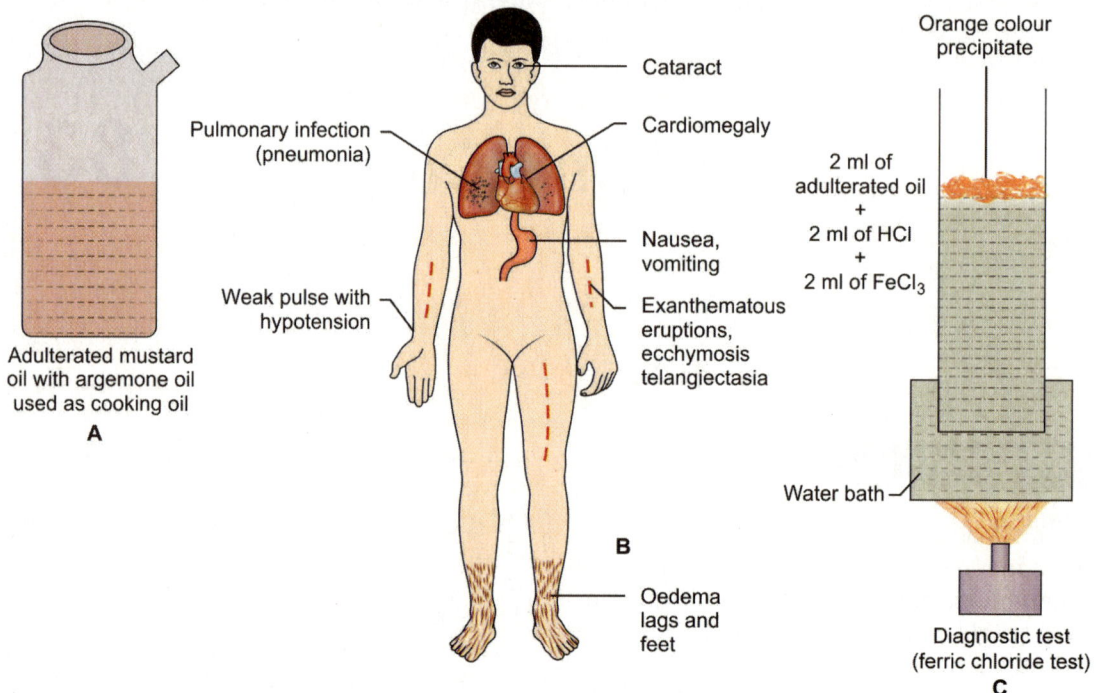

Fig. 83.1: Acute severe argemone oil poisoning—(A) adulterated mustard oil, (B) clinical features and (C) diagnostic test

bounding but in severe cases maybecome irregular and feeble due to arrhythmias. There is cardiomegaly and pericardial effusion may also be seen. There is significant degree of anaemia and patient may develop noncardiogenic pulmonary oedema and pleural effusion. There may corneal oedema and retinal haemorrhages.

Diagnosis

It is based on:
  i. History of consumption of adulterated edible oil.
 ii. History of outbreak. Many persons of a family or a community or in an area may be involved.
iii. Clinical features.
 iv. Detection of argemone oil contamination in edible oil.

Investigations

• Anaemia, leucopenia, thrombocytopenia

• Impairment of renal and hepatic functions
• Hypoalbuminemia is present
• Chest X-ray may reveal pleural effusion, pulmonary oedema and pneumonia
• Pulmonary function tests reveal restrictive lung functions
• Echocardiogram reveals noncardiogenic pulmonary oedema

Tests Used to Detect Argemone Oil

1. **Nitric acid test (Fig. 83.2):** 5 ml of oil is shaken with an equal amount of nitric acid. On standing, the acid layer turns yellow, orange yellow or crimson depending on the amount of argemone oil. It is a sensitive test but not specific because of a high false positive rate, hence, if positive, must be confirmed by other tests.
2. **Ferric chloride test (Fig. 83.1C):** 2 ml of oil and 2 ml of concentrated HCl are mixed and heated in a water bath at 33–35°C for 2 minutes.

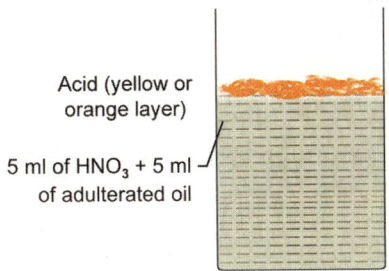

Acid (yellow or orange layer)

5 ml of HNO₃ + 5 ml of adulterated oil

Fig. 83.2: The nitric acid test

Then add 8 ml of ethyl alcohol and mixture is heated in the water bath for 1 minute. Now 2 ml of ferric chloride solution is added and the tube is heated in the bath for further 10 minutes. The appearance of orange-red precipitate indicates presence of argemone oil.

3. **Paper chromatographic method:** It is most sensitive and specific method, can detect even low concentration of argemone oil adulteration up to 0.0001%.

Management

1. Removal or withdrawal of contaminated edible oil from the diet.

2. **Supportive treatment:** To relieve oedema and congestive heart failure if present, diuretics, digitalis, ACE inhibitors and salt and fluid restriction are cornerstones of treatment.

3. The pulmonary oedema (ARDS) may be treated by invasive ventilation.

4. Calcium, Vit. C and Vit. E have been used for restoration of damaged capillaries.

5. Steroids have been sometimes useful in severe cases. For hypotension, inotropic agents may be employed.

Hair Dye Poisoning

Hair dye ingestion is uncommon in West but it is not uncommon in some parts of the world such as East Africa and Indian subcontinent. Hair dyes are either oxidative (permanent) or direct (semi-permanent or temporary) and are metal salts and natural salts. Most of the dyes have two components that are mixed prior to use and generate dye on application of hair by oxidative chemical reaction. The main toxic components of hair dye include, i.e. paraphenylenediamine (PPD), paratoluenediamine (PTD), sodium EDTA, resorcinol and liquid paraffin. PPD is added to hydrogen peroxide and this combination is highly allergic and toxic.

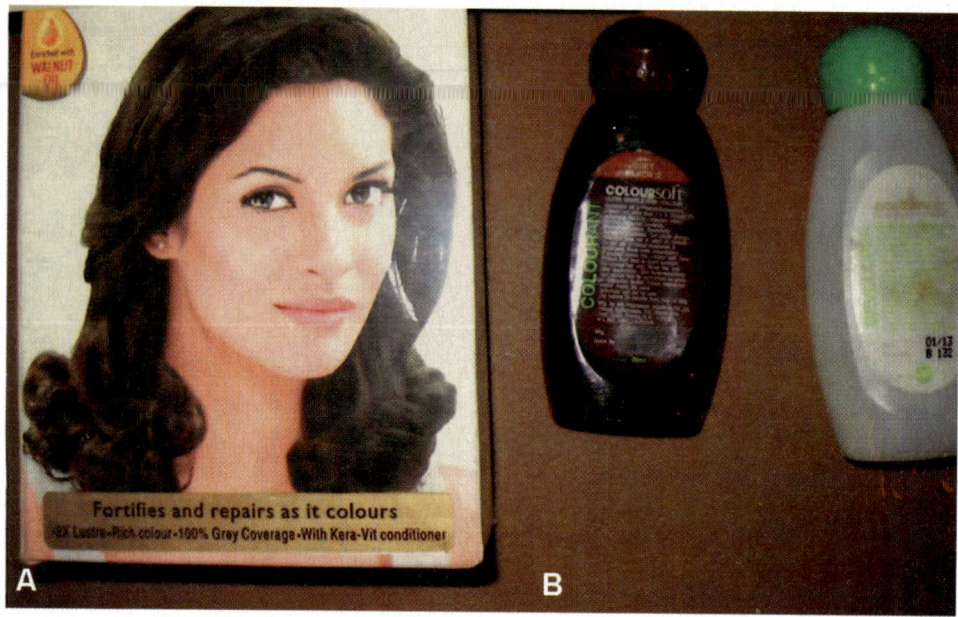

Fig. 84.1: Hair dye poisoning. (A) Use of hair dye by a woman, (B) contents of the hair dye (colourant bottle containing colouring solution the phenylenediamine and resorcinol, etc. and another bottle is a developer containing hydrogen peroxide)

Clinical Features

The poisoning is mainly ingestional for suicidal intent. Symptoms appear within few hours. The main symptoms include angioedema of face, neck, larynx leading to acute breathing problem. There is chocolate brown coloured urine. This is a toxic effect of PPD. This is followed by bone pains and tender muscles due to rhabdomyolysis and acute renal failure which may set in due to hypovolemia and intravascular hemolysis or by direct nephrotoxicity of PPD and may even lead t death. Other effects of PPD are liver failure, altered sensorium, convulsions, GI symptoms, etc.

The other component resorcinol is corrosive, produces methaemoglobinemia and renal toxicity. The sodium EDTA can produce hypocalcaemia and retany.

Investigations

Investigation include complere haemogram, blood urea, serum creatinine, electrolytes (Na⁺, K⁺, Ca⁺⁺, Mg⁺⁺) CPK, ECG and blood methaemoglobin and myoglobinuria for rhabdomyolysis. Liver function rests must be done.

Treatment

- Emergency tracheostomy for laryngeal oedema.
- I.V. fluids, O_2 inhalation, gastric lavage and activated charcoal.
- Antihistaminics and sreroids.
- Calcium and K⁺ replacement if there is hypocalcaemia and hypokalaemia
- Monitor vitals
- Dialysis for renal failure.

Organophosphates (Organophosphorus)

ORGANOPHOSPHATES

Definition

Organophosphorus compounds are widely used as agricultural, industrial and domestic insecticide. The poisoning may occur in isolation or in, epidemics after ingestion of contaminated foodstuffs. Most of these compounds are available either as organophosphates (malathion, parathion, methylparathion, isomalathion, diazinon, dichlorvos, mipafox, tricholorophon and monocrotophos (Fig. 85.1A), etc. or carbamates (carbaryl, matacil, etc.).

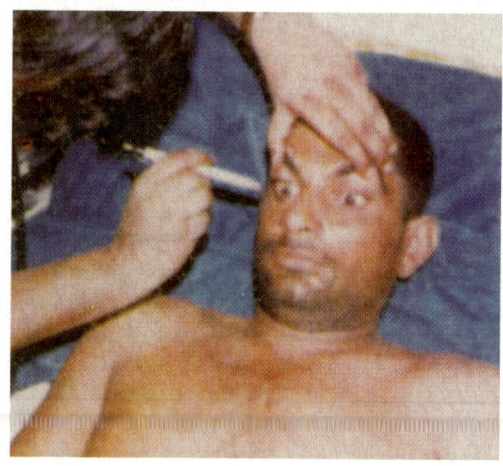

Fig. 85.1B: Looking for the signs of atropinisation during the treatment of OP poisoning. The signs of atropinisation include mid-dilated pupils and clearing of pulmonary secretions (e.g. lungs become dry)

Most chemical warfare 'nerve agents' such as GA (tabun), GB (Sarin), GD (Soman) and VX are organophosphates.

Most of these compounds are poorly water soluble, are available with an aromatic hydrocarbon solvent such as xylene and are used as sprays. The formulations available contain 1–95% of an active ingredient s their toxicity varies widely.

Mode of Action (Fig. 85.2)

Organophosphorus compounds are potent inhibitors of acetylcholinesterase (AChE)

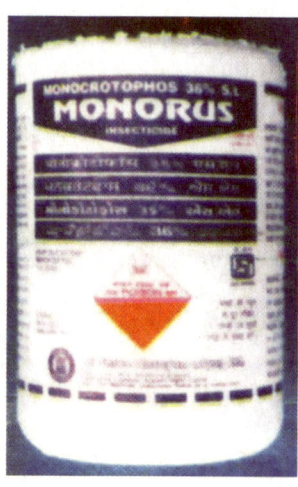

Fig. 85.1A: Monocrotophos—a common OP compound involved in poisoning

and pseudocholinesterase (Pseudo-ChE). In man, true ChE (AChE) is present in CNS and RBC's; while pseudocholinesterase is present in liver, plasma and serum. The inhibition of these enzymes is, due to irreversible binding of phosphate radical of organophosphates to active sites of enzymes. In case of carbamates this binding is reversible. The pharmacological and toxicological effects are due to accumulation of acetylcholine at nicotinic and muscarinic receptors and CNS. The *nicotinic effect* is initial stimulation followed by paralysis of neurotransmission at cholinergic synapses. The cholinergic synapses are present in CNS, somatic nerves, autonomic ganglion, parasympathetic nerve endings and some sympathetic nerve endings like in sweat glands. The *muscarinic effect* is due to cholinergic effect on other systems and glands (Table 85.1).

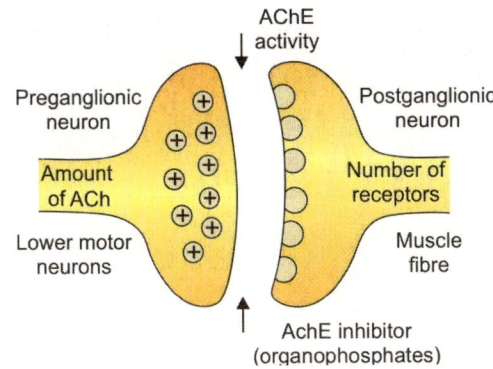

Fig. 85.2: Mechanism of action of AChE (acetyl cholinesterase) and its inhibitor at neuromuscular junction

Absorption, Distribution, Metabolism and Excretion

Organophosphorus insecticides are absorbed through skin, lungs and gastrointestinal tract. The absorption through skin is slow but becomes rapid at high temperature (hot season) or in the presence of dermatitis. It is difficult to remove the poison from skin completely, hence, its absorption is prolonged.

The involvement of CNS shows that these compounds cross the blood brain barrier. Their distribution varies directly with water soluble partition characteristics. The knowledge of their distribution is important and useful for clinical picture and duration of poisoning. After half an hour of absorption, they are accumulated to highest degree in cervical brown fat and salivary glands; to a marked degree in liver, kidneys and adipose tissue; to fairly high degree in gastric and intestinal walls, thyroid, spleen, lungs and to lesser degree in CNS, muscles and bone marrow. After 4 to 5 hours, the concentration in adipose tissue and urine rises. The early relapse of poisoning indicates continued absorption; while late relapse is related to release from storage sites, i.e. fat or adipose tissue.

Metabolism of organophosphorus compounds occurs particularly by oxidation, hydrolysis and by transfer of a portion of the molecule to glutathione. Hydrolysis by the enzymes is the only efficient method of its detoxification in mammals including man. After primary metabolic processes, they are excreted as phosphorus containing residues in the urine and faeces. There is no evidence of incorporation of residues into DNA, hence, no genetic damage occurs.

Clinical Manifestations

Acute organoposphorus poisoning is second common cause of poisoning throughout India. The cases occur after skin exposure (uncommon) during mixing of powder with the solvent or while spraying (Fig. 84.1); after inhalation of fumes or vapours, after ingestion (most common) of compound itself or contaminated foodstuffs. About 70–80% of the poisoning is *accidental* and 20–25% cases are suicidal. The poisoning is more common in agricultural, industrial and domestic workers and chemists. No age is immune to this poisoning. In children it is mostly *accidental* and *homicidal*. The poisoning is more common in men than women (2:1). The severity of poisoning is highly variable. Majority of cases seem to belong to mild to moderate intoxication, hence accounting for low mortality (8–10%). Severe cases of poisoning occur after ingestion or inhalation. The signs and symptoms are due to muscarinic and nicotinic effects (Table 85.1), appear within few minutes to few hours (average 6–8 hours). The critical period is first 24 hours. The effects occur in varied combinations and also vary in time of onset, sequence and duration depending on the chemical, dose, duration and route of exposer. The classification of toxicity is based on clinical symptomatology (Table 85.1) and degree of inhibition of enzyme activity. In mild-to-moderate intoxication, the inhibition of the enzyme is significant to produce muscarinic and nicotinic effects but insignificant to produce respiratory depression, pulmonary oedema or cardiac arrhythmias.

Intermediate Type II Syndrome

These are usually neuropathic syndromes characterized by cranial nerves palsies and weakness of proximal limbs, neck and respiratory muscles. These syndromes usually develop 1–4 days after ingestion of pesticide with severe manifestations. The incidence reported in India is 15%. Recovery occurs within 4–10 days. Death is usually due to respiratory paralysis.

Diagnosis

Diagnosis is based on:
1. History and circumstances leading to exposure.
2. Presence of clinical manifestations (bronchoconstriction, pin-point pupils, fasciculations, etc.).
3. Clinical and therapeutic response to atropine and oximes.
4. Confirmation of diagnosis by measurement of anticholinesterase enzyme in RBC's or plasma pseudocholinesterase enzyme. The enzyme activity is suppressed by 50% below the baseline in severe poisoning.
5. Chemical analysis of body fluids (urine, blood, gastric lavage).

Management

All cases of poisoning should be sent to hospital as quickly as possible. Although symptoms

Table 85.1 Clinical manifestations of acute severe organophosphorus poisoning

Organ/system	Signs and symptoms
A. Muscarinic effects	
• GI tract	Nausea, vomiting, diarrhoea, abdominal colic, involuntary defecation, increased peristalsis
• Salivary glands	Excessive salivation
• Eye (pupils, ciliary body and lacrimal gland)	Lacrimation, blurring of vision, miosis, papilloedema
• Respiratory (bronchial tree)	Bronchorrhoea, breathlessness, crackles, rales, pulmonary oedema, respiratory depression, suffocation
• Heart	Bradycardia, cardiac arrhythmias, cardiac arrest, heart block of varying degree
• Skin (sweat glands)	Hyperhidrosis
• Nose	Rhinorrhoea
• Urinary bladder	Involuntary urination and bed wetting
B. Nicotinic effects	
• Striated muscles	Muscle twitchings, fasciculations, weakness, flaccid paralysis
• Sympathetic ganglion	Pallor, tachycardia, elevation of BP
• CNS manifestations	Giddiness, anxiety, restlessness, emotional lability, insomnia, nightmares, headache, tremors, apathy, withdrawal and depression, difficulty in concentration, drowsiness, confusion, slurred speech, ataxia, absence of reflexes, convulsions, Cheyne-Stokes breathing. Depression of cardiac and respiratory centres leading to fall of blood pressure, dyspnoea and cyanosis. Rarely acute Guillain Barré syndrome reported.

may develop rapidly, delay in onset or steady increase in severity may be seen up to 24 hours after ingestion. The therapy may be graded according to severity of intoxication.

a. **Latent poisoning (serum ChE activity 50–90% of normal value):** There are n clinical manifestations. The diagnosis is based on reduction in serum ChE activity by 10–20%. No treatment is required and observation for few hours is necessary. Prognosis is excellent.

b. **Mild poisoning (serum ChE activity 20–50% of normal value):** Treatment includes atropine 1–2 mg I.V. and pralidoxime (PAM) 1 g I.V. The prognosis is good.

c. **Moderate poisoning (serum ChE activity 10–20% of normal value):** Muscarinic and nicotinic effects are widespread without pulmonary oedema or respiratory paralysis. Atropine in doses of 1–2 mg, I.V. every 20–30 minutes is given till signs and symptoms of poisoning disappear or the signs of atropinization like mid-dilated pupils, clearing of rales and drying of pulmonary secretions appear. Pralidoxime 1 g, I.V. stat is repeated if necessary. The treatment with atropine continues for 2–3 days with same dose but the interval between doses is increased.

d. **Severe poisoning (serum ChE activity less than 10% normal value):** The treatment modalities are as follows:

I. *Steps to remove the unabsorbed poison:* If insufficient amount of poison has been ingested, the unabsorbed poison should be removed and simultaneous steps taken to retard its absorption. The success of these measures depends on time since ingestion and speed of absorption of poison; steps to be taken are:

i. *Evacuation of stomach*
- Do gastric lavage through hyle's tube with lukewarm water or sodium chloride.
- Administer a slurry of activated charcoal (20 to 200 g with water or sorbitol) for adsorption of poison.
- Give magnesium or sodium sulphate to enhance excretion in faeces.

ii. *Prevention of absorption from other sites*
- Wear protective gloves and remove the contaminated clothings.
- Meticulous washing of skin with soap or shampo and water is recommended. Dilute hypochloride solution (e.g. household bleach diluted 1:10) is reported to help break down the organophosphorous and nerve agents on equipment or clothing.
- In the event of inhalation, extensive eye irrigation with water or saline should be given and patient removed to fresh air.

II. *Supportive measures*
- Maintain open airway by oropharyngeal suction, endotracheal tube intubation.
- Maintain respiration by Ambu bag or mechanical means.
- Monitor blood gas analysis and respiratory rate.
- Administer intravenous fluids.
- Monitor pulse, blood pressure, urine output and ECG.
- Give antibiotics if necessary for pulmonary infection after culture and sensitivity.
- If convulsions are not controlled with a tropine and PAM, give diphenyl-hydantoin.
- Sedate with diazepam, 5–10 mg, intramuscular.

III. *Administration of specific antidote*

i. *Intermittent atropine therapy:* Atropine reverses muscarinic effect. Atropine is given in the dose of 2 mg,

I.V. in adults after every 5–10 minutes till parasympathetic manifestations are controlled or early signs of atropinization appear (clearing of rales, drying of pulmonary secretions and mid-dilated pupils) (Fig. 83.1B). Tachycardia and pupillary dilatation are indicators of over atropinization. The maintenance dose is given intermittently as 1–2 mg with increase in the duration between doses; continued for 3–5 days and slowly withdrawn on 6th or 7th day. Sudden withdrawal may produce relapse or exaggeration of signs and symptoms.

Alternatively, atrophine can be given by low dose (0.02–0.08 mg/kg/hr infusion to overcome muscarinic effect, then dose is slowly reduced.

ii. *High dose continuous administration of atropine:* Some studies have shown that high doses of atropine (150 mg in 5% dextrose) drip over a period of 6 hours has been shown to be equally effective as intermittent therapy.

iii. *Glycopyrronium bromide* has been used for muscarinic effects in place of atropine. Its effects are similar to atropine but side effects are less as it does not cross blood–brain barrier.

iv. *Oximes (cholinesterase enzyme reactivators):* Pralidoxime (2–PAM) is a specific antidote that reverses organophosphorus binding to cholinesterase enzyme, therefore, it should be effective at the neuromuscular junction against nicotinic as well as muscarinic effects. It should be given early in the poisoning to prevent permanant binding of OP compound to cholinesterase receptors. However, clinical trials are conflicting regarding the efficacy of PAM.

Administer 1–2 g I.V. as a loading dose followed by a continuous I.V. infusion (200–500 mg/hr titrated to clinical response). Continue PAM infusion as long as there is any evidence of acetylcholine excess. Pralidoxime is not effective in carbamate (Bagyon spray) poisoning as carbamate have transient effect.

Paraquat Poisoning

CHAPTER 86

PARAQUAT POISONING

Paraquat, a herbicide belonging to a bipyridyl group, is used to kill the unwanted weeds. It is available in granular form and as well as water soluble brown odourless liquid (10–20% sol). The poisoning is suicidal and accidental. Common brand names include weedol granules, gamoxon solution and uniquat. Paraquat is a growth regulator, is commonly used on field crops, fruit and nut crops and in gardens in commercial and domestic sectors (Fig. 86.1).

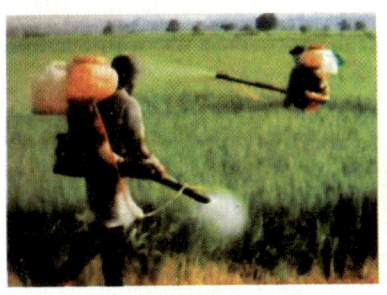 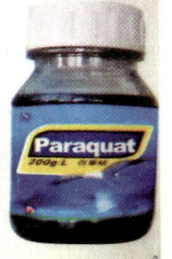

Fig. 86.1: Paraquat and its use

Mode of Action

It produces oxygen reactive species such as *hydrogen peroxide, hydroxyl radicals, superoxide radicals* in the presence of sunlight which disrupts cell membranes. The part of the plant that lies above the ground in sun dies out quickly. The paraquat gets inactivated by adsorption to the soil. Oxygen enhances the toxicity of paraquat and vice versa.

Following ingestion, paraquat is rapidly absorbed from the small intestine. Peak concentration reaches within 1–2 hours and it gets widely distributed throughout the body and gets excreted through the kidneys into urine. Absorption through skin and lungs (inhalation) is negligible.

Clinical Features

The clinical manifestations depend on the dose of paraquat ingested and duration of poisoning (Table 86.1). Higher the dose, higher is the mortality. The lethal dose is 10–15 ml of water soluble compound or 20–40 mg–kg paraquat ion (this is equivalent to 7.5–15 ml of 20% w/w paraquat concentrate).

Management

As poison is most toxic and lethal, hence, early diagnosis and management is mandatory. Treatment is mainly supportive.

Aims of Management

- To maintain circulation and breathing.
- Prevention and treatment of complications and renal failure
- Treatment of secondary infections.

System involved	Symptoms and signs
Table 86.1 Clinical Features of paraquat poisoning	
1. *Gastrointestinal system*	Pain in mouth, corrosions and ulceration of oral mucosa, odynophagia, nausea, vomiting, diarrhoea, pain in abdomen, hematemesis, dysphonia, oesophageal and gastric erosions/ perforation, pancreatitis, jaundice (hepatic necrosis and cholestasis).
2. *Respiratory system*	Cough, expectoration, hemoptysis, pulmonary hemorrhage, pneumothorax and interstitial lung fibrosis and respiratory failure.
3. *Cardiovascular system*	Tachycardia, arrhythmias, cardiogenic shock
4. *Hematopoietic system*	Anaemia, leucocytosis
5. *Central nervous system*	Seizure, cerebral oedema and coma
6. *Renal system*	Azotemia (acute tubular necrosis), acute oliguric and nonoliguric renal failure
7. *Endocrine*	Rarely adrenal insufficiency
8. *Skin and mucous membrane of nose and eyes*	Dermatitis, nail damage (bands/ridges), corneal ulceration, band keratopathy, nasal ulceration.

Supportive Treatment

* Maintain patent airway, endotrocheal intubation and assisted ventilation.
* O_2 therapy to overcome hypoxia should be given. It is administered cautiously only when there is respiratory failure (PaO_2 <50 mmHg). Remember that O_2 therapy potentiates paraquat toxicity.
* **Fluids:** I.V. fluids under CVP monitoring should be given to compensate fluid losses.
* **Relief of local mouth pain** by ice-cold water/ drinks, local anaesthetic spray and lozenges. Analgesic may be given in severe cases.

Specific Treatment

I. **Removal of poison from GI tract:** Decontamination is done by:
  * Gastric lavage should be done only if patient reaches hospital within 1 hour of poisoning
  * Emetics and cathartic are contraindicated.
  * Activated charcoal (50–100 g) is given to adsorb the poisons. Sodium polystyrene is an alternative to activated charcoal.

> **Note:** Pregnant woman should receive same treatment measures as discussed above.

II. **Skin and eye decontamination**
  * Remove the clothing if patient has vomited. Skin should be washed meticulously with soap and water.
  * For eye contact, ocular irrigation must be carried out with plenty of water for 10–15 minutes. For corneal injury, refer the patient to ophthalmologist.

III. **Methods to enhance elimination**
  * Charcoal hemoperfusion is quite effective if done early within 6–8 hours of poisoning.
  * Hemodialysis is effective in enhancing the renal clearance of paraquat in the presence of impaired renal perfusion.
  * Treatment with I.V. N-acetylcysteine and hemodialysis is more effective in severe poisoning.
  * Hemofiltration is also quite effective.

> **Note:** Some other methods such as use off at or recombinant single chain antibody, administration of polyamities, cyclophosphamide to increase egress of paraquat from lungs, administration of antioxidants such as vitamins (E and C), selenium, niacin and N-acetylcysteine, corticosteroids and immunosuppressive agents, inhalation of uitric oxide to minimise lung injury have been tried with variable benefits.

Lung injury can be treated with pulse therapy consisting of cyclophosphamide and methyl prednisolone.

Aluminium and Zinc Phosphide Poisoning

ALUMINIUM PHOSPHIDE POISONING

Definition

Aluminium phosphide (AlP) is an ideal solid fumigant pesticide because of being efficacious, easy to use and low cost. It is available as tablets, (celphos, quickphos, alphose (Fig. 87.1), each weighing 3.0 g liberates 10 g of phosphine gas (PH_3). PH_3 being gaseous in nature diffuses uniformly throughout the stored grains, however, it does not affect the food value of grains. After fumigation, non-toxic residues left in the grains are phosphite and hypophosphite of aluminium. The poisoning involves younger generation and is mostly suicidal, occasionally accidental usually in children and rarely homicidal. It occurs in post-harvest season mostly in rural areas. The important factors for poisoning due to this agent is its easy availability in open market combined with easy accessibility at home especially that of farmers. Recently, cases of poisoning with exposed compound and its combined toxicity with alcohol have been reported. The zinc phosphide is used as rodenticide. It is a 10 g packet containing black coloured powder (Fig. 87.2).

Properties of Phosphine (PH$_3$)

Aluminium phosphide and zinc phosphide liberate toxic phosphine gas upon contact with

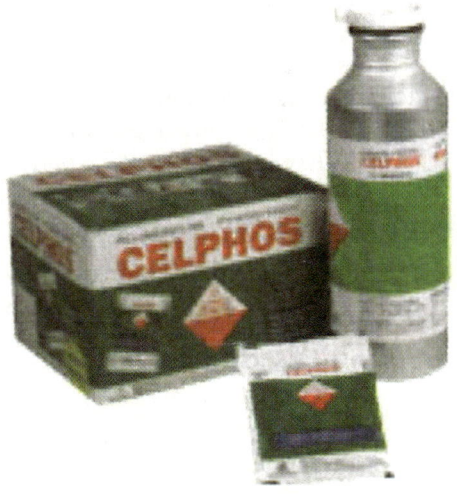

Fig. 87.1 : Available packs of aluminium phosphide

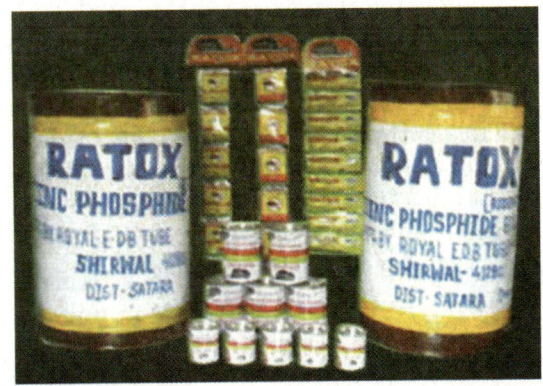

Fig. 87.2: Black-grey powder of zinc phosphide with 10 g packet

water or HCl of stomach, which is responsible for its toxic effects. Each formulation of AlP contains 56% as active ingredient and 44% $(NH_4)_2 CO_3$.

$$AlP + 3H_2O \rightarrow Al(OH)_3 + PH_3$$
$$AlP + 3HCl \rightarrow AlCl_3 + PH_3$$

Absorption, Distribution and Metabolism

Phosphine upon inhalation is freely absorbed by the lungs; the tablet when ingested releases phosphine rapidly which is absorbed through the gastrointestinal tract. A small amount of AlP is absorbed unchanged and deposited in the liver. The release of PH_3 from this unchanged absorbed AlP is slow which explains the extended toxicity of PH_3. After absorption, some phosphine is excreted through lungs and urine. Zinc phosphide is not water soluble but is lipid soluble, hence is slowly absorbed.

Mechanism of Action

Studies carried out on different animals showed non-competitive binding of cytochrome oxidase by phosphine leading to valency change of the heme iron and conformational change of prosthetic group. Later it was found that there is significant inhibition of catalase than cytochrome leading to accumulation of hydrogen peroxide (H_2O_2), an oxyreactive species. Recent experimental studies showed extramitochondrial release of H_2O_2 and liberation of oxygen free radicals. Recently, it has been claimed that inhibition of catalase and induction of superoxide dismutase (SOD) in humans lead to free radicals stress which brings out lipid peroxidation and protein denatuoration of cell membrane leading to hypoxic cell damage. However, the exact mode of action is still unclear.

Acute Poisoning in Humans

AlP poisoning is either inhalational or ingestional while zinc phosphide is only ingestional. The clinical toxicity is more or less the same in both metal phosphide (AlP and Zn_3P_2) poisoning irrespective of the mode of poisoning except slight variation in initial symptoms. The signs and symptoms depend on the dose and severity of poisoning. Nausea and vomiting occur early in zinc phosphide poisoning.

Inhalation Toxicity

Mild exposure to PH_3 produces acute respiratory distress and irritation of mucous membrane. These may be associated with other symptoms such as dizziness, chest discomfort, nausea, vomiting, easy fatigue, headache, etc. More severe toxicity produces ataxia, numbness and paraesthesia, tremors, diplopia, jaundice, muscular weakness, paralysis and muscular incoordination. Severe toxicity is accompanied by shock, cardiac arrhythmia, congestive heart failure, ARDS, pulmonary oedema, convulsions and coma. Acute hepatorenal damage occurs much later. At a level of 400–600 ppm, it is lethal within half an hour.

Ingestional Toxicity

It could be mild or moderate to severe. It is common with both metal phosphides (AlP and Zn).

Mild Ingestional Toxicity

Marked systemic signs and symptoms do not occur except nausea, vomiting, headache, abdominal pain or discomfort. These symptoms are early and more prominent with zinc phosphide poisoning. These usually subside without any treatment except fluid replacement. The prognosis is good.

Moderate to Severe Poisoning

Systemic features appear early, are progressive and mostly fatal. Toxic dose of AlP in humans is 500 mg/70 kg. The time interval between ingestion and death reported is 1–106 hours (average 31 hours). The critical period of poisoning is first 24–36 hours. The systemic manifestations are given in Table 87.1.

Diagnosis

The diagnosis of AlP poisoning is based on (a) history of ingestion of AlP compound, (b) clinical manifestations including shock, (c) foul or decaying fish-like smell and (d) the ECG changes (Fig. 87.3) and metabolic acidosis. The confirmation is done either by qualitative silver nitrate impregnated paper test (Fig. 87.4) or by chemical analysis of blood or gastric fluid for phosphine.

Table 87.1	Systemic manifestations of moderately severe AlP or zinc phosphide poisoning in humans
System affected	*Symptoms and signs*
GI tract	Nausea, vomiting, burning epigastrium, abdominal pain, diarrhoea and excessive thirst
CVS	Hypotension or shock, cardiac arrhythmias, myocardial ischemia, myocarditis, pericarditis, congestive heart failure
Respiratory	Cough, dyspnoea, crackles and rales, type I and II respiratory failure
Hepatobiliary	Jaundice, hepatomegaly, raised transaminases
Renal	Oliguric and nonoliguric renal failure
CNS	Anxiety, fear, apprehension, restlessness, convulsions and terminally coma

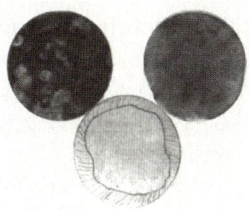

Fig. 87.4: Bedside positive silver nitrate paper test. (A) Positive with gastric lavage, (B) positive with breath and (C) normal control

Investigations

See **Box 1**.

Box 1	Investigations in metal (Al and Zn) phosphide poisoning
Investigation	*Result*
• Serum electrolytes	Serum K^+ and Mg^+ levels low
• Blood urea/creatinine	Normal, raised if ARF develops
• Blood gas analysis	Hypoxaemia, hypocarbia
• Serum HCO_3^- level and pH	Low, metabolic acidosis
• Serum cortisol	Low
• Blood phosphine levels (liquid gas chromatography)	High
• ECG	Changes of myocarditis, arrhythmias
• Echocardiogram	Global hypokinesia
• Chest X-ray	Noncardiogenic pulmonary oedema may be present

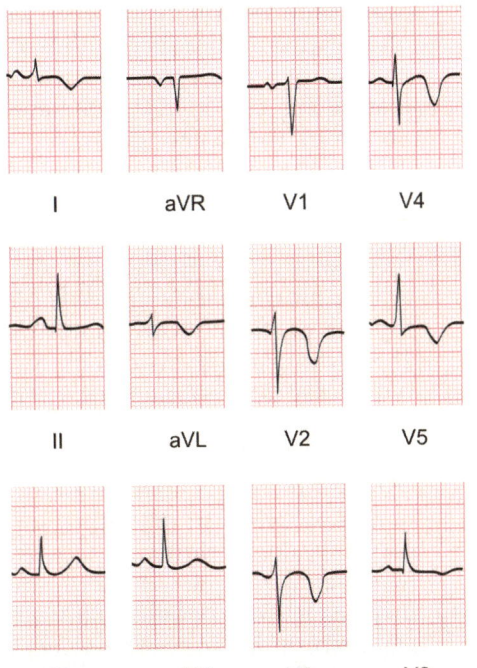

Fig. 87.3: ECG showing toxic myocarditis in a patient who presented with shock

Management

The main aim of management is to sustain life with appropriate resuscitative measures till PH_3 is excreted from body. Hence, early recognition and early institution of therapy are mandatory. The steps to reduce the mortality during first 24 hours include:

1. **To delay absorption of phosphine through GI tract**
   a. Meticulous gastric lavage with $KMnO_4$ (1:1000) to be repeated twice or thrice so as to remove or oxidized unabsorbed poison.
   b. A slurry of activated charcoal (50–100 g) to be given to adsorb PH_3.
   c. Judicious use of antacid orally and H_2–blocker intravenously for symptomatic relief or gastrointestinal manifestations of PH_3.
   d. Medicated liquid paraffin or magnesium sulphate may be given to accelerate its excretion through gut.

II. **Steps to reduce organ toxicity:** In the absence of an antidote and high affinity of PH_3 for enzyme systems, the organ toxicity develops rapidly. Heart is most vulnerable to PH_3 toxicity. Most of the organ toxicity is hypoxic and is due to oxidant injury produced by PH_3. Recently magnesium sulphate has been claimed to be an antioxidant and its use led to significant reduction in the mortality. Magnesium sulphate in addition to an antioxidant effect, is also useful as an antiarrhythmic and antihypoxic agent in this poisoning, hence, acts as a double-edged weapon for protection of the cells in the presence of hypoxia. A dose of Ig of $MgSO_4$ I.V. stat is given followed by Ig every hour for next 3 hours and fmally 1.0–1.5 g after every 4–6 hours for 3–5 days or till final outcome of these patients.

iii. **To enhance PH_3 excretion:** Phosphine is stable and partially water soluble. It is excreted through breath and urine, therefore, adequate hydration and renal perfusion by low dose dopamine 1–3 g/kg/min must be maintained. Diuretics are not useful in the presence of profound shock. However, if blood pressure is stable around 80 mmHg, then frusemide (20 mg I.V.) may be tried.

iv. **Supportive measures**
   a. *Hypoxia:* It is managed by O_2 inhalation, patent airway by endotracheal intubation or assisted ventilation if necessary. Blood gas analysis should be monitored.
   b. *Shock:* Intravenous fluids (4–5 L out of which 50% should be saline) should be given during first 3–6 hours guided by CVP, PCWP and monitoring of electrolytes. Blood pressure should be maintained above 70 mmHg. Low dose dopamine (1–3 g/kg/min) combined with dobutamine (2.5–15 g/kg/min) and intravenous hydrocortisone (200–400 mg after 4–6 hours) have been found effective. Steroids combat shock, reduce dose of dopamine and dobutamine, check the capillary leakage in the lungs (ARDS) and potentiate the responsiveness of shock to catecholamines and restore the low steroid levels.
   c. *Arrhythmias:* Conventional antiarrhythmic drugs such as digoxin, xylocaine are ineffective. Atropine has not been found useful in bradyarrhythmia. Magnesium sulphate has been found effective in both bradyarrhythmias and tachyarrhythmia due to its membrane stabilising effect. Amiodarone has been tried with some success.
   d. *Metabolic acidosis:* Moderate to severe metabolic acidosis is frequent in AlP poisoning. Intravenous sodium bicarbonate 50 mEq may be given if arterial bicarbonate is <15 mM/L, to be repeated to keep bicarbonate around 18–20 mmol. Dialysis can be carried out in case metabolic acidosis persists in haemodynamic stable patients.
   e. *Adult respiratory distress syndrome (ARDS):* 100% O_2 is delivered by face masks or masks fitted with reservoir bag at moderate flow rate of 5–10 L to achieve PaO_2 of 60–70% with lowest inspired fraction of O_2 (FiO_2). Mechanical respiratory support and positive end expiratory pressure (PEEP) therapy are not recommended as patients remain in shocked state.

Zinc Phosphide Poisoning—Diagnosis and Management

Zinc phosphide, a black coloured power, available by different names, e.g. ratol 10 g packet (Fig. 87.2), Fasco filed rat powder, kilrat, mouse con, Rometan, etc. is used as rodenticide. The toxic effects are due to liberation of a toxic phosphine (PH_3) gas. The clinical picture is similar to aluminium phosphide poisoning with following exceptions:

1. It is a fat-soluble not water soluble, remains in the stomach for longer time, hence, local irritative symptoms such as nausea, vomiting, burning in epigastrium are early, more marked and more prolonged.
2. The poisoning is suicidal and ingestional only. The clinical parameters, symptoms and signs, and ECG characteristic observed in a study are depicted in Table 87.2.

It is a lethal poison. Mortality is less than aluminium phosphide because of following factors:

- Not water soluble, hence, absorption is slow.
- Vomiting is early.
- Manifestations are less marked.

The treatment is supportive and symptomatic, is on the same lines as that of aluminium phosphide.

Table 87.2 Clinical features and electrocardiographic changes in 20 patients with zinc phosphide poisoning

1. **Clinical parameters**		
• Mean age (yrs)	26	
• Sex ratio (F:M)	2:1	
• Amount ingested	7.5 g (5–20 g)	
• Mean duration of onset of symptoms (range)	30 minutes (20–40)	
• Interval between ingestion and hospitalisation	4.3 hours (1–8)	
• No. of cases with attempted suicide (%)	13 (65)	
• Accidental intoxication (%)	7(35)	
2. **Symptoms and signs**	**No. of patient**	**%**
• Profuse black-coloured vomitus	20	100
• Restlessness, anxiety	20	100
• Palpitation, sweating	16	80
• Dyspnoea, tachypnoea	15	75
• Metabolic acidosis	12	60
• Shock (unrecordable BP and pulse)	8	40
• Hypotension (SBP<90 mmHg)	3	15
• Pulmonary oedema	2	10
• Hepatomegaly (jaundice)	2	10
3. **ECG changes**		
• SVT or VT or ST segment change (ST↑ or Si↓)	2	10

Organochlorines

ORGANOCHLORINES

With advancement in agriculture production and widespread use of insecticides/pesticides in agriculture sector during the last 3 decades led to acute poisoning with these compounds. Poisoning with these compounds may be occupational (occupational workers) and partly due to their misuse accidentally (Fig. 88.1) or with suicidal intent. These types of mishaps are common in agricultural rural population and are attributed to illiteracy, ignorance, unemployment, mutual disputes and their ready availability in the home.

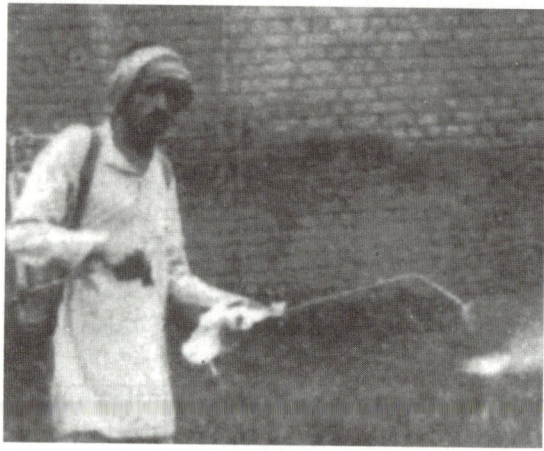

Fig. 88.2: Agriculture worker spraying the compound throughout the day, developed toxicity (mild) by ignoring preventive measures such as gloves were not worn. This patient developed seizures in the evening after 12 hours of exposure. The cause of poisoning was leaking spray nozzle and the plastic container carried on the back resulting in skin exposure

In fact, this is one of the most common poisoning encountered throughout India and other developing countries where agriculture is the main profession.

Classification

The organochlorine compounds are classified into following 4 major groups depending on the biological activity and chemical composition.

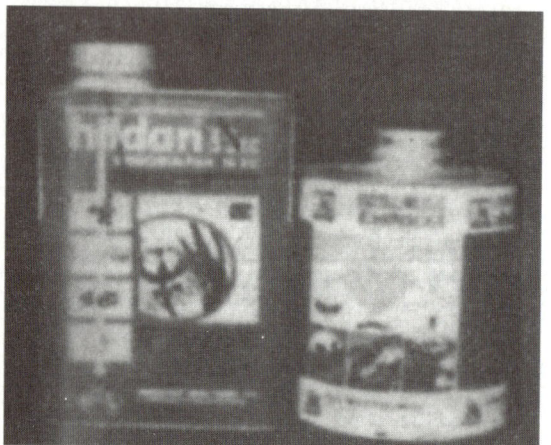

Fig. 88.1: Commonly used agents involved in organochlorine poisoning (endosulfan is available in tins)

1. **Chlorinated ethane derivatives** such as DDT and its analogs methoxychlor, etc.
2. **Hexachlorocyclohexane** such as benzene hexachloride (BHC), lindane.
3. **Cyclodiene derivative** such as chlordane, aldrin, dieldrin, endosulphan (Fig. 88.1) heptachlor.
4. **Chlorinated camphenes** such as toxaphene.

Organochlorines are synthetic compounds that are soluble in lipids and other solvents but not in water. Their main route of entry is through skin (during spray Fig. 88.2), GI tract (following ingestion) and lungs (following inhalations as aerosols). Their toxicity varies considerably and may be modified to a great extent by the toxicity of dissolving agent. The organochlorines are not much used now-a-days, hence, only few compounds are available in the market such as endosulphan and lindane (Fig. 88.1). They are safe and less toxic than organophosphorus compounds.

Mode of Action

The principal site of action is nervous system. They produce initial CNS stimulation followed by depression or paralysis.

Clinical Features

Acute toxicity follows after accidental or suicidal ingestion. Toxic dose is 10 mg/kg body weight. The initial symptoms are gastrointestinal (nausea and vomiting), which occur within 30 minutes to few hours followed by features of CNS stimulation such as hyperexcitability, headache, paraesthesias of lips and face, tremors and touic-clonic seizures. Later, features of CNS depression such as paralysis, coma and respiratory failure may occur in severe cases leading to death.

Chronic toxicity due to repeated prolonged exposure in industrial workers occurs with neurological symptoms such as seizures (endosulphan) have been reported. Liver tumours, neuroblastoma in children and blood dyscrasias have been also reported in workers after prolonged exposure.

Management

There is no specific antidote to this poisoning, hence, management is entirely symptomatic.

1. **Removal of the compound**
   - Repeated skin washings with soap and water to remove the poison from the surface of skin, if it is the route of poisoning.
   - Gastric lavage and induced vomiting: Gastric lavage with 2–4 L of plain water followed by administration of activated charcoal to adsorb the unabsorbed compound.
   - Induced catharsis may rapidly excrete the poison through GI tract.

2. **Supportive treatment**
   - Give respiratory support if there is respiratory failure.
   - Hyperactivity and convulsions may be controlled by diazepam (10 mg I.V. slowly). The dose can be repeated if necessary. Anti-convulsants are usually not needed.

Plant Poisoning (Dhatura, Oleander and Mushrooms

POISONING BY DHATURA AND AND OTHER RELATED PLANTS

Definition

It is poisoning produced by ingestion of fruits or seeds of a poisonous plant, i.e. *D. stramonium* (Jimpson seed), commonly called Dhatura plant (Fig. 89.1). It exists in two forms—white flowered and deep purple flowered plants. All parts of the plant are toxic but seeds and fruits are most toxic.

Other related plants include atropa bella-donna (deadly night-shade) and *Hyoscyamus niger*.

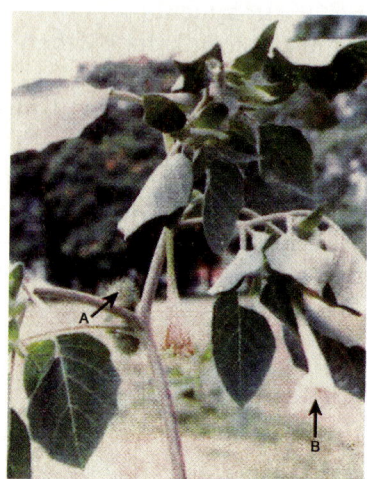

Fig. 89.1: (A) Dhatura plant with fruit, (B) Dhatura flower indicated by arrows

Mechanisms of Toxicity

Ingestion of fruits or seeds of the plants produces toxic effects mainly due to anticho-linergic properties. The active toxins in these plants are atropine and scopolamine, which block the acetylcholine receptors (muscarinic effects) at post-ganglionic synapses of cholin-ergic nerve endings.

Clinical Features

Symptoms of toxicity appear immediately after ingestion usually within half an hour to one hour which persist up to 24 to 48 hours. The clinical features are given in Box 1.

Management

1. **Removal of the poison from GI tract:**
   - Gastric lavage.
   - Activated charcoal administration to adsorb the unabsorbed poison.
2. **Symptomatic treatment:**
   - Urinary catheterization for retention of urine.
   - External cooling for hyperthermia.
   - Benzodiazepines (diazepam) for sedation and control of agitation.
3. **Role of physostigmine:** It is a cholines-terase inhibitor, appears to be useful for severe anticholinergic syndrome (severe poisoning). It may reverse coma, delirium and seizures. Dose is 0.5–1 mg slowly I.V.

Box 1	Clinical features of dhatura poisoning
Organ/System	Symptoms/Signs
Mouth	Dryness of mouth, tongue, mucous membranes and bitter taste.
GI tract	Burning pain in epigastrium, vomiting, difficulty in swallowing, distention and decreased bowel movements (constipation).
CVS	Tachycardia, hypertension initially followed by hypotension.
Urinary	Urinary retention, distended bladder
Eye	Dryness of eyes, red conjunctivae, dilated pupils.
CNS	Delirium, visual hallucinations, ataxia, disorientation, psychosis, extrapyrimidal features. In fatal cases, stupor, convulsions and coma supervene.
Skin	Dry flushed skin, hyperthermia.

over 5 min with ECG monitoring, repeat the dose as needed to a total dose of not more than 2 mg. It has been found to precipitate cholinergic crisis, bradyarrhythmias and asystole, hence cardiac monitoring should be done.

YELLOW OLEANDER POISONING

Poisoning by yellow oleander (*Cerebra thevetia or Thevetia peruviana*) and white or pink oleander (Nervium) has been reported from South India. The kernels of the seeds of these plants are most toxic. The poisoning occurs following ingestion of the seeds or crushed / chewed fruit. These plants contain several glycosides which resemble digitoxin in action. These include peruvoside, ruvoside, thevetin A and B, gerebrin, thevetocin and oleandrin.

Clinical Features

Patient may be asymptomatic even after ingestion of a large number of seads. They occur within 2–3 hours of ingestion. The toxic effects are due to toxic glycosides present in the seeds. The toxicity like digitalis occurs due to inhibition of Na$^+$/K$^+$ ATPase of cell membrane leading to excitability. The systemic effects are given in Box 2.

Management

1. **Gastric lavage and activated charcoal** (50 g is given stat, can be repeated to remove the poison from stomach.
2. **Fluid, electrolyte and acid-base balance:** Fluids should be given to correct dehydration and to prevent renal failure. Hyperkalaemia may require infusion of glucose with insulin. Acidosis may be corrected by sodium bicarbonate.
3. **Monitoring of the patients for cardiac rhythm**
   - Bradycardia and its related arrhythmia may be treated with atropine and transvenous pacing.
   - Lidocaine is effective against ventricular tachy arrhythmias.
4. **Role of digoxin-specific fab-antibody:** It has been employed as 1200 mg single dose intravenously in life-threatening oleander poisoning with encouraging results. It rapidly reverses arrhythmia, bradycardia and hyperkalaemia.

MUSHROOMS POISONING

There are many poisonous mushrooms (*A. phalloides Amanita ocreata, Amanita veera* and Galerina species) that can be confused with edible fungi and may be eaten by mistake. More

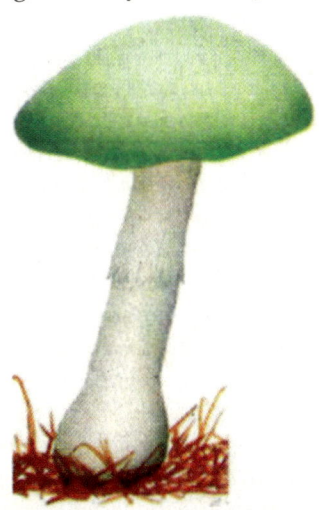

Fig. 89.2: *Amanita phalloides* (death cap-mushroom)

Box 2	Clinical features of yellow oleander poisoning
System affected	**Symptoms and signs**
GI tract	Nausea, vomiting, abdominal pain, diarrhoea, dry mouth
Pupils	Dilatation of pupils
CVS	Bradycardia, hypotension, AV blocks arrhythmias. The ECG shows ST-T changes, prolongation of PR interval, AV dissociation, ventricular ectopics, VT and VF.
Liver	Jaundice
Renal	Renal failure, hyperkalaemia.
Nervous system	Tingling and numbness, restlessness altered sensorium

than 95% of the fatalities due to mushroom ingestion are caused by the ingestion of *Amanita phalloides* (the death-cap mushroom). The mushroom *Amanita phalloides* (Fig. 89.2) contains phallotoxins and amatoxins, which are thermostable toxins, interfere with cell metabolism. *Amanita phalloides* ("death cap") has an olive green cap, white gills and a skirt like ring on the strip. The ingestion of even a portion of one mushroom of a dangerous species may be sufficient to cause death. Cooking the mushroom does not destroy toxin.

Clinical Features

In general, the sooner the symptoms occur, the less serious is the poisoning. There are three stages of the poisoning.

I. Initially nausea, vomiting, abdominal cramps, diarrhoea and profuse sweating appear within 2–3 hours of ingestion.

II. After 12 hours, patient complains of headache, dizziness and severe vomiting. This stage is marked by clinical improvement after volume replacement and lasts for 2–24 hours. During this stage, severe hepatocellular damage (hepatic encephalopathy) and renal damage becomes evident with rising blood urea, creatinine and liver enzymes.

III. The final stage (after 72 hours) is characterised by *acute renal failure* and *massive hepatic necrosis* (*hepatic encephalopathy*) with hypocalcaemia, sepsis and coma.

Monomethyl hydrazine poisoning (Gyromitra and Helvella species) is more common following ingestion of uncooked mushrooms as toxin is water soluble. G.I. symptoms hepatic necrosis convulsions, coma and hemolysis occur after a latent period of 8–12 hours.

Diagnosis

It is made on:
- Clinical history of ingestion.
- Identification of the mushroom, if possible.
- Measurement of amatoxin in blood by radio-immunoassay.

Management

- Gastric lavage may be performed even in the late phases of poisoning because toxins have been demonstrated in duodenal aspirate as long as 36 hours of ingestion. It is claimed to be of not much benefit.
- Activated charcoal may be given to absorb the poison.
- Supportive treatment by I.V. fluids to replace massive fluid loss. The electrolytes, liver enzymes, blood urea, creatinine are to be monitored.
- Thioctic acid, penicillin and silymarin (antidots) inhibit uptake of amatoxin by liver cells, hence, have been associated with reduced mortality.
- The value of thioctic acid—a Krebs' cycle coenzyme is doubtful.
- Interruption of enterohepatic circulation of the amtoxin by the administration of activated charcoal or by cannulation and damage of the bile duct may be of value in removing the toxin based on animal studies and isolated case reports.
- Liver transplant may be the only hope for survival in gravely ill patients.

POISONING BY SEA FOOD

Please read bacterial and toxin-induced food poisoning by fishes.

Snake, Lizard and Spider Bites

SNAKEBITE

Snakebite is a common problem in rural areas throughout the tropics including India. The field workers, i.e. farmers, hunters, rice-pickers are particularly at risk. About 50 species of poisonous snakes are recognised but bites by few snakes are important clinically and create an emergency requiring prompt medical treatment. Poisonous species are given in Box 1 with their identification.

Cobra and kraits are found all over India, the Russell's viper is more prevalent in the south and the saw-scaled viper is commonly found in the North and the West. Most bites are on the limbs because they are used by the person during his/her occupation.

> Common snakes seen in India are vipers (Russell's viper, scaled viper), cobra and the common krait (Fig. 90.1).

Immunological techniques have been developed for species identification of the snakes involved in the bites. An enzyme-linked immunoassay (ELISA) can be used to identify a specific type of snake venom in a victim's blood, wound aspirate, or urine and this method has found place in clinical application throughout the world but is not used still in India.

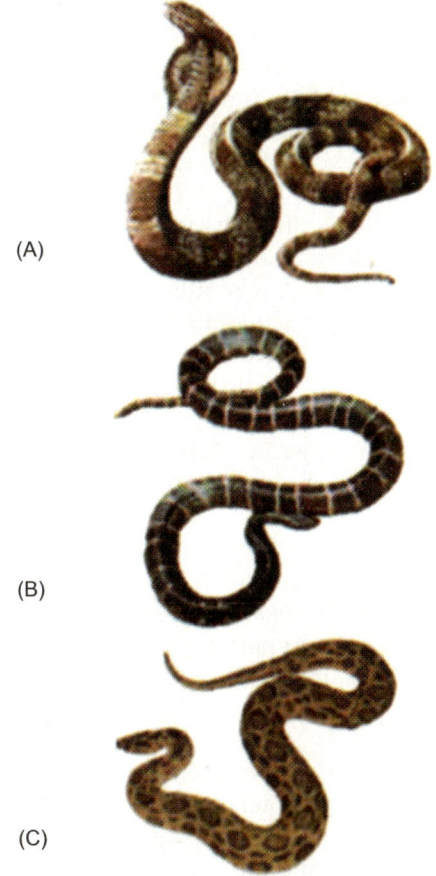

(A)

(B)

(C)

Fig. 90.1: Common poisonous snakes. (A) Indian cobra (*Naja naja*), (B) common krait and (C) Russell's viper

Snake Venoms and their Effects

Snake venom is a complex mixture of several chemical compounds such as enzymes, polypeptides, monoacids, amines, carbohydrate and lipids. They exert their effects in different ways:

- **Elapidae (coral cobra) neurotoxins** produce neuromuscular paralysis by preventing the release of acetylcholine (ACh) or its action either pre or post-synaptically. Death may occur due to respiratory paralysis. Cobra venom is cardiotoxic (induces arrhythmias, AV blocks cardiogenic shock), neurotoxic (ptosis, bulbar palsy, respiratory arrest), hematotoxic (bleeding) and cytotoxic.
- **Viper venom (Russell's viper, European-Adder, bit vipers)** produces cytotoxicity and coagulopathy at several points, Russell's viper venom activates coagulation factors such as factors V, IX, X, XIII, platelets and protein C. This effect causes fibrinolysis, thrombocytopenia and DIC. It also contains a hemorrhaging that renders the vasculature leaky and produces local and systemic bleeding. Various proteolytic enzymes that cause tissue necrosis, also affect the coagulation pathway at various steps or impair organ function; myocardial depressant factors reduce the cardiac output. Saw-scaled vipers activate prothrombin, plasminogen and factor X and produce bleeding.
- **Sea snake venoms** contain neurotoxins and myotoxin which result in muscle necrosis, myoglobinuria, hyperkalaemia and early acute renal failure.

Clinical Features

About one-third of patients bitten by poisonous snake do not exhibit serious envenomation, because the amount of venom injected via a bite is highly variable and maiuly depends on the length of the time since the snake had last bite and its aggression at the time of bite. However, most of the patients present with features of apprehension and fear of intoxication, friends and relatives will frequently bring the snake with the patient for identification.

Local symptoms suggesting an effective bite include:
- Two clear-cut fang marks (Fig. 90.2B).
- Pain and swelling at the site of the bite (Fig. 90.2C).

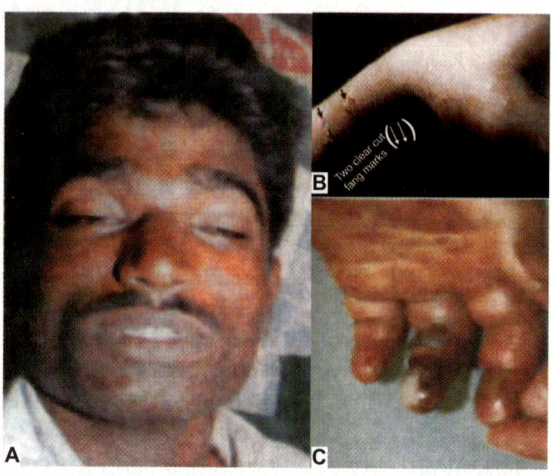

Fig. 90.2: Bite of cobra (*Naja naja*). (A) A patient with bilateral ptosis and ophthalmoplegia. (B) Note the two clear fang marks in upper limb, swelling with local blistering and early signs of impending necrosis of upper limb (lower figure). (C) Local necrosis of fingers in a patient bitten by a snake

Box 1	Common poisonous snakes and their identification
Types of snake	*Identification*
1. *Elapidae* (e.g. coral snake, cobras, Australian snake)	Coral snakes can be identified by red, yellow (or white) and black bands that completely encircle the body.
2. *Crotalidae* (pit vipers, e.g. rattle snake and moccasins)	The heat sensing pits (foveal organs) are present between each eye and nostril. Rattle snakes produce sound by rattling the tail on the ground.
3. *Viperidae* (e.g. Russell's viper, European Adder)	They are characterised by their triangular heads, elliptical pupils, enlarged maxillary tongs and a single scale running over the full width of tail.
4. *Hydrophidae* (e.g. sea snakes)	They occur in coastal areas and bite in the presence of water.
5. *Colubridae* (e.g. mangrove snake)	

- Painful regional lymph node eulargement.
- Nausea, vomiting, headache, faintings and abdominal pain, may be due to over-reaction to the bite or earliest manifestations before envenomation, must be looked with highest degree of suspicion.

The clinical features of various snakebites are given in Table 90.1.

Table 90.1 Clinical features of variouis snakebites

Elapid bite (Cobra and kraits) causative factor-neurotoxin, cardiotoxin, cytotoxin, hematotoxin	Viper bite (Russell's viper; bit vipers), causative factors—hemotoxin and haemorrhagins	Hydrophidae bite (sea snake), causative factors— myotoxin and neurotoxin, hemotoxin

- **Severe local reactions** with pain and blisters formation, and tissue necrosis appear within 1–2 hours
- **Systemic effects:** The venom after absorption stimulates the autonomic nervous system within 20–30 minutes and leads to abdominal colic, sweating, vomiting, bradycardia and hypertension, subsequently neuroparalysis occurs within 6 hours but may be delayed up to 12 hours.
The **symptoms and signs** are divided into preparalytic and paralytic syndromes. In addition, cobra bite produces cardiotoxicity (AV blocks arrhythmias and cardiogenic shock)
1. **Preparalytic syndrome:** It includes vomiting, blurring of vision, drowsiness, heaviness of eyes and paraesthesias around the mouth
2. **Paralytic syndrome:** It manifests with ophthalmoplegia, bilateral ptosis and spreads to involve muscles of palate, pharynx, tongue, jaw to produce dysphagia and limb paresis/paralysis. Finally, respiratorymuscles may be involved producing generalised paralysis. Consciousness is maintained till respiratory depression. The syndrome is reversible either spontaneously or with antivenin over few days
	- **Local swelling, pain and oedema** become obvious within few hours. Painful lymphadenopathy of the drainage area of the bitten part
	- Two clear-cut fang marks are seen
	Systemic effects: These result due to hypofibrinogenaemia, extravasation of blood and consumptive coagulopathy. The symptoms and signs are
	1. Perioral tingling, metallic taste, nausea,vomiting and hypotension
	ii. **Bleeding from the fang marks,** blistering and necrosis become established within 24 hours
	iii. **Bleeding may be obvious from the gums, nose, GI tract, urinaty bladder.** This is due to effect of haemorrhagins and DIC
	iv. Consequently to *bleeding, hypo volaemia, shock* and acute renal failure may develop
	v. *ECG changes and cardiac rhythm disturbances* can occur
	  - In Russell's viper bite neurotoxin(ptosis, bulbar palsy ophthalmoplegia, respiratory paralysis) have been reported from Kerala and Sri Lanka
	  The features may reverse spontaneously or rapidly with specific antivenin therapy
		- **Local tissue reactions** are not seen
		- Soon after bite there is severe *muscle pain,* *tenderness over muscles* followed by paralysis of muscles
		- **Paralytic features** resemble that of elapid bite including respiratory muscle paralysis
		- Myotoxins produce *rhabdomyolysis, myoglobinuria,* and *acute renal failure* supervenes within 6–8 hours

	GRADING OF VIPER BITES (Table 90.2) Clinical features are as discussed above. Local swelling and necrosis are less marked. The preparalytic syndrome is more marked with rapid onset of paralysis	

Investigations

Establish a physiological baseline profile for the following to monitor the progress and to act as a guide to the therapy.

1. **Coagulation profile:** It includes complete haemogram, bleeding time, clotting time, PTTK and fibrinogen degradation products (FDPs). Serial estimations may be done before antivenin therapy and after every 4 hours following antivenin because clotting defect produced by envenomation varies in duration and so is the restoration of the clotting time to normal due to antivenin therapy and resultant clearance of venom from the blood.

2. **Renal profile:** It includes urine examination, blood urea, serum creatinine to detect renal involvement as early as possible and to institute appropriate therapy.

3. **Arterial blood gas analysis:** It is done especially for elapid snakebite to detect impending respiratory failure and to plan the management.

4. **Routine EKG and X-ray chest** may be done to detect arrhythmias and cardiac involvement and / or respiratory infections.

5. **Creatine phosphokinase (CPK)** is greatly elevated in sea snakebite.

6. **ELISA** can be done rapidly and reliably at the bed side to identify a specific type of snake venom in a victim's blood, wound aspirate or urine. Venom levels by ELISA would give an estimate of the venom hours. This method has found clinical application throughout the world but unfortunately is not available in India.

Diagnosis

Diagnosis is based on:

1. **Reliable history of snakebite and identification of the killed snake:** Patients usually give a history of snakebite but this may be lacking in krait bite victims. Although *fang marks* are considered essential for fatal envenomation, but occasionally fatal envenomation can occur *without fang marks*.

The development of severe local reactions with pain, swelling and necrosis is strongly suggestive of envenomation. In India, the killed snake is seldom brought for identification; immunodiagnostic methods are not developed and monovalent antivenom is not available. Hence, the identification of the snake is seldom done enthusiastically.

2. **Clinical features:** These have been discussed according to the snakebite (Table 90.1). Neuroparalytic features with or without local reactions occur due to cobra and kraits, respectively. Viper bites are characterised by local reactions, bleeding and DIC (Fig. 90.3).

3. **Investigations:** They are useful to diagnosis of specific envenomation. Whole blood clotting time is a good bed side test that can be repeated frequently. If blood does not clot for 20 minutes at room temperature, it indicates systemic envenomation by viper bites. CPK is elevated in sea snakebite along with development of acute renal failure. Arterial blood gas analysis can identify the impending respiratory failure. Confirmation of the diagnosis is done by ELISA test for specific envenomation.

Complications

1. Extensive skin necrosis, gangrene, tetanus, secondary infection.
2. Shock, sepsis and organ system failure.
3. Acute adrenal insufficiency due to acute pituitary necrosis. Survivors develop the *Sheehan's syndrome*.
4. Cardiac arrhythmias, heart failure and hypotension
5. Acute renal failure (acute tobular necrosis).
6. Respiratory failure.
7. Abortion in pregnant females.

Management

Aims of Treatment

- To retard the absorption of venom from the site of the bite

- To neutralise the venom as quickly as possible.
- To prevent complications, tetanus, secondary infections.

The management is divided into general and specific measures. General measures are directed against all types of snakebite, while specific are related to the toxicity observed and to the species involved.

Pre-hospital (Field) Management— General Measures

It includes "Do's" and "Don'ts":

A. *"Do's" (to be done)*
   i. All patients with suspected envenomation should be observed for up to 12 hours to rule out dry bite and to confirm envenomation.
   ii. *First Aid:*
      - Reassure the patient. Allay the anxiety and apprehension.
      - Immobilise the bitten area in neutral position by a splint to minimise, pain, bleeding and the venom spread. An absorption delaying compression bandage preferably crepe bandage starting from the bite site extending up to the limbs prevents the lymphatic spread of the venom. Immobilise the limb by splinting during transportation. Avoid unnecessary manipulation of the bitten area.

B. *Important Don'ts (rejected/Controversial Measures)*
   - Avoid manipulation of the bitten area
   - Cruciate incision and suction.
   - Local administration of antisnake venom.
   - Ice packs. It may cause ischaemia and tissue damage, hence, contraindicated.
   - Do not give alcoholic beverage to the victim.
   - Do not apply tourniquet.

Hospital Management

i. Once in the hospital, the victim should be monitored closely for vital signs, i.e. cardiac rhythm, oxygen saturation and urine output while a history is being recorded. A brief and thorough physical examination performed to evaluate presenting symptoms and signs.

ii. **Gather informations** regarding the event, approximate time of the bite, first aid measures, previous episodes of bites and therapy received for that, known allergies and last date of tetanus immunization.

iii. **The level of erythema/swelling in bitten extremity** should be marked and the circumference measured at several locations and 10 cm proximally every 2–4 hours till swelling has stabilised.

iv. **Large-bore intravenous access** in two unaffected extremities should be obtained, or establish a CVP line early since these patients may develop sudden hypotension and may collapse.

v. **Take blood for routine haemogram,** clotting profile (BT, CT, PTTK, FDPs, etc.) and for cross-matching and blood grouping. Perform urgent urinalysis for blood or myoglobin. In severe cases or in the face of significant comorbidity, arterial blood gas analysis, ECG and X-ray chest may also be got done.

vi. **For relief of pain,** use meperidine (pethidine) or any other analgesic. Aspirin should not be used as this may aggravate bleeding.

vii. **Supportive therapy:** Since snake venom contains clostridia, anaerobes and gram-negative organisms, patients should be given a combination of penicillin, metronidazole and aminoglycoside when local infection is very severe.

viii. All patients should receive **tetanus immunoglobin/toxoid since** the wound can act as a portal of entry.

ix. **Care of the bite wound** includes dry sterile dressing, and splinting of the extremity with padding between digits.

x. **All vital signs** (pulse, BP, respiration, urine output, etc.) and laboratory parameters (coagulation profile, arterial blood gas analysis, renal and hepatic functions) should be monitored as hypotension, anaphylactic shock, renal failure and respiratory distress may all develop rapidly without any warning. Patient should be observed for at least 24 hours for signs of systemic envenomation, e.g. difficulty in swallowing and respiration.

Specific Measures
(Anti-Snake Venom—ASV)

The specific management of snakebite envenomation is outlined in Fig. 90.3.

Anti-snake venom is life-saving. Unfortunately monovalent antibodies (Fab antibodies now available in USA) for use and ELISA facility to diagnose specific snake venom are not available in India, therefore, polyvalent anti-snake venom (ASV) is used. Since this is an equine serum, reactions are common. However, the benefits of antivenom are so great that the patients with a severe or progressive local reaction or clinical or biochemical

features of systemic envenomation should receive it as quickly as possible depending on the grading of envenomation of different snakebite (Tables 90.2 and 90.3).

Adrenaline must be made available in the bedside emergency tray to manage anaphylaxis. Antihistamines and hydrocortisone must also be available to take care of immediate allergic reactions. If the patient develops an acute reaction to antivenom, the infusion must be stopped. Administer adrenaline I.M. and antihistamines and steroids intravenously.

The hydrophides bites (sea snakebite) needs up to 1000 ml of monospecific antivenin initially for adequate neutralisation of venom.

Other Measures

1. Wound debridement and aspetic dressing applied to wound once coagulation is restored; vesicle and blebs not to be punctured. If they rupture, debridement with aseptic technique to be done.
2. **Neuroparalytic features** due to elapid bites (cobra bites only) may be treated with anticholinesterases (acetylcholinesterase

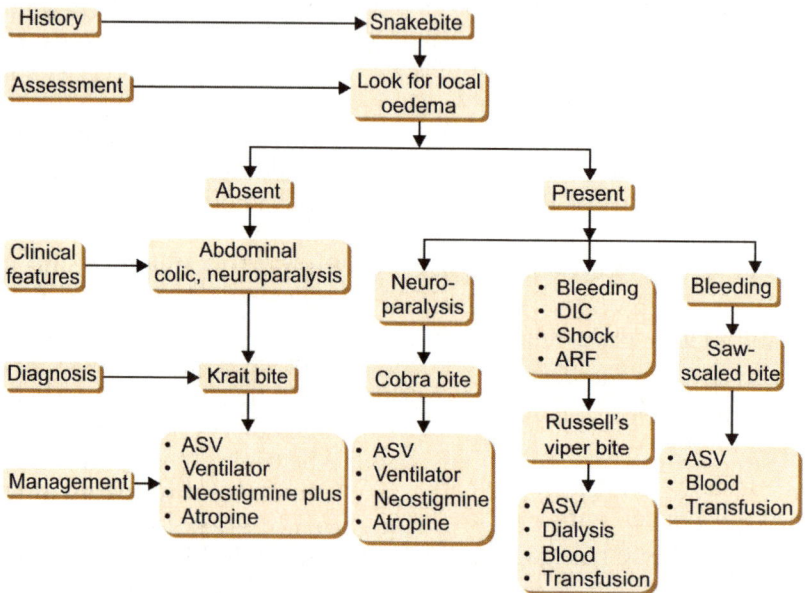

Fig. 90.3: Flowchart for management of venomous snakebite. ASV, anti-snake venom

inhibitors). Edrophonium test positive patients should receive neostigmine 50–100 g/kg every 4–6 hours or 25 g/kg/hour infusion. Atropine sulphate 0.6 mg by infusion I.V. be given intermittently to relieve the side-effects of therapy.

3. **Treatment of hypotension and shockfollowing viper bites (Russell's viper):** Early hypotension is due to pooling of blood in the pulmonary and splanchnic vascular bed, but later haemolysis and loss of intravascular volume contribute to it. Fluid

Table 90.2 Grading of vipers and allied bites and their respective management

Grading of bite	Clinical features	Management with polyvalent ASV
I. Mild	Fang marks plus local swelling, paraesthesias	50 ml (5 vials) of ASV crotalid antivenin infused I.V. in normal saline is insufficient
II. Moderate	Fang marks plus local swelling limited to hands and/or feet. No systemic envenomation	100–150 ml of ASV infused I.V. in 250–500 ml of normal saline over 2 hours
III. Moderately severe	Progression of the swelling beyond the site of the bite. Systemic reactions and laboratory changes present. History of bite by a toxic species or a large snake	150–200 ml of ASV as an infusion in 250–500 ml of saline as described above. Dose, if necessary can be repeated
IV. Severe	Pronounced and rapid progression of swelling, ecchymosis, severe systemic envenomation (signs and symptoms of toxicity plus abnormal laboratory parameters) and history of multiple bites by a large snake and/or highly toxic species	200 ml of ASV as an infusion in the manner described above. Repeated doses are necessary depending on the clotting time which is monitored

Caution: One must be sure of envenomation before antivenin therapy, as a dry bite which does not need treatment is not of uncommon occurrence.

Note:
- Repeat 50 ml doses every 4–6 hours for at least 48–72 hours. Studies have shown that clotting abnormalities may re-appear up to 72 hours after their apparent correction. This is attributed to delayed venom absorption from the site of the bite.
- Lyophilized ASV is polyvalent, hence, is effective against bites of cobra, krait, Russell's viper and saw-scaled viper, lyophilised bowered ASV needs (pre-use reconstitution).
- Heparin worsens coagulopathy, hence, is not recommended.
- The ASV may be administered as long as 10 days to several weeks if signs of envenomation persist.
- Before starting antivenin therapy, enquiry must be made about any history of allergy and an intradermal sensitivity test performed by injecting 0.02 ml of saline diluted antiserum at a site distant from the bite. The injection site is then observed for at least 10 minutes for redness, pruritis or other adverse effects.
- In USA, instead of polyvalent ASV (discontinued production), the antivenom CroFab or Fougera Melvilli NY are current drug of choice for management of pit-vipers envenomation.

Table 90.3 Grading of elapid bites and its management

Grading of bite	Symptoms and signs	Management of ASV
IA.	• No neuroparalytic features • Only local symptoms and signs	**For cobra bite:** An initial high dose (100–150 ml) of ASV is preferred. 100 ml may also be effective. Large doses are required for large snakes
II.	• Ophthalmoplegia and ptosis with or without local symptoms and signs	**For king cobra:** 100 ml of monospecific ASV may be required and should be given early
III.	• Grade II plus palatal, pharyngeal and limb paresis/paralysis	

resuscitation with normal saline or Ringer's lactate should be started immediately. If volume resuscitation fails to improve tissue perfusion, vasopressors (dobutamine, dopamine) may be administered. Intensive hemodynamic monitoring (CVP and/or pulmonary arterial pressures) can be helpful in such cases. Glucocorticosteroids may be useful to reverse adrenal insufficiency leading to shock. Diuretics may be used in case of fluid overload.

4. **Respiratory support:** Repeated pharyngeal suction, intubation and mechanical ventilation are important life-saving measures that should be used energetically. A rise in respiratory rate or fall in single breath count rather than arterial blood gas analysis should be the basis for mechanical ventilation. Where ventilators are not available, Ambu bags bave been successfully employed for several hours.

5. **Renal failure:** Acute renal failure may be one of the gravest complication of viper bite, which is not reversed by ASV. Sea snakebite also produces rabdomyolysis and acute renal failure due to myoglobinuria. Immediate and early treatment of ARF on usual lines with high doses of diuretics (frusemide) and/or dialysis should be instituted.

6. **Bleeding and DIC:** Blood loss, hypovolaemia and DIC should be corrected by fresh blood transfusion, or fresh frozen plasma and volume expansion. These products should only be given after adequate antivenin administration. Heparin should not be used as discussed earlier.

7. **Treatment of compartmental syndromes:** If swelling in the bitten extremity causes subfacial oedema leading to impending tissue perfusion (muscle-compartment syndrome), surgical consultation may be sought to relieve it by possible fasciectomy while anti-snake venom continues. I.V. mannitol may be given to relieve muscle oedema. Compartmental syndromes are, however, rare after snakebites.

8. **Physiotherapy:** It should be started as soon as pain is relieved. This will belp to prevent long term loss of function of an extremity.

9. At discharge, victims of venomous snake-bite should be warned about wound infection and serum sickness. In that eventuality, they should consult doctor.

Prevention

1. **Primary:** Avoidance of contact with a snake by wearing protective knee length foot wear and thick gloves.

2. **Secondary**
   - *Venoms toxoid:* It is being used to immunise farmers in Japan. Elsewhere there has been progress with venoids to protect against the Russell's viper bite.
   - The production and modification of venom antigens by genetic engineering is an exciting new development in invention of snake venom vaccines.

LIZARD BITES

Bites from two venomous species of lizards (the gila monster, *Heloderma suspecturn* and the Mexican beaded lizard, *Heloderma horridurn* are encountered infrequently. The bites usually follow when attempts are made to capture or handle these creatures.

The venom contains proteases, phospholipases which are responsible for systemic effects.

Clinical Features

1. **Local symptoms and signs:** There is local pain, soft tissue oedema at the site of bite due to local venomous effects and mechanical trauma. Broken teeth may be embedded in the wound. Occasionally, local cyanosis and ecchymosis may develop.

2. **Systemic effects:** They include hypotension and shock, weakness, dizziness and diaphoresis.

Investigations

They are done to evaluate the venomous effects and to plan the treatment. These are:

- Complete blood count.
- Coagulation proftle (BT, CT, platelet count, FDPs).
- Electrolytes estimation.
- Blood grouping and cross-matching.
- Urinalysis for renal involvement (blood, myoglobin).
- Electrocardiography (ECG).
- Soft tissue radiography of the bite to identify retained teeth.

Treatment

1. First aid measures for these bites are similar to snakebite (read snakebite poisoning).
2. If the biting lizard is still attached to the victim, it should be detached by mechanical means (opening of its jaws).
3. Local pain is treated by analgesics (opiates).
4. The extremity should be splinted and elevated.
5. Cleansing and irrigation of the wound repeatedly.
6. Tetanus prophylaxis by immunoglobulin toxoid.
7. If soft tissue radiography shows retained teeth, which should be removed by probing under local anaesthesia.
8. **Supportive treatment:** Fluids (intravenous normal saline or Ringer's lactate) should be given for hypotension and shock, blood transfusions be given if bleeding occurs. Pain can be relieved by opiates and regional nerve blocks.

9. Antibiotics have no role.
10. No commercial antivenin exists. Mortality is low with supportive treatment.

SPIDER BITES

The toxin of most of the species, i.e. *black widow spider* and *brown recluse spider* produce only local pain, redness and swelling. In addition, the more venomous black widow spiders (*Latrodectus mactans*) causes muscular pains, muscle spasms and rigidity of limbs. The brown recluse spider (*Loxoscells reclusa*) produces progressive local necrosis and haemolytic reactions.

Management

A. **Treatment of black widow spider bites:**
- Pain can be relieved by parenteral morphine/pethidine or muscle relaxants, e.g. methocarbamol 15 mg/kg.
- For muscle rigidity, calcium gluconate (10%, 0.1–0.2 ml/kg) intravenously may be effective.
- *Antivenin:* Latrodectus antivenin is given after sensitivity testing as it can cause hypersensitivity reactions because of which it is often reserved for very young and elderly people or those who do not respond to above measures.

B. **Treatment of blown recluse spider bite:**
- Relief of pain by analgesic
- Corticosteroids for local oedema.
- Early excision of the bite site to remove necrotic area
- Success has been claimed with dapsone and colchicine treatment. All of these treatments remain of unproved value.

Scorpion, Bees and Wasps Sting

SCORPION STING

Out of 1000 scorpion species known worldwide, only few are toxic to humans. In India, two species *Mesobuthus tamulus* (Indian red scorpion) (Fig. 91.1) and *Palmaneus gravi-manus* (black scorpion) are of medical importance. Most of the cases of scorpion sting by *Mesobuthus tamulus* have been reported from South India.

Farmers, farm workers, labourers, young children are at high risk. They are usually hit or stung while handling debris, paddy husk

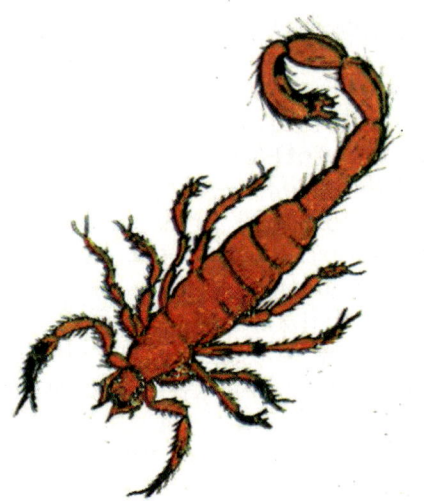

Fig. 91.1: *Mesobuthus tamulus* (Indian red scorpion). Its claws are red-colored. It has a sharp semi-curved stinger

and harvesting grass without using protective measures (shoes) and scorpion stings human beings only when disturbed. Scorpions feed at night and remain hidden during the day in crevices or burrows or underwood, loose bark or logs of wood on the ground. They usually seek cool spots/places under building and often enter houses where they get entry into shoes, clothing or bedding or enter bath-tubs and sinks in search of water.

Venom

Scorpion venom contains neurotoxins (polypeptides) that cause sodium channels to remain open and neurons to fire repetitively. The venom also contains enzymes (hyaluronidase) and serotonin which produce local reactions.

Clinical Features

Clinical effects of envenomation depend on the species of scorpion, the dose of venom injected and the state of venom glands (empty or full) at the time of sting.

1. **Local symptoms and signs:** These occur with stings by less poisonous scorpion or with scorpion with empty venom glands called *telson*. Pain, oedema and sweating appear at the sting site (Fig. 91.2A). The pain may radiate along the involved dermatome and may be severe. The

paraesthesia and hyperparaesthesia or pain may be present, can be accentuated by tapping on the affected area (the tap test). These symptoms may subside within 24 hours without any systemic effects or may soon spread to other locations to produce systemic effects which are described below.

2. **Systemic effects (Fig. 91.2B):** Local effects may be followed by systemic effects due to spread of envenomation to other locations within few hours. Autonomic storm (both sympathetic and parasympathetic stimulation) is the hallmark of poisoning by scorpion sting. It comprises:

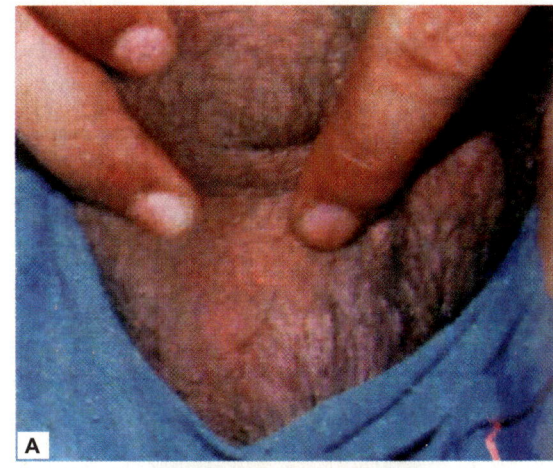

i. *Transient cholinergic parasympathetic manifestations:* These are:
   - Nausea and vomiting.
   - Profuse sweating all over the body.
   - Hypersalivation, lacrimation and rhinorrhoea.
   - Mydriasis (dilatation of pupils).
   - Priapism (painful erection of penis).
   - Bradycardia, hypotension, brady-arrhythmias, ventricular premature beats with bigeminal pattern).
     These manifestations occur within few hours (4–5) and subside within a day or two.

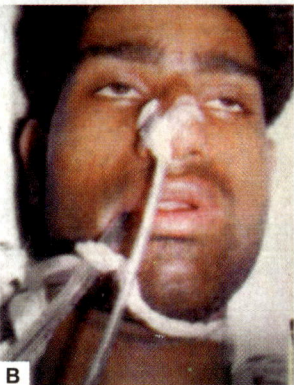

ii. *Transient adrenergic sympathetic manifestations:*
   - Puffy face, propped up eyes, oculo-gyric crisis, parasternal systolic lift, pansystolic or late systolic murmur due to papillary muscle dysfunction due to coronary vasospasm.
   - Cold extremities.
   - Perioral or generalised paraesthesias, muscle twitchings.
   - Patients can have hypertensive crisis (BP 200/140 mmHg) with sinus bradycardia (HR <60/min).
   - Convulsions, transient hemiplegia, bilateral plantar extensor response can occur.
   - At times acute pulmonary oedema (30%).

Fig. 91.2: Scorpion sting. (A) The site of bite is scrotum. Note the red scrotal area. It was tender, (B) the patient developed cholinergic (oculogyric crisis) and adrenergic crisis (blood pressure 180/130 mmHg) within 6 hours of the bite
Note: The patient recovered following treatment

3. **Complications:** Complications include tachycardia, arrhythmias, hypertension, hyperthermia, rhabdomyolysis and acidosis. Fatal respiratory arrest is common among young children and the elderly. Acute pancreatitis with severe pain abdomen has also been reported.

4. **Late features:** Asymptomatic hypotension (BP 70–90 mmHg) with bradycardia with warm extremities are seen in recovered patients (18–36 hours of hospitalization); are due to exhaustion of tissue catecholamines as a result of autonomic crisis, which persist for 3–5 days.

5. **Electrocardiographic manifestations** (Fig. 91.3): Tall tented T-waves, bradycardia, P-R prolongation, coronary sinus rhythm, VPCs in isolation or in runs can be observed.
   - Occasionally, ST segment elevation similar to acute MI may be observed due to vasospasm.
   - Conduction defects, e.g. bundle branch block, fascicular block, complete heart block may appear transiently.
   - Prolonged QTc with broad base, rounded top T waves are seen within 24 hours of poisoning.
6. **Echocardiographic manifestations:** Global hypocontractility, low ejection fraction and decreased systolic performance and mitral regurgitation may be present. There may be abnormal diastolic filling.

Investigations

They may reveal:
- Leucocytosis.
- Raised myocardial injury enzymes (CPK MB).
- Low calcium and high potassium.

- Hyperglycaemia with reduction in serum insulin levels.
- Chest X-ray may show pulmonary oedema (batwing appearance of lung fields)

Management

1. **Pre-hospital or home management**
   - Identification of the offending scorpion aids in planning treatment.
   - Because most victims only experience local pain and discomfort, can be managed at home and asked to report to casualty and emergency department if signs of clinical envenomation, i.e. cranial nerve or neuromuscular dysfunction develop.
   - Keep the patient calm and apply pressure dressings and ice cold packs to the sting site to reduce the absorption of the venom.
   - Pain can be relieved by local measures and by analgesics. Local anaesthesia can be given in case of intolerable pain which can be repeated. Oral diazepam is necessary to relieve anxiety.
2. **Hospital management:** Patient with cranial nerve or neuromuscular manifestations

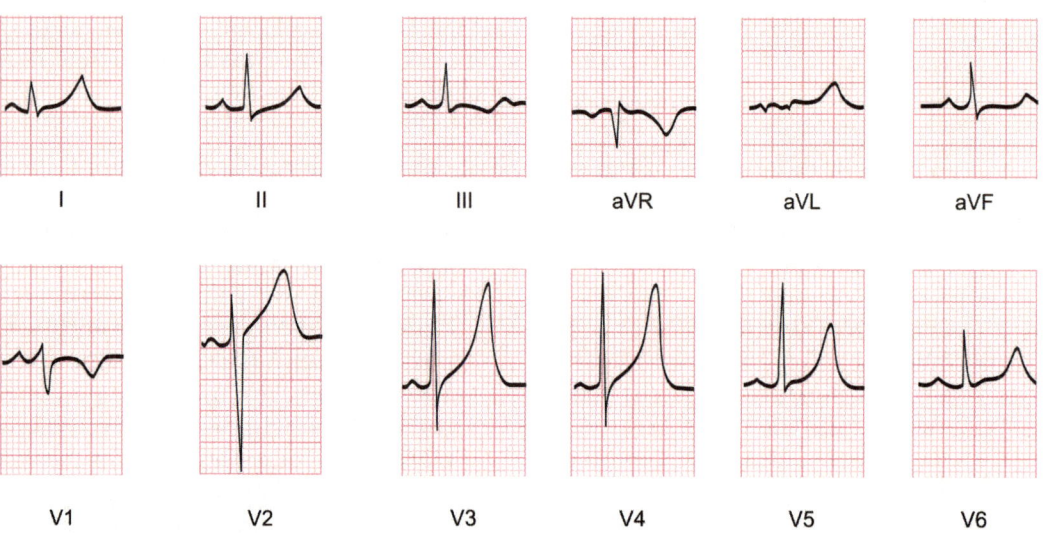

Fig. 91.3: Scorpion sting bite. The ECG recorded from a patient with scorpion bite shows tall tented T waves resembling hyperkalaemia

need immediate hospitalisation and aggressive support care and judicious use of antivenom to reduce mortality.

i. *Correction of dehydration:* Dehydration resulting from vomiting, salivation, diaphoresis should be corrected by continuous oral rehydration solution. This helps to correct initial hypotension and shock. Parenteral crystalloid solutions or nasogastric feeding may be necessary in a confused agitated child. Electrolyte balance must also be corrected with fluid therapy.

ii. *Scorpion antivenom:* Antivenom is available in India. Intravenous antivenom (30–100 ml) rapidly reverses cranial nerve dysfunction and muscular symptoms but does not affect local pain and paraesthesias. However, it does not prevent or protect the victim from development of adrenergic manifestations. Early use of scorpion antivenom combined with prazosin hasten the recovery. No pretesting is required as anaphylaxis with antivenom is rare because of already high level of circulating catecholamines.

iii. *Supportive care:*
   • *Control of restlessness and anxiety:* Although narcotics and sedatives can control restlessness and anxiety, these agents interfere with protective airway reflexes and should not be used in patients with neuromuscular symptoms unless endotracheal tube is inserted. A continuous I.V. infusion of midazolam controls agitation and involuntary movements produced by scorpion stings. A close monitoring for respiratory arrest is needed when this drug is being used in presence of neuromuscular symptoms.
   • *Control of hypertension/hypertensive crisis:* Various drugs like nifedipine, nitroprusside, hydralazine or prazosin have been used with success. Prazosin, a selective alpha-I adrenergic receptor blocker has found wide acceptance due to its pharmacological properties to antagonise the hemodynamic, hormonal and metabolic toxic effects of scorpion venom. Dose is 125–250 g/kg in children and 500 g/kg in adults, to be repeated 3–4 hourly until the signs of improvement appear.
   • *Treatment of cardiac arrhythmia:* Bradycardia or bradyarrhythmias can be controlled with atropine. Runs of VPCs or VPCs with R on T phenomenon and VT respond to intravenous xylocaine and mexiletine. Intravenous amiodarone should be used with caution in patients with myocardial involvement and in presence of pulmonary oedema as it may further precipitate oedema.

3. **Other therapies**
   • DIC, subdural haematoma may be treated with fresh blood transfusions.
   • Noncardiac pulmonary oedema or ARDS is rare with scorpion sting, may require prop up position, I.V. diuretics, oral prazosin. I.V. nitroglycerine, tracheal intubation and oxygen administration.

Prevention

In scorpion-infested areas—shoes, clothing, bedding and towels should be shaken and inspected before being used. Removal of wood, stones, and debris from yards and composites help to remove the biding sites for scorpion. Household spraying of insecticides can deplete their source of food.

BEE AND WASP STINGS

Honeybees and wasps belong to order *hymenoptera,* sting to defend their colonies. Their venoms contain amines, peptides and enzymes that are responsible for local and systemic reactions.

The familiar honeybees *(Apis melliferia)* remain in colonies and attack only when their hives/colonies are disturbed. Honeybee's stings are not uncommon in Africa, America and India. Honeybees usually lose their stinging apparatus and venom sacs during the act of stinging and subsequently die, therefore, their stings are usually not fatal.

Wasps sting in defence of their nests which they build near human dwellings and suspend from plasters onto the walls or caves or shrubbery, or burrow into the wood or soil. As these wasps feed on sugary substances and decaying meal, hence, they are abundant at recreation sites and around the garbage in the month of late summer and fall.

Venom

Their venoms contain:

A. Low molecular weight compounds, e.g. serotonin, bistamine, acetylcholine and kinins.

B. Polypeptide toxins present in venom of honeybees contain, mellitin (damages cell membrane), histamine (from mast cell degranulation), apantine (neurotoxin) and adolapin (anti-inflammatory substance).

C. Enzymes, e.g. hyaluronidase, phospholi-pases which allow spread of the venom.

Clinical Features

1. **Local reactions:** Pain, a wheal and flare, oedema and swelling appear at the site of sting and subside within few hours. Large local reactions spread > 10 cm around the sting site over 24 to 48 hours, are pruritic and produced by hypersensitivity to sting venom. Such reactions recur on subsequent stings. There is no anaphylaxis. Skin tests for type I hypersensitivity are positive.

2. **Systemic reactions:** Multiple stings can lead to diarrhea, vomiting, dyspnoea, hypotension and collapse. Acute renal failure develops due to rhabdomyolysis and haemolysis. Serious reactions produce laryngeal oedema, bronchospasm and shock. Such reactions usually begin within 10 minutes of the sting and can be fatal due to large amount of venom released following 300–500 honeybee stings.

Management

1. **Emergency care:** 'ABC' of patient resuscitation and care take precedent.
   Airway patency is primary concern if any evidence of potential airway obstruction from angioedema manifestated as stridor, pooling of secretion Breathing assessed for rate depth and adequacy of ventilation by pulse oximetry and auscultation. Circulation assessed by B.P. nail bed capillary refill, patients mental status.

2. **Local wound care:** Apply ice to keep area comfortable and reduce swelling.

3. **Urticaria:** Antihistamines mainstay of treatment oral diphenhydramine or hydroxyzine; oral steroid can be added to regimen depending on severity of symptoms.

4. **Bronchospasm:** Nebulisation with beta agonist (albuterol).
   If severity increases epinephrine can be used parenterally.

5. **Hypotension**
   • I.V. fluids
   • Epinephrine (1 mg in 250 ml NS added if condition at 0.5–1 ml/min) not improving.

Sedative and Hypnotic Poisoning
(Benzodiazepine Non-benzodiazepine) and Amphetamines and Cocaine Poisoning

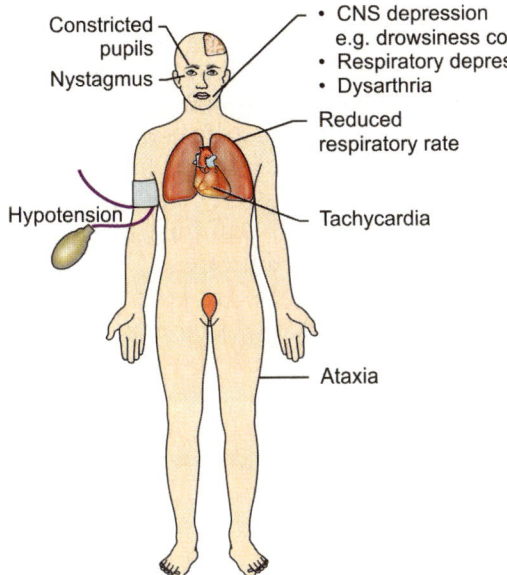

- Constricted pupils
- Nystagmus
- CNS depression e.g. drowsiness coma
- Respiratory depression
- Dysarthria
- Reduced respiratory rate
- Hypotension
- Tachycardia
- Ataxia

Fig. 92.1: Clinical manifestations of benzodiazepine poisoning

SEDATIVE AND HYPNOTIC POISONING

Sedative and hypnotic poisonings include:
- Benzodiazepines.
- Non-benzodiazepines.
- Barbiturates.

Benzodiazepine Poisoning

Benzodiazepines are the commonly used sedatives and anxiolytic drugs in clinical practice. They are consumed in overdoses with suicidal intent.

However, they are comparatively safe drugs even when taken in large doses. Mortality rates are low with this poisoning.

Mode of Action

Benzodiazepines potentiate the inhibitory effects of GABA on CNS neurons by binding to GABA receptors resulting in opening of chloride channels. The drugs included in the group are given in Box 1.

Box 1 Commonly used benzodiazepines		
Long-acting	*Short-acting*	*Ultra-short acting*
• Chlordiazepoxide	• Alprazolam	• Estazolam
• Clonazepam	• Lorazepam	• Midazolam
• Diazepam	• Oxazepam	• Temazepam
• Flurazepam		• Triazolam
• Nitrazepam		
• Prazepam		
• Quazepam		

Clinical Features

All benzodiazepines are well absorbed and exhibit good protein binding (85–99%) and act as weak acids. They are metabolised in the liver and some have pharmacologically active metabolites. Metabolites are generally excreted in the urine along with the small amount of parent compound. Half life varies from 2 hours (short-acting agents) to 8 days (long acting drugs).

The toxic effects (Fig. 92.1) are evident within half an hour of an overdose and include:

- Weakness, hypotonia, hypotension.
- Ataxia, dysarthria.
- Constricted pupils.
- Bradycardia, hypothermia
- Drowsiness, respiratory depression and coma in severe intoxication.
- Paradoxical excitation may occur early in course of poisoning.

Diagnosis

It is based on:

1. Clinical history of intake and suggestive symptoms and signs.
2. Identification of metabolites in urine.
3. A response *to flumazenil* (an antidote) is a more sensitive diagnostic test.

Management

1. *Removal of unabsorbed drug* by repeated gastric lavage and administration of activated charcoal.
2. *Respiratory support:* Supplement oxygen, maintain the patent airway and intubate if there is altered sensorium and/or respiratory depression.
3. *Circulatory support:* Maintain circulation and monitor BP.
4. *Use of an antidote (flumazenil):* Flumazenil, a competitive benzodiazepine-receptor antagonist, can reverse CNS and respiratory depression. It is given in dose of 0.2 mg I.V. over 30 to 60 seconds followed by 0.3 mg at one minute and 0.5 mg at two minutes intervals until the desired effects are achieved or a total dose of 3 to 5 mg has been given. Patients must be monitored for relapse as flumazenil has short duration of action. Should relapse occur, the treatment can be repeated (at intervals of 20 minutes with a maximum dose of 3 mg/hour).

Note: Flumazenil may induce seizures in a patient with pre-existing seizure disorder, benzodiazepine addiction or concomitant tricyclic antidepressant overdose. If seizures occurs, diazepam and benzodiazepine will not be effective. Failure to respond to flumazenil rules out benzodiazepine as the cause of poisoning. Flumazenil should not be used if mixed poisoning or tricyclic antidepressant poisoning is suspected.

Non-benzodiazepine Compound Poisoning

These compounds are taken alone or under the effect of alcohol:

1. **Buspirone:** It is a sedative, has less effect than diazepam. It interacts less with alcohol. Common manifestations of toxicity include drowsiness, dysphoria, hypotension, bradycardia, paraesthesias, seizures, GI upset, dystonic reactions and priapism. Treatment is by gastric lavage, activated charcoal administration and meticulous supportive care.

2. **Zolpidem:** Its effects are potentiated by consumption of alcohol. Common manifestations of toxicity include nausea, vomiting, dizziness amnesia, drowsiness, respiratory and CNS depression. Supportive care, gastric lavage and activated charcoal are mainstay of treatment. Flumazenil has been found effective.

AMPHETAMINE AND COCAINE POISONING

1. **Ecstacy (amphetamines):** Amphetamines or a neural 'designer' amphetamine (MDMA-3, 4 methylenedioxymethamphetamine, ecstasy) and cocaine are euphorigenic and hallucinogenic in their effects. Effects occur within one hour of ingestion or injection or smoking of the drug and last for 4–6 hours following doses up to 150 mg but up to 48 hours after ingestion of doses between 150 and 300 mg. Due to tolerance to these compounds, most users take the large doses.

The clinical features are given in Box 2.

Both amphetamines and cocaine are CNS stimulants and produce euphoria and hallucinations

Box 2   Clinical features of ecstasy and their management

- Tachyarrhythmias, e.g. supraventricular and ventricular tachycardia, hypertension
- Anxiety, tremulousness, agitation
- Perspiration, dehydration, hyponatraemia (dilutional)
- Nausea, muscle pain
- Hyper-reflexia, jaw clinching (trismus), muscular hyperactivity may lead to metabolic acidosis and rhabdomyalysis.
- Dilated pupils, blurred vision and visual hallucinations

Severe intoxication is characterised by convulsions, hypertension, coma and cardiac arrhythmias. A hyperthermic (5 HT like) syndrome may develop, characterised by rigidity, hyper-reflexia and hyperpyrexia leading to hypotension, metabolic acidosis, acute renal failure, DIC, hepatocellular necrosis, ARDS and cardiovascular collapse.

Investigations

- Complete blood count.
- Renal and liver function tests.
- Blood glucose.
- Creatinine kinase (CK).
- ECG
- Blood gas analysis.
- The diagnosis is confirmed by finding amphetamine or cocaine metabolite in urine.

Management

1. Gastric lavage and activated charcoal administrations within one hour of ingestion are useful.
2. Patent airway and assist ventilation if necessary must be secured before attempts are made to remove the poison from the stomach.
3. Intravenous fluids and electrolytes should be given to correct dehydration, hypotension and to prevent acute renal failure.
4. Monitor ECG, blood glucose, blood pressure and temperature. Rapidly lower the temperature by external cooling in patients who are hyperthermic.
5. The complications that are likely to be developed are given in Box 3 with appropriate treatment.

Box 3   Complication of ecstasy and their management

Complications	Management
• Hypertension, hypertensive encephalopathy, infarction/stroke	• Phentolamine (1–5mg I.V). I.V. nitrates or sodium nitroprusside, or labetalol (10–20 mg I.V.). Avoid β-blockers which cause hypertension due to unopposed alpha stimulation
• Supraventricular tachycardia	• I.V. esmolol (25–100 µg/kg/min infusion).
• Amphetamine-induced angina	• I.V. or sublingual nitrates. Avoid β-blockers
• Acute MI	• Avoid thrombolysis because MI is due to vasospasm • Nitrates
• Hyperthermia	• Cool I.V. fluids, cold sponging • Dantrolene • Paralyse and ventilate the patient if above measures fail
• Agitation orpsychosis	• Intravenous diazepam (5–10 mg) or lorazepam (2–3 mg). Avoid phenothiazines and haloperidol as they may precipitate convulsions. Phenobarbitoro I.V. 15 mg/kg may be added for persistent convulsions.
	• Anticonvulsants
• Seizures	• User ailing-bed

Barbiturate Poisoning

BARBITURATE POISONING

Barbiturates were the most frequently used anti-epileptic drugs during seventies, hence,poisoning was common during that period. It has declined remarkably due to introduction of legislation by the Government of India to dispense the drug when prescription in triplicate is produced to the chemist. They are used as a sedative, hypnotic and as an antie-pileptic.

Barbiturates are classified according to their duration of action as follows:

1. **Long-acting (6–12 hours),** e.g. phenobarbi-tone, barbital,pyrimidone.
2. **Intermediate-acting (3–6 hours),** e.g. amlo barbital and butabarbital.
3. **Short-acting (1–3 hours)** e.g. hexabarbital, secobarbital andpentobarbital.
4. **Ultra-short acting (<30 minutes),** e.g. metho-hexital and thiopental.

Clinical Features

The initial features are mainly due to CNS depression followed by features of respiratory depression and hypotension.

1. **CNS depression:** Confusion, lethargy, depressed mental activity, decreased responsiveness to external stimuli, dilated pupils, depressed tendon reflexes and extensor plantar response are seen.

2. **Respiratory depression:** It causes Cheyne Stoke's respiration, apnea, aspiration pneumonia and respiratory acidosis.
3. **Other features** include hypotension, shock, hypothermia, acute renal failure and a characteristic bullous rash seen on pressure points like elbow or malleolus after 2–3 days.

Investigations

A complete haemogram, renal and liver function tests, ECG, X-ray chest are routinely done in the poisoning. Serum barbiturate levels are mandatory to confirm the diagnosis, to judge its severity and to plan the treatment.

Management

1. **To remove the unabsorbed drug** from the stomach by gastric lavage, activated charcoal 50 g every 4 to 6 hours.
2. **To excrete the drug** through stool by catharsis.

Each cycle consists of 1000 ml of dextrose saline +10 ml of KCl and 100 ml of NaHCO$_3$ followed by 1000 ml of 5% dextrose + 10 ml of KCl and 350 ml of mannitol in 60 kg adults. About 3–6 cycles are required depending on the severity. Urine output is to be measured, if it does not match with intake, a bolus dose of 40 mg frusemide may be given I.V. CVP line should be put and fluid balance is maintained.

3. *To enhance urinary excretion by forced alkaline diuresis in cycles.* It is useful for long-acting barbiturate poisoning.

   Complications of forced-alkaline diuresis include circulatory overload, pulmonary oedema, electrolyte disturbance and mannitol, induced acute tubular necrosis.

4. *Removal of drug by extracorporeal means, e.g. peritoneal or haemodialysis.* Haemodialysis is useful in poisoning due to long and short-acting barbiturates and haemoperfusion in short-acting one. The indications are given in Box 1.

5. *Respiratory support:* Maintain a patent airway. Intubate if assisted ventilation is required.

Box 1 Indications of dialysis
1. Deep coma with areflexia, hypotension and respiratory depression.
2. Blood levels, e.g. >9 mg/dl of long acting and >3.5 mg/dl for short-acting barbiturates.
3. Presence of renal failure and pulmonary oedema.

6. *Other measures:* Maintain electrolytes balance, temperature and BP.

Opiate Poisoning

OPIATE POISONING

Opiates

The opiates, i.e. morphine and codeine are derived from the juice of poppy flower—a plant that is grown throughout the world including India (Fig. 94.1). The semisynthetic drugs produced from morphine or thebaine include hydromorphine, heroin (diacetylmorphine) and oxycodone. The synthetic opiates and their cousins include meperidine, propoxyphene, fentanyl, tramadol, methadone and pantazocine.

Acute and Chronic Effects of Opiates

There are three receptors subtypes which influence opiates effects (Table 94.1).

All these opiates decrease CNS activity and sympathetic outflow by acting on opiates receptor in the brain.

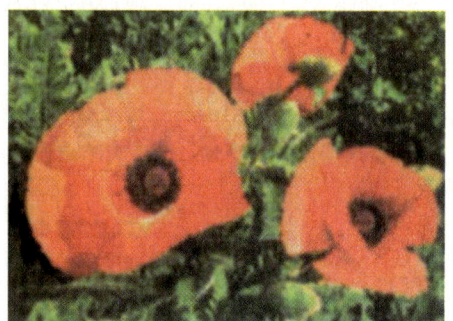

Fig. 94.1: Poppy flower from which opium is obtained

Table 94.1	Opiates receptors and their effects
Receptor	*Effects*
Mu (/L)(e.g. morphine)	1. CNS: Analgesia, euphoria, sedation) decreased pain perception 2. *GI tract:* Nausea, vomiting, appetite suppression, constipation 3. *Respiratory:* Cough suppression and respiratory 4. *Endocrinal:* Decrease in corticotrophin releasing factor, CRF, LH, FSH, TSH and increase in prolactin
Kappa (κ) (e.g. butorphenol)	Decreased dysphoria, decreased gut motility, decreased appetite decreased respiration, psychotic symptoms, analgesia, sedation and diuresis
Delta (δ) (e.g. etorphine)	Hormone changes, decreased appetite, dopamine release

Opiate Toxicity/Poisoning

As opiates are used in medicine as narcotic analgesics, their use disorder can develop in any one. The misuse and dependence can result in following three groups of persons and lead to frequent hospitalisation for overdose.

1. A small number of patients, who consume prescribed opiates for relief of pain, abuse them frequently due to euphoria (sense of well being) and become dependent on them. Once physical dependence develops

then any drop in opiates blood levels can intensify pain and promote continue drug intake. These patients can be treated by avoiding the frequent use of drug, shifting to non-narcotic analgesics, behaviour modification techniques (muscle relaxation and meditation).

2. The **second group** includes doctors and paramedical staff (chemist, pharmacist nurses) who have easy access to opiates, use them initially for sleep or to relieve pain/aches or stress and then escalate doses as tolerance develops. All physicians are advised not to prescribe opiates for themselves or family members or para-medical staff.

3. The **third group** are those persons/politicians who buy illicit drug to get high position in society. Sometimes, opiates are used in "local parlance" and are offered to guests to keep euphoric high during marriage party or in election to woo the voters. This is common practice in Rajasthan (India). In the beginning, they take occasionally, later they derive pleasure from their use, consume them frequently and even escalate the dose to get more pleasure and ultimately become dependent.

Clinical Features

High doses of opiates (oral or I.V.) can result in overdosage or poisoning. This occurs in 50% opiates dependent persons especially with the use of more potent drugs such as fentanyl. Toxic symptoms appear when it is consumed 20 times the required dose. The typical symptoms of intoxication syndrome occur immediately after I.V. overdose. The symptoms and signs include euphoria, depressed respiration (slow and shallow breathing), constriction of pupils (pupils get dilated if brain damage occurs), hypotension, bradycardia, hypothermia and stupor or coma. If not treated immediately then respiratory depression, pulmonary oedema, cardiorespiratory arrest and death can occur.

Methadone has been associated with prolonged QT interval and torsades de pointes. Tramadol, propoxyphene, dextromethorphan and meperidine can cause seizures. The duration of effect of opiate varies from few hours (heroine) to days (methadone).

Treatment

A. Emergency and Supportive Measures

1. Gastric lavage to remove the unabsorbed poison if oral intake is the cause. Activated charcoal 50–100 g may be used.
2. Meticulous use of I.V. fluids to overcome dehydration and hypotension.
3. Inotropic agents are used to raise the BP.
4. Endotracheal intubation and O_2 inhalation mechanical support used if need.
5. Monitor vital signs, e.g. pulse, B.P., respiration and temperature.
6. Care of unconscious patients as usual.

B. Specific Antidote

A narcotic antagonist *naloxone* is given 0.4– 1.2 mg I.V. stat then 1.2–2 mg may be repeated after every 5 minutes till the response (dilated pupils, improved consciousness) occurs or a maximum dose of 10 mg has been used. Remember that the duration of effect of naloxone is only about 2–3 hours, hence, repeated doses may be necessary for patients intoxicated by long acting opiates, i.e. methadone. If there is no response, poisoning due to multiple drugs may be considered. One must remember that opiate dependent individnals do not give up their intake of other drugs which they have been using either concomitantly or have used them during withdrawal. Therefore, the use of alcohol, cocaine and benzodiazepine is not uncommon during opiate poisoning, thus make the poisoning as multiple drug poisoning.

C. Other Measures

1. Treatment of cardiac arrhythmia and convulsions by anti-arrhythmic and anti-convulsant drugs.
2. Prevention and treatment of aspiration pneumonia.
3. Treatment of bacterial endocarditis which develops in I.V. drug abuser due to septic embolization. Stroke can develop.

Emergencies in Internal Medicine

- Systemic Anaphylaxis
- Hyperpyrexia
  (Heatstroke, Heat Exhaustion, Malignant Hyperpyrexia)
- Hypothermia
- High Altilude Related Emergencies
- Electrical and Lightning Injuries
- Drowning and Near Drowning
- Hanging and Strangulation

Systemic Anaphylaxis

Definition

Anaphylaxis is a systemic and life-threatening response of a sensitized human to an antigen, appears immediately within minutes of administration of specific antigen. It is characterized clinically by respiratory distress followed by vascular collapse or shock without antecedent respiratory difficulty. In fact, it is an antigen induced IgE mediated immune reaction, occurs due to a variety of antigens.

Anaphylactoid reaction on the other hand occurs in an unsensitized person and is not IgE-mediated but there is mast cell degranulation. Both anaphylaxis and anaphylactoid reactions produce similar symptoms and signs. Rarely, the life-threatening anaphylactoid reactions may occur during anaesthesia due to muscle relaxants such as alcuronium and pancuronium.

Exercise-induced Anaphylaxis

It is a unique form of allergy in which flushing sensation, a feeling of warmth and urticarial wheals develop in association with vigorous exercise. These symptoms do not occur with passive exercise or warming up.

Predisposing Factors

The patients having history of atopy, allergy and asthma are more prone to develop this reaction. This is due to release of histamine and other mediators (kinins) following the interaction of antigen with antibody (IgE) produced by B lymphocytes and bound to cell membranes of mast cell or circulating basophils leading to their degranulation (Fig. 95.1). The predisposing factors are given in Box 1.

Anaphylaxis may be caused by ingestion, inhalation or parenteral injection of an antigen that sensitizes the predisposed individuals.

Clinical Features

The symptoms and signs vary usually, appear immediately within few seconds to minutes after introduction of the antigen through injection but are late following ingestion and inhalation. These are:

1. **Respiratory manifestations**
    i. *Acute bronchial obstruction:* There may be upper and lower airway obstruction leading to feeling of tightness in the chest with audible wheeze (bronchospasm)
    ii. *Laryngeal oedema:* It is characterized by feeling of a 'lump' in the throat, hoarseness or stridor.
2. **Cutaneous manifestations:** A characteristic feature is urticarial eruptions (well-circumscribed cutaneous wheals with erythematous, raised serpiginous

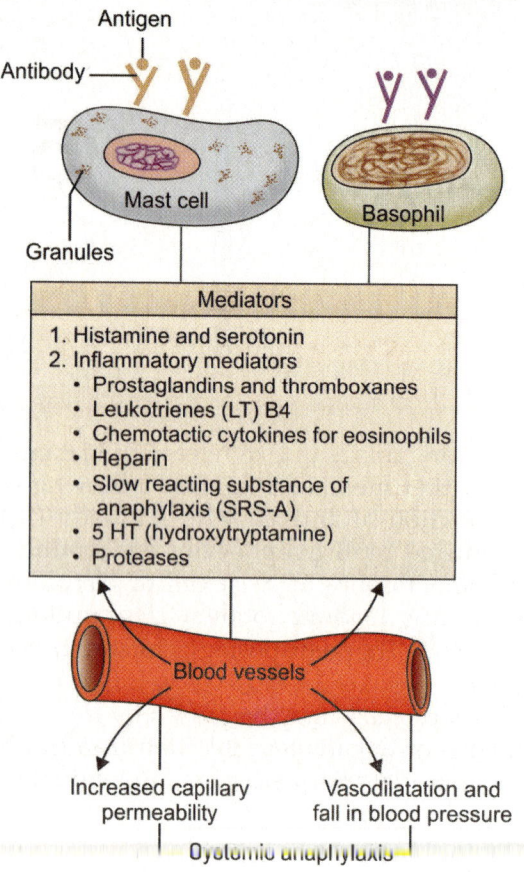

Antigen

Antibody

Mast cell

Basophil

Granules

Mediators

1. Histamine and serotonin
2. Inflammatory mediators
   • Prostaglandins and thromboxanes
   • Leukotrienes (LT) B4
   • Chemotactic cytokines for eosinophils
   • Heparin
   • Slow reacting substance of anaphylaxis (SRS-A)
   • 5 HT (hydroxytryptamine)
   • Proteases

Blood vessels

Increased capillary permeability

Vasodilatation and fall in blood pressure

Systemic anaphylaxis

Fig. 95.1: Pathogenic mechanisms of anaphylaxis

borders and branched centres) which are intensely itchy and may be localized or generalised. They seldom persist beyond 48 hours.

A localized, nonpitting oedema, angioedema may also be present. It may be asymptomatic or may cause burning or tingling sensation.

3. **Cardiovascular manifestations:** Syncope, hypotension and tachycardia may occur before cardiovascular collapse.

4. **Gastrointestinal:** Nausea, vomiting and diarrhea may occur or shock.

The associated ECG abnormalities with or without infarction may be noted in these patients, reflect either a primary cardiac event or can be due to critical reduction in blood volume.

Diagnosis

The diagnosis of anaphylaxis depends on:

i. A reliable accurate history of administration of an antigen followed by acute onset of appropriate symptoms and signs.

ii. Radioimmunoassay for detection of IgE antibodies. These assays require purified antigens.

iii. Elevation of tryptase levels occurs due to mast cell activation, in an adverse systemic reaction, and are particularly informative with episodes of hypotension during general anaesthesia or when there has been a fatal outcome. Elevated tryptase levels have been associated with systemic mastocytosis and anaphylactoid reactions (mast cell degranulation) in addition to anaphylaxis.

Box 1	Predisposing factors for anaphylaxis
1. Drugs	
	• Penicillin, cephalosporins, amphotericin B
	• Local anaesthetics, e.g. procaine, lidocaine
	• Vitamins, e.g. thiamine, folic acid
	• Contrast medium agents
	• Occupational related agent, e.g. ethylene oxide
	• Antisera, dextran, albumin
	• Cyclosporine
	• Opiates
	• NSAIDs and azo dyes
2. Hymenopetra venoms	
	• Hornets, wasp, honeybee, ants
3. Heterologous proteins	
	• Hormones, e.g. insulin, vasopressin, paratharmone
	• Enzymes, e.g. trypsin, chymotrypsin, penicillinase
4. Foods	
	• Eggs, sea food, nuts, grains, beans
5. Pollen extracts	
	• Ragweed, grass, trees
6. Nonpollen extracts	
	• Dust mites, cot dander
7. Idiopathic	
	• Blood transfusion (immune complex mediated), e.g. whole blood, plasma and immunoglobulins.

Management

Early diagnosis and early institution of treatment is mandatory since death may occur within minutes to hours after the first symptom. Ideally ABC of cardiopulmonary resuscitation should be achieved at the earliest in severe cases.

1. **Subcutaneous or intramuscular adrenaline (epineprine):** Adrenaline (0.2 to 0.5 ml of 1: 1000) dil), is given subcutaneously or I.M. with repeat dose at 20 minutes interval. Mild to moderate symptoms can be controlled with single dose. If the patient does not improve with subcutaneous dosing, then 2–5 ml of epinephrine diluted in 1:10,000 may be given I.V. through an intravenous infusion line. In extreme cases or in whom I.V. line is not accessible, then adrenaline can be introduced via endotracheal route. In co-operative patients, nebulised epinephrine is effective.

2. **To retard the absorption of injected antigen:** If an antigenic material has been administered through an injection (insect stinger) into an extremity, its rate of absorption can be reduced by an application of a tourniquet proximal to injection site, administer 0.2 ml of 1: 1000 epinephrine into the site, and remove without compression an insect stinger if insect bite is the cause of reaction.

3. **Intravenous glucagon:** 1 mg of glucagon I.V. over 5 minutes may be useful in epinephrine resistant cases especially patients receiving beta-blockers.

4. **Volume expansion:** Volume expanders such as normal saline or Ringer's solution and vasopressor agents (e.g. dopamine) may restore vascular volume. Increased capillary leakage may require several litres of saline. About 90% patients respond to this therapy.

5. **Respiratory support:** Oxygen via a nasal catheter or IPP breathing of oxygen with 0.5 ml of isoproterenol diluted in 1:200 in saline may be helpful. Either endotracheal intubation or tracheostomy is mandatory for oxygen therapy in severe cases if progressive hypoxia develops.

6. **Other measures:** Parenteral antihistaminics and aminophylline are useful to control allergic symptoms and bronchospasm respectively. Steroids are not effective during an acute event but may alleviate the recurrence of bronchospasm, hypotension, and urticaria. When long term oral steroids and antihistamines are used in combination.

Prevention

1. If there is a definite history of past anaphylaxis with any known agent or procedure, even though mild, it is advisable to select another agent or procedure. A knowledge of cross-reactivity amongst the substances is crucial.

2. **A skin test** must be performed with allergenic extracts or when the nature of the past adverse reaction is unknown. Skin testing is of no value for non-IgE-mediated reactions.

3. One should use special precautions while giving drugs to patients with history of hay fever, asthma and other allergic disorders.

4. Those who are known to be sensitive to insect bite should avoid visit to areas where such insects are likely to be present. Protective garments must be worn if they visit such areas, and they must be trained to inject adrenaline and antihistamine on the first symptom of anaphylactic reaction. Desensitization of such individuals may be necessary.

5. Venom immunotherapy to achieve venom specific IgG titres above 3.0 g/ml in serum is recommended in persons having sting sensitivity. A 5 years treatment induces a state of resistance.

Hyperpyrexia
(Heatstroke, Heat Exhaustion, Malignant Hyperpyrexia)

HYPERPYREXIA

Hyperpyrexia is defined as body temperature of greater than 40°C (106°F) and when it occurs due to exposure to high environmental temperature, then it is called *'heat hyperpyrexia'. Acclimatisation* is an effective protective mechanism against the effects of hot climate. In acclimatised individuals, the concentration of sodium chloride in sweat is very low and this helps in the conservation of sodium chloride in hot climate. In contrast to this, unacclimatised individuals are predisposed to the effects of heat leading to *"heat hyperpyrexia* or *heat syndromes"*.

HEATSTROKE

Definition

It is a catastrophic condition which results from complete breakdown of thermoregulatory mechanism and is characterised by **a triad** consisting of *high grade fever* usually >41°C (>106°F), *absence of sweating* and *disturbance in consciousness*.

> *Absence of sweating is the cardinal feature of heat stroke.*

Predisposing Factors (Box 1)

It occurs in unacclimatised individuals in whom sweating is either absent or minimal.

Box 1   Predisposing factors for heat stroke

- High environmental temperature
- Hot and humid condition/ atmosphere
- Old age
- Debility
- Obesity
- Diabetes
- Alcoholism
- Dehydration or lack of water intake
- Heavy exercise/work
- Associated infection
- CVA

Clinical Features (Fig. 96.1)

Exertional heat stroke occurs in unacclimatized young persons particularly athletes, soldiers or labourers who perform strenuous work/ task in hot and humid climate, while classical or nonexertional heat stroke occurs among elderly, debilitated persons often in epidemic fashion during heat waves of hot season. The elderly bedridden, persons taking anticholinergics or anti-Parkinsonian drugs or diuretics are most susceptible.

All the body tissues are susceptible to heat injury. High temperature >41°C raises the BMR exuberantly and results in enzyme denaturation, protein coagulation and lipid liquefaction. The systems involved are cardiovascular, CNS, renal and hepatic.

1. **Neurological manifestations:** Altered mental status, seizures, confusion, disorientation, stupor and coma may occur. Some patients who develop severe neurological features and survive may be left with permanent neurological complications, i.e.

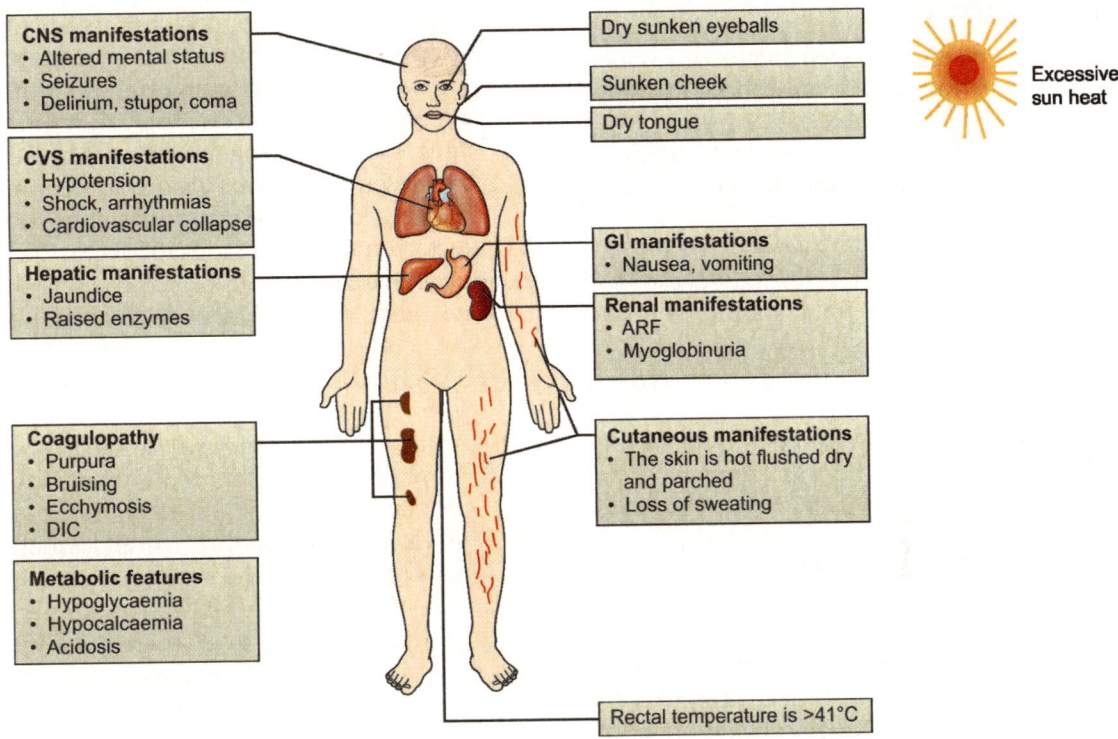

CNS manifestations
- Altered mental status
- Seizures
- Delirium, stupor, coma

CVS manifestations
- Hypotension
- Shock, arrhythmias
- Cardiovascular collapse

Hepatic manifestations
- Jaundice
- Raised enzymes

Coagulopathy
- Purpura
- Bruising
- Ecchymosis
- DIC

Metabolic features
- Hypoglycaemia
- Hypocalcaemia
- Acidosis

Dry sunken eyeballs

Sunken cheek

Dry tongue

Excessive sun heat

GI manifestations
- Nausea, vomiting

Renal manifestations
- ARF
- Myoglobinuria

Cutaneous manifestations
- The skin is hot flushed dry and parched
- Loss of sweating

Rectal temperature is >41°C

Fig. 96.1: Dry hot man due to heatstroke

cerebral (amnesia, dementia, hemiparesis), cerebellar (dysarthria, ataxia) and spinal cord (polyneuropathy).

2. **Cardiovascular manifestations:** Initially, the pulse is good volume and bounding (high cardiac output), becomes weak and feeble due to development of shock, hypotension or cardiovascular collapse due to thermal myocardial injury and hypoxia. Cardiac arrhythmias and nonspecific ECG changes suggest myocardial damage and electrolyte disturbance. Death may occur due to circulatory collapse or sudden cardiac arrest.

3. **Renal manifestations:** Acute renal failure (tubular necrosis) is common, as a result of ischaemia or myoglobinuria due to rhabdomyolysis.

4. **Gastrointestinal manifestations:** Nausea, vomiting are common due to mucosal heat injury.

5. **Hepatic manifestations:** Elevations of bilirubin and SGPT are frequently encountered.

6. **Coagulopathy:** Heart injury results in early coagulopathy leading to petechiae and ecchymosis. Thrombocytopenia can occur. Disseminated intravascular coagulation is seen only in severe cases.

7. **Metabolic/electrolyte manifestations:** Metabolic acidosis occurs leading to acidotic breathing. Hypocalcaemia, hypoglycaemia and hypokalaemia may occur.

8. **Skin manifestations:** The skin is hot and dry. Patient is dehydrated.

9. **Pulmonary manifestations:** Pulmonary dysfunction leading to hypoxaemia is frequent. Pneumonitis, acute respiratory failure can occur.

Laboratory Findings

- Haemoconcentration, leucocytosis.
- Urine is concentrated, may show proteins, casts, myoglobin, RBCs.
- Acid-base disturbance, e.g. lactic acidosis respiratory alkalosis, low K^+, N^+, Ca^{++} and phosphorus.
- Blood gases, i.e. $PaCO_2$ may be <20 mmHg
- Coagulation profile, e.g. thrombocytopenia, DIC. After cooling patient should be investigated for DIC.
- Liver profile show raised aminotransferases and bilirubin.
- Renal profile shows raised BUN, creatinine.
- ECG shows nonspecific ST-T changes.

Management

Steps of management include:

1. **To reduce the temperature as quickly as possible by**
   - *Evaporative cooling* is a noninvasive, effective, quick and easy way to reduce temperature. This method is done by placing the undressed patients in lateral recumbent position or supported in a hand-and-knees position to expose maximum skin surface to the air. Large fans circulate the room air while the entire body is sprayed with lukewarm water (20°C) or cold wet sheets are applied to the undressed body, inhalation of cool air or oxygen is also effective.
   - *Conductive based cooling (immersion cooling):* It involves immersion into ice water or cool water. Ice bath (1–5°C) is effective but usually an impractical method due to its limitations (space, patient access and monitoring). Cold water immersion includes cool baths, localized ice or ice packs application (groin, axillas, neck), and cool gastric and bladder lavage, and infusion of cool intravenous fluids, intravascular heat exchange catheter systems as well as hemodialysis using cool dialysate.

   Shivering must be avoided because it inhibits the effectiveness of cooling.

Medications that can be used to suppress shivering ioclude magnesium, quickacting opioid analgesic, benzodiazepines, and quick-acting anesthetic agents. Skin massage is recommended to prevent cutaneous vasoconstriction. Cooling should be continued until the rectal temperature drops to 39°C.

2. **Supportive care**
   a. *A patent airway* should be established by endotracheal tube, if necessary. Adequate oxygenation is done by giving 100% oxygen. In comatosed patient with severe respiratory depression, assisted ventilation may be needed.
   b. *Fluid replacements* are usually small as compared to heat exhaustion. It consists of 1200–1500 ml of saline/dextrose saline to be given under CVP monitoring in old persons and 2–3 L in adults. 50 ml of sodium bicarbonate is given to combat acidosis. Hypocalcaemia, if occurs may be treated appropriately. Hypoglycaemia is treated by glucose infusion.
   c. *Role of corticosteroids* though controversial, may be used to combat shock, cerebral oedema and adrenal insufficiency. Antipyretics have no effect on environmental hyperthermia hence, are contraindicated.
   d. *Urine output improves after external cooling and fluid replacement.* If urine output falls, mannitol 1.5 g/kg is given. Prolonged oliguria is an indication of dialysis.
   e. *Coagulopathy,* if develops may be treated with fresh frozen plasma and platelets infusion.

HEAT EXHAUSTION

Definition

It is an another catastrophic condition of dysregulation of body temperature characterised by water and/or salt depletion due to profuse sweating. It is commoner than heat stroke. The thermoregulatory control and CNS functions are normal. The core temperature is elevated, but generally less than 40.5°C (<105°F).

Types

1. **Pure water depletion heat 'exhaustion:** It results from excessive sweating and inadequate water replacement by drinking. It occurs in athletes, labourer and military personnel exerting themselves in hot weather without adequate fluid intake. The patients present with excessive thirst with signs of dehydration. As salt is not lost in sweat proportionately, therefore, there is rise in serum osmolarity. Mental confusion, impaired sensorium, delirium, coma and death may occur. There is rise in body temperature (38–40°C).

2. **Pure salt depletion heat exhaustion:** It is slow in onset, occurs in people working in hot and humid environment, especially in unacclimatized people (troops landed in hot climate) in whom salt loss in sweat is very high with replacement of water. The thirst is absent in this type. The skin is dry and inelastic. The **symptoms** pertain to dehydration and salt loss, i.e. *fatigue, weakness, painful muscle cramps, nausea, vomiting* and *headache. Dehydration* and hypotension develop subsequently. There is slight rise in body temperature. *Confusion, delirium, coma* supervene due to shock and cerebral oedema.

3. **Combined type of heat exhaustion:** It is the most common type, presents with clinical picture of both pure types (a mixed picture).

Clinical Features and Diagnosis

The diagnosis is based on

1. **High core temperature** around 40°C with rapid pulse and moist skin.
2. **GI tract manifestations,** e.g. nausea, vomiting, malaise, myalgia, thirst, and weakness.

3. **Neurological manifestations,** e.g. headache, dizziness, fatigue, anxiety paraesthesias, impaired judgement. These are mild. More significant neurological manifestations suggest heat stroke or CNS infections rather than heat exhaustion.

4. **Metabolic disturbance** due to accumulation of lactic acid (lactic acidosis) and hyperventilation leading to respiratory alkalosis.

Management

1. **Treatment irrespective of its types:** Shift the patient to a shaded and a cool environment.

2. **Treatment of specific type:**
   i. *Pure water depletion type* needs judicious replacement of fluids, i.e. 1–2 L over 2–4 hours. About 6–8 L of fluid should be given in first 24 hours and fluid therapy is continued until urine output is normal. The 5% dextrose is ideal when the patient does not take orally. Oral hydration with water may be needed in mild cases.

   ii. *Salt depletion type* is characterised by hyponatraemia, needs replacement of fluid and salts by salted drinks orally (fruit drinks with 7 g of salt per litre, soups, etc.). In unconscious patient, isotonic saline (2–4 liters) I. V. may be given within 24 hours and continued till urine output is normalised and sodium and chloride levels return to normal. Monitor sodium and chloride.

   iii. Active cooling with fans, cool packs until their core temperature comes down to 39°C.

   iv. Rest for at least 24 hours for rehydration.

MALIGNANT HYPERPYREXIA

Definition

It is an inherited abnormality of skeletal muscle sarcoplasmic reticulum that causes rapid increase in intracellular calcium levels in response to halothane or other inhalational anesthetics or to succinylcholine.

Clinical Features

- Elevated temperature (hyperpyrexia).
- Muscle rigidity.
- Rhabdomyolysis.
- Acidosis.
- Cardiovascular instability, i.e. tachycardia or rapid ventricular arrhythmias.

Treatment

- Cessation of anaesthesia.
- Administration of dantrolene to control rigidity.

The recommended dose of dantrolene is 1 to 2.5 mg/kg of body weight given I.V. after every 6 hours for at least 24–48 hours or until oral dantrolene can be given, if needed.

- Procainamide should also be administered to patients with malignant hyperthermia (hyperpyrexia) because of likelihood of ventricular fibrillation in this syndrome.

Neuroleptic Malignant Syndrome

It occurs either due to use of neuroleptic agent (antipsychotic phenothiazines, haloperidol, prochlorperazine, metoclopramide) or withdrawl of dopaminergic drugs. This disorder is caused by inhibition of dopaminergic/receptors in hypothalamus which results in increased heat production and decreased heat loss.

It is characterised by hyperthermia, lead-pipe rigidity, extrapyrimidal signs and autonomic disturbance.

It is treated by dantrolene in the same dosage as used for malignant hyperpyrexia. The other treatment options include use of bromocriptine, levodopa, amantadine, nifedipine and/ or induction of muscle paralysis by curare or pancuronium

Hypothermia

Definition

Hypothermia is defined as a core body temperature (rectal temperature) of 35°C or less. It is classified as *mild* (temp, between 35°C and 32°C), *moderate* (< 32°C to 28°C) or *severe* (<28°C). This is depicted in Fig. 97.1. The hypothermia is mostly accidental, may be *primary* (direct exposure of a healthy person to cold) or *secondary*.

Pathogenesis

Hypothermia represents a loss of balance between heat production and the heat loss. Heat is generated in all the tissues and is lost by *radiation, respiration, evaporation, conduction* and *convection*. The balance between heat production and heat loss is regulated by the hypothalamus (preoptic and posterior region). Cold exposure activates the cold receptors in the

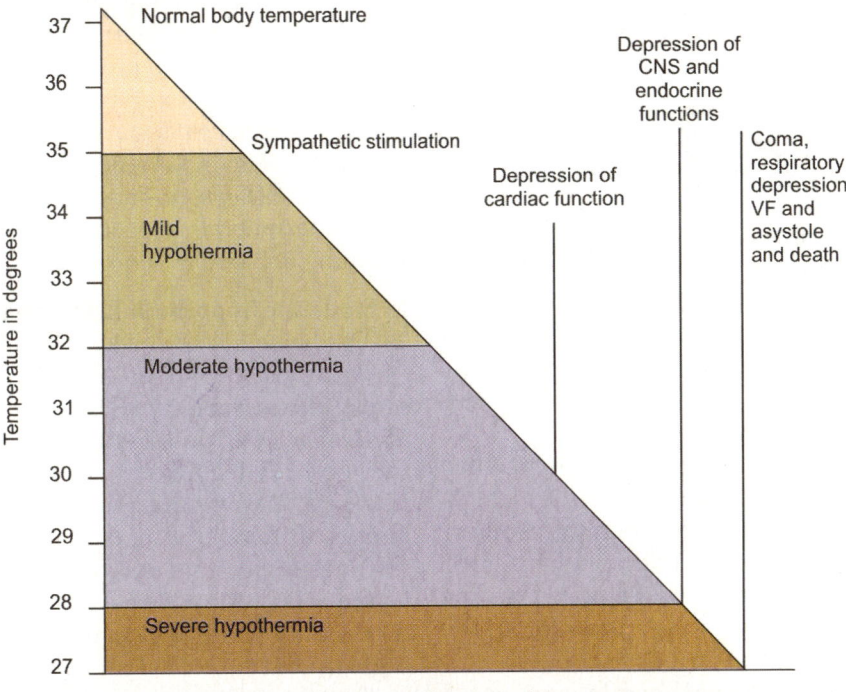

Fig. 97.1: Systemic effects of cold exposure

skin and transmits the signal to hypothalamus via lateral spinothalamic tract. The hypothalamus (posterior region) activates the sympathetic nervous system to increase muscle tone and causes shivering. The shivering, in turn, increases the metabolic rate from normal level (40 to 60 kcal/h) to as high as 300 kcal/h. Shivering tries to conserve heat to overcome ambient temperature gradient, hence, is protective mechanism. Even at maximum metabolic rates, heat loss from the body can exceed heat production. As the body temperature drops to 30°C, metabolic process slows and shivering stops, thereby accelerating the development of hypothermia. When the skin temperature falls to 25°C, tissue demand for O_2 is greater-than what is supplied and the area becomes cyanotic. At 15°C, tissue damage occurs due to marked reduction in tissue metabolism and oxyhemoglobin dissociation. Tissue damage may result from ischemia and thromboses of small vessels.

Causes

Extreme environmental conditions can cause hypothermia in healthy individuals. It may be *primary* (from exposure to cold or extremely low temperature) or *secondary* (thermoregulatory dysfunction or both. Most severe hypothermia occurs in persons with underlying medical conditions either due to excessive heat loss (environmental exposure) or inadequate heat production or both processes are involved (Table 97.1). It is hereby stressed that body temperature never falls below the environmental temperature.

1. **Iatrogenic hypothermia:** It can occur when semiconscious or unconscious patients are left uncovered in hospital room or during surgical procedures where large body surface areas are exposed to low temperature for long periods in the operating room.
2. **Intentional hypothermia,** i.e. cold cardioplegia in cardiopulmonary bypass surgery.

3. **Accidental hypothermia:** Most environmental exposures are accidental. It can also occur due to altered thermoregulation and drugs. *In the home environment* in cold climates hypothermia occurs due to poor heating, inadequate or wet clothing and poor nutrition. *In the hospital,* accidental hypothermia occurs due to prolonged postoperative hypothermia or infusion of large amounts of refrigerated blood products, rapid infusion of I.V fluids, and prolonged exposure of an undressed patient during resuscitation or operative procedures.

The *outdoor hypothermia* also involves climbers, skiers, arctic and anarctic travellers due to exposure to extreme low temperatures. Physical exhaustion and inadequate clothing are contributory.

Clinical Features

In mild hypothermia (core temp. 35°C to 32°C), there is *shivering* and *feeling of intense cold.* The subject is alert and usually takes appropriate actions to rewarm, e.g. huddling, extraclothing or exercise. There is *tachycardia, increased cardiac output* and *hypertension* secondary to sympathetic stimulation. There may occur *tachypnoea, shivering* and *cold diuresis* due to peripheral vasoconstriction leading to shunting of blood to central circulation.

In moderate hypothermia (core temp. 32°C to 28°C), the ability to shiver is lost and cardiac conduction is depressed. There is sinus *bradycardia, dilated pupils* and *slowed reflexes. Atrial fibrillation* with slow ventricular conduction may occur. The *ECG* may show slow ventricular rate, T wave inversion and QT prolongation. At temperature of 28–30°C, Osborne 'J' waves (a positive upward deflection with J point elevation) appear at the junction of descending limb of R wave (QRS) with ST segment.

The neurological manifestations are diverse. At temperature of 32°, there is confusion and lethargy. As the temperature falls further (at

Table 97.1 Causes of hypothermia

I. Excessive heat loss
a. Environmental exposure
- Accidental with high wind velocity wind chill factor) or direct contact with cold surface
- Iatrogenic, e.g. cold weather injury, inadequate clothing

b. Increased continuous blood flow
- Bum, psoriasis, toxic epidermal necrolysis.

II. Inadequate heat production
a. Inadequate metabolism
- Malnutrition and/or starvation
- Hypothyroidism, adrenal insufficiency
- Hepatic failure
- Diabetic ketoacidosis and hypoglycaemia.

b. Altered thermoregulation
- Sepsis
- Uraemia and hepatic dysfunction
- Hypothalamic dysfunction, e.g. head trauma, stroke, tumour
- Spinal cord injury—T 1 or above
- *Shapirco's syndrome* (episodic spontaneous hypothermia with hyperhidrosis)

c. Drug-induced
- Barbiturates, phenothiazincs, opiates, lithium, benzodiazepines anesthetics, neuromuscular blockers
- Alcohol.

Investigations

Investigation may show:

1. Haemoconcentration (raised Hb and PCV).
2. Cold-induced granulocytopenia.
3. There may be evidence of hepatic (raised enzymes) and renal impairment (raised urea and creatinine).
4. Serum cortisol level may be low.
5. Coagulation profile may show depressed platelet function and DIC.
6. Arterial blood gas analysis may show hypoxaemia and metabolic acidosis.
7. Serum K^+ may be elevated.
8. X-ray chest and abdomen are important in patients with immersion hypothermia to see the evidence of aspiration.
9. BEG and evoked potentials. Evoked potentials show increase in latency and decrease in amplitude of visual, auditory and somatosensory potentials. Severe hypothermia may be associated with isoelectric EEG which should not be taken as brain death and it is reversible.
10. ECG for Osborne 'J' waves and cardiac arrhythmias.

Management

30°C), violent behaviour, confusion, disturbance of vision, ataxia, dysarthria may follow. Staggering, falling and faintings are common. Below 30 to 28°C, there is depression of all the cerebral functions. Pulse and respiration become slow. There are slow pupillary as well as tendon reflexes.

In severe hypothermia (core temp. <28°C), there is loss of consciousness and patient becomes blue and deeply comatosed at <25°C. As the coma increases, pupils become dilated and fixed, metabolic acidosis, coagulopathy and pulmonary oedema leading to hypoxemia develop. The reflexes become lost and generalised rigidity simulating rigor mortis appears and patient may be mistaken as a dead man. Ventricular fibrillation and asystole may develop as temperature falls below 20°C and are the leading causes of death.

It is a medical emergency and requires energetic and immediate management to bring the core body temperature slowly to normal while correcting metabolic abnormalities and treating cardiac arrhythmias. A common dictum quoted in the treatment of hypothermia is *"the person is not dead until it is warm and dead"* stresses the need of rewarming before a person is declared dead.

Initial assessment should be done by accurately recording the rectal, esophageal and bladder temperature (probe). Oral and axillary temperatures are unreliable. Patient should also be evaluated by blood sugar estimation (hypoglycaemia), trauma, drug levels and thyroid function tests. Renal and hepatic function should be assessed. ECG monitoring is done.

Steps of Management

Resuscitation begins with assessment and support of airway, breathing and circulation, initiation of rewarming and prevention of further heat loss. The steps are:

1. Rewarming (active or passive, internal or external).
2. Supportive treatment for volume depletion, hypotension, hypoxia and arrhythmias.
3. Treatment of underlying cause when patient becomes stable. Underlying hypothyroidism must be looked for, if present, must be treated. Avoid the precipitating factors.
4. Monitor temperature (core body), vital signs (pulse, BP, respiration, urine output), biochemical parameters (arterial blood gas, pH), ECG and electrolytes.

Rewarming

It is done to increase the body temperature by 0.5°C to 2°C/hr. Rewarming techniques can be active or passive, internal or external.

i. *Passive external rewarming:* It is the easiest and safest method. It involves removal of cold wet clothing, dry them and covering the patient with blankets and clothing in a warm environment to allow the endogenous heat production to correct the hypothermia. It is important to keep the head covered because up to 30% heat is lost from the head. A single layer of cotton blanket decreases the heat loss by 30%. Three layers of blankets reduce the heat loss by 50%.

ii. *Active external rewarming:* It involves direct application of heat sources (hot water bottles, heat packs, heating blankets, heat lamps, submersion in a tank of hot water) to external body surfaces. This procedure may be hazardous as it may cause hypotension, or "*rewarming shock*" and cause temperature to drop (after drop) There is a risk of bum injury due to application of direct heat, therefore, active rewarming should be done only on a young

previously healthy person. Direct heat to be applied only to the thorax if active rewarming is used to avoid after drop.

Recently field treatment with insulating covers have been used with minimal loss of heat. It has also been observed that carbon fibre rewarming has resulted in a rapid rise in core temperature. Convection warmers have been used in operation theatres for management of perioperative hypothermia.

iii. *Active internal rewarming:* The simplest method is airway rewarming in which the patient inspires humidified oxygen heated to 42°C via face mask or endotracheal tube and this technique raises the core temperature by 1 to 2°C/hr.

Warmed intravenous fluid (42°C) and lavage of the stomach, bladder or colon with warmed fluids have a limited warming effects, may not be of much help when rapid rewarming is needed. Heated peritoneal and pleural lavage induce rapid rewarming (2–4°C/hr), should be used only in moderate to severe hypothermia with cardiovascular instability or when external rewarming is ineffective.

The most efficient rewarming technique is via *haemodialysis* or *cardiopulmonary bypass*. Both methods require continuous removal of blood that is circulated and warmed externally before being reinfused. These methods are used for rapid rewarming in severe hypothermia when other methods are ineffective.

Supportive Measures

1. *Correction of volume depletion:* Warmed normal saline or 5% dextrose saline may be given intravenously. Lactate Ringer's solution should be avoided.
2. *Physical manipulation of the patient* should be minimized. Central venous line, nasogastric tube and endotracheal tube should be inserted carefully because of likelihood of cardiac arrhythmia.
3. *Treatment of hypotension:* If hypotension does not respond to fluids and rewarming, low dose dopamine may be given.

4. *Treatment of sepsis:* If it is a possibility (leucocytosis, positive culture) then a broad-spectrum antibiotics is employed before a culture or sensitivity report is received.

5. *Correction of hypokalaemia:* Rewarming alone corrects hypokalaemia.

6. *Correction of hyperglycaemia:* Rewarming often corrects hyperglycaemia, if persists a small dose of insulin may be used.

Monitoring

1. Monitoring of temperature by rectal thermometer.
2. Continuous cardiac monitoring is required for arrhythmias. Atrial arrhythmias are common and reverse with rewarming alone. Ventricular arrhythmias are usually refractory to drugs and to defibrillation. Bretylium tosylate (5 g/kg I.V.) is the agent of choice.

When cardiac arrest is present, active internal rewarming and cardiopulmonary resuscitation (CPR) should be initiated simultaneously.

Treatment of Underlying Cause

Treatment or removal of underlying cause/precipitating cause once the patient becomes stabilised after rewarming. A careful search should be made for myxoedema, if found to be the cause, should be treated. Alcohol should be avoided in future.

High Altitude Related Emergencies

HIGH ALTITUDE RELATED ACUTE DISORDERS

High altitude environment is different than the environment at ground level. It is characterised by hypobaric hypoxia, low temperatures and increased radiation (ultraviolet and ionising) and most of high altitude disorders are attributed to hypoxia.

Altitudes above 2700 m is defined as *high altitude.* Most low-landers on reaching these heights develop biophysiological changes related to acclimatization to these heights. Failure of acclimatization or acute effects of these biophysiological changes lead to diseases found at these heights. Altitude above 5500 m is termed as *extreme altitude.* At extreme altitude, permanent adaptation or acclimatization of man does not occur.

Physiological Changes to High Altitude

1. **Hyperventilation:** It is mediated via peripheral chemoreceptors due to hypoxia and is the earliest change that occurs on ascent to high altitude.

2. **Hyperventilation is followed by hypocapnia** that leads to respiratory alkalosis and dehydration which is compensated by renal bicarbonate excretion.

3. **Hypoxia** leads to pulmonary vasoconstriction.

4. **Secondary polycythaemia** occurs as a response to hypoxia, is mediated through erythropoietin production. Although, it is a physiological response and increases O_2 carrying capacity of blood but leads to an increase in blood viscosity which can be deleterious specially at extreme heights. It may lead to venous thrombosis and may predispose to pulmonary embolism.

5. **There is decrease in partial pressure** of oxygen and barometric pressure with increasing heights (Fig. 98.1). At 5000 m height, the partial pressure of O_2 is reduced to 50%. The oxygen saturation falls with increase in altitude. Below 2500 m, the reduction in O_2 saturation is small and no symptoms other than exertional dyspnoea appear. All syndromes of high altitude appear at heights >2700 m.

6. **Other changes** include an increase in sympathetic tone, and long-term changes of increase in capillary density and intracellular oxidative enzymes.

Risk Factors

Risk factors for altitude related illnesses are:
1. Rate of ascent and previous history of high altitude illness.
2. Exertion, younger age groups, women.
3. Debilitating fatigue.
4. Neck radiation, surgery damaging the

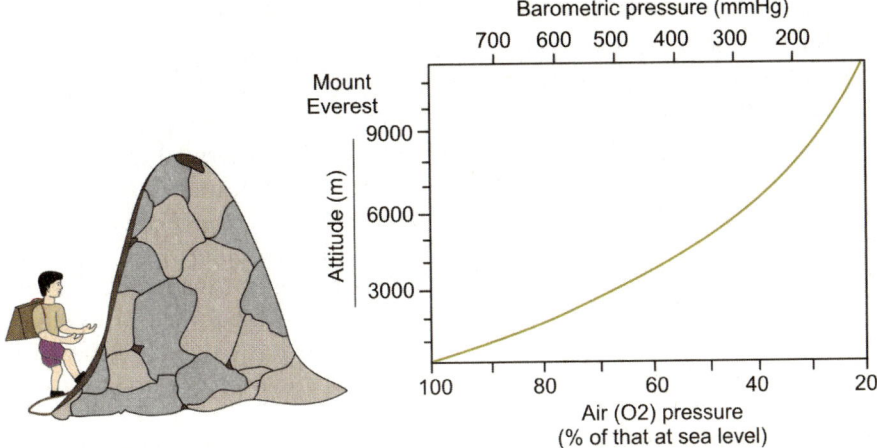

Fig. 98.1: Diagram showing the decrease in oxygen and barometric pressure with increasing heights

cartoid bodies, respiratory tract infections and dehydration.

Classification

Depending on the onset of manifestations, high altitude disorders may be classified into *acute, subacute* and *chronic* (Table 98.1). Here, only acute disorders will be discussed. Most of the high attitude illnesses occur in travellers and mountaineers.

Table 98.1 Classification of high altitude disorders
1. **Acute**
• Benign form, e.g. acute mountain sickness
• Malignant forms
• High altitude pulmonary oedema
• High altitude cerebral oedema
2. **Subacute**: Infantile or adult mountain sickness
3. **Chronic**: Chronic mountain sickness
4. **Others**
• High altitude pulmonary arterial hypertension
• High altitude retinopathy
• Thrombotic episodes
• Gastrointestinal problems

ACUTE MOUNTAIN SICKNESS

It is a benign and reversible condition, occurs in travellers ascending to altitude of 3000 m (40–50%).

Hypoxia, stimulation of renin-angiotensin aldosterone and ADH release resulting in fluid retention are the underlying pathogenic mechanisms. Hypoxia leads to cerebral vasodilation with increased blood flow. Fluid retention leads to oedema.

Clinical Features

The symptoms develop within 6 to 24 hours of an ascent and vary in severity from trivial to incapacitating (uncommon). *Headache* is the predominant presenting symptom which is generally frontal, throbbing, aggravated by exertion and is more severe in the morning. It is due to cerebral vasodilatation induced by hypoxia.

In severe cases, *headache* is associated with *malaise, anorexia, giddiness, insomnia, nausea, irritability, pallor* and *vomiting*. There may be *visual* and *auditory, disturbances* (*tinnitis, vertigo*), *Cheyne-Stoke breathing* and *weakness. Dyspnoea ataxia, pulmonary oedema* (*cyanosis*) and *encephalopathy* may appear in more severe cases.

In minority of cases, more serious sequelae such as *high-altitude pulmonary oedema* (*HAPO*) and *high-altitude cerebral oedema* (*HACO*) may also occur.

Management and Prophylaxis

1. Immediate descent is the definite treatment. If immediate descent not possible,

providing portable hyperbaric O_2 chambers will give symptomatic relief.

2. In mild cases, rest and an analgesic are just adequate. Symptoms resolve after 12–48 hours at a stable altitude but may recur with further ascent. Give 100% low flow O_2 (1–2 L/min) for acute symptoms.

3. Persistent symptoms or severe form of illness respond to acetazolamide in the dose of 250 mg 8 hourly for 2–3 days. Acetazolamide is a carbonic anhydrase inhibitor, hence response to it indicates alkalosis as the probable cause of these symptoms. Dexamethasone (8 mg stat) 4 mg 6 to 8 hourly may be useful if symptoms persist. Both are recommended for treatment as long as symptoms persist in severe cases.

4. Patients with severe form need to be monitored closely for evidence of HAPO as minority of cases may develop it.

5. Acclimatizing by ascending gradually is the best prophylaxis.

ACUTE HIGH ALTITUDE PULMONARY OEDEMA (HAPO)

Definition

High altitude pulmonary oedema is a serious condition that occurs rarely due to exposure to high altitude (>3000 m) in association with severe physical exertion in unacclimatized yet otherwise healthy young persons.

Predisposing Factors

Rapidity of ascent, young age (<25 years), heavy exertion and the presence of mountain sickness are common precipitating events.

An incidence of 1–4% at altitude of 4000 m has been reported. It is more common in highlanders who re-enter high altitude after a short journey to low altitudes. Recent data shows that acclimatized high-altitude natives also develop this syndrome on return to high altitude after a brief stay at lower altitude.

Pathophysiology

The mechanism for high-altitude pulmonary oedema is obscure. It is an example of noncardiogenic pre-arteriolar high-altitude pulmonary oedema characterised by increase in cardiac output and pulmonary arterial pressure that decreases the O_2 uptake and saturation while pulmonary capillary wedge pressure and left atrial pressures are normal. There is increased capillary permeability of alveolar capillary membrane due to mismatch perfusion (areas of over and under perfusion lead to stress failure) induced by hypoxia. Higher incidence of HAPO in re-entrants to high altitude indicates larger hypoxic pulmonary response to ascent to further heights after brief stay at lower altitudes.

Clinical Features

HAPO develops within 2–4 days after arrival at high altitude. The *clinical manifestations* usually start within 6–36 hours with symptoms suggestive of *acute mountain sickness* followed by *dry mouth, incessant dry cough, breathlessness* and *headache*. The cough later on becomes productive with frothy sputum which may be *blood-stained* (*haemoptysis*). The *chest pain* or *discomfort, tachypnoea* and *wheezing* may also occur.

On examination, patient looks ill, tachypnoea and tachycardia are present. BP is normal. There may be mild to moderate pyrexia. *Central cyanosis* occurs late. Optic fundi may show retinal hemorrhage in 10–15% of cases. Presence of *papilloedema* indicates associated cerebral oedema. There are signs of *noncardiogenic pulmonary oedema*, i.e. rales and rhonchi are heard on both lung fields.

Investigations

There may be leucocytosis. **X-ray chest** shows bilateral or unilateral diffuse haze due to alveolar oedema mostly involving the midzones and lower zones of the lungs but Kerley's B lines and bat-wing appearance are not seen (*noncardiogenic pulmonary oedema*). The cardiac size is normal. The pulmonary artery is dilated and prominent. **ECG** shows right axis deviation, right ventricular strain or hypertroph and sinus tachycardia. **Arterial blood gas analysis** may show hypoxaemia with hypocapnia or normocapnia, alkalosis.

Management

Unless recognized and treated rapidly, this may lead to cardiorespiratory failure, collapse and death.

Steps of Treatment

1. **Descent to lower altitude:** It should take place as early as possible. Even 500 to 1000 m descent may produce relief in symptoms.
2. **Rest** in head raised (semi-Fowler) position. Avoid exertion.
3. **Reversal of hypoxia by oxygen:** 100% oxygen should be administered at high flow rates (4–6 L/min) with a face mask, if possible. In mild to moderate cases, this is sufficient. Later on low flow rates (2–4 L/min) may be used if necessary.
4. **Recompression in portable Gamow bag:** Hyperbaric O$_2$ therapy in a portable pressure chamber can be used in patients where descent to lower altitude is not feasible; usage of this bag can effectively reduce the altitude by about 1800 m for the patient inside.
5. **Diuretics** have a limited role, can be used only in severe cases. Frusemide (20–40 mg) may be given intravenously.
6. **Inhaled β-agonists** to relieve bronchospasm are effective.
7. **Oral nifedipine** (10 mg initially then 30 mg slow release tablets every 12 hourly) can be given to reduce pulmonary arterial pressure and subsequently to relieve oedema.
8. **Nitric oxide (15 ppm)** combined with oxygen has been shown to have excellent beneficial effect.
10. **Role of steroids** is controversial. However, dexamethasone 4 mg 6 hourly is recommended by some physicians if CNS symptoms are present.

The mortality rate in untreated or inadequately treated patients is as high as 50%. When treated early the mortality is less than 10%.

HIGH ALTITUDE CEREBRAL OEDEMA (HACO)

It is the least common high altitude associated disorder but is a serious and potentially fatal condition like HAPO, and most of times is associated with acute mountain sickness and HAPO.

The pathophysiology is similar to acute mountain sickness and HAPO. Worsening hypoxaemia leading to severe cerebral vasodilatation combined with increased capillary permeability contributes to it.

Clinical Features

It occurs at moderate height of 3500–4000 m in sensitive individuals.

It usually follows acute mountain sickness and HAPO, hence, their features are usually present. In addition, patients present with rapidly progressive **cerebral symptoms** such as *hallucinations* or *behavioural change, confusion, blurring of vision, headache, dizziness, vomiting* and *ataxia. Speech* is often slurred. *Alteration in consciousness* and *truncal ataxia* are characteristic features; *coma* appears in severe cases. *Focal neurological signs (haemiparesis), abnormal plantar response can also occur.* The *optic fundi* may show retinal haemorrhage and papilloedema (*high altitude retinopathy*).

Management

1. **Rapid descent to lower altitude:** Descent should be at least 2000 feet and should continue until symptoms improve. Use the portable hyperbaric chamber where descent is not possible and 100% *oxygen therapy* by mask are mainstay of treatment.
2. **Decongestive therapy:** High dose parenteral steroids (dexamethasone 4 mg hourly), mannitol and diuretics have been used successfully as decongestive therapy, but their efficacy is difficult to judge as these treatment are usually given in field conditions.

Electrical and Lightning Injuries

ELECTRICAL AND LIGHTNING INJURIES

Definition

Injuries inflicted by an electrical current of low voltage, high voltage and lightning are called *electrical injuries*. These occur when comes in contact with live wires or electrical gadgets. The severity and distribution of electrical injury depend on:

i. **Type of current (direct or alternating):** At low voltage, alternate current (supplied for household use) produces ventricular fibrillation (VF) while high voltage produces respiratory depression, and AC current is dangerous than DC. At higher voltages, both alternate current (AC) and direct current (DC) are equally dangerous or lethal (Fig. 99.2).

ii. **Amount and voltage of current:** High voltage current produces violent muscular contractions and may throw the patient away from the source of current, but even a small contact may be lethal. On the other hand, a low voltage current causes spasms in the muscles and person may remain in contact with the source causing extensive injuries or death.

iii. **Resistance offered by the body:** Human body is a bad conductor of electricity, but wet perspiring soft skin makes it more vulnerable by lowering its resistance. If resistance offered by the body is high, then local tissue destruction results only; while at low resistance, systemic effects on the heart and brain appear.

iv. **Pathway of the current:** Whenever current flows through a conductor, heat is generated and skin being the most resistant tissue of the body gets the most heat at the point of entry as well as at exit. The two danger zones for electrical injury are brain and the heart where immediate effects of heating become evident.

v. **Duration of current:** The prolonged the contact, the more serious is the effect.

Lightning injury is direct current of short duration and most of the current flashes over the outer surface of the body (Fig. 99.1). Lightning differs from high-voltage electrical shock in that lightning is massive high voltage electric flash lasting for short period. The passage of lightning electricity from arm to arm or arm to leg is most likely to involve the heart (asystole) or spinal cord. It may cause immediate effect by heating the nervous system, while delayed spinal cord syndrome is due to secondary vascular occlusion. About 30% victims seriously injured by lightning die; while 70% may have permanent sequelae.

Clinical Features

The AC current being more dangerous than DC can cause immediate death due to ventricular

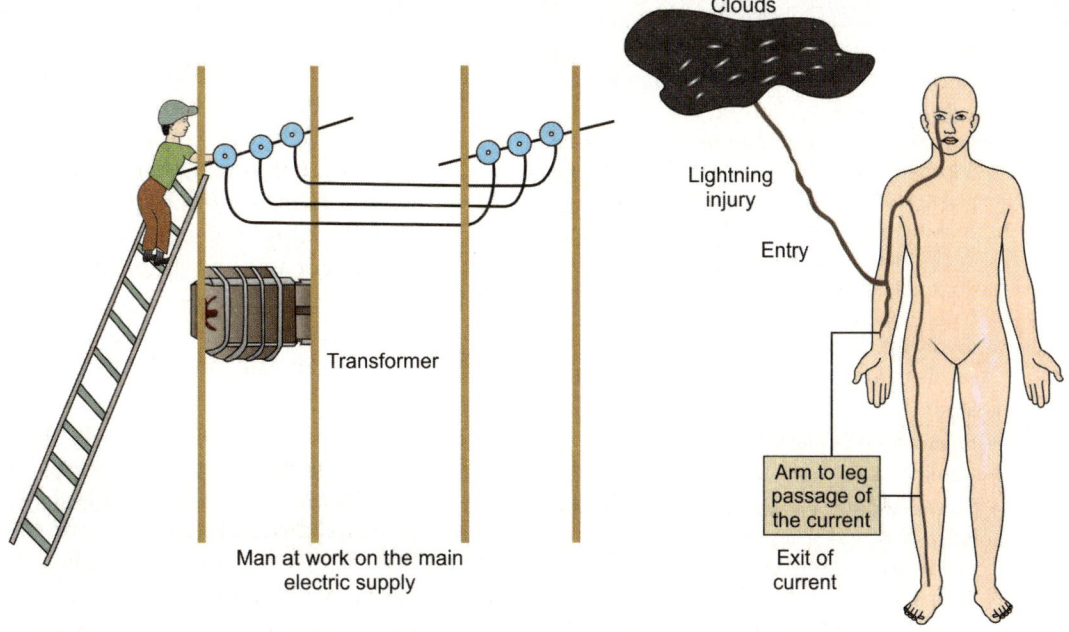

Fig. 99.1: Sources of electrical injury (AC current) and lighting injury

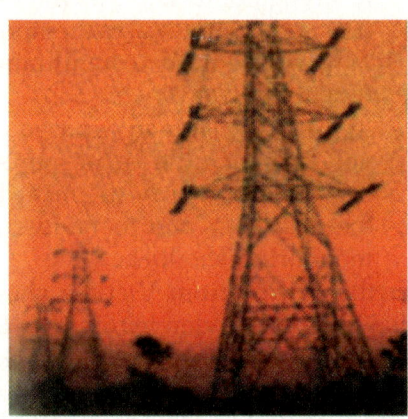

Fig. 99.2: Crossing of high-tension wire over the residential area—a potential risk for public

fibrillation and respiratory arrest. The clinical features can be divided into immediate and remote or late effects. They are given in Box 1.

Management

1. **Basic measures:** The victim should be freed from the current at once after switching off the mains. A dry pole or a stick of wood, leather belt or rubber should be used during separation. If there is fire, it should be extinguished with sand only. Do not use water or other liquids.

2. **Initial hospital evaluation:** Initial assessment involves airway, breathing, and circulation. I.V. line should be procured and fluid administration is started. In the meantime, collect blood samples for blood count, electrolytes, renal profile (urea, creatinine), bilirubin and liver enzymes, serum creatinine kinase, and cardiac enzymes.

   Urinalysis and urine for myoglobin should also be done. Cardiac monitoring is done and intermittent ECG may also be done.

3. **Cardiopulmonary resuscitation:** Immediate cardiopulmonary resuscitation may be life-saving, hence, should be started at once. Breathing and circulation should be supported in an unconscious patient using mouth-to-mouth respiration and external cardiac compression. Airway should be maintained. Ventricular fibrillation should be treated with defibrillation.

Box 1   Clinial features of eletrical and lighting injuries

1. *Immediate:* They usually appear within few hours and may affect the various systems as follows:

   i. *Local heat effects:*
- Local burns, i.e. flash (arcing) burn or flame (clothing). Burn or direct heating effect burn at the point of entry and exit.
- Sinking of hair, blisters, fissures, charring, ecchymosis and lacerations. Skin injury does not correlate with degree of injury.
- Deep extensive tissue damage (rhabdomyolysis), oedema with compression and focal neuropathies or plexus lesions.

   ii. Features due to fall
- Fracture, dislocation, head injury.

   iii. Systemic features
- Cardiovascular, e.g. shock, ventricular fibrillation and cardiac arrest.
- Respiratory, e.g. hypoxia and asphyxia.
- Neurological, e.g. consciousness may be lost with electrical injury either from syncope or from immediate concussion or cerebral oedema. Other features include visual disturbance, headache, amnesia, speech disturbance, tingling and muscular contractions, convulsions, motor paralysis and stroke. Temporary tinnitus and deafness may be experienced.
- Renal, e.g. acute renal failure.

2. *Remote or late effects:* They are usually permanent.
- Neurological, e.g. seizures, myelopathy, neuropathy, causalgias, motor neuron disease like features, tetanus.
- *Visual:* Cataract is an occasional late sequel to the electrical flash and may appear as late as 2 years of injury.

All patients with cardiac arrhythmias should be monitored in intensive care unit for 48 hours.

Artificial respiratory support with an oxygen supply should be started. Assisted ventilation may be used, if required.

4. **Other measures**
   i. Pain management before during and after initial treatment with NSAIDs and opiates.

   ii. *Treatment of shock:* Intravenous fluids should be given in cases with deep extensive burns and tissue damage leading to shock. Usual fluid used is Ringer's lactate 0.5 ml/kg/hr. Fluid and electrolyte balance is maintained to prevent acute renal failure.

   iii. *Tetanus prophylaxis:* Tetanus toxoid should be given. Penicillin and other-broad-spectrum antibiotics are used as clostridia may infect the tissue.

   iv. *Treatment of burn and local tissue damage:* High voltage injury with deep tissue damage may require surgical exploration, debridement of necrotic tissue. Amputation may be needed with extensive damage,

   v. *Acute renal failure:* It may occur due to shock or rhabdomyolysis leading to myoglobinuria. Adequate hydration and in some cases, hemodialysis may be required to maintain renal functions.

   vi. In pregnant women exposed to high voltage injury, the foetus may sustain intrauterine growth retardation, foetal distress and foetal loss. Foetal monitoring, should be done.

5. **Further evaluation:** Victims should be evaluated for hidden injury (eye, ENT or muscle) organ injury (heart, liver, kidney, pancreas), blunt trauma, dehydration, skin burns, hypertension, acid-base disturbance and neurological damage.

Complications

- Sepsis.
- Gangrene requiring amputation of limb.
- Disability due to neurologic, cognitive or psychiatric dysfunction.

Drowning and Near Drowning

Definition

It is an unexpected submersion injury in which a previous healthy person dies or is exposed to severe cerebral hypoxia (asphyxiation), aspiration, acidemia and suffers permanent brain damage.

Near drowning: It refers to a condition from which a person is rescued alive.

Dry drowning: Drowning without aspiration of water into the lungs is called *dry drowning*.It occurs in 10% of cases. Airway obstruction is the cause of hypoxaemia. Death follows intense laryngospasm and airway obstruction.

Wet drowning: It refers to entry of water or foreign matter into the lungs. It occurs in 90% cases. Ventilation-perfusion mismatch is the cause of hypoxaemia.

Pathophysiology (Fig. 100.1)

1. Consequent to submersion, breath holding occurs for a variable period till the accumulating CO_2 stimulates the respiratory centre sufficiently enough to force an inspiration which results in aspiration of water into the lungs (wet drowning). In about 10% of cases, death may occur due to asphyxia without any entry of water into the lungs (dry drowning). Airway obstruction the cause of hypoxaemia and laryngospasm are the causes of asphyxia and death.

2. About 90% of drowning victims aspirate the water into the lungs. Fresh water aspiration alters the surface tension properties of the alveolar surfactants and makes the alveoli unstable which causes a decreased ventilation-perfusion ratio with hypoxaemia and development of diffuse pulmonary oedema. Hypertonic sea water pulls extra amount of fluid from plasma into the lungs with the result alveoli become fluid-filled with normal perfusion. This event also causes right-to-left shunting with venous admixture in the lungs. With both types of water, pulmonary oedema occurs.

3. Freshwater in the alveoli is hypotonic, and is rapidly absorbed, impairs alveolar surfactant function and leads to alveolar collapse which promotes intrapulmonary right-to-left shunting (pulmonary venous admixture).

4. About 85% of patients of near-drowning aspirate 22 ml/kg of water or less which does not significantly affect blood volume or serum electrolytes concentration. When a large amount of freshwater is aspirated, it causes haemodilution, acute hypervolaemia and severe haemolysis, but this development has been reported rarely. With rapid redistribution of water and development of pulmonary oedema, even freshwater victims frequently demonstrate

hypovolaemia by the time they reach the hospital.

5. Aspiration of grossly contaminated water may lead to severe pulmonary infection.
6. Occasionally, death may occur due to injury to head or cervical spine, as in the case of divers.

Severe degree of near drowning produces respiratory failure, pulmonary oedema, hypoxic encephalopathy, shock, cerebral oedema and cardiac arrest.

Causes

Drowning is particularly common in children. Drowning may be a secondary event during swimming, may occur due to unrelated factors such as sudden occurrence of an epileptic fit or a stroke or myocardial infarction. The initiating event is usually unknown. The causes of drowning in various age groups are given in Box 1.

Clinical Features

Those who are rescued alive (near drowning), are often semiconscious or unconscious and not breathing. Some victims may be awake, restless, apprehensive, complain of headache, vomiting, cough, dyspnoea and chest pain. Hypoxaemia, hypocarbia and metabolic acidosis are invariable features. The oral cavity may contain a foreign body which may be

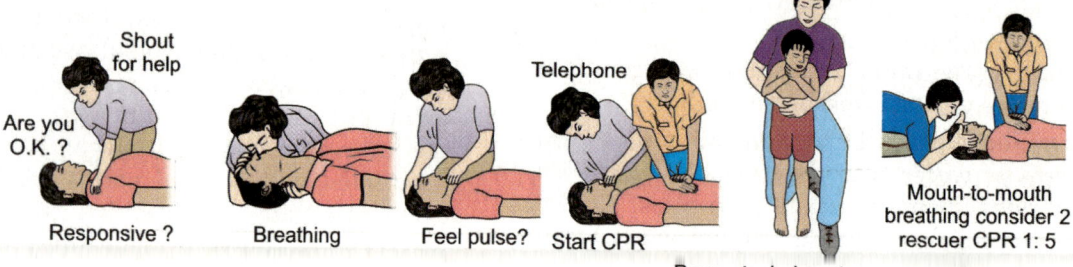

Are you O.K. ? — Responsive ?
Shout for help — Breathing
Feel pulse?
Telephone — Start CPR
Mouth-to-mouth breathing consider 2 rescuer CPR 1: 5

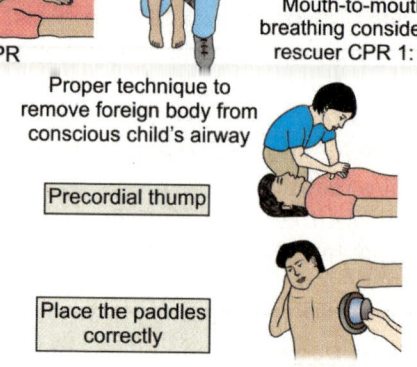

Proper technique to remove foreign body from conscious child's airway

Precordial thump

Place the paddles correctly

If ECG tracing flat, check switches, electric supply and connections

Give oxygen

Endotracheal intubation

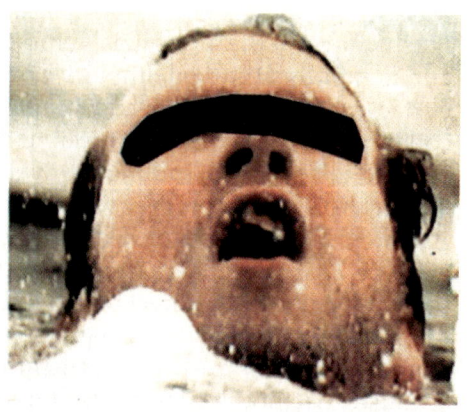

Fig. 100.1: Sudden immersion in an unacclimatised subject in ice cold water results in reflux hyper ventilation and tachycardia, often with supraventricular ectopic beats and hypertension, a condition known as *"cold shock"*, drowning is likely to occur immediately unless a buoyancy aid is used. The clinical picture is one of asphyxiation, often with pulmonary oedema due to water inhalation. Cardiopulmonary arrest is a feature of near drowning, hence resuscitation is mandatory

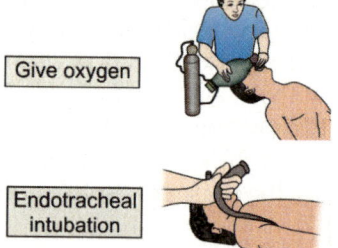

- Use of alcohol or other drugs (25% cases of adult drowning is due to it)
- Extreme fatigue
- Intentional hyperventilation
- Sudden acute illness (e.g. seizure, hypoglycaemia, arrhythmia, attack of asthma, myocardial infarction)
- Spinal cord/head injury sustained during diving
- Stings by venomous aquatic animals
- Decompression sickness in deep water diving
- Carbon monoxide exposure from boat motors
- Dangerous water conditions, e.g. temperature and turbulence

inhaled and lead to respiratory obstruction and asphyxia.

Some recover spontaneous ventilation and consciousness rapidly. There may be features of acute lung injury such as wheezes, tachypnoea, tachycardia, cyanosis and pink frothy sputum due to pulmonary oedema (ARDS). The acute lung injury recovers within 48–72 hours unless complicated by infection. Cardiovascular features include hypotension/shock, arrhythmias and cardiac arrest.

Early complications include:

- Dehydration.
- Gastric distension.
- Hypotension.
- Haemoptysis.
- Cardiac arrhythmias.
- Hypothermia (submersion in cold water). It may be protective and recovery have been reported after prolonged immersion in cold water in children.

It must be remembered that survival may be possible after submersion for a period of up to 30 minutes in very cold water without brain damage. The outcome depends on duration of immersion, intensity of acidosis, presence of cardiac arrest and time-delay before resuscitation.

Management

Regardless of the conditions surrounding a drowning or near drowning, following steps of treatment (Fig. 100.2) must be adhere to:

1. Retrieve or remove the victim from the water and stabilise his/her head and neck if trauma is being suspected.

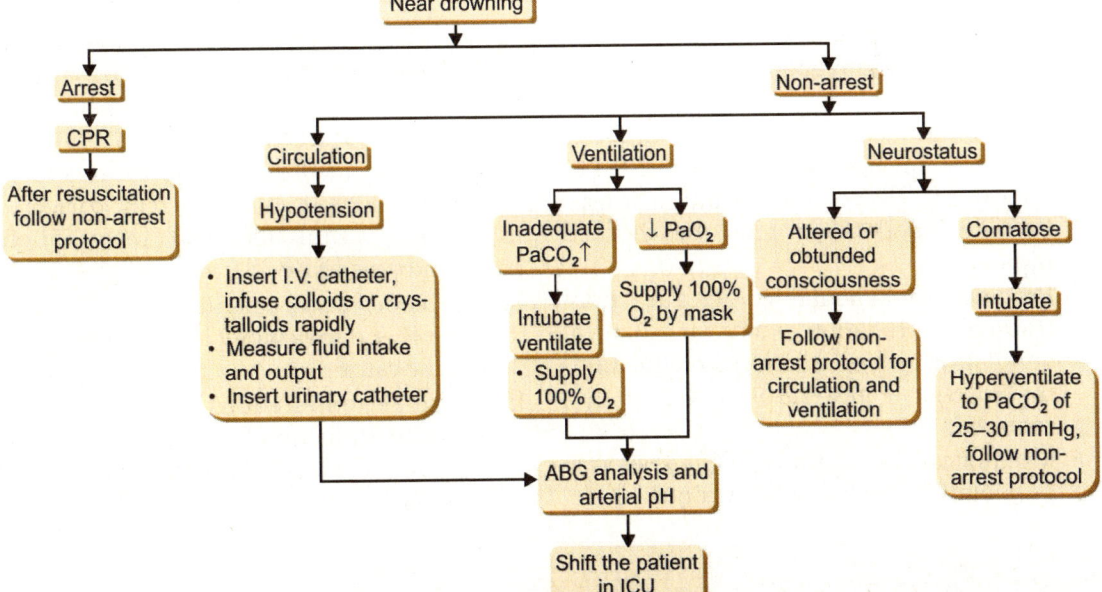

Fig. 100.2: Algorithm for a near drowned victim to be followed in order of priorities—Guidelines only; assume victim had normal arterial blood gas values (ABGs) before near drowning

2. ABC (airway, breathing and circulation) or CAB of cardiopulmonary resuscitation (CPR) must be instituted immediately, even in the water, if this does not danger the rescuer.

3. If the patient is unconscious, clean the oral cavity off debris or any foreign body and protect the airway as needed for endotracheal intubation and ventilatory support, if required subsequently.

4. Rescuer should not attempt to drain water from the victim's lung. The American Heart Association as well as Special Committee of Institute of Medicine (1994) have recommended that an abdominal thrust should not be used routinely in victims of submersion because of two reasons:

   i. It may lead to regurgitation of gastric contents into the lungs or aspiration of the vomitus.

   ii. It may further delay ventilatory and circulatory resuscitation.

   Therefore, abdominal thrust should only be used when the airway is obstructed with a foreign body or when victim fails to respond to mouth-to-mouth breathing.

5. Establish an intravenous line as early as possible.

6. Samples for arterial blood gas analysis should be taken to known the degree of hypoxemia, hypercapnia and acidosis. Bedside blood sugar must be checked rapidly.

7. Provide supplemental oxygen and endotracheal intubation and mechanical ventilation to overcome hypoxaemia until the blood gas analysis proves it is no longer required.

8. Monitor cardiac rhythm by ECG as soon as possible. Get cardiac markers done.

9. Monitor body temperature and restore it to normal.

10. If spontaneous breathing patient has persistent respiratory insufficiency, continuous positive airway (CPAP) breathing is useful in maintaining arterial oxygenation. Oxygen saturation should be maintained at 90% or higher. Positive end-expiratory pressure (PEEP) is also effective for treating respiratory insufficiency. Assisted ventilation may be necessary for pulmonary oedema, respiratory failure, aspiration, pneumonia and CNS injury. Bronchodilator may be used for bronchospasm. Antibiotics are not to be used prophylactically but if there is evidence of an infection, they may be prescribed. Patient should be monitored by serial chest X-rays and physical examination to detect atelectasis, pneumonitis and pulmonary oedema.

11. If patient has cardiovascular instability, evaluate cardiac output and effective circulatory volume by CVP/PCWP monitoring, and measure serum electrolytes. After adequate hydration, for low cardiac output use pressure agents and for pulmonary oedema, use diuretics.

12. Evaluate renal function (urinalysis, urea, creatinine) and cerebral status as indicated.

13. Metabolic acidosis which is invariably present is automatically get corrected through ventilation and oxygenation. Monitor lactate levels.

14. Get blood count, coagulation profile, and alcohol and toxicology levels done to find out the cause.

15. Residual complications of near drowning may include intellectual impairment, seizure disorder and pulmonary or cardiac disease.

Hanging and Strangulation

Definition

Hanging is a form of asphyxia produced by suspension of the body by a ligature around the neck which constricts the neck by the weight of the body (Fig. 101.1). In hanging, the ligature runs from the front above the thyroid cartilage symmetrically upwards on both sides of the neck to the back (occipital region).

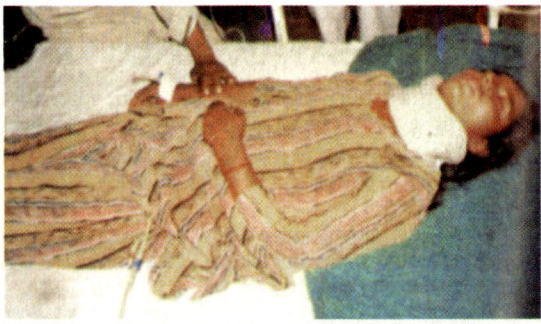

Fig. 101.2: Dislocation of cervical spine due to hanging for which neck collar has been applied

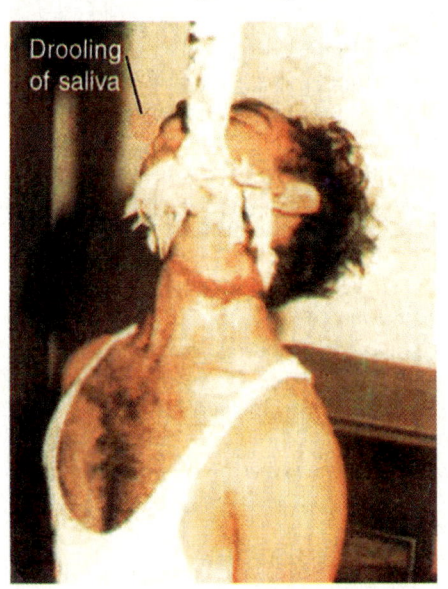

Fig. 101.1: Hanging

A ligature mark around the neck is diagnostic of hanging.

In partial hanging, the bodies are partially suspended; the toes or feet touching the ground or are in a sitting, kneeling, lying down prone or any other position. The weight of the head acts as constricting force instead of the body.

Strangulation: Strangulation is also a form of asphyxia similar to hanging caused by constriction of the neck by a ligature without suspending the body. The ligature is U-shaped pulled by the manual force around the front and back of neck and person stands behind the body. Strangulation can be attempted using both hands around the neck called throttling.

Ligature used: The ligature used include a rope, metallic chains, wire, leather strap or belt, bedsheet, scarf, dhoti, sari, turban, etc. It must be remembered that these cases are medicolegal cases, hence, every physician is duty-bound to complete the medicolegal formalities including medicolegal report (MLR). A doctor who examines the patient first of all should note the following:

1. Ligature used.
2. Ligature mark on the neck. One should note whether it corresponds to the material used for hanging.
3. One should ascertain the length and texture of the ligature and to verify whether it was sufficient to hang the victim.
4. Before removing the ligature; one should ascertain the width, nature and composition, mode of application and type of the knot used during hanging.

    Sometimes, the rope may break and becomes detached and the victim will be found lying on the ground with a ligature around the neck.

5. A suicidal note may be present at the site of hanging, if it is suicidal hanging. The note should be procured and handed over to the police.

Clinical Features

The symptoms and their pathogenesis are described in Table 101.1.

Diagnosis

It is based on:
 i. Ligation mark running around the neck, i.e. obliquely in hanging and transverse in strangulation.
 ii. Presence of abrasions, ecchymosis and redness around the ligation mark.
 iii. Dribbling or drooling of saliva from the angle of the mouth.
 iv. Ecchymoses of larynx or epiglottitis.
 v. Symptoms and signs of asphyxia.

Table 101.1 Symptoms of hanging and strangulation

Causes/mechanisms	Symptoms
1. **Stretching of neck** by constricting force	• The neck is elongated and head is turned to the side opposite to knot. • Pain in the neck due to fracture or dislocation of cervical vertebrae (Fig. 101.2).
2. **Cerebral anoxia** due to constriction of carotid arteries. Asphysia develops rapidly due to sudden compression of windpipe	• Face is pale. There is loss of power and sensory disturbances, such as flashes of light, ringing and hissing noises in the ears, mental confusion, disturbance in consciousness and convulsion. Death may occur rapidly as patient can do nothing to help himself or herself.
3. **Venous congestion** due to constriction of jugular veins and rise in venous pressure in the head	• Congestion of head and neck. When the constricting force is great, then face becomes puffy, oedematous, congested and cyanotic. • The eyes are wide open, bulging and suffused. The pupils are dilated. • The tongue is swollen, protruding and often bruised. • Patechial haemorrhages are common in the skin of eyelids, conjunctivae, face, forehead. • Bloody froth may escape from the mouth and nostrils. Bleeding may occur from the nose and ears. • The hands are clenched. • The genital organs may be congested and there may be discharge of urine, faeces and semen. *These asphyxial signs may be absent if death occurs quickly.*
• Stimulation of cervical sympathetic by the ligation knot. It may occur sometimes	• The pupil is dilated and the eye on the same side may remain open. It indicates antemortem hanging (*le facie sympatheique*).
• Increased salivation due to stimulation of salivary glands by the ligature	• Drooling of saliva from the angle of the month when the head is dropping forward.

Management

I. **Pre-hospital management:** When you witness a victim:

- Cut the ligature and remove it. Keep the ligature for inspection of forensic expert.
- Make the patient to lie flat with cervical spine supported.
- Loosen all his/her clothes and allows him/her to breath fresh air.
- If the patient is unresponsive, call for help and activate emergency medical services (phone and call for van).
- Start ABC of cardiopulmonary resuscitation.

II. **Treatment in the hospital**

- O_2 inhalation.
- Procure I.V. line and start glucose drip.
- Endotracheal intubation and breathing by ambu bag, if there is or has been respiratory arrest.
- Removal of secretions by intermittent suction.
- Continue rescue breathing.
- Complete the medicolegal formalities.
- Use anticonvulsants for control of convulsions. If convulsions not controlled by anticonvulsants, use midazolam, assisted ventilation and neuromuscular blockade.
- Use mannitol or I.V. steroids to reduce raised intracranial tension though its benefit is debatable.
- Take the emergency X-ray of the cervical spine and seek orthopedic consultation for any cervical injury. If necessary, a cervical collar may be used to support the cervical spine.

III. **Treatment in respiratory intensive care unit (RICU)**

- If there is respiratory difficulty or arrest or anoxic encephalopathy, shift the patient to RICU for respiratory support.
- Respiratory stimulants may be used.

Causes of Death

- Asphyxia.
- Venous congestion and raised cerebral venous pressure.
- Combined asphyxia and venous congestion.
- Reflex vagal inhibition.
- Fracture or dislocation of cervical vertebrae.

Complications

- Aspiration pneumonia.
- Pulmonary oedema.
- Infections.
- Oedema of larynx.
- Hypoxic encephalopathy. Cerebral infarction.
- Brain abscess.

Sequelae/After Effects

- Hemiplegia.
- Epileptiform convulsions.
- Amnesia (loss of memory).
- Dementia.
- Cervical cellulitis.
- Retropharyngeal abscess.
- Parotitis.
- Persistent coma.
- Cerebellar ataxia, myoclonus.
- Korsakoff's amnesic state.
- Choreoathetosis.

Emergencies Related to Acid–Base and Electrolyte Disturbance

Acid–Base Disturbance

METABOLIC ACIDOSIS

Metabolic acidosis is characterised by:
- Reduction in plasma HCO_3^-.
- Rise in H^+ ion and fall in pH.
- $PaCO_2$ is reduced secondarily by hyperventilation.

Metabolic acidosis is classified by the anion gap, either normal or increased (Table 102.1). The anion gap is the difference between readily measurable cation and anion. Normal anion gap is 12 ± 4 mEq/L.

Aetiology

The physiological disturbances that give rise to metabolic acidosis include either an addition of exogenous acids or there is failure of acid excretion leading to high anion-gap acidosis.

On the other hand, metabolic acidosis that results due to loss of HCO_3 results in normal anion gap. The disturbances leading to metabolic acidosis are given in Box 1. In most situations, metabolic acidosis is accompanied by sodium and water depletion.

Box 1 | Disturbances associated with metabolic acidosis

- Overproduction of acids other than H_2CO_3 by disordered metabolism
- Addition of exogenous acid (ingestion of acids)
- Failure to excrete acids other than H_2CO_3 at a rate equal to their generation
- Loss of bicarbonate in the urine or through GI tract

The first step is to identify whether acidosis is due to retention of HCl or to another acid. This is achieved by calculating the anion gap. The calculation of anion gap is simple as follows:
- The normal cations in plasma are Na^+, K^+, Ca^{++} and Mg^{++}.
- The normal anions in plasma are Cl^- and HCO_3^-, negative charges present on albumin, phosphate, sulphate, lactate and other organic acids.
- The sum of the positive and negative charges are equal.
- Measurement of Na^+, K^+, Cl^- and HCO_3^- are usually easily available.

Anion gap = (Unmeasured cations) − (Unmeasured anions).

Clinical tip: A useful mnemonic for causes of a raised anion gap recalls Kussmaul:

K for ketosis (diabetes, alcoholism, malnutrition)
U for uraemia
SS for salicylate poisoning M for methanol poisoning
A for ethylene (formerly spelt as ethylene glycol poisoning)
U for uraemia
L for lactic acidosis

Normal Anion Gap Acidosis

Renal Tubular Acidosis (RTA)

It includes a group of conditions characterised by hypercholeraemic metabolic acidosis. Any

Table 102.1   Differential diagnosis of metabolic acidosis

Mechanisms	Conditions	Accumulating acid
I. High anion gap metabolic acidosis		
i. Addition of excessive acids to extracellular fluid		
a. Organic acids (metabolic anions)	• Ketoacidosis, e.g. diabetes, alcoholism and starvation • Lactic acidosis	• Acetoacetic acid • β-hydroxybutyric • Lactic acid
b. Poisoning (drugs or chemical anion)	• Methanol poisoning • Ethylene glycol poisoning • Salicylate poisoning	• Formic acid • Glycolic and oxalic • Salicylic and lactic acid
ii. Failure to excrete acid at a normal rate		
• Decreased GFR and inadequate renal NH_4 production	• Acute on chronic renal failure	• Sulphuric, phosphoric and hydrochloric acid
II. Normal anion gap metabolic acidosis		
i. Loss of bicarbonate		
• In urine	• Proximal renal tubular defect • Acetazolamide • Hyperparathyroidism • Tubular damage due to drugs heavy metals	• Hydrochloric acid • Hydrochloric acid
• From gastrointestinal tract	• Diarrhoea, fistulae, ileostomy and ureterosigmoidostomy	• Hydrochloric acid
ii. Failure to excrete acid at a normal rate		
• Failure of the distal tubular H^+ secretory system	• Distal renal tubular acidosis	• Hydrochloric acid

condition affecting tubular function can lead to RTA. Three variants are described:

1. **Proximal hypokalaemic RTA (former type II)** is caused by failure of sodium biocarbonate reabsorption in the proximal tubule. It is characterized by acidosis, hypokalaemia, an inability to lower the pH of urine below 5.5 despite systemic acidosis and bicarbonate loss in urine.

2. **Distal hypokalaemic RTA (former type I)** is due to failure of H^+ excretion in the tubule. It is characterised by acidosis, hypokalaemia, inability to lower urinary pH less than 5.5 despite systemic acidosis and low urinary ammonium production.

3. **Distal hyperkalaemic RTA (fromer type IV)** is caused by defective hydrogen ion secretion. There is hyporeninaemia and hypoaldosteronism. It is characterised by hyperkalaemia, acidosis in a patient with

mild chronic renal insufficiency usually caused by tubulointerstial disease.

Increased Anion Gap Metabolic Acidosis

1. **Lactic acidosis:** One of the most common types of metabolic acidosis is lactic acidosis in which lactic acid production from pyruvate in the muscle, skin, brain and RBCs exceeds its removal by the liver and kidneys. The causes of lactic acidosis (types A and B) are given in Box 2.

2. **Diabetic ketoacidosis** (read it as an emergency).

Clinical Features of Metabolic Acidosis

1. **Respiratory manifestations:** Severe metabolic acidosis usually manifests with stimulation of respiration leading to hyperventilation (Kussmaul's respiration), respiratory distress and air hunger.

Box 2 Causes of lactic acidosis	
Type A	*Type B*
Conditions associated with tissue hypoxia	*Impaired mitochondrial function*
• Shock due to any cause (septic shock is the most common) • Respiratory failure • Carbon monoxide and cyanide poisoning • Severe anaemia	• Diabetes mellitus • Hepatic failure • Severe infection • Drugs (metformin, isoniazid, salicylates) • Toxins (ethanol, methanol) • Congenital enzyme defects

2. **Cardiovascular features:** Severe acidosis may lead to myocardial depression resulting in reduced cardiac output, fatigue and hypotension. Cardiac arrhythmias may occur.
3. **Cerebral features:** There may be confusion, drowsiness and fits.
4. **Miscellaneous features:** Insulin resistance, hyperkalaemia and increased protein catabolism.
5. **Features of underlying disorder:** In many cases, features of underlying disorder and presence of sodium and water depletion may dominate.

Laboratory Findings

- Blood pH, serum bicarbonate and $PaCO_2$ are decreased
- Anion gap may be normal (hyperchloremic) or increased (normochloremic)
- Serum potassium levels are high.

Management

A. **Increased anion gap acidosis:** Treatment is directed at the underlying cause such as insulin and fluid therapy for diabetic ketoacidosis (read diabetic ketoacidosis as an emergency). Volume resuscitation should be done to restore tissue perfusion. Supplemental HCO_3 is indicated for hyperkalaemia and some forms of normal anion gap acidosis but has been controversial for treatment of increased anion gap acidosis.

In addition, alkali ($NaHCO_3$) administration exacerbates lactic acidosis via enhanced lactate production. Ketogenesis is also augmented by alkali therapy.

In salicylate poisoning, alkali, therapy must be started unless blood pH is already alkaline by respiratory alkalosis (hyperventilation). In alcoholic ketoacidosis, thiamine (B_1) should be given with glucose to avoid Wernicke encephalopathy. In methanol poisoning, ethanol may be used. In renal failure, $NaHCO_3$ may be required.

$$HCO_3^- \text{ deficit} = 0.5 \times \text{body wt(kg)} \times (24 - HCO_3^-)$$

Half of the calculated deficit should be administered within first 3–4 hours.

B. **Normal anion gap acidosis:** Treatment of renal tubular acidosis (RTA) is mainly administration of alkali 10–15 mEq/kg/day either as bicarbonate or citrate. Sodium and potassium salts of bicarbonate are preferred. Potassium supplementation may be necessary if hypokalaemia develops.

In type IV RTA, dietary potassium and potassium retaining drugs should be withheld. In some cases, alkali supplementation (1–3 mEq/kg/day) may be required.

METABOLIC ALKALOSIS

It is characterised by an increase in plasma bicarbonate ($HCO_3^- > 25$ mmol/L) and pH (>7.40).

It is less common than metabolic acidosis. It is usually a response to an HCl, KCl and NaCl deficit. In health, when plasma (HCO_3^-) rises above normal, urinary excretion of (HCO_3^-) increases rapidly. It is, therefore, very unusual to observe metabolic alkalosis in the presence of normal renal function.

Aetiology and Pathogenic Mechanism

A number of factors stimulate bicarbonate reabsorption and hydrogen ion secretion because of altered renal function (Box 3).

Box 3 Conditions which sustain metabolic alkalosis

1. Strong stimulus to reabsorb sodium (i.e. hypovolaemia) particularly in the presence of low plasma chloride
2. Increased (H^+) ion secretion by renal tubules
   - Increased delivery of Na^+ to distal tubule (e.g. loop diuretics)
   - High $PaCO_2$ due to chronic respiratory failure
   - Potassium depletion
   - Excess mineralocorticoids

There are important relationship between tubular handling of Na+, K+ and H+ ions. In the distal tubule where there is final composition of urine, reabsorption of Na+ generates an electromechanical gradient which derives both K+ and H+ ions from the tubular cells into the lumen. Thus, if kidneys are avidly retaining sodium due to any cause (aldosterone and other mineralocorticoids), it cannot retain K+ and H+ ion. If the intracellular K+ concentration is already low because of K+ depletion, there is obligatory rise in secretion of H+ ions.

Sodium is reabsorbed from nephron either with chloride or with bicarbonate. If chloride is deficient, then there is preferential reabsorption of bicarbonate which will worsen the alkalosis and will prevent the additional excretion of bicarbonate by the distal tubule which is necessary to correct an established metabolic alkalosis.

The causes of metabolic alkalosis given in Table 102.2, are divided into saline-response and saline unresponsive alkalosis. Saline-responsive metabolic alkalosis is characterised by normotension, extracellular fluid depletion. Hypotension may also be seen. Vomiting and nasogastric aspiration initiates alkalosis.

Saline-unresponsive metabolic alkalosis is characterised by excessive total body bicarbonate with either normovolemia or hypervolemia.

The classical pradigm sustaining metabolic alkalosis due to vomiting and administration diuretics is presented in Fig. 102.1.

Table 102.2 Common causes of metabolic alkalosis

I. Saline-responsive (normotensive extracellular volume contraction and hypokalemia)

A. Excessive body bicarbonate content
  i. Renal alkalosis
     - Diuretic therapy
     - Drugs, e.g. carbenicillin, penicillin, sulphate, phosphate
     - Posthypercapnia
  ii. Gastrointestinal alkalosis
     - Vomiting or nasogastric aspirations
     - Diarrhoea (chloride loss)
     - Sodium citrate, lactate, gluconate, acetate
     - Transfusions
     - Antacids
B. Normal body bicarbonate content
  - Contraction alkalosis

II. Saline-unresponsive (normotensive or hypertensive normovolaemia or hypervolaemia)

A. Excessive body bicarbonate content
  i. Normotensive
     - Severe potassium depletion
     - Bartter syndrome
     - Refeeding alkalosis
     - Hypercalcemic and hypoparathyroidism
  ii. Hypertensive
     - Hyper-reninism, primary aldosteronism
     - Liddle syndrome
     - Exogenous alkali
     - Exogenous mineralocorticoids
     - Liquorice use

Clinical Features

Patients of metabolic alkalosis may be asymptomatic or may complain of symptoms related to volume depletion or hypokalaemia.

1. **Symptoms due to volume contraction/depletion:** Weakness, muscle cramps and postural dizziness.
2. **Symptoms due to hypokalaemia:** Polyuria, polydipsia and muscle weakness
3. **Symptoms of cerebral dysfunction:** Altered mental status, apathy, confusion and drowsiness.
4. **Acute alkalosis:** Acute severe alkalosis may cause:
   - Respiratory depression.

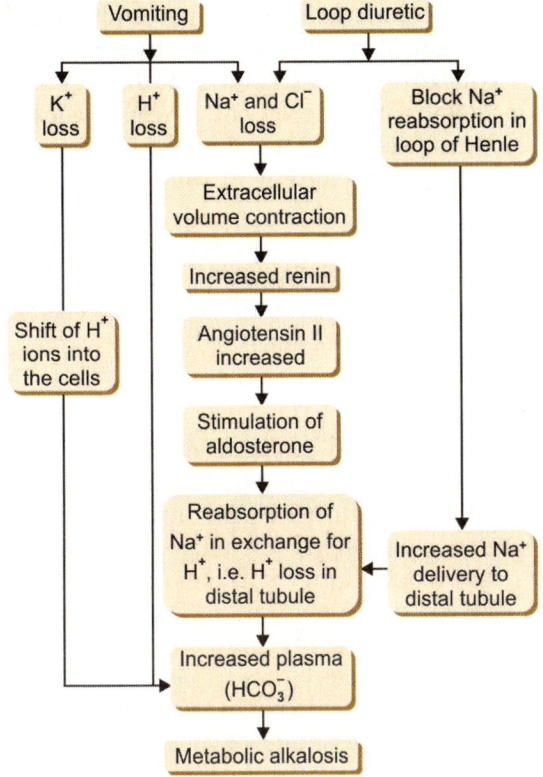

Fig. 102.1: Schematic representation of pathogenesis of saline-responsive metabolic alkalosis. Vomiting or loop diuretic initiates the process

- Cardiac arrhythmias (supraventricular or ventricular).
- Tetany due to lowered ionised calcium (Trousseau's sign positive).

5. **Severe long-standing alkalosis** may be associated with reduced renal function and uraemia.

Investigations

- Arterial pH and bicarbonate are elevated
- Serum potassium and chloride are decreased. They may be increased anion gap.
- Urine chloride can differentiate between saline response (<25 mEq/L) and unresponsive (>40 mEq/L) metabolic alkalosis.

Management

1. Mild to moderate alkalosis may not require any treatment.

2. **Treatment of saline-responsive metabolic alkalosis:** In patients without renal disease, restoration of ECF (extracellular fluid) volume and the plasma chloride and K⁺ concentration will remove the stimulus to renal (H⁺) secretion and allow renal excretion of excess bicarbonate. In patients who have lost gastric contents, e.g. in pyloric outlet obstruction, should be replaced with isotonic (0.9%), NaCl solution (3–6 litres/day) and sufficient KCl to restore K⁺ deficit (40–60 mmol/day). Patients who are on continuous gastric aspiration should also have the volume of aspirate replaced by I.V. infusion of an equal amount of isotonic saline solution containing KCl (20 mmol/L). Alkalosis associated with K⁺ deficiency is corrected by stopping the diuretics (potassium losing) and administration of sufficient KCl to restore body K⁺ to normal.

3. **Treatment of saline-unresponsive metabolic alkalosis:** The cases, termed saline-resistant are associated with marked K⁺ deficits (>1000 mmol), Mg⁺⁺ deficiency such as, Batter's syndrome, or primary hypermineralocorticoid states. Therapy in these cases must be directed toward the underlying pathophysiological problem. It includes removal of a mineralo-corticoid producing tumor or blockage of aldosterone effect with ACE inhibitor or spironolactone. Primary hyperaldosteronism is treated by K⁺ therapy.

4. **Treatment of severe alkalosis:** If associated conditions preclude infusion of saline or alkalosis is severe (pH >7.55), HCO₃⁻ loss can be accelerated by use of acetazolamide (250–500 mg orally or I.V.). Dilute HCl (0.1 N) or NH₄Cl may be used as acidifying agent. If renal function is impaired, haemo-dialysis against dialysate low in (HCO₃⁻) and high in (Cl⁻) can be effective.

RESPIRATORY ACIDOSIS

Respiratory acidosis results when the effective alveolar ventilation fails to keep pace with the rate of CO_2 production. As a result, there is retention of CO_2 leading to rise in $PaCO_2$ and H^+ ion, and of HCO_3^-.

Predicted Physiological Response

1. In acute respiratory acidosis, the plasma HCO_3^- will rise by 1 nmol/L with 10 mm rise in $PaCO_2$.
2. In chronic respiratory acidosis, the plasma HCO_3^- will rise by 4 nmol/L with 10 mmHg rise in $PaCO_2$.

The kidneys respond by increased H^+ secretion, so that urine becomes acidic and bicarbonate is added to the blood. The distinction between respiratory acidosis and metabolic alkalosis can be made by the fact that urine (H^+) ion is characteristically raised in respiratory acidosis and reduced in metabolic alkalosis. A chronically raised $PaCO_2$ is compensated by renal retention of HCO_3^- and the (H^+) ion returns to normal. A constant arterial HCO_3^- concentration then usually becomes established within 5 days. This represents primary respiratory acidosis with compensatory metabolic alkalosis.

Causes

Respiratory acidosis results due to hypoventilation as a result of severe pulmonary disease, respiratory muscle fatigue, or abnormalities in ventilatory control (depression of medullary respiratory centre) and is due to the increase in $PaCO_2$. The causes are enumerated in Table 102.3.

Clinical Features

The clinical features vary according to severity and duration of the respiratory acidosis, the underlying disease, and whether there is accompanying hypoxaemia.

1. A rapid rise in $PaCO_2$ (acute hypercapnia) may cause anxiety, dyspnoea, confusion, psychosis and hallucinations and may progress to coma called acute hypercapnic encephalopathy.
2. Lesser and slowly rising $PaCO_2$ (chronic hypercapnia) leads to sleep disturbances, loss of memory, daytime somnolence, personality changes, impairment of coordination and motor disturbances such as flapping tremors and myoclonic jerks. Headache and signs of raised intracranial pressure including papilloedema may occur.
3. Cardiovascular effects of respiratory acidosis include increased cardiac output, normal or increased BP, warm skin, bounding pulse and diaphoresis.

Investigations

1. Arterial blood gas analysis shows rise in $PaCO_2$ and H^+ ions with fall in blood pH.
2. Pulmonary function tests include spirometry, diffusion capacity for carbon monoxide, lung volumes and arterial $PaCO_2$ and O_2 saturation. These tests help to determine if respiratory acidosis is due to lung disease.
3. Non-pulmonary causes need appropriate tests for assessment of chest wall, pleura and neuromuscular functions.
4. Measurement of haematocrit in each and every case.

Management

1. **Acute respiratory acidosis:** It can be life-threatening and measures to reverse the underlying cause should be undertaken simultaneously with restoration of adequate alveolar ventilation. These are:
   - Prompt removal of underlying cause.
   - Establish patent airway.
   - Administer O_2 carefully which should be titrated in patients of COPD with CO_2 retention. O_2 can be given at 6 L/min if $PaCO_2$ is less than 65 mmHg.
   - Improvement of pulmonary functions by using bronchodilators, clearing of bronchial secretions, treatment of infection and avoiding fluid overload.
   - When patient is in coma or has extreme hypercapnoea ($PaCO_2$ >80 mmHg) or severe acidosis (pH <7.1) tracheal

intubation with assisted ventilation may be needed. If opiate overdose is the cause, give I.V. naloxone.

2. **Chronic respiratory acidosis:** It is frequently difficult to correct as one can rarely remove the underlying cause. Measures taken are aimed at improving lung functions such as cessation of smoking, use of O_2, bronchodilator, gluco corticoids, diuretics and controlling infection. Excessive O_2 and sedatives are to be avoided. Acute exacerbation of chronic hypercapnia may need mechanical ventilation.

RESPIRATORY ALKALOSIS

Respiratory alkalosis occurs when alveolar hyperventilation results in excessive loss of CO_2 (fall in $PaCO_2$) and fall in H^+ ion and rise in pH.

Predicted physiological response

1. In acute respiratory alkalosis, HCO_3^- will fall by 2 mmol/L with 10 mm fall in $PaCO_2$.

2. In chronic respiratory alkalosis, HCO_3^- will fall by 4 mmol/L with 10 mmHg fall in $PaCO_2$.

Causes

The causes are given in Box 4.

Clinical Features

They are due to hyperventilation and hypoxaemia. Paraesthesias, circumoral numbness, chest wall tightness or pain, light-headedness, dizziness, inability to take an adequate breath and rarely tetany or convulsions may occur. In digitalised patients, cardiac arrhythmias and cardiac arrest may occur.

Investigations

1. Arterial blood gas analysis demonstrates an acute or chronic rise in pH, often with hypocapnia, e.g. $PaCO_2$ in the range of 15 to 30 mmHg and no hypoxaemia. Arterial pH is high.

Table 102.3 Causes of respiratory acidosis (acute and chronic)

	Acute	Chronic
1. *Depression of respiratory centre in medulla, i.e. ventilatory control*	• Drugs, e.g. opiates, anaesthetics, sedatives • Cardiac arrest • Stroke • Central sleep apnoea • Infection	• Extreme obesity (pickwickian syndrome) • CNS lesion (rare)
2. *Diseases of chest wall and respiratory muscles*	• Myasthenic crisis • Guillain-Barré syndrome • Severe hypokalaemia • Drugs, e.g. aminoglycosides, organophosphorus compound, curare succinylcholine • Periodic paralysis	• Poliomyelitis • Multiple sclerosis • Amyotrophic lateal sclerosis • Diaphragmatic paralysis • Scoliosis • Myxoedema • Thymoma
3. *Airway obstruction*	• Asthma • Aspiration of foreign body or vomitus • Obstructive apnoea • Laryngospasm	• Tonsillar hypertrophy • Paralysis of vocal cords • Aortic aneurysm
4. *Disorders of lung parenchyma*	• Severe asthma or pneumonia • Acute exacerbation of chronic lung disease • Pneumothorax • ARDS • Acute cardiogenic pulmonary oedema	• COPD • Pulmonary emphysema • Interstitial fibrosis
5. *Mechanical ventilation*	• Improperly adjusted and not supervised	• Large increase in alveolar dead space

Box 4	Common causes of respiratory alkalosis

1. Hypoxia due to acute attack of bronchial asthma pulmonary oedema, pulmonary embolism and acute circulatory failure. Chronic hypoxia occur in cyanotic heart disease, high altitude and pulmonary fibrosis.
2. CNS disorders (e.g. CVA, brain tumour, encephalitis).
3. Pregnancy
4. Gram-negative septicaemia or endotoxaemia.
5. Hepatic failure
6. Drugs, e.g. salicylate and xanthine poisoning.
7. Anxiety-induced hyperventilation
8. Pain
9. Excessive mechanical ventilation

2. The plasma (K^+) is often reduced and the (Cl^-) increased. In acute hyperventilation syndrome, ionised calcium level may be reduced.
3. In chronic respiratory acidosis and alkalosis, the kidneys return H^+ towards normal by transiently increasing or decreasing the rate of NH_4^+ excretion and thereby increasing the plasma HCO_3^- in chronic respiratory acidosis or decreasing the plasma HCO_3^- in chronic respiratory alkalosis.

Management

When diagnosis of respiratory alkalosis is made, its cause should be investigated. The diagnosis of hyperventilation syndrome (common cause) is made by exclusion. In difficult cases, it may be important to rule out other conditions such as pulmonary embolism, coronary artery disease and hyperthyroidism.

The treatment of respiratory alkalosis is directed towards the alleviation of the underlying cause. If respiratory alkalosis complicates ventilator management, changes in dead space, tidal volume, and frequency can minimize the hypocapnia. In chronic respiratory alkalosis, measures to treat respiratory alkalosis itself are generally not required.

In patients with anxiety-hyperventilation syndromes, reassurance of the patient or sedation, or sometime rebreathing into a closed system (a paper bag) during symptomatic attacks and attention to underlying psychological stress may be beneficial. Antidepressants are not recommended. Beta blockers may ameliorate the anxiety-induced hyperadrenergic state.

In severe alkalaemia, along with the treatment of primary disorder, skeletal muscle paralysis and assisted mechanical ventilation may be required.

Hypokalaemia, a common accompaniment must be corrected.

MIXED ACID-BASE DISORDERS

Definitions

Mixed acid–base disorders are defined as independently coexisting disorders (Table 102.4), not merely compensated responses, are often seen in critically ill patients in critical care units. The diagnosis of mixed disorder should be considered in the clinical context.

Mixed respiratory and metabolic acidosis or mixed respiratory and metabolic alkalosis can

Table 102.4	Common causes of mixed acid-base disorders

1. **Metabolic acidosis and respiratory acidosis (common)**
   - Cardiopulmonary arrest
   - Severe pulmonary oedema
   - Sedative and salicylate poisoning
   - Pulmonary disease with renal failure or sepsis
2. **Metabolic acidosis with respiratory alkalosis**
   - Salicylate overdose
   - Recent alcoholic binge
   - Combined hepatic and renal insufficiency
3. **Metabolic alkalosis with respiratory alkalosis**
   - Chronic respiratory disease with diuretic therapy, steroid therapy, severe vomiting, reduction of hypercapnia by ventilation
4. **Metabolic acidosis and metabolic alkalosis**
   - Severe vomiting in patients with underlying renal failure, diabetic ketoacidosis and alcoholic ketoacidosis

lead to dangerous extremes of pH. A patient first of all may have simple acid-base disturbance due to underlying cause, develops second acid-base disorder as a result of complication. For example, a patient with diabetic ketoacidosis (metabolic acidosis) may develop a respiratory problem leading to respiratory acidosis or alkalosis.

When metabolic acidosis and metabolic alkalosis coexist in the same patient, the pH may be normal or near normal. When the pH is normal, an elevated anion gap denotes the presence of a metabolic acidosis. A diabetic patient with ketoacidosis may develop metabolic acidosis due to renal dysfunction.

Management

Management involves the treatments described above for each element of the disturbance.

Disorders of Sodium Balance

HYPONATRAEMIA

Definition

A plasma Na⁺ concentration less than 135 mEq/L is called *hyponatraemia*. Acute symptomatic *hyponotraemia* is a medical emergency. Acute severe *hyponatraemia* is often iatrogenic (excess hypotonic fluid infusion in postoperative patient), or exercise induced or use of recreational drugs molly and ecstasy.

The hyponatraemia is almost always due to disturbance in water metabolism, i.e. water imbalance or abnormal water handling not sodium imbalance indicating the primary role of ADH in pathophysiology of hyponatraemia.

Isotonic hyponatraemia or spurious or pseudo-hyponatraemia: The plasma osmolality remains normal. The Na⁺ ion concentration measured by Na⁺-sensitive glass electrode remains normal. This type of hyponatraemia is of little significance, needs evaluation of the underlying cause such as hyperproteinaemia and hyperlipidaernia.

Classification

Depending on the serum osmolality, hypona-traemia causes isotonic, hypotonic and hyper-tonic (Fig. 103.1). Hypotonic hyponatraemia

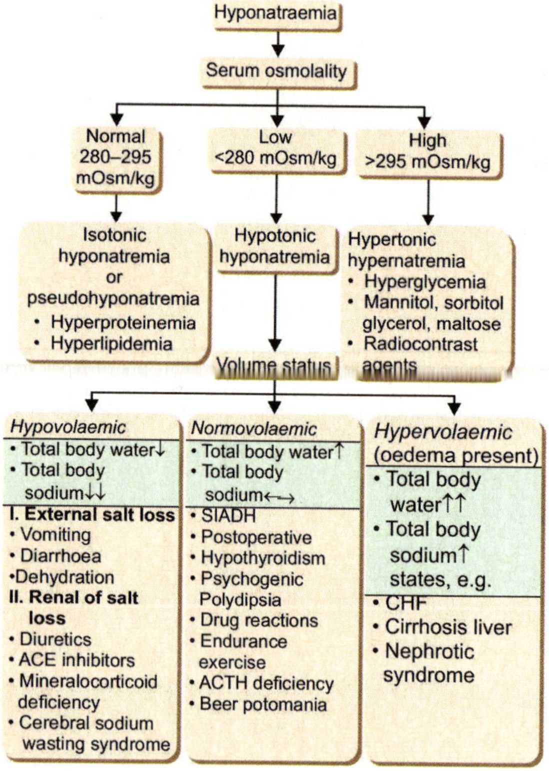

---

* Serum osmolality $= (2 \times Na) + \dfrac{BUN}{2.8} + \dfrac{Blood\ sugar}{18}$

Fig. 103.1: Classification of hyponatraemia based on serum osmolality* and fluid volume status

depending on blood volume status is further classified into hypovolaemic, normovolaemic and hypervolaemic.

Hypotonic or dilutional hyponatraemia may complicate transuretheral resection of the prostate or bladder because large volumes of iso-osmotic (mannitol) or hypo-osmotic (sorbitol or glycine) bladder irrigation solution can be absorbed resulting in dilutional hyponatraemia. The metabolism of absorbed sorbitol or glycine to CO_2 and water may lead to hypotonicity of the accumulated fluid and solutes are not rapidly excreted.

Hypertonic hyponatraemia: It is characterised by increased plasma osmolality, is seen in hyperglycaemia and intravenous administration of mannitol. This is due to the fact that, during uncontrolled or poorly controlled diabetes, the glucose being an effective osmole draws water from the muscle cells resulting in hyponatraemia. Plasma Na^+ concentration falls by 1.4 mmol/L for every 100 mg/dl rise in plasma glucose.

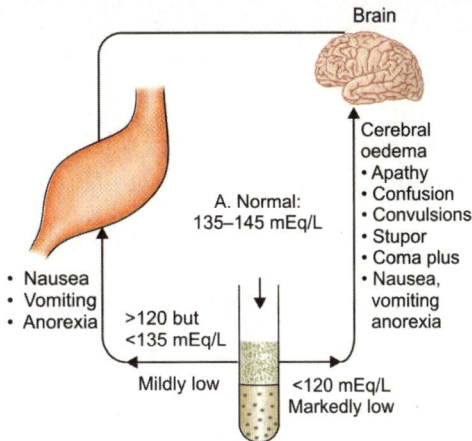

Fig. 103.2: Clinical effects of hyponatraemia

CLASSIFICATION, CAUSES AND CLINICAL FEATURES

The causes of hyponatraemia are given in Table 103.1 along with clinical features and respective treatment.

Clinical Features

Clinical features depend on rate of change and severity of hyponatraemia.
1. At plasma sodium level above 120 mEq/L gastrointestinal manifestations occur (Fig. 103.2)
2. At plasma sodium concentration below 120 mEq/L, neurological manifestations will occur in addition to GI manifestations (Fig. 103.2)

Investigations

1. **Plasma osmolality:** Most patients with hyponatraemia have low plasma osmolality (<275 mOsm/kg). If plasma osmolality is normal with hyponatraemia, then pseudohyponatraemia must be ruled out.
2. **Urine osmolality:** Urine osmolality and specific gravity of less than 100 mOsm/kg

and 1.003, respectively occurs in patients with primary polydipsia. If this is not low, then ADH release due to pain, nausea, drugs or physiological response to haemodynamic stimuli may be suspected or it may be SIADH.

3. **Urine Na^+ concentration:** Volume depletion (hypovolaemia) with normal renal functions results in a urine concentration of Na^+ less than 20 mmol/L due to extrarenal losses i.e. vomiting, diarrhoea, burns, trauma, pancreatitis, etc. because Na^+ is reabsorbed from the tubules. The finding of a urine Na^+ concentration greater than 20 mmol/L indicates a salt-wasting nephropathy, diuretic therapy, hypoaldosteronism or occasionally vomiting.

4. **Serum sodium levels:** Low levels less than 135 mEq/L indicate hyponatraemia irrespective of its cause.

Management (Read Table 103.1 Also)

Regardless of the patient volume status, restrict free water and hypotonic fluid intake to less than 1 to 1.5 L/day.

Hypovolaemic hyponatremic patients require adequate fluid resuscitation by isotonic fluids (either normal saline or Ringer lactate solution).

Table 103.1   Pattern of hyponatraemia its causes, clinical features and management

Disturbance	Causes	Clinical features	Management
1. Hypovolaemic, hypotonic hyponatraemia (Fig. 103.1)	i. Extra-renal • Vomiting • Diarrhoea • Burns • Sweating • Pancreatitis ii. Renal-loses • Excess of diuretics, ACE inhibitor • Osmotic diuresis (e.g. hyperglycaemia, tubulo-interstitial disease • Salt-wasting nephropathy • Hypoaldosteronism	i. Low jugular/central venous pressure ii. Feaures of ECF depletion • Thirst • Concentrated urine • Dizziness, weakness, oliguria • Postural, hypotension • Apathy, confusion • Tachycardia • Cold extremities • Redued skin turgor	• Volume replacement with isotonic saline—normal saline • If severe, use colloid initially • Avoid excess water intake
2. Normovolaemic hypotonic hyponatraemia (Fig. 103.1)	iii. Cerebral salt wasting • Psychogenic water drinking • Iatrogenic water excess, i.e. I.V. dextrose solution, postoperative • Hypothyroidism • Drug idiosyncracy • SIADH (dilutional hyponatraemia) • Beer potomania	• Normal JVP • No signs of ECF depletion or excess	• Water restriction (e.g. 500 ml/day) • Severe cases may require hypertonic saline with extreme care and expert advice
3. Hypervolemic hypotonic hyponatraemia (Fig. 103.1)	Odematous states such as: • CHF • Nephrotic syndrome • Liver cell failure • Renal failure	• There is pitting oedema of face, extremities • JVP is raised in CHF and renal failure • Other features of cardiac, renal and liver disease	• Diuretic therapy • Salt restriction

Patients with cerebral salt wasting may require hypertonic saline or fludrocortisone.

Hypervolemic patients may require loop diuretics or dialysis or both, while normovolemic hyponatremic patients respond to free water restriction alone.

Pseudohyponatraemia does not require any therapy.

Symptomatic and severe hyponatraemia requires hospitalisation for careful monitoring of weight, fluid balance, sodium estimation and treatment. Inciting medications should be stopped.

There is no concensus about optimal rate of sodium correction in symptomatic hyponatraemia patients but 10–12 mEq/L/day is reasonable in mild to moderate hyponatrernic patients. A more aggressive rate can be employed in severely symptomatic patients. Sodium levels must be monitored during saline therapy because overcorrection can lead to volume overload and pulmonary oedema.

In severely symptomatic patients, sodium deficit should be calculated and 3% hypertonic saline at an appropriate rate may be given (a rate of 0.5 ml/kg/hr). Sodium should be continuously monitored.

For patients who cannot restrict free water or have an inadequate response to conservative measures, demeclocyline (350–600 mg orally twice a day) is recommended for inhibiting ADH response.

Vasopressin antagonists: They have revolutionised the treatment of normo and hypervolemic hyponatraemia. Lixivaptan, tolvaptan and satavaptan are oral selective vasopressin-2 receptors antagonists. The V2 receptors mediate the diuretic effect of ADH. For patients with normovolemia SIADH, conivapton infusion may be given, but these drugs are not available in India.

SYNDROME OF INAPPROPRIATE SECRETION OF ADH (SIADH)

Definition

It is characterised by a defect in osmoregulation of ADH (vasopressin) from posterior pituitary. Nonnally, water overload, hyponatraemia and a low plasma osmolality would suppress ADH and produce a very dilute urine, but in this syndrome, all these factors cannot suppress ADH, hence, there is inappropriate or persistent secretion of ADH either from posterior pituitary, or there is ectopic produc tion of ADH by a tumour. The presence of ADH leads to inappropriate concentration of the urine (urine osmolality above that of plasma) and retention of water (i.e. there is normovolemia). Serum urea concentration is often low because of dilution by retention of water.

Causes

The causes of SIADH are listed in Table 103.2.

Clinical Features

They are same as discussed under hypona-traemia.

Table 103.2 Causes of inappropriate secretion of ADH (SIADH)

1. **CNS disorders**
   - Meningitis
   - Encephalitis
   - Brain abscess
   - Brain tumour
   - Delirium tremens, psychosis
   - CVA (stroke)
   - Hydrocephalus
   - Head trauma
   - Guillain-Barré syndrome

2. **Pulmonary disorders**
   - Pneumonias (viral or bacterial)
   - Lung abscess, bronchiectasis
   - Tuberculosis
   - Cystic fibrosis

3. **Neoplasm**
   - Carcinoma of bronchus (small cell), pancreas, duodenum, urinary tract, lymphoma, thymoma and mesothelioma

4. **Drug-induced**
   i. *Hypoglycaemics*, e.g. chlorpropamide, tolbutamide
   ii. *Antidepressants*, e.g. amitriptyline, fluoxetine
   iii. *Major tranquillisers*, e.g. haloperidol, fluphenazine
   iv. *Anti-epileptics*, e.g. carbamazepine
   v. *Chemotherapeutic drugs*, e.g. cyclopho-sphamide, vincristine, vinblastine
   vi. *Thiazide diuretics*, e.g. hydrochlorthiazide
   vii. *Opiates,* e.g. morphine
   viii. *NSAIDs*

5. **Miscellaneous**
   - Pain, stress
   - Severe nausea
   - Postoperative period
   - Pregnancy

Diagnosis

The diagnosis is based on the fact that the patients with SIADH have normovolaemia with hyponatraemia (dilutional hypona-traemia) (dilutional hyponatracemia) and there is no evidence of cardiac, renal, hepatic and endocrinal cause to explain impaired water excretion. The diagnostic criteria are depicted in Box 1 and an approach to diagnosis is illustrated in Fig. 103.3.

Management

1. Restriction of fluid intake to 800 to 1000ml/day. Since this fluid intake is always less than urinary output plus insensible

Box 1   Diagnostic criteria for SIADH
1. Essential
• Plasma osmolality low, i.e. less than 280 mOsm/ kg H₂O (normal is >280 mOsm/kg)
• Plasma urea low (<10 mg/dl (normal 20–40 mg/ dl)
• Uric acid level is low (<4 mg/dl)
• Plasma sodium low, i.e. about 124 mmol/L (normal 135–145 mmol/L)
• Urine osmolality is higher than plasma, i.e. about 430 mOsm/kg (should be <150 mOsm/kg in face of low plasma osmolality)
• Elevated urinary sodium excretion >20 mEq/L
• Clinical normovolaemia
• Absence of endocrinal (thyroid, adrenal), renal, hepatic and cardiac failure
2. Supplemental
• Abnormal water load test. Patient is unable to excrete at least 90% of a 20 ml/kg water load in 4 hours and/or failure to dilute urine osmolality to <100 mOsm/kg
• Plasma vasopressin (ADH) levels are elevated inappropriate to the plasma osmolality
• Improvement of plasma Na⁺ levels with fluid restriction

fluid loss, a negative water balance ensues that results in gradual daily reduction in weight, a progressive rise in serum Na⁺ concentration and osmolality, and symptomatic improvement. Fluid restriction to be continued until serum Na⁺ exceeds 135 mmol/L.

2. The underlying cause should be corrected wherever possible. Fluid restriction to be continued until the cause is corrected.

> *Plasma osmolality, serum Na⁺ and body weight should be monitored daily or frequently until serum Na⁺ exceeds 135 mmol/L*

3. If water restriction is poorly tolerated or ineffective, demeclocycline—a potent inhibitor of ADH, may be given in doses of 900–1200 mg/day. Patient receiving demeclocycline should be followed carefully to detect any evidence of renal failure, bacterial superinfection, or excessive drug-induced water loss.

4. When syndrome is very severe, hypertonic saline (300 ml of 3 or 5% sodium chloride) should be infused intravenously over 3–4 hours. To avoid the possibility of inducing central pontine myelinolysis, the serum sodium concentration should not be raised too rapidly. Frusemide may be used along with it to reduce the chances of congestive heart failure state.

5. Vasopressin antagonist (conivaptan, lixivaptan and tolvaptan) inhibit the diuretic effect of ADH hence are useful in SIADH syndrome but are still not available.

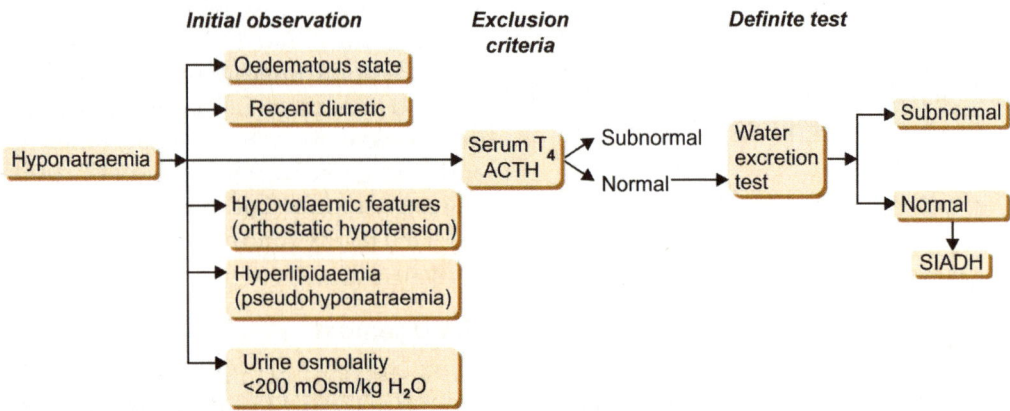

Fig. 103.3: An approach to the diagnosis of SIADH

HYPERNATRAEMIA

Definition

Hypernatraemia is defined as plasma sodium concentration greater than 145 mEq/L. Hyper natraemia in fact is hyperosmolar state because Na^+ is a major effective ECF osmole and a major detertminant of osmolality.

Hypematraemia may be due to primary Na^+ gain or water deficit. Thus hypematremic patients are usually hypovolaemic, while hypervolemia is frequently seen as iatrogenic complication in hospitalised patients with impaired access to free water. The two physiological responses to hyper natraemia are increased water intake stimulated by thirst and excretion of concentrated urine reflecting ADH secretion in response to an increased osmolality.

Causes

Hypematremia could be hypovolaemic, normovolemic and hypervolemic (Table 102.3).

In practice, hypematraemia results either due to decreased water intake or increased water loss or both. It commonly occurs in elderly patients with intercurrent illnesses.

These causes are given in Table 103.3.

Clinical Features

The clinical manifestations are as a result of hypertonicity which shifts water out of the cells leading to contraction of ICF (intracellular fluid) volume. A decreased brain cell volume results in CNS features and increases the chances of brain haemorrhage. The *symptoms and signs* are:

Table 103.3 Causes and management of hypernatraemia

Disturbance	Total body sodium	Causes	Urinary finding	Management (central,
1. Pure water losses (normovolaemic hypernatraemia)	Normal	1. Extra-renal losses • Skin (sweating, fever) • Respiratory (tachypnoea)	Hypertonic urine	• To restore water dificit by water replacement
		2. Renal losses • Diabetes insipidus (central, nephrogenic)	Hypo or Iso or hypertonic urine	• Treat diabetes insipidus • Replace Na^+ deficit by isotonic saline
2. Sodium and water deficit (hypo-volaemic hypernatraemia)	Low	1. Extra-renal losses • GI tract (diarrhoea), lactulose • Skin (burns, sweating)	Hypertonic urine (urine Na^+ <10 mEq/L)	
		2. Renal losses • Osmotic diuresis (glycosuria, urea, mannitol) • Postobstructi ve diuresis	Iso or hypotonic urine (urine Na^+ >20 mEq/L)	• Diuretics and water replacement
3. Addition of Na^+ (Hypervolaemic hypernatraemia)	Increased	• Primary hyperaldosteronism • Cushing's syndrome • Excessive saline administration	Isotonic or hypertonic urine	• Replacement of ADH
		• Central diabetes insipidous	Dilute, hypotonic urine	

1. **CNS involvement**
   - Altered mental status, restlessness, lethargy, weakness.
   - Neuromuscular irritability, e.g. muscular twitchings, hyperreflexia, tremulousness, ataxia.
   - Focal neurological deficits.
   - Occasionally seizures and coma.
   - Polyuria and excessive thirst.
2. **Volume depletion**
   - Severe thirst.
   - Dryness of tongue, loss of skin turgor.
   - Tachycardia, hypotension (low BP).
   - Oliguria, concentrated urine, raised urea and Na^+.
3. **Vascular consequences:** There are increased chances of intracerebral and subarachnoid haemorrhage leading to irreversible neurological sequalae.

Investigations

- Urine osmolality >400 mOsm/kg if renal water conserving ability is functioning (intact ADH)
- Urine osmolality <250 mOsm/kg indicate central diabetes insipidous due to loss of ADH. There will be hypematremia with dilute urine.

Management

The treatment of hypematraemia depends on two important determinants—ECF volume status and rate of development of hypematraemia (Table 103.3).

1. **Hypovolaemic hypernatraemia:** The main aim is to restore ECF volume by isotonic saline infusion; and plasma osmolality is corrected by half saline or 5% dextrose.
2. **Hypervolaemic hypernatraemia:** Diuretics and water replacement is needed to reduce hyperosmolality (Table 103.3). In the presence of renal insufficiency, dialysis may be required.
3. **Normovolaemic hypernatraemia:** It is treated by water replacement either orally or parenterally with 5% dextrose. Water ingestion will result in the excretion of excess of sodium in the urine. Calculation of water replacement is as follows:

   Desired total body water =

   $$\frac{\text{Actual plasma Na}^+}{\text{Desired plasma Na}^+} \times \begin{array}{l}\text{Actual total}\\\text{body water}\end{array}$$

   Water replacement = Desired total body water – Actual total body water
4. **Treatment of diabetes insipidus:** Read textbook of medicine.

Acute Disturbance of Potassium Balance (Dyskalaemia)

ACUTE POTASSIUM IMBALANCE (DYSKALAEMIA)

The total body potassium is 3500 mEq. Potassium is the major intracellular cation. Only 2% is found in the extracellular fluid (ECF). The ratio of intracellular to extracellular potassium concentration is 38:1, and, changes in the normal potassium concentration have an important influence on the neuromuscular transmission and resting membrane potentials, most significantly in the heart (Fig. 104.1).

Regulation of Potassium Balance

The two mechanisms are:

1. **Distribution of potassium** between intracellular and extracellular fluid.
2. **Excretion of K⁺ by the kidneys mainly and to some extent in the stool and sweat.** Potassium is pumped into cells in exchange for sodium by Na^+/K^+ ATPase, in a ratio of 3 sodium to 2 potassium ions. The intracellular K^+ concentration remains constant at around 150 mmol/L because of passive leakage from cells through non-selective K^+ channels. Certain drugs, i.e. β-adrenergic agonists and insulin shift the K^+ from extracellular compartment into the cells through Na^+/K^+ ATPase stimulation, hence, are useful for treatment of hyperkalaemia.

Acidosis, exercise, digoxin and hypertonicity have reverse effect, i.e. they shift K^+ out of the cells into extracellular compartment by inhibiting the Na/K^+ ATPase mechanism. Hyperkalemia is commonly seen in metabolic acidosis. The plasma potassium is therefore most vulnerable to factors influencing the shift of K^+ between extracellular and intracellular compartments.

3. **Potassium excretion:** Most of the dietary K^+ is excreted through kidneys. In the kidneys, about 90% of filtered K^+ is reabsorbed actively in the proximal tubule and thick ascending limb. About 10% escapes the reabsorption which is sufficient to maintain K^+ balance in the presence of normal renal function. This is the reason that hyper-kalaemia does not occur in the presence of normal GFR. However, if GFR is reduced, then active secretion of K^+ by the distal tubule is necessary to avoid progressive accumulation of K^+ and eventual hyperkalaemia. The active secretion of potassium is mediated by aldosterone, which stimulates Na^+/K^+ ATPase to facilitate sodium reabsorption and potassium secretion. In health, plasma levels of aldosterone rises parallel to increase in plasma potassium. The other stimulus to aldosterone is angiotensin II, thus, any factor which inhibits angiotensin

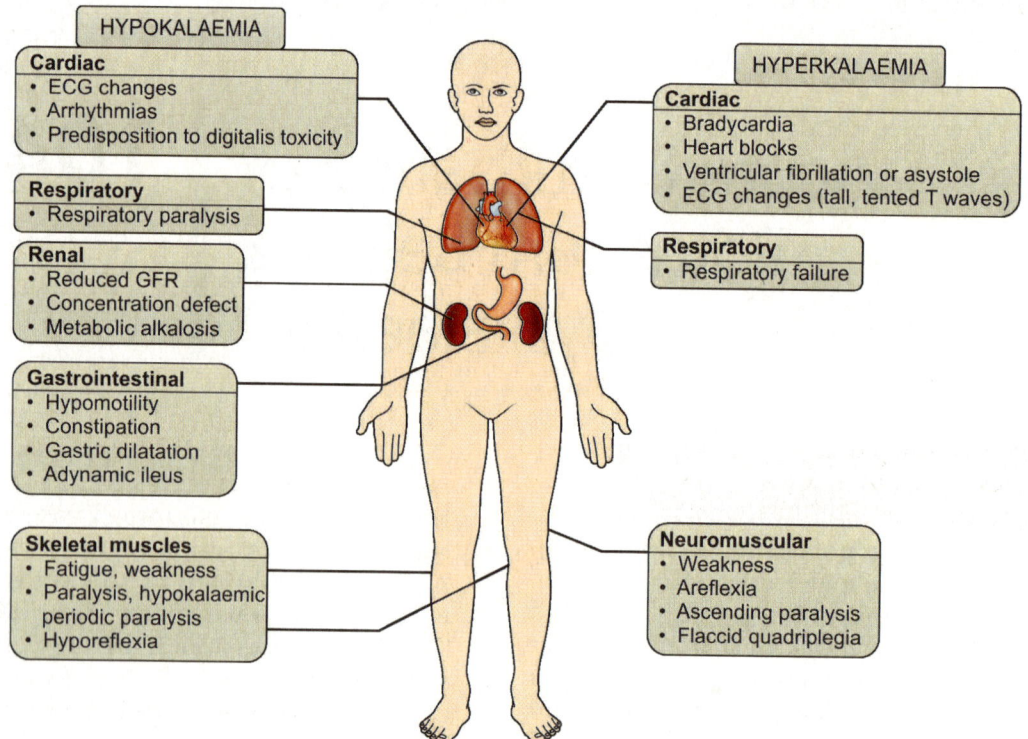

Fig. 104.1: Clinical manifestations of potassium disturbance (hypokalaemia and hyperkalaemia)

production will rouse potassium level This is the reason of hyperkalaemia due to ACE inhibitor therapy, NSAIDs therapy and beta blockers that inhibit renin-angiotensin system. Drugs which block the action of aldosterone (e.g. spironolactone, amiloride) also cause hyperkalaemia particularly in the presence of renal failure.

HYPOKALAEMIA

Definition

It is defined as serum potassium level less than 3.5 mEq/L. It is a common and serious problem in sick hospitalised patients especially on diuretics.

Aetiopathogenesis

Hypokalaemia may result from:
  i. Decreased net potassium intake.

  ii. Shift of K^+ into the cells, and / or
 iii. Increased net loss of potassium

Diminished dietary intake: It cannot be a sole cause of hypokalaemia because the amount of K^+ in the diet almost always exceeds that excreted in the urine. However, it is made clear that decreased dietary intake can exacerbate the potassium depletion secondary to increased loss through the gastrointestinal tract and kidneys. An usual cause of decreased intake is ingestion of clay (geophagia) which binds dietary K^+ and iron. It was customary among African Americans.

Movement of potassium into the cell: The intracellular shift of K^+ into the cells may transiently decrease the K^+ concentration. Metabolic alkalosis, uncontrolled hyperglycaemia treatment of diabetic ketoacidosis with insulin results in hypokalaemia due to intracellular shift of K^+. Stress induced catecholamines release and use of beta-adrenergic agonists, anabolism also promotes cellular uptake of K^+

(Fig. 104.2). Massive transfusion with thawed washed RBCs, may cause hypokalaemia. This is called *iatrogenic hypokalaemia*. *Spurious hypokalaemia (pseudohypokalaemia)* is seen with leucocytosis which can be avoided by storing the blood sample on ice or by rapidly separating the plasma or serum from cells.

Increases net loss : Excessive sweating causes loss of K+ through skin. Hype raldosteronism enhances K+ excretion in the urine. Profuse diarrhoea, WDHA syndrome, laxative abuse cause loss of K+ through the stool. Most cases of chronic hypokalaemia are due to renal K+ wasting. Increased renin and aldosterone levels lead to renal K+ wasting and hypoka-laemia. Primary hyperaldosteronism (Conn's syndrome) or adrenocortical hyperplasia, and renin-secreting tumours of juxtaglomer-ular apparatus (Bartter's syndrome), renal cell car cinoma, Ovarian and Wilms' tumour may produce hypokalaernia due to hyperren-inaemia.

Renal K+ wasting is seen in Liddle' syndrome (an autosomal dominant disease).

The causes of hypokalaernia are given in Table 104.1.

Clinical Features

The clinical manifestations vary from patient to patient even with same degree of hypoka-laernia, and their severity depends on the degree of hypokalaemia . Symptoms seldom occur unless serum K+ concentration falls below 3 mEq/L. Paralytic ileus and cardiac arrhythmias are usually seen in hypokalaemia with serum K+ level < 2.5 mEq/L. The clinical features are enumerated in Box 1 and Fig. 104.1.

Diagnosis and Differential Diagnosis

An approach to differential diagnosis is depicted in Fig. 104.2. The diagnosis of hypokalaemia depends on:
  i. History of decreased K+ intake and K+ loss (medications, vomiting and diarrhoea).
  ii. Physical examination, e.g. hypertension, diabetes.

iii. Laboratory tests:
  • Urinary K+ is low (<20 mEq/L) or inappropriately high (>40 mEq/L)
  • Plasma and urine osmolarity.
  • ECG (Fig. 104.3)

Table 104.1 Causes of hypokalaemia
1. Reduced intake
• Inadequate dietary intake • Starvation • Clay ingestion • Potassium free I.V. fluids
2. Shift of K+ into the cells
• Metabolic alkalosis • Insulin effect • β-adrenergic agonists and alpha-adrenergic antagonists • Anabolic state • Others such as hypothermia, hypokalaemic periodic paralysis, pseudohypokalaemia, barium toxicity
3. Increased loss

a. Losses from gastrointestinal tract
  • Vomiting and diarrhoea
  • Aspiration of upper GI contents
  • Fistulae
  • Villous adenoma of colon
  • Ureterosigmoid anastomósis
  • Laxative abuse
b. Losses from the kidneys
  • Recovery phase of ATN (diuretic phase)
  • Following relief of urinary tract obstruction
  • Proximal renal tubular acidosis (RTA)
  • Drug-induced tubular damage, e.g. amphotericin
  • Loop and thiazide diuretics
  • Uncontrolled diabetes (osmotic diuresis)
  • Bartter's syndrome
  • Gitelman's syndrome

4. Aldosteronism
• Primary hyperaldosteronism (Conn's syndrome) • Secondary aldosteronism, e.g. renal artery stenosis, renovascular hypertension, liver cirrhosis, cardiac failure and nephrotic syndrome • Cushing's syndrome or steroids therapy • Carbenoxolone, liquorice use.
5. Miscellaneous
• Hypomagnesemia • Carbenicillin, penicillin

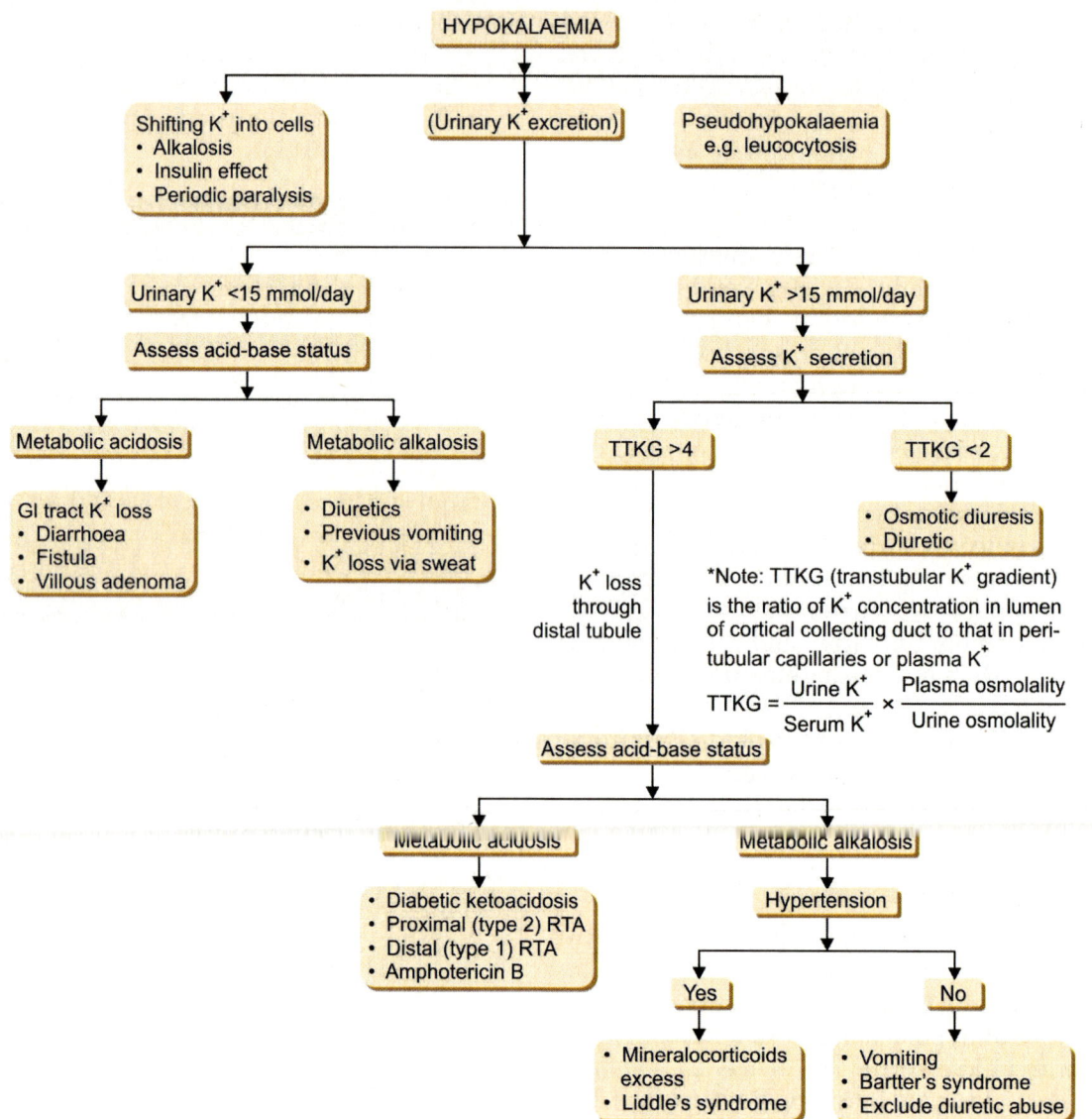

Fig. 104.2: A clinical approach to diagnosis of hypokalaemia

- Acid-base status
- Transtubular K⁺ gradient >4 suggest renal K⁺ loss with increased distal K⁺ secretion. In such cases plasma renin and aldosterone measurement is useful in differential diagnosis
iv. Exclusion of spurious hypokalaemia. Spurious hypokalaemia (pseudo-hypokalaemia) seen with leucocytosis (>50,000/mm³) and redistribution of K⁺ seen in certain clinical settings must be excluded before evaluating K⁺ deficit/depletion.

Management

Aims and objectives

- To correct the K⁺ deficit.
- To minimise ongoing losses.

Box 1	Clinical features of hypokalaemia

1. Cardiac

- The EKG abnormalities (Fig. 103.3)
  - Appearance of U wave
  - Prolongation of QTc or QU interval
  - Flattening of T wave/inversion
  - ST segment depression
  - Prolongation of P-R interval
  - Widening of QRS
- Arrhythmias
  - Atrial and ventricular ectopics
  - Ventricular tachycardia, torsades de pointes, ventricular fibrillation
- Predisposition to digitalis toxicity and digitalis-induced arrhythmias

2. Neuromuscular

- Gastrointestinal
  - Hypomotility
  - Constipation
  - Adynamic ileus
- Genitourinary
  - Dilatation of bladder
- Striated muscle
  - Fatigue, weakness, muscle cramps, tetany
  - Rhabdomyolysis
  - Transient paralysis-hypokalaemic periodic paralysis
  - Hyporeflexia
- Respiratory
  - Respiratory paralysis, hypercapnia

3. Renal

- Decrease in GFR
- Concentration defect (diabetes insipidous)
- Metabolic alkalosis

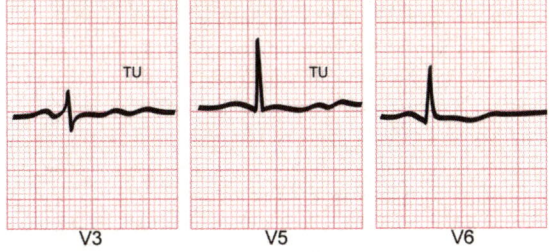

Fig. 104.3: Hypokalaemia. Note prominent U wave, prolonged QTU interval , ST segment depression and T wave inversion

1. *Correction of potassium deficit:* It is safer to correct hypokalaemia via oral route with exception of periodic paralysis. The degree of potassium depletion does not correlate well with plasma K$^+$ concentration, plasma K$^+$ concentration should be monitored frequently. Potassium chloride is usually the preparation of choice for hypokalaemia. Ulcers in the small bowel are reported with enteric coated KCl tablets.

In the setting of abnormal kidney function and diuretic therapy, 20 mEq/L of oral potassium is sufficient. In some cases 40–100 mEq/L over a period of few days may be needed to treat hypokalaemia and to replenish potassium stores.

Patients with severe hypokalaemia or those unable to take any thing by mouth require intravenous replacement therapy with KCl. For intravenous therapy, the maximum concentration should not exceed 60 mEq/L and rate of infusion should not exceed 20 mEq/h. In emergency situation, in patients with paralysis, digitalis intoxication or hepatic coma, K$^+$ can be infused rapidly (<40 mEq/h) with EKG monitoring in ICU. Fluids with K$^+$ concentration >40 mEq/L should be administered through a large vein to avoid phlebitis.

Note: KCl should be mixed in normal saline since dextrose solutions may initially exacerbate hypokalaemia under the effect of insulin.

Hypomagnesaemia and hypokalaemia occur concomitantly in most of the conditions responsible for hypokalaemia. Magnesium deficiency is the most overlooked electrolyte abnormality in the intensive care setting. Tissue magnesium deficit is an important cause of refractory hypokalaemia. Lack of response to potassium replacement suggests the need for magnesium replacement even in the presence of normal Mg^{++} level. It is very difficult to administer large quantities of magnesium orally because magnesium salts produce diarrhoea. With repletion of magnesium losses, the renal potassium wasting resolves.

In addition to potassium salts, supplementation therapy with potassium-sparing diuretics (spironolactone, triamterene, amiloride) may be helpful.

2. **To minimise ongoing losses:** If there is an identifiable and correctable cause of K$^+$ loss, then it should be rectified to stop or minimise ongoing losses. Avoid glucose containing fluid.

HYPERKALAEMIA

Definition

Serum potassium concentration more than 5.5 mEq/L is called *hyperkalaemia*. It occurs as a result of either K$^+$ release from the cells or decrease renal loss.

Iatrogenic hyperkalaemia: May result from over enthusiastic parenteral K$^+$ replacement or in patients with renal insufficiency.

Pseudohyperkalaemia or spurious hyper kalemia: An artificially elevated K$^+$ concentration due to K$^+$ movement out of cells immediately prior to or following venepuncture is called pseudohyperkalaemia. The various contributing factors are:
• Prolonged use of a tourniquet with or without repeated fist clenching.
• Haemolysis.
• Marked leucocytosis or thrombocytosis. The clot formation results in release of K$^+$ from the cells.

Pseudohyperkalaemia should be suspected in an otherwise asymptomatic patient with no obvious underlying cause. If proper venepuncture technique is used and plasma K$^+$ instead of serum if measured will be found to be normal.

Causes

The causes of hyperkalaemia are listed in Table 104.2. In diabetic ketoacidosis, hyperkalaemia is relatively common because of metabolic acidosis (extracellular shift of K$^+$), hypoinsulinaemia and hypovolaemia (impaired K$^+$ excretion) despite an overall K$^+$ deficit accumulating during the preceding

Table 104.2 Causes of hyperkalaemia
1. **Increased K$^+$ intake**
• Overzealous intravenous K$^+$ replacement
• High K$^+$ containing foods or drugs
2. **Release of intracellular K$^+$ following cell death**
• Bleeding into GI tract, soft tissues or body cavities with lysis of RBCs
• Intravascular haemolysis
• Rhabdomyolysis or tissue damage by crush injuries
• Tissue necrosis due to ischaemia/hypoxia/infection
• Catabolic states, e.g. fasting
3. **Shift of K$^+$ out of cells (extracellular shift)**
• Metabolic acidosis
• Hypoinsulinaemia (diabetic ketoacidosis)
• Drugs, e.g. beta blockers, digoxin (in toxic doses)
• Hypoaldosteronism and hyporeninaemia
• Hypertonicity of ECF
• Strenuous exercise, tissue hypoxia
• Hyperkalaemic periodic paralysis
4. **Impaired renal excretion of K$^+$**
a. Reduction in GFR
• Acute renal failure and chronic renal failure
• Urinary tract obstruction
b. Reduced renal blood flow
• Hypovolaemia and circulatory failure
c. Impaired tubular secretion of K$^+$
i. Primary hypoaldosteronism
• Adrenal insufficiency (Addison's disease)
• Adrenal enzyme deficiency
ii. Secondary hypoaldosteronism
• Hyporeninaemia • Beta blockers
• ACE inhibitors or ARBS
• Cyclosporin • NSAIDs
• Heparin
• Gordon's syndrome
iii. Resistance to aldosterone
• Pseudohypoaldosteronism
• Tubulointerstitial disease
• Transplanted kidneys
• Amyloidosis
• Sickle-cell disease
• Drugs (e.g. K$^+$ sparing diuretics, trimethoprim, pentamidine)
5. **Spurious hyperkalaemia (pseudohyperkalaemia)**
• Tissue damage during venepuncture
• Incorrect blood sampling and improper handling
• Haemolysis
• Marked leucocytosis or thrombocytosis
• Repeated fist clenching during phlebotomy with release of K$^+$ from the muscles

period of osmotic diuresis. With treatment, hyperkalaemia rapidly resolves and may be followed by significant hypokalaemia.

Spurious hyperkalaemia is caused by release of K$^+$ *in vitro* from abnormal or damaged cells such as abnormal WBCs in leukaemia, haemolysis and incorrect blood sample collection or poorly handled blood specimens that have been left for too long at room temperature before separation and analysis.

Chronic hyperkalaemia is virtually associated with decreased renal K$^+$ excretion due to either impaired secretion or diminished distal solute delivery.

Clinical Features

Since the resting membrane potential is related to the ratio of the ICF to ECF potassium concentration, hence, hyperkalaemia prolongs depolarization of the cell membrane. Prolonged depolarisation impairs membrane excitability leading to neuromuscular and cardiac manifestations. Clinical features usually appear when serum K$^+$ is 6.5 mEq/L. The manifestations include:

1. **Neuromuscular manifestations:** They include tingling, paraesthesias, muscle weakness, areflexia, ileus, flaccid paralysis (Gullain-Barré like and respiratory paralysis.
2. **Cardiac manifestations:** There may be bradycardia which may progress to complete heart block, ventricular fibrillation or asystole. The ECG manifestations correlate well with rise in plasma K+ level. There may be tall, tented T waves (Fig. 104.4), ST segment depression, first degree AV block, and QRS widening. Finally, a biphasic sine wave (representing fusion of widened QRS and T waves) develop signalling imminent ventricular standstill which is a terminal event in hyperkalaemia.

Diagnosis and Investigation

The diagnosis should be confirmed by repeat laboratory testing to rule out spurious hyperkalemia especially in the absence of medications known to lead hyperkalemia.

Management

Aims and Objectives

1. To counteract cardiac toxicity.
2. To shift K$^+$ into the cells.
3. To remove the excessive K$^+$ burden from the body.

Therapeutic approach to hyperkalaemia depends on the clinical setting, the ECG changes and serum potassium levels. Aggressive anti-hyperkalaemic therapy should be immediately initiated if serum potassium concentration exceeds 6.5 mEq/L or at any level of hyperkalaemia if EKG abnormalities are present such as absent P wave, widened QRS or a ventricular arrhythmia. Potentially fatal hyperkalemia rarely occurs unless K$^+$ level exceeds 7.5 mEq/L. It is wise to overtreat this disorder rather than undertreatment. The therapeutic measures employed are depicted in Box 2. They are:

1. **To counteract cardiac toxicity:** Administration of calcium gluconate decreases membrane excitability thus antagonises the effects of hyperkalaemia on cardiac conduction and has an immediate onset of action. In the setting of hypotension or cardiac arrest, calcium chloride should be preferred because it releases calcium ions into circulation immediately without requiring prior hepatic deconjugation of the parent compound. Calcium is useful to counteract the arrhythmic effects of hyperkalaemia on heart by increasing the threshold potential and thereby exerting an anti-arrhythmic action.
2. **To promote intracellular shift of K$^+$:** Insulin causes K$^+$ to shift into cells by mechanisms already discussed, and lowers the serum K$^+$ levels. Although glucose alone will stimulate insulin release from normal β-cells of pancreas but for a more rapid response, exogenous insulin is administered with glucose (glucose neutralised

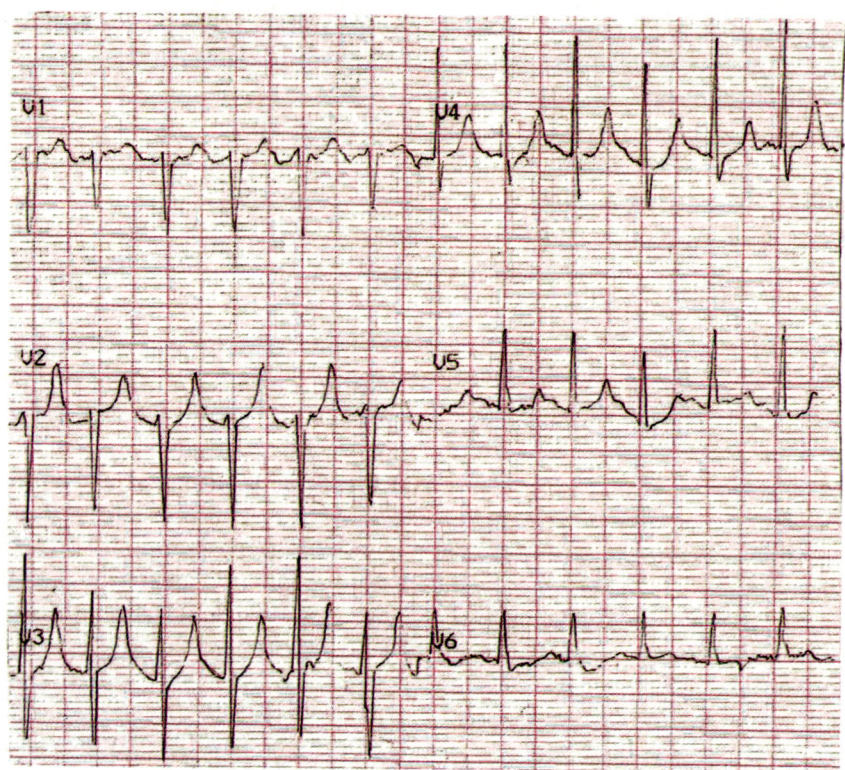

Fig. 104.4: Hyperkalaemia: Note tall tented T waves

drip) to prevent hypoglycaemia. A commonly recommended combination is 10 to 20 IU of insulin with 25 to 50 g of glucose.

Alkali therapy with I.V. $NaHCO_3$ can also shift the K^+ into the cells. This is safest when administered as an isotonic solution of 3 ampoules per litre (134 mmol/L $NaHCO_3$). Alkali therapy is reserved for severe hyperkalaemia associated with metabolic acidosis.

Calcium gluconate and $NaHCO_3$ should not be mixed as they can precipitate from a solution.

Patients with end stage renal disease (ESRD) do not tolerate Na^+ and volume overload. Nebulised β-adrenergic agonists, i.e. albuterol promotes cellular uptake of K^+ in such patients.

3. **Removal of the excessive potassium burden from the body:** Excessive potassium burden can be removed by diuretics (loop and thiazide diuretics). Withhold exogenous potassium from every source.

A cation-exchange resin promotes the exchange of Na^+ for K^+ in the gastrointestional tract and lowers K^+ concentration by 0.5 to 1.0 mmol/L within 1 to 2 hours and last for 4–6 hours. The cation-exchange resin is used in sodium phase (sodium polystyrene sulphonate) either orally or by enema. Definite therapy for hyperkalaemia is removal of K^+ by *haemodialysis*. This should be reserved for patients with renal failure and those with life-threatening hyperkalaemia unresponsive to other measures.

4. **Treat the underlying cause of hyperkalaemia,** if found. This may involve dietary modification, correction of metabolic acidosis, volume expansion, etc.

Box 2   Therapies for acute hyperkalaemia

Treatment	Mechanism of action	Onset of action	Duration of action
1. Calcium gluconate (10–30 ml of 10% solution I.V.)	Antagonises membrane effect, counteracts cardiac toxicity	Few minutes	30–60 minutes
2. Glucose 50 g, i.e. 500 ml of 10% dextrose with 10 units of regular insulin infusion	Shifts the potassium into the cells	15–30 minutes	4–6 hours
3. Nebulised salbutamol or albuterol (10–20 mg in 4 ml normal saline as nebulised aerosol)	Stimulates, Na^+, K^+ pump, redistributes K^+ into the cells	15 minutes	2 hours
4. Sodium bicarbonate (44–132 mEq I.V.)	Shifts K^+ into the cells	30 minutes	4 hours
5. Cation-exchange resin (sodium poly-styrene sulphonate)	There is removal of K^+ by exchange of Na^+		
• Oral 40 g in 20 ml of 70% sorbitol to avoid constipation		120 minutes	
• Enema (50–100 g)		60 minutes	4–6 hours
6. Dialysis	Removal of K^+ from circulation	Few minutes after start	Variable
• Haemodialysis			
• Peritoneal dialysis			

Skin Emergencies

CHAPTER

105

Acute Urticaria and Angioedema

ACUTE URTICARIA AND ANGIOEDEMA

Definition

Acute urticaria is defined as transient urticarial (hives) pruritic lesions consisting of a central wheal surrounded by an erythematous halo lasting for more than 24 hours (Fig. 105.1A and B). Urticaria is due to dilatation of dermal vessels whereas *angioedema* (Fig. 105.2) results due to dermal oedema as well as subcutaneous oedema. Angioedema occurs alone or in combination with urticaria (e.g. urticarial vasculitis and physical urticaria). Angioedema may also involve respiratory and G.I. tract. Urticaria and angioedema may be part of a life-threatening anaphylactic reactions.

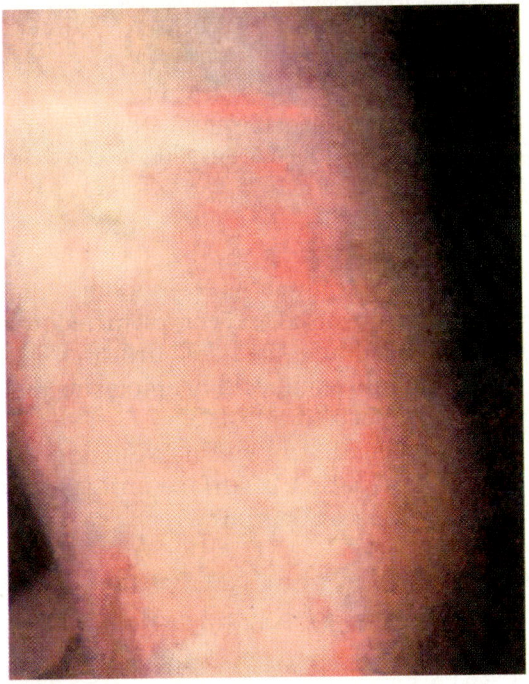

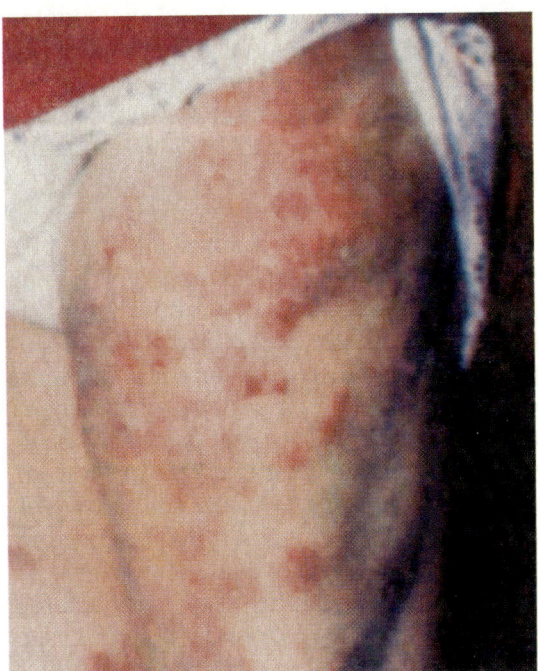

Fig. 105.1A: Acute urticaria: Following exposure to a drug

Fig. 105.1B: Papular urticaria: Papular urticaria following an insect bite

Causes

Acute urticaria has a wide variety of allergic aetiologies i.e. immune mediated, IgE mediated and non-immune mediated (Box 1), but it is difficult to ascertain its cause in emergency situations. However, cause is not needed in the management of urticaria. A significant number of patients have no identifiable cause.

Pathophysiology

In urticaria, the immunologic mechanism is most common and is mediated by IgE. Another mechanism involved is activation of complement cascade (serum sickness).

Clinical Picture

The patient usually presents with pruritus and circumscribed, raised, erythematous lesion (wheals). They are raised because of dermal oedema which may extend deep into the tissue resulting in subcutaneous swelling called angioedema. Hence, urticaria and angioedema may occur in any location together or individually. The sites of involvement include, i.e. the eyelids (Fig. 105.2), lips, tongue, larynx palms-soles, genitalia and GI tract as well as subcutaneous tissue.

The immune complex-induced urticaria associated with serum sickness like reaction occurs 6–12 days after first exposure.

The *wheals (lesions)* appear suddenly and are itchy, do not last longer than 48 hours, but may continue to occur for indefinite periods. Several attacks may be associated with *laryngeal oedema, diarrhoea, abdominal pain, hematuria, vomiting, dizziness, syncope, hypotension* or *shock, arthralgias* and *broncho-spasm* called *anaphylactic syndrome.* Laryngeal involvement may be potentially fatal if not treated urgently.

In children urticaria may be associated with fever or pain abdomen (*worm infestation*).

In cholinergic urticaria triggered by a rise in core body temperature (hot showers, exercise) *wheals* are 2–3 mm in diameter with a large surrounding red flare. **Cold urticaria**

is acquired or inherited and triggered by exposure to cold and wind.

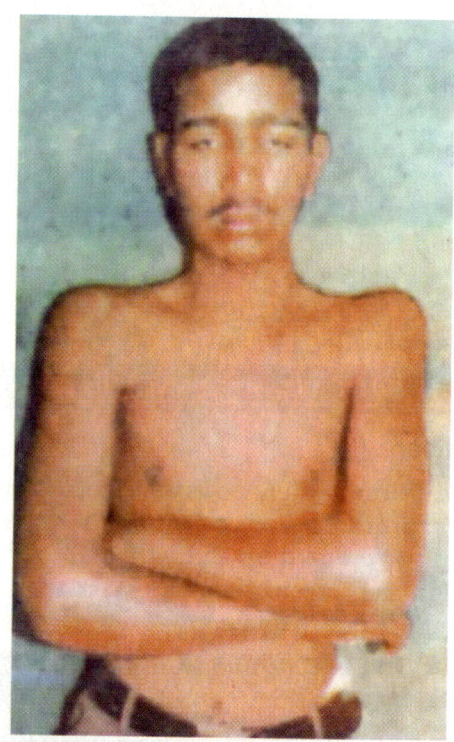

Fig. 105.2: Angioedema. Note the erythematous skin with oedema around the eyelids, face and subcutaneous tissue

Investigations

- TLC and DLC may show eosinophilia.
- IgG levels are raised and complement levels are low in immune-mediated urticaria.
- "Cryoglobulins and cold haemolysins may be detected in cold urticaria.
- Stool examination for worm infestations.
- LE cells, hepatitis B surface antigens for systemic causes of purpura.

Treatment

1. Patient should avoid triggering factor listed in Box 1.
2. **Antihistamines** are the mainstay of treatment in acute urticaria. In adequate doses, antihistamines alone are sufficient to control the symptoms and

Box 1 Common causes of acute urticaria and angioedema

Immune mediated	Non-immune causes

• Atopy
• Physical urticaria (e.g. dermatographism, solar, cold and cholinergic urticaria caused by hot showers and exercise)
 	
• Antigen sensitivity, e.g. feathers, animal danders pollens, foods (milk and its products, egg, nuts, chocolate and shellfish), drugs, (ACE inhibitor and ARBs) and helminths
 	
• Hereditary angioedema
• Arthropod bites, e.g. insect bites and bee stings
• Serum sickness, vaccine
• Blood transfusion reactions
• External contactants, e.g. chemicals, cosmatics
• Necrotising vasculitis
• Hepatitis B infection
	1. Mast cell releasing agents
	  • Mastocytosis
	  • Food additives, e.g. tartrazine
	  • Opiates, radiocontrast agents, antibiotics
	2. Prostaglandin inhibitors
	  • Aspirin
	  • NSAIDs
	  • Azo dyes
	  • Benzoates

corticosteroids are not needed. Similarly parenteral antihistamines are usually not indicated.

- *A sedative H_1 antihistamine* is preferred at night such as long-acting chlorpheniramine maleate (8–12 mg) or bromopheniramine 12–24 mg or hydroxyzine HCl 10–50 mg.

- *Non-sedative H_1 antihistamines* such as terfenadine (60 mg bid) or astemizole (10 mg daily) or Loratidine (10 mg/day) or cetrizine (10 mg daily) are useful for daytime use.

- *Hydroxyzine HCl or cyproheptadine HCl* have wider spectrum of action than routine H_1 receptor-blocking agents. Angioedema will often rash and better with these agents.

- *Combination treatment:* Antihistaminics (H_1 blockers) may be used in combination with H_2 receptors blockers (ranitidine, famotidine).

- *Corticosteroids* are indicated in acute and chronic urticaria orally or parenterally only when the antihistamines fail to control the symptoms.

- *Cyclosporine* (3–5 mg/kg/day) may be effective in severe cases of autoimmune urticaria.

- Adrenalin is life saving measure.

Subcutaneous adrenaline (1:1000 dil) is used for anaphylaxis to control the laryngeal oedema and hypotension, can be repeated safely after 15–20 minutes if there is no tachycardia. Other measures such as tracheostomy, infusion of saline, dopamine and I.V. steroids may be employed as already discussed in the management of anaphylactic shock.

Most patients with acute urticaria recover completely from the acute attack and may remain well throughout their lives.

Erythroderma and Exfoliative Dermatitis

Definition

Erythroderma is a nonspecific inflammatory condition characterised by redness of the skin surface involving more than 90% of the body surface. There may be associated scaling, erosions, pustules as well as shedding of hair and nails.

Aetiology

Males are more commonly affected (2–3 times) than females. The causes are given in Table 106.1.

Clinical Features

Erythroderma developing in primary eczema or dermatitis, underlying malignancy and following drug intake is often sudden. The cutaneous inflammation is seen as erythema (redness) and scaling within few days. The scalp and body hair may fall along with nails in erythroderma of few weeks duration, secondary changes such as erosions and pustules may be associated. The mucosae are spared.

Drug-induced erythroderma (exfoliative dermatitis, Fig. 106.1) often begins as morbilliform eruption or it may arise as diffuse erythema. Fever and eosinophilia often accompany the eruption and occasionally there is an associated interstitial nephritis.

Potential systemic manifestations include fever, itching, chills, hypothermia, reactive

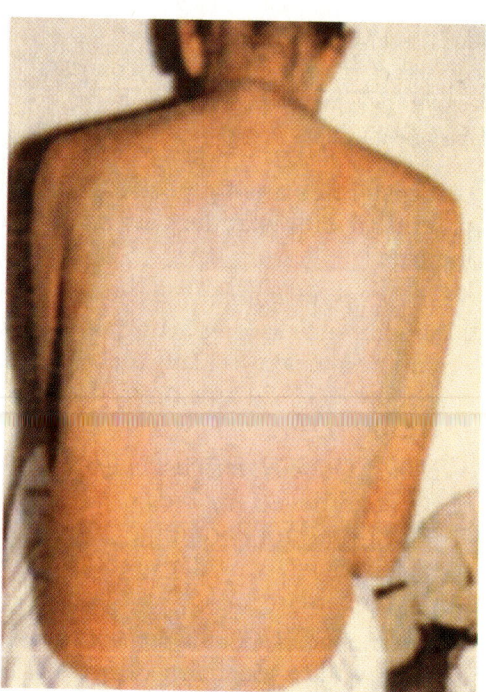

Fig. 106.1: Erythroderma (exfoliative dermatitis)

lymphadenopathy, peripheral oedema, hypoalbuminaemia and high output cardiac failure.

Investigations

- TLC and DLC for leucocytosis, eosinophilia.
- ESR may be raised.
- Urea and electrolytes may be monitored.

Table 106.1 Causes of erythroderma

1. **Primary cutaneous disorders**
   - Psoriasis.
   - Dermatitis (atopic, stasis, contact, seborrhagic)
   - Pityriasis rubra pilaris.
2. **Drugs,** e.g. sulphonamides, salicylates, penicillins, hydantoin, thioacetazone, gold, allopurinol, captopril carbamazepine.
3. **Systemic diseases**
   - Cutaneous T cell lymphoma.
   - Lymphoma.
4. **Idiopathic**

- Skin biopsy may show changes of inflammatory dermatitis or cutaneous T cell lymphoma or leukemia.

Complications

- Disturbance of temperature regulation due to diffuse involvement of skin leading to hypothermia.
- High output cardiac failure due to vasodilatation.
- Dehydration due to water loss and there may be dyselectrolytemia.

Treatment/Management

- Hospitalization and bed rest.
- Nutritional supplements, e.g. high protein intake, multivitamins and mineral.
- Stop the drug if it is the underlying cause.
- Check and treat secondary infections with appropriate antibiotics.
- Physiological saline compresses for 30 minutes 4 times a day is helpful in removing the scales, debris and bacteria.
- Emollients (liquid paraffin) after short lukewarm bath is helpful. Sedative antihistamines may be used to control pruritus, sometimes, low potency steroid creams or ointments may be used except in psoriatic erythroderma. Systemic steroids may show dramatic improvement in severe or fulminant cases except in psoriatic erythroderma.
- Treat appropriately the complications such as high output state, hypoalbuminaemia, hypothermia and water and electrolyte imbalance.
- Specific treatment for psoriasis or malignancy may be instituted if it is the underlying cause.
- For psoriatic erythroderma or pityriasis rubrapilaris, either acitretin or methotrexate may be indicated. Erythroderma due to lymphoma/leukemia need systemic chemotherapy.

PEMPHIGUS

Definition

Pemphigus is the most common autoimmune blistering (bullous) disorder involving the skin and the mucous membrane.

Types

Histologically, there is **acantholysis** (loss of cohesion between epidermal cells) and *cell separation* and *intradermal blister formation*.

Depending on the cleavage level within epidermis and different clinical patterns, two forms are recognized, each with a variant (Fig. 107.1).

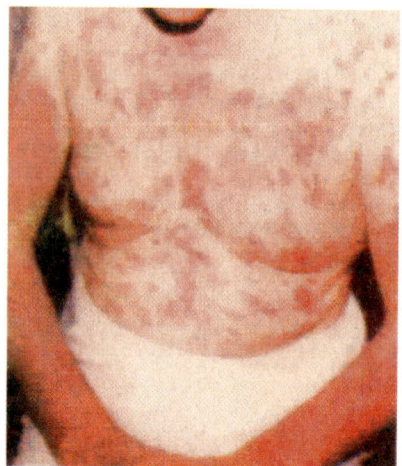

Fig. 107.1: Bullous pemphigus

1. **Pemphigus vulgaris** and its variant pemphigus vegetans.
2. **Pemphigus foliaceous** and its variant pemphigus erythematosus.

Aetiology

The IgG class of autoantibodies directed against intracellular cement substance of the epidermal keratinocytes identified as desmogleins lead to formation of clefts (acantholysis and cell separation) in the epidermis. Similar antibodies have also been demonstrated in patients with burns, bullous pemphigoid and penicillin-induced eruptions. Pemphigus like eruptions can be produced by some drugs, e.g. captopril, d-penicillamine and rifampicin. Rarely pemphigus may be associated with thymoma, myasthenia gravis, SLE, carcinoma and lymphoproliferative diseases.

Clinical Features

Pemphigus vulgaris: It is very common mucocutaneous blistering disease in India, involves younger persons in the age groups of 20–40 years.

It presents commonly with *oral erosions* followed by *skin lesions* such as generalized *flaccid blisters* (*vesicles*) or *bullae* usually on normal looking skin, that quickly rupture to leave large denuded areas which crust and continue to spread without further blistering at the same area.

The sites of oral lesion are buccal and palatine mucosae. The lesions are painful, tender and heal slowly. Other uncommon sites are conjunctivae, pharyngeal, laryngeal and anorectal mucosae. The sites of blisters are scalp, face, trunk, axillae and groin. Skin lesions heal without scarring except at sites complicated by secondary infections or trauma. Post-inflammatory hyperpigmentation is present for some time.

Nikolsky's sign is positive which means tangential pressure (sliding pressure) on the unaffected skin may cause separation of the epidermal layers and denudation of the skin.

Asboe-Hansen sign indicates bulla spreading or blisters spreading by lateral and perpendicular pressure applied on intact blisters.

Pemphigus vegetans: It is a variant of pemphigus vulgaris, is a much milder form of the disease which may begin either as vesicles or blisters that eventually develop hypertrophic granulation or vegetative granulation. Oral lesions may occur. Intertriginous involvement is common. The initial moist vegetative lesions turn dry later on.

Pemphigus foliaceous: It is a less common disease and lesions are superficial blisters and erosions that appear on the face, neck and upper trunk. Oral lesions are rarely seen. The course of the disease is more or less similar to pemphigus vulgaris. Sun exposure is an aggravating factor.

Drugs-induced pemphigus (e.g. pencillamine, captopril, enalapril) resembles PF rather than phemphigus vulgaris.

Pemphigus erythematosus: It is a variant of pemphigus foliaceous. Erythematous, scaly, hyperkeratotic dry plaques (lesions) are seen in butterfly distribution over the face starting from the nose spreading over the cheeks. Oral mucosa is rarely involved. Though it resembles SLE but systemic involvement never occurs.

Diagnosis and Investigations

The diagnosis is made by:
1. **Tzanck smear:** The blister is ruptured and the base is scrapped with the scalpel and smear is made on a glass slide. Staining with Giemsa reveals acantholytic cells with large dense nuclei and a rim of cytoplasm.
2. **Skin biopsy from a fresh blister and its histopathology:** Histopathology shows intradermal cleft which is subcorneal in pemphigus foliaceous and its variant but is suprabasal in pemphigus vulgaris and its variant. Acantholytic cells are seen in clefts. In pemphigus vegetans, hyperkeratosis, acanthosis and intradermal eosinophilic abscesses are seen. Blister cavities contain acantholytic epidermal cells.
3. **Immunofluorescence:** Direct immunofluorescence microscopy of lesional or intact skin reveals deposition of IgG in the intercellular space of both involved and uninvolved skin. Deposits of IgG on keratinocytes are derived from circulating autoantibodies to cell surface autoantigens which are detected by ELISA. Less commonly IgM and IgA may be found. Indirect immunofluorescence shows IgG antibodies which corresponds with the severity of the disease.
4. **ELISA:** Recently, ELISA tests that can detect IgG autoantibodies to desmoglein-1 and 3 have been developed that will help for rapid diagnosis.

Treatment

A. **General measures**
   - Hospitalisation and bedrest
   - General supportive measures include compresses with $KMnO_4$ or simply with soap and water.
   - Anaesthetic troches used before eating ease painful oral lesions.
   - Maintain fluid and electrolyte balance I.V. feedings if indicated.
   - Treatment of infection by antibiotics.
B. **Systemic measures**
   - *Immunosuppression:* Systemic steroids (prednisolone 1–2 mg/kg/day orally) either alone or along with cytotoxic agents like cyclophosphamide or azathioprine (1 mg/kg/day) are the main drugs used

in the treatment of pemphigus. Cyclo-phosphamide pulse therapy or cyclo-phosphamide plus steroid pulse therapy have been employed for severe cases and have been beneficial. Azathioprine (100–200 mg daily) or mycophenolate mofetil (1–1.5 g twice daily) is used most frequently. **Plasmapheris** is may be used for severe treatment resistant disease.

Rituximab may be given in refractory cases. If this fails, IVIG monthly at a dose of 2 g/kg I.V. over 3 days, with rituximab is most beneficial regimen.

C. **Local measures**
  • Topical or intralesional steroids help the mild limited disease. Topical $AgNO_3$ (0.5%) may be used to promote healing.

Skin Infections **108**

SKIN INFECTIONS

Skin infection is very common in clinical practice. Every physician shall see some form of cutaneous infection in his day-to-day practice. It is stressed here, that sometimes, the serious and/or potentially serious skin infection may pose an emergency situation, therefore, it is imperative for the physician to know the site of their localisation, degree of involvement and presence of toxaemia/septicaemia. The following skin infections may pose as an emergency.

Staphylococcal Scalded Skin Syndrome (SSSS, Fig. 108.1)

1. It is a severe form of blistering skin disease produced by exotoxins elaborated by *S. aureus* of phase group.
2. It affects infants and young children, is characterised by diffuse/extensive erythema, fever, tenderness of central face, neck, trunk, intertriginous zones followed by wide-spread flaccid bullae formation and exfoliation. Crusted areas may develop. The raw areas are extremely tender but not purulent. There is significant fluid and electrolyte loss. A rapid diagnosis of SSSS can be made by frozen section of blister roof or exfoliative cytology of blister contents. The cutaneous lesions in SSSS are sterile. Secondary infection is common. The entire illness resolves within 10 days.

It can be, however, fatal in 2–3% cases due to hypovolemia and sepsis.

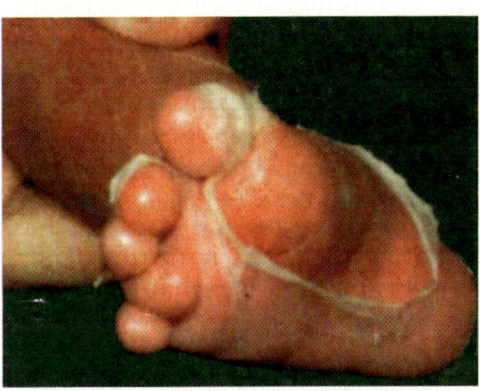

Fig. 108.1: Staphylococcal scalded skin syndrome (SSSS). Note the peeling of the skin preceded by redness and tenderness in an infant. The skin lesions are similar to toxic epidermal necrolysis

Treatment

1. Local care of denuded skin.
2. Replacement of fluids and electrolyte to correct hypovolaemia and electrolyte imbalance. The electrolytes should be monitored.
3. *Antibiotics:* The antistaphylococcal antibiotics are most useful. Parenteral cloxacillin is the treatment of choice.

II. **Toxic Shock Syndrome (TSS):** It is an acute life-threatening intoxication or endotoxaemia produced by toxin-producing strains of *S. aureus*. It is characterised by fever, hypotension, rash, multiorgan dysfunction (at least 3 organs must be involved) and desquamation during the early convalescent period. The disease was recognised with a large outbreak in menstruating women because menstruation is the most commnon setting for TSS but non-menstruation cases also occur frequently (50%).It affects both sexes and all ages. It is common in menstruating women using tampons.

The toxins responsible for TSS include toxic shock syndrome toxin 1 (TSST-1), pyrogenic exotoxin C and endotoxin F.

The syndrome in non-menstrual cases complicate skin lesions of many types including burns, insect bites, varicella lesions and surgical wounds. Postoperative disease develops hours to days following a surgical procedure.

Clinical Features

- Patient is toxic and ill-looking. There is tachypnoea and tachycardia.
- General symptoms, e.g. nausea, vomiting abdominal pain, diarrhoea, muscular pains and headache.
- Features of hypotension, e.g. dizziness, vertigo, low urinary output and perspiration.
- **Rash:** The macular erythematous rash develops over first 2 days of illness. It is usually generalised. There may be conjunctival suffusion, periorbital oedema.
- **In menstruating women**, there may be purulent vaginal discharge and vaginal mucosa is red.
- A strawberry tongue develops in 50% cases.
- There is involvement of multiple organs, e.g. brain, kidneys, lungs, liver, GI tract, etc. Mental status is clear.

Diagnosis

The diagnosis of TSS is based on clinical criteria and three of the involved *mucocutaneous sites* (i.e. diffuse erythema of the skin, desquamation of the palms and soles 1–2 weeks after the onset of illness and involvement of mucous membrane.)

Investigations

- TLC, DLC may show neutrophilic leucocytosis.
- There may be anaemia, thrombocytopenia.
- Urine may show pyuria, haematuria, proteinuria.
- There may be hypoalbuminaemia, raised blood urea and creatinine.
- Raised SGOT and SGPT levels.
- There may be hypocalcaemia and hypophosphatermia.
- Creatinine phosphokinase (CK) levels are elevated.
- Blood cultures are usually negative.

Treatment

- Decontamination of the site of toxin production, e.g. removal of tampons and debridement of surgical wounds.
- Correction of fluids and electrolyte balance. Liberal administration of fluids including saline should be used to resuscitate shock. Pressure agents, e.g. dobutamine may be used to resuscitate shock unresponsive to fluids. The dose of dobutamine is same as described in management of peripheral circulatory failure.
- Electrolytes particularly hypocalcaemia and hypomagnesaemia may be corrected and maintained.
- *Antibiotics:* Semisynthetic penicillins (nafcil lin, oxacillin) or vancomycin are the drugs of choice. In serious infection, clindamyin 900 mg I.V. 8 hourly alone or with vancomycin have been used.
- Infusion of neutralizing antibody to TSST-1 (immunoglobulin) as a single dose of 400 mg/kg generates a protective level of antibody.

Complications

- *Multiple organ failure* due to hypoperfusion.
- *Massive oedema* due to hypoalbuminaemia.
- *Adult respiratory distress syndrome.*

Stevens-Johnson Syndrome

Definition

The Stevens-Johnson syndrome describes a severe erythema multiforme (erythematous maculopapular lesions) with widespread blisters developing on dusky or purpuric macules associated with oral and genital ulceration and marked consti tutional symptoms (Fig. 109.1).

Causes

1. **Infections:**
   - Viral, e.g. herpes simplex

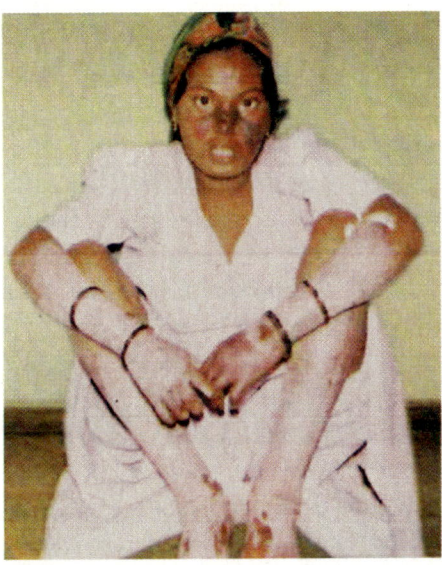

Fig. 109.1: Stevens-Johnson syndrome

   - Mycoplasma
   - Yersinia, tuberculosis, histoplasmosis
2. **Drugs:**
   - Sulphonamide
   - Nevirapine
   - Allopurinol
   - Lamotrigene
   - Codeine
   - Thiacetazone
   - Carbamazepine
   - Phenytoin
   - Phenobarbitone
3. **Connective tissue disease:** A rare precipating factor.
4. **Topical applications**

Clinical Features

1. **Constitutional symptoms:** The onset is acute with mild fever, sore throat, conjunctivitis, malaise and prostration.
2. **Skin lesions:** Extensive bullous eruption of the skin and mucous membranes. The skin lesions are distributed symmetrically on the dorsum of hands, feet, forearms, legs, face and neck. Total percent of body surface area detachment is less than 10% which differentiates it from another potentially fatal condition called toxic epidermal necrolysis where >30% of the body area shows detachment of skin.
3. **Systemic manifestations** include iritis, urethritis, gastritis, arthritis and

haemorrhages, e.g. haemoptysis. There may be difficulty in respiration. Dehydration occurs due to fluid and sodium loss. Hypotension can occur. Frozen section skin biopsy helps in diagnosis.

Treatment

The disease has usually a spontaneous resolution subsiding within few weeks. Stevens-Johnson syndrome can be recalcitrant and can be fatal. The emergency measures include:

1. **Immediate**
   - Removal of the cause, e.g. infection, drug, etc. All drugs the patient was taking must be stopped immediately. If that is not possible, substitute them with chemically unrelated drug.
   - Symptomatic treatment with antihistamines and calamine lotion. The antihistamines can be used intravenously. Calamine lotion is used locally.

2. **Specific emergency treatment**
   - Maintenance of a patent airway.
   - Good nutrition supplementation.
   - Proper fluid and electrolyte administration to correct hypovolaemia and electrolyte disturbance. BP and electrolytes should be monitored.
   - Prevention of secondary skin infection of skin lesion by appropriate antibiotic therapy.
   - Care of mouth and eyes.
   - Good nursing care.
   - Systemic corticosteroids: A short course of steroids (prednisolone 60–80 mg daily then gradually tapered of) may be used to overcome acute phase and to relieve constitutional symptoms. Cyclosporine may also be possible therapy. IVIG (I.V. immunoglobulin) has no role.

Index

Emergency Medicine